W9-BFT-356

Handbook of Neuroradiology:
Brain and Skull

HANDBOOKS IN RADIOLOGY SERIES

Other Volumes in This Series

Genitourinary and Gastrointestinal Radiology
STEPHEN R. ELL, M.D., Ph.D.

Head and Neck Imaging, Second Edition
H. RIC HARNSBERGER, M.D.

Interventional Radiology and Angiography, Second Edition
MYRON WOJTOWYCZ, M.D.

Nuclear Medicine, Second Edition
FREDERICK L. DATZ, M.D.

Skeletal Radiology
B.J. MANASTER, M.D., Ph.D.

Handbook of Neuroradiology: Brain and Skull

Anne G. Osborn, M.D., F.A.C.R.
Professor of Radiology
University of Utah School of Medicine
Salt Lake City, Utah
and
Nycomed Visiting Professor in Diagnostic Imaging
Armed Forces Institute of Pathology
Washington, D.C.

Karen A. Tong, M.D.
Senior Fellow in Neuroradiology
University of Utah School of Medicine
Salt Lake City, Utah

SECOND EDITION

with 100 illustrations

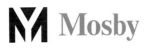 Mosby

St. Louis   Baltimore   Boston   Carlsbad   Chicago   Naples   New York   Philadelphia   Portland
London   Madrid   Mexico City   Singapore   Sydney   Tokyo   Toronto   Wiesbaden

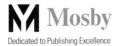

Mosby

Dedicated to Publishing Excellence

A Times Mirror
Company

Publisher: Anne S. Patterson
Managing Editor: Elizabeth Corra
Project Manager: Linda Clarke
Senior Production Editor: Allan S. Kleinberg
Editing and Production: Graphic World Publishing Services
Designer: Carolyn O'Brien
Manufacturing Manager: Tony McAllister

SECOND EDITION

Copyright © 1996 by Mosby–Year Book, Inc.

Previous edition copyrighted 1991.

All rights reserved. No part of this publication may be reproduced, stored in a retrieval system, or transmitted, in any form or by any means, electronic, mechanical, photocopying, recording, or otherwise, without prior written permission from the publisher.

Permission to photocopy or reproduce solely for internal or personal use is permitted for libraries or other users registered with the Copyright Clearance Center, provided that the base fee of $4.00 per chapter plus $.10 per page is paid directly to the Copyright Clearance Center, 27 Congress Street, Salem, MA 01970. This consent does not extend to other kinds of copying, such as copying for general distribution, for advertising or promotional purposes, for creating new collected works, or for resale.

Printed in the United States of America
Composition by Graphic World Inc.
Printing/binding by Maple-Vail/York

Mosby–Year Book, Inc.
11830 Westline Industrial Drive
St. Louis, Missouri 63146

ISBN: 0-8151-6593-5

96 97 98 99 00 / 9 8 7 6 5 4 3 2 1

We dedicate this handbook to all the residents, fellows, and practicing radiologists whose enthusiastic reception of the first *Handbook of Neuroradiology* inspired and energized us. We hope you will find the practice of neuroradiology an enjoyable adventure and this *Handbook* a useful guide to the exciting world of neuroimaging.

Anne G. Osborn, M.D.
Karen A. Tong, M.D.

Preface

The second edition of *Handbook of Neuroradiology* extensively revises and updates the information initially presented in the 1991 edition. We have completely reorganized the *Handbook,* adding dozens of new drawings, tables, and charts that summarize important concepts for the reader. We have also updated the selected references through September 1995 to provide the newest available perspectives on neuropathology and neuroimaging.

Other significant changes include the expanded focus on skull and brain pathology in the second edition. Spine and spinal cord will be covered separately in a follow-up companion volume, *Handbook of Neuroradiology: Spine and Cord.* For otolaryngologic imaging, the reader is referred to H. Ric Harnsberger's second edition of his superb text, *Handbook of Head and Neck Imaging* (Mosby–Year Book, 1995).

This edition of the *Handbook of Neuroradiology: Brain and Skull* is also intended to serve as a companion volume to the comprehensive textbook *Diagnostic Neuroradiology* (Mosby–Year Book, 1994). By using the updated outlined *Handbook* text in combination with the extensive illustrations of imaging studies and pathology in *Diagnostic Neuroradiology,* the reader will have an up-to-date comprehensive compendium of neuroradiology.

We have designed this new edition of *Handbook of Neuroradiology* to provide a comprehensive, yet easy-to-read, summary of the essentials in neuroimaging. Both basic and more advanced topics are included so that residents, fellows, and practicing radiologists will have a conveniently sized, highly readable reference for the day-to-day practice of clinical neuroradiology.

We hope you will find the book useful; we had fun writing it. Enjoy!

Anne G. Osborn, M.D.
Karen A. Tong, M.D.

Contents

I. Normal Anatomy   1

    1   Scalp and Skull   3

    2   Meninges, Meningeal Spaces, Ventricles, Cisterns, and CSF   15

    3   Aortic Arch, Great Vessels, and External Carotid Artery   29

    4   Internal Carotid Artery   39

    5   Circle of Willis and Cerebral Arteries   49

    6   Posterior Fossa Arteries   65

    7   Intracranial Venous System   72

    8   Brain   83

    9   Cranial Nerves   101

II. Brain Development and Congenital Malformations   119

    10   Normal Brain Development and Classification of Congenital Malformations   121

    11   Neural Tube Disorders and the Chiari Malformations   125

    12   Cephaloceles and Corpus Callosum Anomalies   133

    13   Holoprosencephaly   141

    14   Sulcation and Cellular Migration Disorders   146

15   Dandy-Walker Complex and Miscellaneous Posterior Fossa
      Malformations   153

16   Neurofibromatosis   163

17   Major Neurocutaneous Syndromes Other Than
      Neurofibromatosis   169

18   Other Neurocutaneous Syndromes   176

III.   Trauma and Intracranial Hemorrhage   181

19   Understanding Intracranial Hemorrhage   183

20   Craniocerebral Trauma: Primary Manifestations   188

21   Secondary Effects of Craniocerebral Trauma   198

22   Vascular Effects of Trauma   206

23   Nontraumatic Intracranial Hemorrhage   213

IV.   Intracranial Neoplasms and Tumor-like Lesions   221

24   Classification   223

25   Astrocytoma   230

26   Astrocytoma Variants   240

27   Nonastrocytic Glial Tumors   252

28   Neuronal, Mixed Neuronal-Glial, and Pineal Parenchymal
      Tumors   262

29   Primitive Neuroepithelial Tumors and Germ Cell Tumors   271

30   Pituitary Adenoma and Tumors of Rathke's Pouch
      Origin   280

31   Meningeal Tumors   289

32   Reticuloendothelial Tumors and Intracranial Metastasis   302

33   Regional Head and Neck Tumors with Intracranial
     Extension   313

34   Nonneoplastic Cysts and Tumor-like Lesions   322

V.   Aneurysms, Vascular Malformations, and Other Vascular
     Lesions   337

35   Intracranial Aneurysms   339

36   Intracranial Vascular Malformations   354

37   Stroke   373

38   Atherosclerosis   386

39   Nonatheromatous Causes of Arterial Stenosis and
     Occlusion   395

40   Venous Occlusions   405

VI. Intracranial Infections and Inflammation   413

41   Congenital and Neonatal Infections   415

42   Infectious Meningitis, Subdural Empyema and Epidural
     Abscesses   425

43   Cerebritis, Abscess, and Ventriculitis/Ependymitis   434

44   Encephalitis and Post-Infectious Syndromes   442

45   CNS Manifestations of HIV Infection   456

46   Granulomatous Diseases   473

47   Fungal and Parasitic Infections   482

VII. Metabolic, White Matter, and Degenerative Diseases   495

48   Normal Myelination   497

49   Inherited Metabolic and Degenerative Brain Disorders:
     Introduction, Overview, and Classification   510

50   Inherited Metabolic and Degenerative Brain Disorders That Primarily Affect White Matter   517

51   Inherited Metabolic and Neurodegenerative Disorders That Affect the Gray Matter   528

52   The Normal Aging Brain   537

53   Acquired Degenerative, Toxic, and Metabolic White Matter Diseases   545

54   Gray Matter Neurodegenerative Disorders   560

VIII.   Disease Processes by Location   571

55   Scalp and Calvarium   573

56   Extraaxial Pathology   585

57   Ventricular Pathology   594

58   Sellar and Juxtasellar Lesions   604

59   Pineal Region   615

60   Cerebellopontine Angle Region   621

61   Skull Base Lesions   630

62   Foramen Magnum Lesions   642

Appendix   Differential Diagnosis of Imaging Patterns   647

A   Morphologic Patterns   649

B   Lesions by Location   652

C   Calcifications   656

D   Enhancement Patterns   660

E   Miscellaneous CT Patterns   664

F   Miscellaneous MRI Patterns   667

SECTION I
Normal Anatomy

1

Scalp and Skull

Key Concepts

1. SCALP serves as mnemonic for the layers (from external to internal): *S*kin, *C*onnective tissue, *A*poneurosis, *L*oose connective tissue, and *P*eriosteum.
2. The outer connective tissue layer and galea aponeurotica layer act as barriers, whereas the loose areolar layer is a potential space for accumulation of blood or spread of infection.
3. Calvarial fontanelles close by 2 years of age, whereas calvarial sutures do not fully close until 30 years of age.
4. There are numerous calvarial foramina that transmit important neurovascular structures.
5. In children the calvarial marrow is actively hematopoetic and demonstrates low signal on T1WI up to age 7, and may enhance on MRI up to age 9 or 10.

I. Scalp.
   A. SCALP serves as mnemonic for the layers (from external to internal): *S*kin, *C*onnective tissue, *A*poneurosis, *L*oose connective tissue, and *P*eriosteum (Fig. 2-1).
   B. Five layers: outer three constitute scalp proper and remain together with peeling of flap.
      1. Skin.
         a. Forms majority of scalp.
      2. Connective tissue.
         a. Dense subcutaneous layer connecting skin to aponeurosis.
         b. Moderate barrier to deeper spread of superficial scalp infections.
      3. Aponeurosis epicranialis or galea aponeurotica.
         a. Sheetlike tendon connecting epicranius muscle (occipitalis and frontalis).
         b. Laterally continuous with fascia over temporalis muscle.
         c. Strength prevents gaping of more superficial lacerations.
         d. Posterior and lateral muscle attachments into bone prevent spread of infection beyond the subaponeurotic space into masticator space and posterior neck.
         e. Anterior attachment of frontalis muscle is directly into skin rather than bone, thereby allowing spread of fluid, blood, or infection into periorbital and nasal area.
      4. Loose connective tissue or areolar tissue or subaponeurotic space.
         a. Cleavage plane between scalp proper and periosteum.
         b. Allows scalp mobility.
         c. Potential space for spread of fluid, blood, or infection.
         d. Infection can be transmitted intracranially via emissary veins that travel through this space.
      5. Periosteum or pericranium.
         a. Dense connective tissue with osteogenic properties.
         b. Attached to outer calvarium by Sharpey's fibers but even more firmly adherent to fibrous tissue at suture.
II. Skull.
   A. Cranial bones (excluding facial skeleton) (Figs. 1-1, 1-2).
      1. Frontal (paired): anterior skull.
      2. Parietal (paired): superolateral skull.
      3. Temporal (paired): inferolateral skull and portions of skull base.
         a. Squamous portion.
         b. Petrous portion.
         c. Tympanic portion.
         d. Mastoid portion.

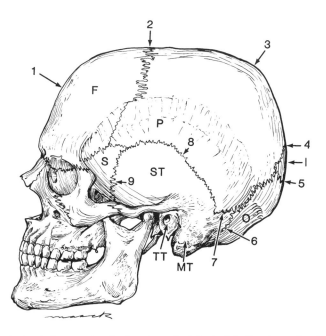

Fig. 1-1   Lateral view anatomic drawing of adult skull indicating calvarial bones and sutures.

Bones:
     F: Frontal bone
     P: Parietal bone
     O: Occipital bone
     I: Inca bone
   ST: Squamous portion of temporal bone
  MT: Mastoid portion of temporal bone
  TT: Tympanic portion of temporal bone
     S: Sphenoid bone

Sutures:
1. Metopic suture
2. Coronal suture
3. Sagittal suture
4. Lambdoid suture
5. Mendosal suture
6. Occipitomastoid suture
7. Parietomastoid suture
8. Squamosal suture
9. Sphenotemporal suture

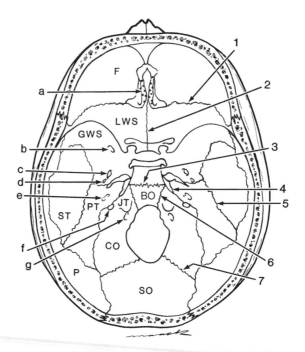

Fig. 1-2 Endocranial skull base anatomic drawing indicating bones comprising skull base, synchondroses, and foramina.

Bones:
F: Frontal
LWS: Lesser wing of sphenoid
GWS: Greater wing of sphenoid
ST: Squamous portion of temporal bone
PT: Petrous portion of temporal bone
JT: Jugular tubercle
CO: Condylar portion of occipital bone
SO: Squamous portion of occipital bone
BO: Basi-occiput
P: Parietal bone

Synchondroses:
1. Frontosphenoid synchondrosis
2. Intersphenoid synchondrosis
3. Basisphenoid synchondrosis
4. Petrobasilar synchondrosis
5. Petrosquamous suture
6. Anterior intraoccipital synchondrosis
7. Posterior intraoccipital synchondrosis

Foramina:
a. Ethmoidal foramina
b. Foramen rotundum
c. Foramen ovale
d. Foramen spinosum
e. Porus acousticus of internal auditory canal
f. Jugular foramen
g. Hypoglossal canal

(Adapted from Harnsberger HR: *Handbook of head and neck imaging,* ed 2, St Louis, 1995, Mosby.)

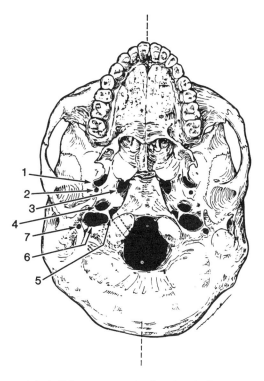

Fig. 1-5   Exocranial skull base anatomic drawing indicating critical apertures.
1. Foramen ovale
2. Foramen spinosum
3. Foramen lacerum
4. Carotid canal
5. Hypoglossal canal
6. Jugular foramen
7. Styloid foramen

(Adapted from Osborn AG, Harnsberger HR, Smoker WRK: Base of skull imaging, *Semin Ultrasound CT MR* 7:91-106, 1986.)

    c. Foramen rotundum: CN V_2, artery of foramen rotundum, emissary vv.

    d. Vidian or pterygoid canal: vidian a., vidian n.

    e. Foramen ovale: CN V_3, emissary vv. (from cavernous sinus to pterygoid plexus), accessory meningeal branch of maxillary artery (variable).

    f. Foramen spinosum: middle meningeal a., recurrent (meningeal) branch of mandibular nerve (variable).

Table 1-1   Major Apertures of the Skull Base

Aperture	Location	Fissure Transmitted Structure(s)	Connects
Cribriform plate	Medial floor of anterior cranial fossa	Olfactory nerve (CN I) Ethmoidal arteries (anterior and posterior)	Anterior fossa to superior nasal cavity
Optic canal	Lesser wing of sphenoid bone	Optic nerve (CN II) Ophthalmic artery Subarachnoid space, cerebrospinal fluid, and dura around optic nerve	Orbital apex to middle cranial fossa
Superior orbital fissure	Between lesser and greater sphenoid wings	CNs III, IV, V$_1$, VI Superior ophthalmic vein	Orbit to middle cranial fossa
Foramen rotundum	Middle cranial fossa floor inferior to superior orbital fissure	CN V$_2$ Emissary veins Artery of foramen rotundum	Meckel's cave to pterygopalatine fossa
Foramen ovale	Floor of middle cranial fossa lateral to sella	CN V$_3$ Emissary veins from cavernous sinus to pterygoid plexus Accessory meningeal branch of maxillary artery (when present)	Meckel's cave to nasopharyngeal masticator space (infratemporal fossa)
Foramen spinosum	Posterolateral to foramen ovale	Middle meningeal artery Recurrent (meningeal) branch of mandibular nerve	Middle cranial fossa to high masticator space (infratemporal fossa)

Foramen lacerum	Base of medial pterygoid plate at petrous apex	Meningeal branches of ascending pharyngeal artery (*not* internal carotid artery)	Not a true foramen; filled with fibrocartilage in life
Vidian canal	In sphenoid bone below and medial to foramen rotundum	Vidian artery and nerve	Foramen lacerum to pterygopalatine fossa
Carotid canal	Within petrous temporal bone	Internal carotid artery Sympathetic plexus	Carotid space to cavernous sinus
Jugular foramen	Posterolateral to carotid canal, between petrous temporal bone and occipital bone	Pars nervosa: inferior petrosal sinuses (CN IX and Jacobson's nerve) Pars vascularis: internal jugular vein, CNs X and XI, nerve of Arnold, small meningeal branches of ascending pharyngeal and occipital arteries	Posterior fossa to nasopharyngeal carotid space
Stylomastoid foramen	Behind styloid process	CN VII	Parotid space to middle ear
Hypoglossal canal	Base of occipital condyles	CN XII	Foramen magnum to nasopharyngeal carotid space
Foramen magnum	Floor of posterior fossa	Medulla and its meninges Spinal segment of CN XI Vertebral arteries and veins Anterior and posterior spinal arteries	Posterior fossa to cervical spinal canal

CN, Cranial nerve.

    6. Ethmoid.
       a. Foramina of cribriform plate: CN I.
       b. Anterior ethmoidal foramen: anterior ethmoidal a., anterior ethmoidal n.
       c. Posterior ethmoidal foramen: posterior ethmoidal a., posterior ethmoidal n.
       d. Foramen cecum (midline): emissary vv. (from veins of frontal sinus and nose to superior sagittal sinus).
  G. Marrow.
    1. Tissue composition varies with age and location.
    2. Less than 1 year: active hematopoetic marrow exists in calvarium and clivus; low signal on T1WI.
    3. In children: active (red) marrow is gradually replaced by fatty (yellow) marrow; high signal on T1WI.
       a. Low-signal marrow in skull or clivus normally persists up to approximately age 7.
       b. Because red marrow is present in varying degrees and at various locations in children, some enhancement on MRI may normally occur up to age 9 or 10.

SUGGESTED READINGS

Bourekas EC, Lanzieri CF: The calvarium, *Semin US CT MR* 15:424-453, 1994.

Harnsberger HR: *Handbook of head and neck imaging,* ed 2, St Louis, 1995, Mosby.

Harnberger HR (guest ed): Extracranial head and neck imaging, *Semin US CT MR* June 1986 (entire monograph).

Laine FJ, Nadel L, Braun IF: CT and MR imaging of the central skull base. I. Techniques, embryologic development, and anatomy, *Radiographics* 10:591-602, 1990.

Mancuso AA, Harnsberger HR, Dillon WP: *Workbook for MRI and CT of the head and neck,* ed 2, Baltimore, 1989, Williams and Wilkins.

Okada Y, Aoki S, Barkovich AJ, et al: Cranial bone marrow in children: assessment of normal development with MR imaging, *Radiology* 171:161-164, 1989.

Schnitzlein HN, Murtagh FR: *Imaging anatomy of the head and spine,* ed 2, Baltimore, 1990, Urban and Schwarzenberg.

2

Meninges, Meningeal Spaces, Ventricles, Cisterns, and CSF

Key Concepts

1. The meninges are made up of 3 layers. The outer pachymenix (G. pachys = thick, meninx = membrane) consists of the thick dura mater. The inner leptomeninges (G. leptos = slender) consist of the arachnoid and pia.
2. The dura forms major supporting septa that also contain dural venous sinuses.
3. Major dural reflections (e.g., falx, tentorium, lateral cavernous sinus walls) normally enhance on CT and MR studies with contrast. Mild leptomeningeal enhancement is normal if:
    a. Thin (less than 1 mm).
    b. Smooth and linear.
    c. Discontinuous or focal, in short segments.
    d. Of minimal intensity, most striking at vertex and anterior temporal lobes.
    e. Less intense than cavernous sinus enhancement.
4. Of the meningeal spaces, only the subarachnoid space exists normally. The epidural and subdural spaces are potential spaces that only manifest with pathology.
5. All ventricles and cisterns intercommunicate.
6. The subarachnoid cisterns contain specific neurovascular structures.
7. The majority of CSF is produced by choroid plexus, the largest and most important being in the lateral ventricles.
8. CSF turns over three times per day, with adult daily production of about 500 cc and total volume of about 150 cc at any given time. Distribution is approximately 20% in ventricles, 50% in intracranial subarachnoid space, and 30% in spinal subarachnoid space.

I. Meninges (Fig. 2-1 and Table 2-1).
   A. Pachymenix (G. pachys = thick; meninx = membrane).
      1. Thick, tough outer layer also referred to as dura mater.
      2. Because it adheres so intimately to the bony calvarium it is said to have two layers.

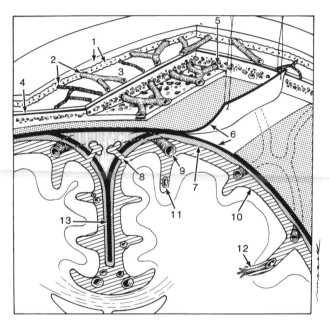

Fig. 2-1 Anatomic drawing depicts the scalp, skull, and meninges.
1. Scalp with subcutaneous fat
2. Scalp arteries and veins
3. Galea aponeurotica
4. Potential subgaleal space and periosteum (shown together as thin black line)
5. Diploic veins in calvarium
6. Dura (outer and inner layers)
7. Arachnoid
8. Arachnoid villi or pacchionian granulations, projecting from subarachnoid space into superior sagittal sinus (SSS)
9. Cortical veins (shown coursing across potential subdural space to enter SSS)
10. Pia mater
11. Pial arteries
12. Perivascular or Virchow-Robin spaces (pial-lined infoldings of CSF around penetrating cortical vessels)
13. Falx cerebri (note potential subdural space adjacent to falx)
(From Osborn A: *Diagnostic neuroradiology,* St Louis, 1994, Mosby.)

   a. Endosteal layer—is actually the internal periosteum or endosteum of the calvarium.
   b. Meningeal layer—is the dura proper and is continuous with the spinal dura.
3. The dura extends inwardly to form four major septa or reflections.
   a. Falx cerebri.
      (1) Large sickle-shaped midline vertical fold within interhemispheric fissure.
      (2) Larger posteriorly than anteriorly.
      (3) Attached to crista galli anteriorly and to internal occipital protuberance and tentorium posteriorly.
      (4) Several dural sinuses are contained within:
         (a) Superior sagittal sinus.
         (b) Inferior sagittal sinus.
         (c) Straight sinus.
   b. Tentorium cerebelli.
      (1) Crescent-shaped horizontal fold between the cerebrum and cerebellum.
      (2) Anterior attachment to anterior/posterior clinoid processes and petromastoid bones. Posterior attachment to occipital bone.
      (3) Contains right and left transverse sinuses.
      (4) Anteromedial free margins form tentorial incisure or notch.
   c. Falx cerebelli.
      (1) Small sickle-shaped vertical midline fold in posterior fossa, immediately inferior to tentorium, projecting

Table 2-1   Meningeal Anatomy

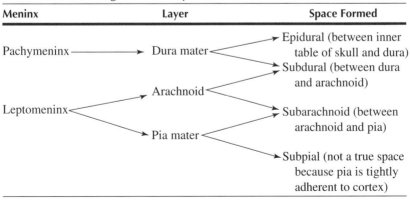

Meninx	Layer	Space Formed
Pachymeninx ⟶	Dura mater	Epidural (between inner table of skull and dura)
		Subdural (between dura and arachnoid)
Leptomeninx	Arachnoid	
	Pia mater	Subarachnoid (between arachnoid and pia)
		Subpial (not a true space because pia is tightly adherent to cortex)

slightly between cerebellar hemispheres posteriorly.
      (2) Contains occipital sinus.
    d. Diaphragma sellae.
      (1) Small circular horizontal fold forming the roof of the
          pituitary fossa.
      (2) Small central opening for passage of pituitary infund-
          ibulum.
  4. Dural reflections such as the falx and tentorium normally are
     slightly hyperdense to adjacent brain on noncontrast CT.
  5. Enhancement of dura (e.g., falx, tentorium, lateral cavernous
     sinus walls) is normal on both CT and MR. Obliquely sectioned
     dural structures can have a bizarre appearance on contrast-
     enhanced studies.
B. Leptomeninges.
  1. Arachnoid mater.
    a. Delicate, transparent membrane forming intermediate brain
       covering.
  2. Pia mater.
    a. Highly vascular thin innermost membrane adhering closely
       to surface of brain including sulci and fissures.
    b. Forms membranous sleeves that follow penetrating vessels
       into the brain parenchyma, resulting in perivascular spaces
       (Virchow-Robin spaces) that may be continuous with the
       subpial or subarachnoid space (controversial).
    c. Also forms tela choroidea of choroid plexus.
  3. Mild leptomeningeal enhancement on contrast-enhanced MR is
     normal and should be:
    a. Thin (less than 1 mm).
    b. Smooth and linear.
    c. Discontinuous or focal, occurring in short segments.
    d. Of minimal intensity, most prominent at vertex and anterior
       temporal lobe; little around sides and base of brain.
    e. Somewhat less intense than cavernous sinus enhance-
       ment.
II. Meningeal spaces (Fig. 2-1 and Table 2-1).
  A. Extradural or epidural space.
    1. Location: superficial to the dura mater; between bony calvarium
       and endosteal layer (internal periosteum).
    2. Is essentially a potential space that becomes real only when
       blood accumulates and pulls dura away from calvarium.
    3. Important related vascular structures: at risk during surgery or
       from adjacent fractures.

       a. Meningeal arteries and veins: ramify on internal surface of the calvarium, often form distinct grooves.

       b. Dural venous sinuses: venous channels located between the internal periosteum and dura proper, drain cortical veins that cross subarachnoid and subdural spaces.

  B. Subdural space.

    1. Location: between dura and arachnoid membranes.

    2. Is essentially a potential space with only a thin film of subdural fluid within.

    3. Important related vascular structures: at risk from shearing forces from trauma.

       a. Bridging veins: between cortical veins and dural venous sinuses.

  C. Subarachnoid space.

    1. Location: between arachnoid and pia.

    2. Contains CSF and is contiguous with ventricular spaces as well as spinal subarachnoid space.

    3. Important related vascular structures: at risk from ruptured aneurysm or vascular malformation.

       a. Cerebral arteries: travel through major cisternal spaces.

III. Ventricles and interventricular communications (Fig. 2-2).

  A. Lateral ventricles.

    1. Paired, complex C-shaped structures.

    2. Components.

       a. Frontal or Anterior horn.

       b. Body.

       c. Trigone or Atrium: junction of body, occipital horn, and temporal horn.

       d. Occipital or Posterior horn.

       e. Temporal horn.

    3. Borders (vary according to part of ventricle).

       a. Superior: mostly corpus callosum.

       b. Lateral: caudate nucleus.

       c. Medial: septum pellucidum anteriorly, fornix posteriorly.

       d. Inferior: stria terminalis (between caudate nucleus and thalamus), thalamus, then hippocampus as it forms floor of temporal horn.

    4. Communicate inferiorly with third ventricle via foramen of Monro.

    5. Contain largest and most important choroid plexus, which are also continuous with the choroid plexus of the third ventricle.

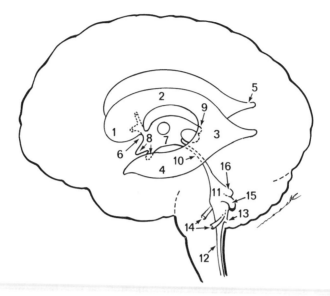

Fig. 2-2   Anatomic drawing of ventricular system (view is from lateral, slightly cephalad aspect).

1. Frontal horn, lateral ventricle
2. Body, lateral ventricle
3. Atrium, lateral ventricle
4. Temporal horn, lateral ventricle
5. Occipital horn, lateral ventricle
6. Foramen of Monro
7. Body, third ventricle
8. Optic and infundibular recesses, third ventricle
9. Suprapineal recess, third ventricle
10. Aqueduct
11. Body, fourth ventricle
12. Obex
13. Foramen of Magendie
14. Lateral recesses of fourth ventricle with foramina of Luschka
15. Posterior superior recesses, fourth ventricle (cap cerebellar tonsils)
16. Fastigium, fourth ventricle

6. Normal variations.
    a. Asymmetric size common.
    b. Coarcted or coapted parts (e.g., frontal or occipital horns) common.
    c. Cavum septi pellucidi.
        (1) Potential CSF space between two leaves of septum.

        (2) Nearly always present in fetus and disappears in childhood, but can occasionally persist into adulthood.

        (3) Occasionally communicates with lateral ventricle.

    d. Cavum vergae.

        (1) Posterior extension of cavum septi pellucidi below corpus callosum and above fornix.

        (2) Almost never seen in absence of cavum septi pellucidi.

B. Foramen of Monro.

  1. Y-shaped aperture connecting lateral ventricles to third ventricle.

  2. Borders.

    a. Anterior: columns of fornix and septum pellucidum.

    b. Posterior: choroid plexus.

C. Third ventricle.

  1. Complex midline thin vertical structure located below bodies of the lateral ventricles.

  2. Components.

    a. Optic recess: V-shaped recess immediately anterosuperior to optic chiasm.

    b. Infundibular recess: shallower V-shaped or U-shaped recess posterior to optic recess; bordered inferiorly by infundibular stalk and posteriorly by tuber cinereum of hypothalamus.

    c. Suprapineal recess: tail-like posterior extension immediately above pineal gland.

  3. Borders.

    a. Superior: fornix, velum interpositum, internal cerebral veins.

    b. Lateral: thalami.

    c. Anterior: anterior commissure, lamina terminalis.

    d. Posterior: posterior commissure, pineal gland.

    e. Inferior: optic chiasm, infundibulum, hypothalamus, mamillary bodies.

  4. Indentations.

    a. By massa intermedia (interthalamic adhesion): centrally.

    b. By infundibulum and optic chiasm: inferiorly.

    c. By anterior and posterior commissures: anteriorly and posteriorly, respectively.

  5. Communicates with:

    a. Lateral ventricles anterosuperiorly via foramen of Monro.

    b. Fourth ventricle posteroinferiorly via aqueduct.

  6. Choroid plexus is located in the roof of the third ventricle and is contiguous with choroid plexus of the lateral ventricles through the foramen of Monro.

D. Cerebral aqueduct of Sylvius.
   1. Connects third ventricle with fourth ventricle.
   2. Borders.
      a. Anterior: periaqueductal grey matter of midbrain (tegmentum).
      b. Posterior: quadrigeminal plate (tectum).
E. Fourth ventricle.
   1. Complex rhomboid structure below third ventricle and cerebral aqueduct.
   2. Components.
      a. Floor: ventral wall.
      b. Roof.
         (1) Anterior or rostral or superior medullary velum.
         (2) Posterior or caudal or inferior medullary velum.
      c. Fastigium: dorsal apex of ventricle between superior and inferior velum.
      d. Lateral recesses: lead to the foramina of Luschka.
      e. Obex: inferiormost aspect, leads to central canal of spinal cord.
   3. Borders.
      a. Anterior: pons, medulla. Nuclei of cranial nerves V through XII are ventral to floor of fourth ventricle.
      b. Posterior: superior and inferior medullary vela and cerebellar vermis.
      c. Lateral: superior, middle, and inferior cerebellar peduncles.
      d. Inferior: cerebellar tonsils (capped by posterior superior recesses).
   4. Communicates with:
      a. Cisterna magna posteroinferiorly via foramen of Magendie.
      b. Cerebellopontine angle and medullary cisterns anterolaterally via lateral recesses and foramina of Luschka.
      c. Is contiguous with central canal of medulla and spinal cord inferiorly via obex, although this is not normally a route of CSF flow.
   5. Choroid plexus is located in the roof of the fourth ventricle and extends into the lateral recesses and possibly through the foramina of Luschka.
F. Foramen of Magendie or median aperture (M for midline).
   1. Midline communication between fourth ventricle and cisterna magna.
G. Foramina of Luschka or lateral apertures (L for lateral).
   1. Paired lateral apertures between fourth ventricle and cerebellopontine angles.

        2. Choroid plexus from fourth ventricle extends through foramina of Luschka to cerebellopontine angle cisterns.

IV. Subarachnoid cisterns (Fig. 2-3 and Table 2-2).
    A. Posterior fossa cisterns.
        1. Medullary cistern: anterior to medulla.
        2. Cerebellomedullary cistern or Cisterna magna: posterior to medulla, inferior to vermis.
        3. Pontine cistern: along ventral and lateral peripontine surfaces.
        4. Cerebellopontine angle cistern.

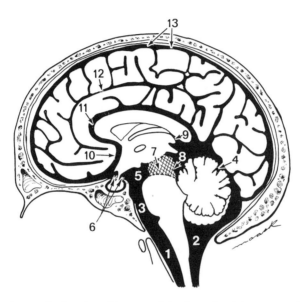

Fig. 2-3 Anatomic drawing of intracranial subarachnoid spaces and cisterns (in black). Wings of ambient cisterns (cross-hatched area) curve around mesencephalon and connect quadrigeminal to basal cisterns.

    1. Medullary cistern
    2. Cisterna magna
    3. Pontine cistern
    4. Superior cerebellar cistern
    5. Interpeduncular cistern
    6. Chiasmatic (suprasellar) cistern
    7. Ambient cistern
    8. Quadrigeminal plate cistern
    9. Velum interpositum
    10. Cistern of lamina terminalis
    11. Pericallosal cistern
    12. Cingulate sulcus
    13. Convexity subarachnoid space

Table 2-2   Major Subarachnoid Cisterns and Their Contents

Cistern	Location	Contents
Posterior Fossa Cisterns		
Medullary cistern	Anterior to medulla	Vertebral arteries; anterior, posterior spinal arteries; CN XII
Cisterna magna	Posterior to medulla	Posterior inferior cerebellar artery; inferior cerebellar veins; CNs IX, X, XI
Pontine cistern	Between pons and clivus	Vertebrobasilar arteries; origins of anterior inferior cerebellar and superior cerebellar arteries; anterior pontomesencephalic venous plexus; CN VI
Cerebellopontine angle cistern	Between petrous temporal bone, cerebellum, pons, and tentorium	Anterior inferior cerebellar artery; sometimes superior petrosal veins; CNs V, VII, VIII
Superior cerebellar cistern	Between tentorium and vermis, cerebellar hemispheres; connects with quadrigeminal cistern anterosuperiorly	Superior cerebellar artery; superior vermian veins
Suprasellar (Basal) Cisterns		
Interpeduncular cistern	Between cerebral peduncles	Basilar artery; origins of thalamoperforating and posterior choroidal arteries; CN III

Chiasmatic (suprasellar) cistern	Above sella	Distal internal carotid artery; origins of anterior and middle cerebral arteries; posterior communicating artery; anterior choroidal artery; proximal basal vein of Rosenthal; optic tracts, chiasm, CN II; hypothalamus infundibulum, mammillary bodies; anterior recesses of third ventricle
Cistern of the lamina terminalis	Anterosuperior extension of chiasmatic cistern	
Cistern of the corpus callosum	Anterosuperior extension of cistern of the lamina terminals	
Mesencephalic Cisterns		
Ambient cistern	Around midbrain; connects suprasellar, pontine, and quadrigeminal cisterns	Posterior cerebral artery; basilar artery; superior cerebellar artery; CN IV; mesencephalic veins
Quadrigeminal cistern	Behind pineal and quadrigeminal plate; connects ambient and superior cerebellar cisterns	Pineal gland; posterior third ventricle; posterior choroidal artery; vein of Galen and basal vein of Rosenthal
Velum interpositum	Above third ventricle; below corpus callosum and fornix: anterior continuation of quadrigeminal cistern	Internal cerebral veins; branches of anterior and posterior choroidal arteries
Lateral Superior Cisterns		
Sylvian cistern	Between insula and opercula; connects medially with suprasellar cistern	Middle cerebral artery and its branches; superficial middle cerebral vein
Convexity subarachnoid spaces	Over surface of hemispheres	Cortical arteries; veins

CN, Cranial nerve.

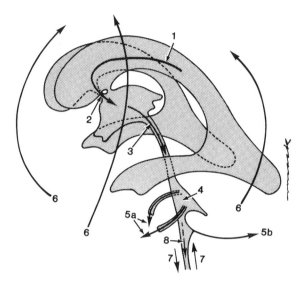

Fig. 2-4   Diagrammatic representation of circulation of cerebrospinal fluid.
1. Formation of CSF in choroid plexus of lateral ventricle
2. Foramen of Monro
3. Formation of CSF in choroid plexus of third ventricle and subsequent passage through the cerebral aqueduct
4. Formation of CSF in choroid plexus of fourth ventricle
5. Exit from ventricular system through openings of fourth ventricle
   a. Foramina of Lushka
   b. Foramen of Magendie
6. Absorption through arachnoid granulations into superior sagittal venous sinus
7. Circulation around spinal cord in subarachnoid space
8. Descent in central canal of spinal cord (minimal)

       5. Superior cerebellar or superior vermian cistern: midline, between tentorium and vermis.
   B. Mesencephalic cisterns.
      1. Ambient cistern: ventral and lateral to midbrain.
      2. Quadrigeminal cistern or cistern of the great cerebral vein: posterior to pineal gland and quadrigeminal plate.
      3. (Cavum) Velum interpositum: anterior continuation of quadrigeminal cistern above third ventricle, below corpus callosum and fornix.
   C. Suprasellar or basal cisterns.
      1. Interpeduncular cistern: between cerebral peduncles.
      2. Chiasmatic or suprasellar cistern.

3. Cistern of the lamina terminalis: anterosuperior extension of chiasmatic cistern.
4. Cistern of the corpus callosum: anterosuperior extension of cistern of the lamina terminalis.
D. Lateral superior cisterns.
 1. Sylvian cistern or cistern of the lateral sulcus: Sylvian fissure, between insula and opercula.
 2. Convexity subarachnoid spaces: over cerebral hemispheres.
V. CSF.
A. Total volume in adult approximately 150 cc.
B. CSF production: approximately 500 cc produced per day.
 1. 85% production is from choroid plexus of ventricles; largest and most important is in lateral ventricles.
 2. 15% production is from ependyma or capillary filtration.
C. CSF circulation: approximately 3 times per day, aided by arterial pulsations (Fig. 2-4).
 1. CSF flows from the lateral ventricles to the third ventricle via the foramen of Monro, which in turn flows to the fourth ventricle via the aqueduct of Sylvius.
 2. CSF exits the fourth ventricles by the median and lateral apertures to the posterior fossa cisterns. CSF does not normally flow through the obex into the central canal of the spinal cord.
 3. Most CSF then flows superiorly through the tentorial incisure to reach the mesencephalic and suprasellar cisterns, and eventually the convexity subarachnoid spaces.
 4. Some CSF from the posterior fossa cisterns continue inferiorly into the spinal subarachnoid space.
 5. Small amounts of CSF also continue into the subarachnoid extensions around the optic nerves.
D. Approximate CSF distribution.
 1. 20% in cerebral ventricles.
 2. 50% in intracranial subarachnoid space.
 3. 30% in spinal subarachnoid space.
E. CSF absorption.
 1. Mostly through arachnoid villi, which are protrusions of arachnoid into the dural venous sinuses, particularly the superior sagittal sinus and transverse sinuses.
 2. Some CSF is absorbed by ependyma.
 3. Some CSF is absorbed through the capillary walls.
 4. Some CSF is absorbed by lymphatics adjacent to cranial and spinal nerves.

SUGGESTED READINGS

Amundsen P, Newton TH: Subarachnoid cisterns. In Newton TH and Potts DG, eds: *Radiology of the skull and brain, ventricles and cisterns,* St Louis, 1978, Mosby, pp 3588-3711.

Greenberg RW, Lane EL, Cinnamon J, et al: The cranial meninges: anatomic considerations, *Semin US CT MRI* 15:454-465, 1994.

Jinkins JR: The cisternal ventricle, *AJNR* 9:111-113, 1988.

Malko JA, Hoffman JC Jr, Green RC: MR measurement of intracranial CSF volume in 41 elderly normal volunteers, *AJNR* 12:371-374, 1991.

Matsuno H, Rhoton AL Jr, Peace D: Microsurgical anatomy of the posterior fossa cisterns, *Neurosurgery* 23:58-80, 1988.

Pappas CTE, Sonntag VKH, Spetzler RF: Surgical anatomy of the anterior aspect of the third ventricle, *BNI Q* 6:2-10, 1990.

3

Aortic Arch, Great Vessels, and External Carotid Artery

Key Concepts

1. Three major branches arise directly from the arch. They are (in order) the innominate artery (brachiocephalic trunk), left common carotid artery, and left subclavian artery.
2. Common anomalies include origin of the left common carotid artery with or from the innominate artery (25%), arch origin of the left verteral artery (5%), and an aberrant right subclavian artery (0.5% to 1%).
3. The common carotid bifurcation usually occurs between C3 to C5 but may be as high as C2 or as low as C6.
4. Immediately after bifurcation the internal carotid artery is usually posterolateral (90%) to the external carotid artery.
5. Initials of external carotid artery (ECA) branches form mnemonic SALFOPSM:
   - S   Superior thyroid.
   - A   Ascending pharyngeal.
   - L   Lingual.
   - F   Facial.
   - O   Occipital.
   - P   Posterior auricular.
   - S   Superficial temporal.
   - M   Maxillary (Internal).
6. Lower cranial nerves (CNs V, VII, IX, X, XI, and XII) are supplied principally by ECA branches, especially the internal maxillary, posterior auricular, and ascending pharyngeal arteries.

I. Aortic arch (Fig. 3-1).
   A. Three major branches (great vessels) arise from the outer curve of the arch (in order).
      1. Innominate artery (brachiocephalic trunk).
      2. Left common carotid artery.
      3. Left subclavian artery.
   B. Common anomalies.
      1. Left common carotid artery arises with or from the innominate artery (25%).
      2. Left vertebral artery arises directly from the arch (5%).
      3. Aberrant right subclavian artery (0.5% to 1%).
II. Innominate artery (Fig. 3-1).
   A. The innominate artery (brachiocephalic trunk) is the first vessel that arises from the arch. Shortly after its origin it bifurcates into the right common carotid and right subclavian arteries. The right vertebral artery is the first branch of the right subclavian artery.
   B. Branches.
      1. Right common carotid artery (CCA).
         a. Normal origin: innominate artery bifurcation, (medial vessel) directed cephalad.
         b. Anomalous origin: If right subclavian artery is aberrant, right CCA has separate origin as first vessel arising from the aortic arch.
      2. Right subclavian artery.
         a. Normal origin: innominate artery bifurcation, (lateral vessel) directed to upper extremity.
         b. Anomalous origin: Aberrant right subclavian artery arises as last brachiocephalic vessel from aortic arch (0.5% to 1%).
         c. Major branches (in order of proximal to distal).
            (1) Right vertebral artery.
            (2) Right thyrocervical trunk.
            (3) Right internal thoracic artery.
            (4) Right costocervical trunk.
      3. Right vertebral artery (VA).
         a. First branch of right subclavian artery.
         b. Anomalous origin: rarely may arise from distal aortic arch, proximal to the origin of the left subclavian artery.
         c. Right vertebral artery is dominant over the left in about 25% of cases.
         d. Vertebral arteries course through transverse foramina from C6 to C2, then turn laterally and superiorly through C1 vertebral foramina before entering foramen magnum.

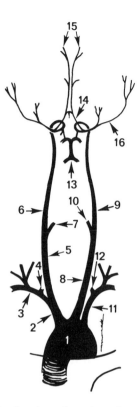

Fig. 3-1   Frontal anatomic drawing of aortic arch and great vessels with major branches.

1. Aortic arch
2. Innominate artery (brachiocephalic trunk)
3. Right subclavian artery
4. Right vertebral artery
5. Right common carotid artery
6. Right internal carotid artery
7. Right external carotid artery
8. Left common carotid artery
9. Left internal carotid artery
10. Left external carotid artery
11. Left subclavian artery
12. Left vertebral artery
13. Vertebral arteries uniting to form basilar artery
14. Circle of Willis
15. Anterior cerebral arteries
16. Middle cerebral arteries

III. Left common carotid artery (CCA) (Fig. 3-1).
    A. Normal origin: second major vessel arising from aortic arch.
    B. Variants.
        1. Common origin with or arising from innominate artery (25%).
IV. Left subclavian artery (Fig. 3-1).
    A. Normal origin: third and last major vessel arising from aortic arch.
    B. Major branches (in order of proximal to distal).
        1. Left vertebral artery.
            a. Normal origin: first branch of the left subclavian artery.
            b. Anomalous origin: directly from the aortic arch, forming fourth and last major brachiocephalic vessel (5%). In these cases the left vertebral artery is usually nondominant.
            c. Left vertebral artery is dominant over right in about 50% of cases.
            d. In remaining 25% of cases, both vertebral arteries are approximately equal.
        2. Left thyrocervical trunk.
        3. Left internal thoracic artery.
        4. Left costocervical trunk.
V. CCA bifurcation (Fig. 3-1).
    A. Normal.
        1. Bifurcation into internal carotid artery (ICA) and external carotid artery (ECA) between C3 to C5.
        2. ICA initially posterolateral to ECA, then courses medial to ECA as it ascends.
        3. No normal extracranial ICA branches in neck.
    B. Variants and anomalies.
        1. Bifurcation may be as high as C2 or as low as C6.
        2. ICA arises medial to ECA in 10%.
        3. Some proximal ECA branches (e.g., ascending pharyngeal and superior thyroid) can arise from distal CCA or CCA bifurcation.
        4. Rarely, ICA and ECA arise separately due to absence of common trunk (e.g., both arise directly from innominate artery on the right, or from aortic arch on the left).
        5. Rarely, nonbifurcating carotid artery gives rise to branch arteries of both ECA and ICA.
VI. External carotid artery (Figs. 3-2, 3-3, and box on p. 35).
    A. Normal anatomy: arises from CCA bifurcation as smaller of the two branches. It initially courses medial and anterior to ICA but eventually courses posterolaterally.
    B. Major branches (in approximate order).
        1. Superior thyroid artery.
            a. Origin: usually arises anteriorly from proximal ECA as first branch; can occasionally arise from CCA (16%).

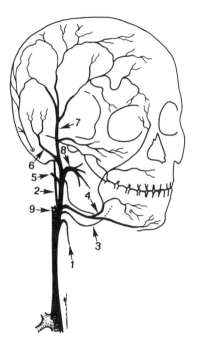

Fig. 3-2   Oblique anatomic drawing of right common carotid bifurcation with external carotid artery and major branches.

1. Superior thyroidal artery
2. Ascending pharyngeal artery
3. Lingual artery
4. Facial artery
5. Occipital artery
6. Posterior auricular artery
7. Superficial temporal artery
8. Maxillary artery
9. Internal carotid artery

b. Supplies: larynx and upper thyroid gland.
c. *Note:* Inferior thyroid gland is supplied by branches of thyrocervical trunk or a small branch of the aortic arch (arteria thyroidea ima).

2. Ascending pharyngeal artery.
a. Origin: is variable but typically arises posteriorly from the CCA bifurcation or the proximal ECA. Occasionally arises from the occipital artery (14%).
b. Branches.
(1) Meningeal branch: enters through F. lacerum.
(2) Muscular branches.

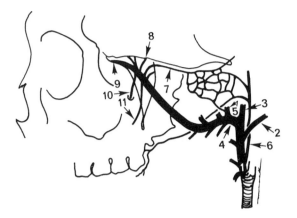

Fig. 3-3 Lateral anatomic drawing of external carotid artery, distal branches, and major branches of maxillary artery.

1. External carotid artery
2. Occipital artery
3. Superficial temporal artery
4. Maxillary artery
5. Middle meningeal artery
6. Ascending pharyngeal artery
7. Vidian artery
8. Artery of the foramen rotundum
9. Infraorbital artery
10. Descending palatine artery
11. Buccal artery

   c. Supplies: nasopharynx, oropharynx, tympanic cavity, CNs IX, X, XI, meninges, musculature.

   d. Anastomoses.

     (1) To vertebral artery via musculospinal branches at C3 level.

     (2) To ICA (petrous and cavernous segments) via meningeal branches connecting to inferolateral and meningohypophyseal trunks.

     (3) To middle meningeal artery via meningeal branch.

3. Lingual artery.

   a. Origin: usually arises directly from ECA but can arise from common lingual-facial trunk (20%).

   b. Branches.

     (1) Deep lingual A.: courses to tip of tongue.

     (2) Sublingual A.: traverses floor of mouth.

Major Extracranial to Intracranial Vascular Anastomoses

1. Maxillary artery to internal carotid artery (ICA) via:
   a. Middle meningeal artery to ethmoidal branches of ophthalmic artery
   b. Artery of the foramen rotundum to inferolateral trunk of ICA
   c. Accessory meningeal artery to inferolateral trunk
   d. Vidian artery to intratemporal ICA
   e. Anterior and middeep temporal arteries to ophthalmic artery via lacrimal, palpebral, or muscular branches
2. Occipital artery to vertebral artery (via muscular and radicular branches) arteries of the first and second cervical spaces
3. Ascending pharyngeal artery to vertebral artery (via musculospinal branches) at C3 level
4. Ascending pharyngeal artery to internal carotid artery (via petrous and cavernous branches)
5. Facial artery to internal carotid artery (via angular branch of facial to orbital branches of ophthalmic artery)
6. Posterior auricular artery to internal carotid artery (via stylomastoid artery)
7. Extracranial-intracranial surgical bypass (typically superficial temporal or occipital artery to middle cerebral); rarely performed

---

      c. Supplies: tongue, floor of mouth, submandibular and sublingual glands, part of mandible.
   4. Facial artery.
      a. Origin: usually arises directly from ECA but can arise from common lingual-facial trunk (20%). Has tortuous course over the mandibular ramus.
      b. Branches.
         (1) Ascending palatine A.
         (2) Glandular branches.
         (3) Submental A.
         (4) Superior and inferior labial arteries.
         (5) Lateral nasal branch.
         (6) Angular artery (termination).
      c. Supplies: face, palate, pharynx, cheek, lip.
      d. Anatomoses.
         (1) To ICA via angular branch connecting to dorsal nasal branch of ophthalmic artery.
   5. Occipital artery.
      a. Branches.
         (1) Meningeal branch.
         (2) Muscular branches.

      b. Supplies: posterior scalp, upper cervical musculature, posterior fossa meninges.

      c. Anastomoses.

         (1) To vertebral artery via muscular and radicular branches at C1 and C2 levels.

6. Posterior auricular artery.

      a. Supplies: pinna, external auditory canal, scalp.

      b. Anastomoses.

         (1) To ICA via stylomastoid artery connecting to petrous ICA.

7. Superficial temporal artery.

      a. One of two distal terminal ECA branches. Has a characteristic hairpin turn where it crosses the zygomatic arch.

      b. Branches.

         (1) Transverse facial A: occasionally arises directly from ECA.

         (2) Zygomaticoorbital A.

         (3) Middle temporal A.

      c. Supplies: scalp, ear. The transverse facial artery supplies the deep face and cheek.

      d. Anastomoses.

         (1) To ICA via frontal branch connecting to supraorbital branch of ophthalmic artery.

8. Internal maxillary artery.

      a. Is largest of two distal terminal ECA branches.

      b. Branches.

         (1) Mandibular portion.

            (a) Anterior tympanic A.

            (b) Deep auricular A.

            (c) Middle meningeal A.

            (d) Accessory meningeal A.

            (e) Inferior alveolar A.

         (2) Pterygoid portion.

            (a) Deep temporal A.

            (b) Pterygoid A.

            (c) Masseteric A.

            (d) Buccal A.

         (3) Pterygopalatine portion.

            (a) Posterior superior alveolar A.

            (b) Infraorbital A.

            (c) Greater (descending) palatine A.

            (d) Artery to foramen rotundum.

            (e) Artery of pterygoid canal or Vidian A.

(f) Pharyngeal A.

(g) Sphenopalatine A.

  c. Supplies: middle and accessory meningeal arteries, muscles of mastication, palate, maxilla, sinuses, nose, and orbit.

  d. Anastomoses.

    (1) To ICA via middle meningeal artery connecting to inferolateral trunk or ethmoidal branches of ophthalmic A.

    (2) To ICA via accessory meningeal artery connecting to inferolateral trunk.

    (3) To ICA via artery of foramen rotundum connecting to inferolateral trunk of ICA.

    (4) To ICA via vidian artery connecting to petrous ICA.

    (5) To ICA via anterior and middle deep temporal arteries connecting to lacrimal, palpebral and muscular branches of ophthalmic artery.

    (6) To ICA via infraorbital artery connecting to dorsal nasal branch of ophthalmic artery.

    (7) To ICA via sphenopalatine artery connecting to ethmoidal branches of ophthalmic artery.

VII. Cranial and peripheral nerve supply: ECA supplies nerves directly via ECA branches or indirectly via dural and transosseous collaterals to ICA branches.

  A. CNs III, IV, V, and VI.

    1. ICA cavernous branches.

    2. Middle and accessory meningeal (pterygomeningeal) arteries of ECA.

    3. Ascending pharyngeal artery (CN VI, gasserian ganglion).

    4. Artery of foramen rotundum (branch of maxillary artery): CN V_2.

  B. CNs VII, VIII.

    1. Anteroinferior cerebellar artery (acoustic branch): supplies CNs VII and VIII.

    2. Middle meningeal artery (petrosal branch): CN VII.

    3. Occipital or posterior auricular arteries (stylomastoid branch): CN VII.

    4. Peripheral CN VII supply is based on territory.

  C. CNs IX, X, XI.

    1. Ascending pharyngeal artery.

    2. Occipital artery.

    3. Anterior cervical arteries (vertebral artery branches).

  D. CN XII.

    1. Ascending pharyngeal artery.

    2. Vertebral artery branches.

SUGGESTED READINGS

Ahn HS, Kerber CW, Deeb ZL: Extra- to intracranial arterial anastomoses in therapeutic embolization: recognition and role, *Am J Radiol* 1:71-75, 1980.

Anderson CM, Haacke EM: Approaches to diagnostic magnetic resonance carotid angiography, *Semin US CT MRI* 13:246-255, 1992.

Beigelman C, Mourey-Gerosa I, Gamsu G, Grenier P: New morphological approach to the classification of anomalies of the aortic arch, *Eur Radiol* 5:435-442, 1995.

Carroll BA: Carotid sonography, *Radiology* 178:303-313, 1991.

Edelman RR, Mattle HP, Atkinson DJ, Hoogewoud HM: MR angiography, *AJR* 154:937-946, 1990.

El Gammal T, Brooks BS: Conventional MR neuroangiography, *AJR* 156:1075-1080, 1991.

Foley WD, Erickson SJ: Color Doppler flow imaging, *AJR* 156:3-13, 1991.

Garcia-Monaco R: Transcranial arterial anastomoses, *Riv de Neuroradiol* 7(suppl 4):63-66, 1994.

Huston J III, Ehman RL: Comparison of time-of-flight and phase-contrast MR neuroangiographic techniques, *Radiographics* 13:9-19, 1993.

Keller PJ, Drayer BP, Fram EK: Magnetic resonance angiography, *Neuroimaging Clinics of North America,* November, 1992 (entire monograph).

Kido DK, Barsotti JB, Rice LZ, et al: Evaluation of the carotid artery bifurcation: comparison of magnetic resonance angiography and digital subtraction arch aortography, *Neuroradiology* 33:48-51, 1991.

Lasjaunias PL, Berenstein A: *Surgical neuroangiography,* vol 1, Baltimore, 1987, Williams and Wilkins, pp 1-153.

Lasjaunias PL, Choi IS: The external carotid artery: functional anatomy, *Riv de Neuroradiol* 4 (Suppl 1):39-45, 1991.

Morimoto T, Nitta K, Kazekawa K, Hashizume K: The anomaly of a non-bifurcating cervical carotid artery, *J Neurosurg* 72:130-132, 1990.

Morvay Z, Milassin P, Barzo P: Assessment of steal syndromes with colour and pulsed Doppler imaging, *Eur Radiol* 5:359-363, 1995.

Osborn AG: *Introduction to cerebral angiography,* New York, 1980, Harper & Row, Chapters 2 to 4.

Ross JS, Masaryk TJ, Ruggieri PM: Magnetic resonance angiography of the carotid bifurcation, *Top Magn Reson Imaging* 3:12-22, 1991.

Russell EJ: Functional angiography of the head and neck, *Am J Radiol* 7:927-936, 1986.

Vitek JJ: Accessory meningeal artery, *AJNR* 10:569-573, 1989.

Wasserman BA, Mikulis DJ, Manzione JV: Origin of the right vertebral artery from the left side of the aortic arch proximal to the origin of the left subclavian artery, *AJNR* 13:355-358, 1992.

Zamir M, Sinclair P: Origin of the brachiocephalic trunk, left carotid, and left subclavian arteries from the arch of the human aorta, *Invest Radiol* 26:128-133, 1991.

4

Internal Carotid Artery

Key Concepts

1. The ICA normally has no branches in the neck (i.e., cervical portion).
2. Aberrant ICA may course through the middle ear.
3. Persistent (embryonic) carotid-vertebrobasilar anastomoses can occur (in descending order of frequency).
   a. Trigeminal artery.
   b. Hypoglossal artery.
   c. Acoustic or otic artery.
   d. Proatlantal intersegmental artery.
4. The intracalvarial ICA can be loosely divided into petrous, cavernous (juxtasellar), and intracranial (supraclinoid) portions. The cavernous portion can be further divided into numbered segments.
   a. C5 or ascending cavernous segment.
   b. C4 or posterior genu.
   c. C3 or horizontal cavernous segment.
   d. C2 or anterior genu.
   e. C1 or remaining intracavernous segment.
5. Major ICA branches occur mostly in the cavernous and intradural cerebral segments (in order of origin):
   a. Meningohypophyseal trunk.
   b. Inferolateral trunk (lateral mainstem artery).
   c. Ophthalmic artery.
   d. Posterior communicating artery.
   e. Anterior choroidal artery.
   f. Anterior and middle cerebral arteries (terminal ICA bifurcation).

I. Cervical ICA (Fig. 4-1).
   A. Normal course.
      1. Originates from CCA bifurcation.
      2. Carotid bulb is proximal dilatation that extends for short 2 to 4 cm segment.
      3. Initially posterolateral to ECA, then courses medially as it runs cephalad (90%) to enter skull base at petrous temporal bone.
   B. Branches.
      1. Normally no branches occur from cervical ICA.
   C. Anomalies.
      1. ICA agenesis.
         a. Rare. May be unilateral or even more rarely bilateral.
         b. May have total or segmental agenesis.
         c. Total or proximal segmental agenesis is associated with absent or hypoplastic carotid canal.
         d. Various vascular rerouting patterns are possible to maintain

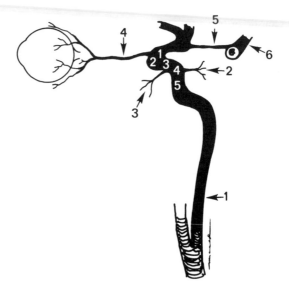

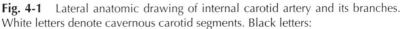

Fig. 4-1   Lateral anatomic drawing of internal carotid artery and its branches. White letters denote cavernous carotid segments. Black letters:
   1. Cervical ICA
   2. Meningohypophyseal trunk
   3. Lateral mainstem artery
   4. Ophthalmic artery
   5. Posterior communicating artery
   6. Posterior cerebral artery

hemispheric arterial supply, including the circle of Willis, anastomoses via persistent embryologic vessels, persistent primitive carotid-vertebrobasilar anastomoses, and complex anastomoses with ECA branches.

e. Associated with increased incidence of aneurysms of the circle of Willis.

2. Nonbifurcating carotid artery.

a. Rare.

b. ICA and ECA branches originate from single carotid trunk.

3. Anomalous branches.

a. Some ECA branches may arise from ICA; such as occipital and ascending pharyngeal arteries.

b. Persistent mandibular artery from cervical ICA.

4. Carotid-vertebrobasilar anastomoses: represent persistent embryonic circulatory patterns linking carotid and vertebrobasilar systems. May be named according to cranial nerves they parallel (Fig. 4-2).

a. Proatlantal intersegmental artery.

(1) Connects cervical ICA or ECA with vertebral artery.

(2) Courses between arch of C1 and occiput.

b. Persistent hypoglossal artery.

(1) Second most common (after trigeminal artery) anastomosis.

(2) Connects cervical ICA with basilar artery.

(3) Courses through hypoglossal canal.

5. Aberrant course.

a. Retropharyngeal course of cervical ICA; can present as pulsatile oropharyngeal submucosal mass.

II. Petrous ICA (Fig. 4-1).

A. Normal course.

1. The carotid canal lies within petrous temporal bone.

2. Short initial portion is vertically oriented and located anterior to jugular fossa and bulb.

3. Turns anteromedially in front of middle ear cavity to run horizontally above foramen lacerum.

4. Emerges from carotid canal at petrous apex.

B. Branches.

1. Anterior and posterior tympanic branches: supply middle ear.

2. Vidian artery (artery of pterygoid canal).

a. Inconstant, seen in 25% of angiograms.

b. Anastomoses with internal maxillary artery (i.e., ICA to ECA connection).

3. Caroticotympanic artery: supplies middle and inner ear.

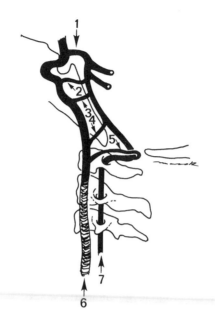

Fig. 4-2 Lateral anatomic drawing of potential embryonic carotid-vertebrobasilar anastomoses.

1. Posterior communicating artery
2. Persistent trigeminal artery
3. Acoustic (otic) artery
4. Hypoglossal artery
5. Proatlantal intersegmental artery
6. Internal carotid artery
7. Vertebral artery

C. Anomalies.
   1. Agenesis of cervical carotid artery resulting in aberrant course of ICA.
      a. Vascular rerouting occurs via the inferior tympanic branch of the ascending pharyngeal artery, anastomosing with the caroticotympanic branch of the petrous ICA. This anastomosis occurs at the site of the primitive hyoid artery. The aberrant artery traverses the hypotympanum and then reunites with the horizontal portion of the petrous ICA.
      b. Associated with absence or hypoplasia of the vertical petrous carotid canal, and enlargement of the inferior tympanic and caroticotympanic canaliculi.
      c. May or may not be associated with persistent stapedial artery (see following discussion).

      d. May cause pulsatile tinnitus and vascular ("blue") tympanic membrane.

      e. Clinical importance: if unrecognized, biopsy or puncture can result in life-threatening hemorrhage or cerebral infarction.

  2. Persistent stapedial artery from petrous ICA.

      a. Caused by intrapetrous embryonic vascular channel (stapedio-hyoid artery).

      b. Originates from petrous ICA and usually enclosed within a bony canal on the cochlear promontory.

      c. Usually terminates as the middle meningeal artery; in these cases the foramen spinosum is absent.

      d. May or may not be associated with aberrant course of ICA (see above).

      e. Clinical significance: may course across or through the footplate of the stapes, complicating prosthetic surgery.

  3. Carotid-vertebrobasilar anastomosis (Fig. 4-2).

      a. Persistent otic artery.

        (1) Extremely rare.

        (2) Connects petrous ICA with proximal basilar artery.

        (3) Clinical significance: projects medially through ICA.

III. Cavernous (Juxtasellar) ICA (Fig. 4-1).

  A. Normal course: Cavernous and supraclinoid ICA segments form S-shaped loop, collectively called "carotid siphon." Cavernous segments can be divided into numbered segments.

    1. C5 or ascending cavernous portion: vertical segment from entrance at petrous apex to posterior genu.

    2. C4 or posterior genu: segment at posteroinferior aspect of juxtasellar region, between ascending and horizontal segments.

    3. C3 or horizontal cavernous portion: between the posterior and anterior genua.

    4. C2 or anterior genu: segment at anterosuperior aspect of juxtasellar region, between horizontal segment and remaining intracavernous ICA.

    5. C1: remainder of intracavernous ICA.

  B. Branches.

    1. Meningohypophyseal or posterior or dorsal trunk.

      a. Although present in 100% of anatomic specimens, it may not be seen on angiography unless high-resolution techniques used.

      b. Arises from C5 portion near junction with C4 segment.

      c. Supplies:

        (1) Posterior pituitary (inferior hypophyseal branch).

        (2) Tentorium (marginal tentorial branch).

           (3) Part of cavernous sinus/clival dura (dorsal meningeal branch).

           (4) Sometimes supplies cranial nerves III to VI.

    2. Inferolateral trunk or lateral mainstem artery or artery of inferior cavernous sinus.

       a. Present in about two thirds of anatomic specimens.

       b. Arises from inferolateral aspect of C3 or C4 segments.

       c. Supplies:

           (1) Cavernous sinus dura.

           (2) Cranial nerves III to VI.

       d. Numerous important anastomoses with ECA branches through foramina ovale, rotundum and spinosum, and superior orbital fissure. (See Chapter 33.)

    3. Capsular branches.

       a. Arise from distal C3 or C2 segments.

       b. Supply:

           (1) Sella.

           (2) Capsule of pituitary gland.

       c. Usually too small to be seen on angiography.

  C. Anomalies.

    1. Persistent trigeminal artery (Fig. 4-2).

       a. Most common carotid-vertebrobasilar anastomosis (85%).

       b. Angiographic incidence of about 0.6%.

       c. Connects intracavernous ICA (usually from C4 segment) with basilar artery (between superior and anterior inferior cerebellar arteries).

       d. Two types.

           (1) Medial type: courses over or through dorsum sellae and perforates dura near clivus.

           (2) Lateral type: courses between sensory root of CN V along lateral aspect of sella to penetrate dura medial to Meckel's cave.

       e. Frequently associated with aneurysms.

       f. Clinical significance: surgical hazard in juxtasellar surgery.

IV. Intracranial (supraclinoid or intradural) ICA (Fig. 4-1).

  A. Normal anatomy.

    1. The ICA pierces the dura adjacent to the anterior clinoid process and ascends for short segment before terminating at bifurcation into anterior and middle cerebral arteries.

  B. Branches (in order of origin).

    1. Ophthalmic artery.

       a. Arises from anterosuperior ICA medial to anterior clinoid process.

    b. Course.
       (1) Exits skull through optic canal, with optic nerve.
       (2) Initially below optic nerve, then crosses superomedially over nerve.
    c. Supplies:
       (1) Globe (central retinal artery, ciliary arteries).
       (2) Orbit and contents (in balance with ECA branches).
       (3) Extraorbital soft tissues (reciprocal with ECA).
       (4) Dura (anterior falcine artery, recurrent meningeal artery).
    d. Numerous anastomoses with ECA (facial, maxillary, and middle meningeal arteries).
    e. Variants.
       (1) Arises from cavernous ICA (i.e., extradural) in 8% to 16% of cases.
       (2) Occasionally gives rise to middle meningeal artery (0.5%).

2. Superior hypophyseal trunk.
    a. Arises from posteromedial aspect of supraclinoid ICA.
    b. Courses across ventral surface of optic chiasm to terminate in the pituitary stalk and gland.
    c. Supplies:
       (1) Pituitary infundibulum and anterior pituitary gland.
       (2) Optic chiasm.
       (3) Hypothalamus.
    d. Numerous anastomoses with contralateral branches form vascular network known as the hypophyseal portal plexus.
    e. Usually too small to be visualized on angiography.

3. Posterior communicating artery (PCoA).
    a. Arises from posterior aspect of intradural ICA.
    b. Course: superolateral to CN III.
    c. Joins ICA with proximal posterior cerebral artery (PCA). Its junction defines the P1 and P2 segments of the PCA.
    d. Supplies (via small perforating branches known as anterior thalamoperforating arteries):
       (1) Parts of thalamus and hypothalamus.
       (2) Parts of optic chiasm and mammillary bodies.
    e. Anomalies.
       (1) Hypoplasia is most common anomaly (33% of anatomic specimens).
       (2) Persistent embryonic configuration is known as "fetal origin" of the PCA, in which PCA arises directly from ICA (20% to 25% of cases).

   (3) Junctional dilatation (infundibulum) of the PCoA origin occurs in 6%.
4. Anterior choroidal artery (AChA).
   a. Arises from posterior ICA just above PCoA.
   b. Two distinct segments.
      (1) Cisternal (proximal) segment: initially courses within suprasellar cistern under optic tract and posteromedially around temporal lobe uncus, then angles sharply laterally ("plexal point") before entering the choroidal fissure of the temporal horn.
      (2) Plexal (intraventricular) segment: courses in choroid plexus of temporal horn, curves posterolaterally around thalamus.
   c. Supply is variable (in reciprocal with lateral and medial posterior choroidal arteries) but usually includes:
      (1) Choroid plexus in the temporal horn and part of the atrium.
      (2) Optic tract.
      (3) Cerebral peduncle, substantia nigra, red nucleus.
      (4) Uncal and parahippocampal gyri of temporal lobe.
      (5) Parts of globus pallidus, caudate, thalamus, hypothalamus, and posterior limb of internal capsule.
   d. Numerous anastomoses with posterior choroidal, PCoA, PCA, and MCA branches.

SUGGESTED READINGS

Bisaria K: Anomalies of the posterior communicating artery and their potential clinical significance, *J Neurosurg* 60:572-576, 1984.

Brant-Zawadzki M: Routine MR imaging of the internal carotid artery siphon: angiographic correlation with cervical carotid lesions, *AJNR* 11:467-471, 1990.

Cali RL, Berg R, Rama K: Bilateral internal carotid artery agenesis: a case study and review of the literature, *Surgery* 113:227-233, 1993.

Chess MA, Barsotti JB, Chang J-K, et al: Duplication of the extracranial internal carotid artery, *AJNR* 16:1545-1547, 1995.

Fortner AA, Smoker WRK: Persistent primitive trigeminal artery aneurysm evaluated by MR imaging and angiography, *J Comp Asst Tomogr* 12:847-850, 1988.

George B, Mourier KL, Belbert F, et al: Vascular abnormalities in the neck associated with intracranial aneurysms, *Neurosurgery* 24:499-508, 1989.

Ghika JA, Bogousslavsky J, Regli F: Deep perforators from the carotid system: template of the vascular territories, *Arch Neurol* 47:1097-1100, 1990.

Grossman RI, Davis KR, Taveras JM: Circulatory variations of the ophthalmic artery, *AJNR* 3:327-329, 1982.

Hamada J-I, Kitamura I, Kurino M, et al: Abnormal origin of bilateral ophthalmic arteries, *J Neurosurg* 74:287-289, 1991.

Helgason CM: A new view of anterior choroidal artery territory infarction, *J Neurol* 235:387-391, 1988.

Kanai H, Nagai H, Wakabayashi S, Hashimoto N: A large aneurysm of the persistent primitive hypoglossal artery, *Neurosurgery* 30:794-797, 1992.

Kikuchi K, Kowada M, Kojima H: Hypoplasia of the internal carotid artery associated with spasmodic torticollis: the possible route of altered vertebrobasilar haemodynamics, *Neuroradiol* 37:362-364, 1995.

Knosp E, Muller G, Perneczky A: The paraclinoid carotid artery: anatomical aspects of a microsurgical approach, *Neurosurgery* 22:896-901, 1988.

Lasjaunias P, Santoyo-Vazquez: Segmental agensis of the internal carotid artery: angiographic aspects with embryological discussion, *Anat Clin* 6:133-141, 1984.

Littooy FN, Baker WH, Field TC, et al: Anomalous branches of the cervical internal carotid artery: two cases of clinical importance, *J Vasc Surg* 8:634-637, 1988.

Mohr JP, Steinke W, Timsit SG et al: The anterior choroidal artery does not supply the corona radiata and lateral ventricular wall, *Stroke* 22:1502-1507, 1991.

Morimoto T, Nitta K, Kozekawa K, Hoshizume K: The anomaly of a non-bifurcating cervical carotid artery, *J Neurosurg* 72:130-132, 1990.

Moyer DJ, Flamm ES: Anomalous arrangement of the origins of the anterior choroidal and posterior communicating arteries, *J Neurosurg* 76:1017-1018, 1992.

Obayashi T, Furuse M: The proatlantal intersegmental artery, *Arch Neurol* 37:387-389, 1980.

Okada Y, Shima T, Nishida M, et al: Bilateral persistent trigeminal arteries presenting with brain-stem infarction, *Neuroradiology* 34:283-286, 1992.

Osborn AG: *Introduction to cerebral angiography,* New York, 1980, Harper & Row, Chapters 4 and 5.

Ohshiro S, Inoue T, Hamada Y, Matsuno H: Branches of the persistent primitive trigeminal artery—an autopsy case, *Neurosurgery* 32:144-147, 1993.

Pahor AL, Hussain SSM: Persistent stapedial artery, *J Laryng Otol* 106:254-257, 1992.

Pedroza A, Dujovny M, Artero JC, et al: Microanatomy of the posterior communicating artery, *Neurosurgery* 20:228-235, 1987.

Quint DJ, Boulos RS, Spera TD: Congenital absence of the cervical and petrous internal carotid artery with intercavernous anastomosis, *AJNR* 10:435-439, 1989.

Quint DJ, Silbergleit R, Young WC: Absence of the carotid canals at skull base CT, *Radiol* 182:477-481, 1992.

Reynolds AF Jr, Stovring J, Turner PT: Persistent otic artery, *Surg Neurol* 13:115-117, 1980.

Richardson DN, Elster AD, Ball MR: Intrasellar trigeminal artery, *AJNR* 10:205, 1989.

Schlenska GK: Absence of both internal carotid arteries, *J Neurol* 233:263-266, 1986.

Schuierer G, Laub G, Huk WJ: MR angiography of the primitive trigeminal artery: report on two cases, *AJNR* 11:1131-1132, 1990.

Silbergleit R, Mehta BA, Barnes RD II, et al: Persistent trigeminal artery detected with standard MRI, *J Comp Asst Tomogr* 17:22-25, 1993.

Takahashi S, Suga T, Kawata Y, Sakamoto K: Anterior choroidal artery: angiographic analysis of variations and anomalies, *AJNR* 11:719-729, 1990.

Tran-Dinh H: Cavernous branches of the internal carotid artery: anatomy and nomenclature, *Neurosurgery* 20:205-209, 1987.

Udzura M, Kobayashi H, Taguchi Y, Sekino H: Intrasellar intercarotid communicating artery associated with agenesis of the right internal carotid artery: case report, *Neurosurgery* 23:770-773, 1988.

5
Circle of Willis and Cerebral Arteries

Key Concepts

1. Less than 20% of persons have a complete circle of Willis.
2. Common normal variants of the circle of Willis are:
   a. Absent or hypoplastic A1 segment (associated with increased incidence of aneurysms).
   b. Duplicated or hypoplastic anterior communicating artery.
   c. Hypoplasia of one or both posterior communicating arteries.
   d. "Fetal origin" of the PCA from the ICA instead of the vertebrobasilar system.
3. The ACA supplies the anterior two thirds of the medial hemisphere as well as a small medial strip of the superior surface of the brain convexity.
4. The MCA supplies the majority of the convexity cerebral cortex and white matter.
5. The PCA supplies the diencephalon, midbrain, posterior one third of the medial hemisphere, and the occipital pole.
6. The three major vascular territories of the cerebral hemispheres are variable among individuals. Minimum and maximum territories have been described.
7. Variants of the ACA include:
   a. Hypoplastic or absent A1 segment with bilateral A2 segments derived from the contralateral ACA (associated with increased incidence of aneurysms).
   b. Bihemispheric ACA in which there are bilateral ACA vessels but one is dominant and sends branches to right and left hemispheres.
   c. Azygous artery is a rare solitary unpaired vessel that arises as a single trunk from the bilateral A1 segments.
   d. Infraoptic origin of the ACA is uncommon but associated with increased incidence of aneurysms.
   e. Duplicated or fenestrated segments are uncommon but associated with increased incidence of aneurysms.
8. Variants of the MCA are uncommon but include fenestration, duplication, single trunk, and accessory arteries.
9. Variants of the PCA include:
   a. "Fetal origin" of the PCA from the ICA instead of the vertebrobasilar system; associated with hypoplastic or absent ipsilateral P1 segment.
   b. Carotid-vertebrobasilar anastomoses may supply the posterior circulation.

I. Circle of Willis (Fig. 5-1).
   A. Normal anatomy.
      1. Anterior communicating artery.
      2. Horizontal (A1) segments of right and left ACAs.
      3. Supraclinoid segments of right and left ICAs.
      4. Right and left posterior communicating arteries.
      5. Horizontal (P1) segments of right and left PCAs.
      6. Basilar artery tip.
   B. Branches.
      1. Medial lenticulostriate arteries.

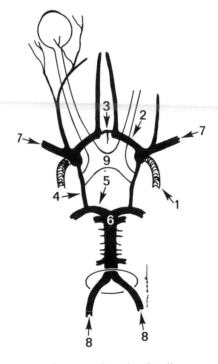

Fig. 5-1   Anatomic drawing of Circle of Willis as seen from above.
   1. Internal carotid artery
   2. Horizontal (A1) segment of anterior cerebral artery
   3. Anterior communicating artery
   4. Posterior communicating artery
   5. P1 segment of posterior cerebral artery
   6. Basilar artery bifurcation
   7. Middle cerebral artery (not part of circle of Willis)
   8. Vertebral arteries (not part of circle of Willis)
   9. Optic chiasm

      a. Arise from A1 segment of ACA.
      b. Supply:
         (1) Head of caudate nucleus.
         (2) Anterior limb of internal capsule.
    2. Thalamoperforating arteries.
      a. Arise from PCoA, basilar tip, P1 segment of PCA.
      b. Supply:
         (1) Thalamus and hypothalamus.
         (2) Posterior limb of internal capsule.
         (3) Midbrain.
    3. Thalamogeniculate arteries.
      a. Arise from proximal PCA.
      b. Supply:
         (1) Medial (and occasionally lateral) geniculate body and pulvinar of thalamus.
         (2) Part of midbrain.
  C. Variants.
    1. Less than 20% of persons have complete circle of Willis.
    2. Hypoplasia of one or both PCoAs (33%).
    3. "Fetal origin" of PCA in which PCA arises from ICA (20% to 25%); usually associated with hypoplasia of ipsilateral P1 segment.
    4. A1 hypoplastic in 10%; absent in 1% to 2%; rarely duplicated.
    5. ACoA hypoplastic in 15%; double ACoA in 30%, triple ACoA in 10%.
    6. PCoA infundibulum.
      a. Infundibula are funnel-shaped junctional dilatations at branch artery origins; most commonly seen at PCoA origin (6%) but also reported at origins of ophthalmic and anterior choroidal arteries.
      b. Not to be confused with true aneurysms.
         (1) Infundibulum is less than 3 mm in diameter.
         (2) Infundibulum is symmetric, funnel-shaped enlargement of PCoA origin.
         (3) Infundibulum has smooth dome with PCoA arising from apex, whereas aneurysm has asymmetric PCoA origin.
         (4) Infundibulum is not lobulated and does not have "tit."
II. Anterior cerebral artery.
  A. Normal anatomy (Figs. 5-2, 5-3).
    1. Formed by the termination and bifurcation of ICA into ACA and MCA. Is the smaller of the two terminal ICA branches.
    2. Segments.
      a. Horizontal (A1) segment: from ICA bifurcation to ACoA.

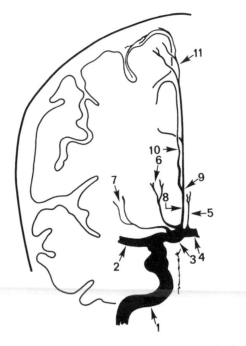

Fig. 5-2   Anteroposterior anatomic drawing of anterior cerebral artery (ACA) and its branches.

1. Internal carotid artery
2. Middle cerebral artery
3. Horizontal (A1) segment of ACA
4. Anterior communicating artery (ACoA)
5. Small ACoA branch to basal ganglia, corpus callosum
6. Medial lenticulostriate arteries
7. Recurrent artery of Heubner
8. A2 segment of ACA
9. ACA bifurcation
10. Pericallosal artery
11. Callosomarginal artery

    (1) Medial lenticulostriate arteries.
        (a) Arise from A1 segment and pass cephalad through the anterior perforated substance.
        (b) Supply: head of caudate nucleus, anterior limb of internal capsule.
    (2) ACoA.
        (a) Unpaired artery that joins right and left A1 segments. Actually part of the circle of Willis but

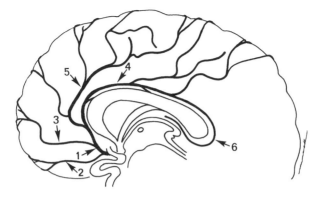

Fig. 5-3   Lateral anatomic drawing of medial surface of cerebral hemisphere showing anterior cerebral artery (ACA) and its major branches.

1. A2 segment of ACA
2. Orbitofrontal artery
3. Frontopolar artery
4. Pericallosal artery
5. Callosomarginal artery
6. Splenial artery

          usually treated as part of ACA complex. Numerous small perforating branches with important distribution.

   (b) Supplies: parts of lamina terminalis and hypothalamus, anterior commissure, fornix, septum pellucidum, paraolfactory gyrus, the subcallosal region, and the anterior part of the cingulate gyrus.

  (3) Recurrent artery of Heubner.

   (a) Is a prominent medial lenticulostriate branch.

   (b) Usually arises from A2 segment near ACoA (50%) but can also arise from A1 segment (44%). Loops back parallel to A1 then courses posterosuperiorly.

   (c) Supplies: head of caudate nucleus, rostral putamen, anterior limb of internal capsule.

 b. A2 segment.

  (1) Segment from ACoA to bifurcation into pericallosal and callosomarginal arteries. Courses cephalad in cistern of the lamina terminalis and curves around the genu of the corpus callosum where it terminates at its bifurcation.

  (2) Branches.

   (a) Recurrent artery of Heubner (see above).

           (b) Orbitofrontal or medial frontobasal A.

           (c) Frontopolar A.

           (d) Callosomarginal A.

           (e) Pericallosal A.

     c. Cortical branches (A3).

        (1) Branches.

           (a) Anterior internal frontal A.

           (b) Middle internal frontal A.

           (c) Posterior internal frontal A.

           (d) Paracentral A.

           (e) Superior internal parietal or superior precuneal A.

           (f) Inferior internal parietal or inferior precuneal or parieto-occipital A.

        (2) Vascular distribution: typically anterior two thirds of medial hemisphere surface as well as a small strip of superior convexity (Fig. 5-4).

        (3) Vascular territory is variable among individuals. Minimum and maximum territories have been described.

  B. Anatomic variants.

    1. Hypoplastic (10%) or absent (1% to 2%) A1 segment with bilateral A2 segments derived from the contralateral ACA.

    2. Bihemispheric ACA in which there are bilateral ACA vessels but one is dominant and sends branches to right and left hemispheres.

    3. Rarely, "azygous" artery occurs as a solitary unpaired vessel that arises as a single trunk from the bilateral A1 segments and supplies both hemispheres. Accidental clipping of this vessel can result in bifrontal infarctions.

    4. Uncommonly may have infraoptic origin of ACA with low bifurcation of ICA (associated with increased incidence of aneurysms).

    5. Also uncommon are fenestrated or duplicated segments (associated with increased incidence of aneurysms).

III. Middle cerebral artery.

  A. Normal anatomy (Figs. 5-5, 5-6).

    1. Formed by the termination and bifurcation of ICA into ACA and MCA. Is the larger of the two terminal branches. Divided into four major segments.

    2. Segments.

     a. Horizontal (M1) segment.

        (1) Courses from origin at ICA bifurcation laterally toward insula, paralleling sphenoid wing.

        (2) Branches: lateral lenticulostriate arteries.

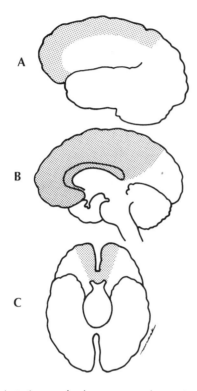

A

B

C

Fig. 5-4   Anterior cerebral artery vascular territory (dotted area).
A. Lateral view
B. Medial view
C. Base view

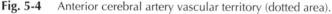

        (a) Deep perforators that course superiorly.
        (b) Supply: lentiform nucleus, part of caudate nucleus, anterior limb of internal capsule.
    b. Insular (M2) segment.
        (1) At genu, MCA bifurcates (78%) or trifurcates (12%) into its insular (M2) branches.
        (2) Branches loop over the insula within the sylvian fissure, forming "sylvian triangle."
    c. Opercular (M3) segment.
        (1) MCA branches emerge from the sylvian fissure and ramify over the hemispheric surface.
    d. Suprasylvian or terminal cortical (M4) branches (two groups).
        (1) Superior group: supplies frontal and parietal lobes.

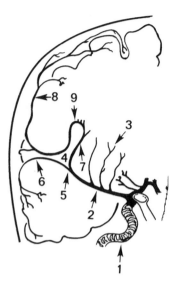

Fig. 5-5 Anteroposterior anatomic drawing of middle cerebral artery (MCA) and its branches.

1. Internal carotid artery
2. Horizontal (M1) segment of MCA
3. Lateral lenticulostriate arteries
4. Sylvian fissure
5. MCA bifurcation
6. Anterior temporal artery
7. M2 (sylvian) segment of MCA
8. M3 (opercular) branches
9. Sylvian point

    (a) Orbitofrontal or lateral frontobasal A.
    (b) Prefrontal A.
    (c) Precentral (sulcus) or prerolandic A.
    (d) Central (sulcus) or Rolandic A.
    (e) Anterior parietal or postcentral (sulcus) A.
    (f) Posterior parietal A.
    (g) Angular gyrus A.
(2) Inferior group: supplies temporal lobe.
    (a) Temporo-occipital A.
    (b) Posterior temporal A.
    (c) Middle temporal or intermedial temporal A.
    (d) Anterior temporal A.
    (e) Temporopolar A.
(3) Vascular distribution.

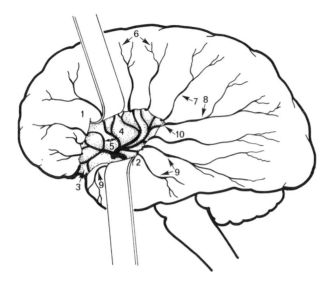

Fig. 5-6   Lateral anatomic drawing of brain showing middle cerebral artery (MCA) and its branches. Retractors have been applied and sylvian fissure widened by pulling apart frontal (1) and temporal (2) opercula. Insula is exposed within depths of sylvian fissure. MCA branches loop over surface of insula, then pass laterally through sylvian fissure to course over surface of brain.

    1. Operculum of frontal lobe
    2. Operculum of temporal lobe
    3. Sylvian fissure (pulled apart)
    4. Insula
    5. Insular (M2) MCA branches
    6. Precentral and postcentral sulcal MCA branches
    7. Posterior parietal artery
    8. Angular artery
    9. Temporal branches
   10. Sylvian point

        (a) MCA and its branches supply most of lateral surface of hemisphere, insula, and anterior and lateral aspects of temporal lobe (Fig. 5-7).
        (b) Vascular territory can be rather variable among individuals. Minimum and maximum territories have been described.
  B. Anatomic variations: MCA anomalies occur less frequently than variations in other major intracranial arteries.
    1. Quadrifurcation of MCA (4%).
    2. Single-trunk MCA (4%).

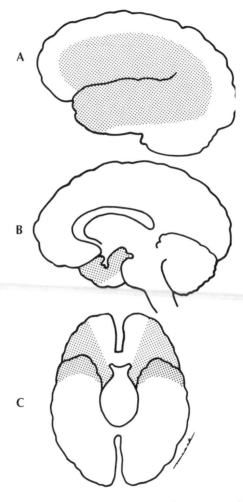

Fig. 5-7 Middle cerebral artery vascular territory (dotted area).
A. Lateral view
B. Medial view
C. Base view

    3. Fenestration or partial duplication (1%).
    4. Accessory MCA (origin from A1 segment of ACA) (1% to 3%).
    5. Duplication (distal ICA gives origin to an MCA branch) (1% to 3%).
IV. Posterior cerebral artery.
    A. Normal anatomy (Fig. 5-8, 5-9).

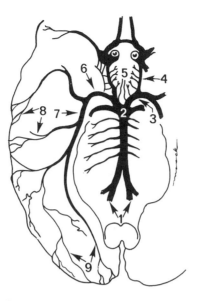

Fig. 5-8   Anatomic drawing of base of brain showing basilar artery, posterior cerebral artery (PCA), and circle of Willis.
1. Vertebral arteries
2. Basilar artery
3. P1 segment of PCA
4. Posterior communicating artery
5. Small branches from circle of Willis and basilar tip that supply base of brain
6. P2 segment of PCA
7. P3 segment of PCA
8. Temporal branches of PCA
9. Occipital branches with calcarine artery (medial arrow)

1. PCA originates from the basilar artery bifurcation.
2. Segments and major branches.
   a. Precommunicating or peduncular (P1) segment.
      (1) Short segment extending laterally from basilar bifurcation to PCA junction with PCoA. Courses above CN III.
      (2) Branches.
         (a) Posterior thalamoperforating arteries.
            i. Arise from basilar bifurcation and P1 segments, course cephalad.
            ii. Supply: medial thalamus and midbrain.
         (b) Medial posterior choroidal arteries.
            i. Can arise from P1 or proximal P2 segments,

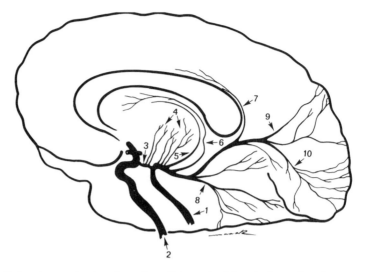

Fig. 5-9 Anatomic drawing of medial cerebral hemisphere showing posterior cerebral artery and its branches to occipital and temporal lobes and basal ganglia.

1. Basilar artery
2. Internal carotid artery
3. Posterior communicating artery
4. Thalamoperforating arteries
5. Medial posterior choroidal artery
6. Lateral posterior choroidal artery
7. Splenial artery
8. Posterior temporal artery
9. Posterior parietal artery
10. Occipital artery

       course anteromedially around midbrain and then forward along roof of third ventricle.

   ii. Supply: colliculi, posterior thalamus, pineal gland, part of midbrain, tela choroidea of the third ventricle.

  iii. Anastomoses with anterior choroidal and lateral posterior choroidal arteries.

  b. Ambient (P2) segment.

    (1) Courses in ambient cistern from PCA-PCoA junction posteriorly around midbrain. Lies above CN IV and tentorial incisura.

    (2) Branches.

      (a) Medial posterior choroidal arteries (see above).

      (b) Lateral posterior choroidal arteries.

      i. Can arise from P2 segment or proximal cortical branches. Courses into choroid plexus of lateral ventricle, over pulvinar of thalamus.

      ii. Supply: posterior thalamus and lateral ventricular choroid plexus.

      iii. Anastomoses with anterior choroidal and medial posterior choroidal arteries.

    (c) Thalamogeniculate arteries.

      i. Arise from the P2 segment.

      ii. Supply: medial geniculate body, pulvinar, brachium of the superior colliculus, crus cerebri, and occasionally the lateral geniculate body.

  c. Quadrigeminal (P3) segment.

    (1) Courses within the quadrigeminal plate cistern, behind the midbrain, then frequently divides in the form of a bifurcation or trifurcation.

    (2) Branches.

      (a) Medial occipital A.

      (b) Lateral occipital A.

      (c) Calcarine A.

      (d) Parieto-occipital A.

      (e) Posterior pericallosal or splenial A.

      (f) Lateral occipital or occipital temporal A.

      (g) Anterior inferior temporal A.

      (h) Middle inferior temporal A.

      (i) Posterior inferior temporal A.

    (3) PCA vascular distribution.

      (a) PCA and its branches supply posterior one third of medial hemisphere, small portion of lateral hemispheric surface, undersurface of temporal lobe, occipital pole, and splenium of corpus callosum (Fig. 5-10).

      (b) Vascular territory is variable among individuals. Minimum and maximum territories have been described.

B. Anatomic variants.

  1. "Fetal origin" of PCA (15% to 20%).

    a. PCA arises directly from ICA (i.e., seen on angiography during ICA injection, and not vertebral injection).

    b. Associated hypoplastic or absent P1 segment.

  2. Carotid-basilar anastomoses (see chapter 4): may result in carotid supply of PCA via persistent embryonic vessel.

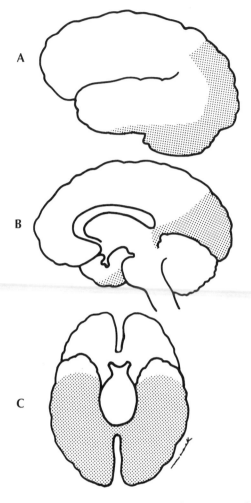

Fig. 5-10 Posterior cerebral artery vascular territory (dotted areas).
A. Lateral view
B. Medial view
C. Base view

SUGGESTED READINGS

Berman SA, Hayman LA, Hinck VC: Cerebrovascular territories. In LA Hayman: *Clinical brain imaging: normal structure and functional anatomy,* St Louis, 1992, Mosby, pp 402-416.

Berman SA, Hayman LA, Hinck VC: Correlation of CT cerebral vascular territories with function. I. Anterior cerebral artery, *AJNR* 1:259-263, 1980.

Berman SA, Hayman LA, Hinck VC: Correlation of CT cerebral vascular territories with function. III. Middle cerebral artery, *AJNR* 5:161-166, 1984.

Bradac GB: Angiography in cerebral ischemia, *Riv Neuroradiol* 3 (suppl 2):57-66, 1990.

Brassier G, Morandi X, Mercier PH, Velut S: The posterior part of the arterial circle of the skull base: caudal division of the embryonic internal carotid artery, *Riv Neuroradiol* 7 (suppl 4):85-89, 1994.

Cennamon J, Zito J, Chalif DJ, et al: Aneurysm of the azygos pericallosal artery: diagnosis by MR imaging and MR angiography, *AJNR* 13:280-282, 1992.

Damasio H: A computed tomographic guide to the identification of cerebral vascular territories, *Arch Neurol* 40:138-142, 1983.

Davis WL, Warnock SH, Harnsberger HR, et al: Intracranial MRA: single volume vs. multiple thin slab 3D time-of-flight acquisition, *J Comp Asst Tomogr* 17:15-21, 1993.

Dunker RO, Harris AB: Surgical anatomy of the proximal anterior cerebral artery, *J Neurosurg* 44:359-367, 1976.

Gibo H, Carver CC, Rhoton AL Jr, et al: Microsurgical anatomy of the middle cerebral artery, *J Neurosurg* 54:151-169, 1981.

Gibbons K, Hopkins LN, Heros RC: Occlusion of an "accessory" distal anterior cerebral artery during treatment of anterior communicating artery aneurysms, *J Neurosurg* 74:133-135, 1991.

Gloger S, Gloger A, Vogt H, Kretschmann H-J: Computer-assisted 3D reconstruction of the terminal branches of the cerebral arteries, *Neuroradiology* 36:173-257, 1994.

Grand W: Microsurgical anatomy of the proximal middle cerebral artery and the internal carotid artery bifurcation, *Neurosurgery* 7:215-218, 1980.

Hayman LA, Berman SA, Hinck VC: Correlation of CT cerebral vascular territories with function: II. Posterior cerebral artery, *AJNR* 2:219-225, 1981.

Marinkovic SV, Milisavljevic MM, Kovacevik MS: Anastomosis among the thalamoperforating branches of the posterior cerebral artery, *Arch Neurol* 43:811-814, 1986.

Mercier PH, Fournier D, Brassier G, et al: The perforating arteries of the anterior part of the circle of Willis: microsurgical anatomy, *Riv Neuroradiol* 7 (suppl 4):79-83, 1994.

Milisavljevic MM, Marinkovic SV, Gibo H, Puskas LF: The thalamogeniculate perforators of the posterior cerebral artery: the microsurgical anatomy, *Neurosurgery* 28:523-530, 1991.

Mitchell DG, Merton DA, Mirsky PJ, Needleman L: Circle of Willis in newborns, *Radiology* 172:201-205, 1989.

Osborn AG: *Introduction to cerebral angiography,* New York, 1980, Harper & Row, Chapters 6-10.

Perlmutter D, Rhoton AL Jr: Microsurgical anatomy of the anterior cerebral-anterior communicating-recurrent artery complex, *J Neurosurg* 45:259-272, 1976.

Perlmutter D, Rhoton AL Jr: Microsurgical anatomy of the distal anterior cerebral artery, *J Neurosurg* 49:204-228, 1978.

Pernicone JR, Thorp KE, Ouimette MV, et al: Magnetic resonance angiography in intracranial vascular disease, *Semin US CT MRI* 13:256-273, 1992.

Ross MR, Pelc NJ, Enzmann DR: Qualitative phase contrast MRA in the normal and abnormal circle of Willis, *AJNR* 14:19-25, 1993.

Ruggieri PM, Masaryk TJ, Ross JS, Modic MT, Magnetic resonance angiography of the intracranial vasculature, *Top Magn Reson Imaging* 3:23-33, 1991.

Saeki N, Rhoton AL Jr: Microsurgical anatomy of the upper basilar artery and the posterior circle of Willis, *J Neurosurg* 46:563-578, 1977.

Sanders WP, Sorek PA, Mehta BA: Fenestration of intracranial arteries with special attention to associated aneurysms and other anomalies, *AJNR* 14:675-680, 1993.

Savoiardo M: The vascular territories of the carotid and vertebrobasilar systems: diagrams based on CT studies of infarcts, *Ital J Neurol Sci* 7:405-409, 1986.

Schick RM, Rumbaugh CL: Saccular aneurysm of the azygos anterior cerebral artery, *AJNR* 10:S73, 1989.

Takahashi S, Fukasawa H, Ishii K, Sakamoto K: The anterior choroidal artery syndrome: I. Microangiography of the anterior choroidal artery, *Neuroradiology* 36:337-339, 1994.

Takahashi S, Hoshino F, Uemura K, et al: Accessory middle cerebral artery, *AJNR* 10:563-568, 1989.

Umansky F, Dujouny M, Ausman JI, et al: Anomalies and variations of the middle cerebral artery: a microanatomical study, *Neurosurgery* 22:1023-1027, 1988.

van der Zwan A, Hillen B, Tulleken CAF, et al: Variability of the major cerebral arteries, *J Neurosurg* 77:927-940, 1992.

Vinansky F, Dujovny M, Ausman JI, et al: Anomalies and variations of the middle cerebral artery: a microanatomical study, *Neurosurg* 22:1023-1027, 1988.

Wismer GL: Circle of Willis variant analogous to fetal type primitive trigeminal artery, *Neuroradiology* 31:366-368, 1989.

Zeal AA, Rhoton AL Jr: Microsurgical anatomy of the posterior cerebral artery, *J Neurosurg* 48:534-559, 1978.

6

Posterior Fossa Arteries

Key Concepts

1. Left vertebral artery is dominant in 50% of cases. Right vertebral artery is dominant in 25% of cases. Both vertebral arteries are approximately equal in 25% of cases. When the left vertebral artery arises directly from the aortic arch, it is usually nondominant in these cases.
2. Abundant anastomoses exist between VA and ECA branches (i.e., occipital, ascending pharyngeal arteries), thyrocervical and costocervical branches.
3. The course of the basilar artery is highly variable and does not consistently delineate the ventral surface of the pons. The anterior pontomesencephalic vein more reliably defines the ventral pontine margin.
4. Near its origin, the AICA is usually crossed by CN VI. Near the IAC meatus the AICA is typically anteroinferior to CNs VII and VIII, and may loop slightly into the meatus.
5. The superior cerebellar arteries (SCA) course below CNs III and IV; course above CN V.
6. Variants and anomalies include:
   a. Left VA may arise directly from aortic arch (5%).
   b. Hypoplastic VA is common (up to 40% of normal angiograms). Aplasia is rare.
   c. VA may be fenestrated or duplicated (associated with increased incidence of aneurysms and vascular malformations).
   d. VA may terminate in posterior inferior cerebellar artery (PICA) (1%).
   e. Persistent embryonic carotid-vertebral anastomoses may occur.
   f. PICA origin may be below level of foramen magnum (18%).
   g. Posterior fossa arteries (SCA, AICA, PICA) can arise from ICA.
   h. If PCA has "fetal origin" then distal basilar artery may be hypoplastic.
   i. Occasionally may have fenestrated basilar artery (associated with increased incidence of aneurysms).

I. Vertebral arteries.
    A. Normal anatomy (Figs. 3-1, 6-1, 6-2).
        1. Origin: from subclavian arteries (95%) or less commonly directly from aortic arch (usually left VA in these cases).
        2. Dominant vessel.
            a. Left vertebral artery is dominant in 50% of cases.
            b. Right vertebral artery is dominant in 25% of cases.
            c. Both vertebral arteries are approximately equal in 25% of cases.
            d. When the left vertebral artery arises directly from the aortic arch, it is usually nondominant in these cases.
        3. Course.
            a. VAs course cephalad from origin to enter the transverse foramina, usually at C6; if VA has arch origin, then enters transverse foramina at C5.
            b. Then pass directly superiorly through consecutive transverse

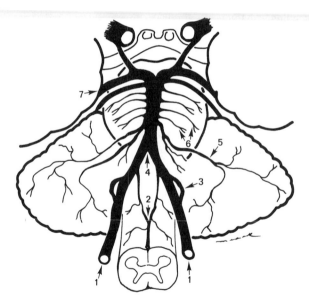

Fig. 6-1 Anteroposterior anatomic drawing of vertebrobasilar circulation.
1. Vertebral artery
2. Anterior spinal artery
3. Posterior inferior cerebellar artery
4. Basilar artery
5. Anterior inferior cerebellar artery
6. Pontine perforating branches
7. Posterior cerebral artery

foramina up to C2, after which they turn laterally, then superiorly again through the transverse foramina of C1.

 c. After looping posteriorly along the atlas, each VA passes superomedially through foramen magnum.

 d. Right and left vertebral arteries unite ventral to medulla to form BA.

4. Branches.

 a. Extracranial.

  (1) Numerous small segmental spinal, meningeal, and muscular branches arise from the VA.

  (2) Abundant anastomoses exist between VA and ECA

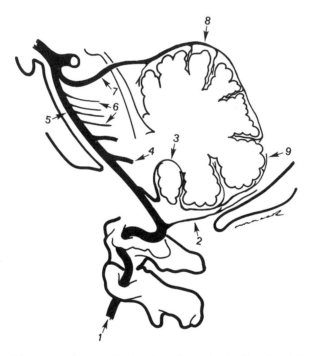

Fig. 6-2 Lateral anatomic drawing of vertebrobasilar circulation.
  1. Vertebral artery
  2. Posterior meningeal artery
  3. Posterior inferior cerebellar artery
  4. Anterior inferior cerebellar artery (cut off)
  5. Basilar artery
  6. Pontine perforating branches
  7. Superior cerebellar artery
  8. Superior vermian artery
  9. Inferior vermian artery

branches (i.e., occipital, ascending pharyngeal arteries), thyrocervical and costocervical branches.
  b. Intracranial.
    (1) Posterior meningeal artery.
      (a) Usually arises from the VA as it courses along the posterior arch of the atlas; occasionally may arise from the occipital artery, ascending pharyngeal artery, or PICA. Initially extracranial but soon enters posterior foramen magnum and courses behind cerebellar vermis.
      (b) Supplies falx cerebelli.
    (2) Anterior spinal artery.
      (a) Usually joins with counterpart on contralateral side to form single trunk. Courses caudally for variable distance in anteromedial sulcus of cervical cord.
      (b) Supplies: ventral medulla (including pyramid and ventral part of olive) and ventral cervical cord.
    (3) Posterior spinal artery.
      (a) May arise from vertebral artery or from PICA. Rarely visualized.
      (b) Supplies: dorsal cervical cord.
    (4) Posterior inferior cerebellar artery (PICA).
      (a) Arises 13 to 16 mm proximal to basilar artery. Courses around medulla and over or across tonsil. Has five segments.
        i. Anterior medullary segment: in front of medulla.
        ii. Lateral medullary segment: courses alongside the medulla caudally to the level of CNs IV-XI.
        iii. Tonsillomedullary segment: courses around the inferior half of the cerebellar tonsil.
        iv. Telovelotonsillar segment: in the cleft between the tela choroidea and inferior medullary velum rostrally and the superior pole of the tonsil caudally.
        v. Cortical or hemispheric branches.
      (b) Supplies: choroid plexus of fourth ventricle, posterolateral medulla, cerebellar tonsil, inferior vermis, and posterioinferior surface of the cerebellar hemispheres.
      (c) Size is variable and depends on size of ipsilateral AICA and contralateral PICA.
B. Variants and anomalies.
  1. Left VA may arise directly from aortic arch (5%).

2. Hypoplastic VA is common (up to 40% of normal angiograms). Aplasia is extremely rare.
3. VA may be fenestrated or duplicated (associated with increased incidence of aneurysms and vascular malformations).
4. VA may terminate in PICA (1%).
5. Persistent embryonic carotid-vertebral anastomoses may occur (see Chapter 4).
6. PICA origin may be below level of foramen magnum (18%).
7. Posterior fossa arteries (SCA, AICA, PICA) can arise from ICA.

II. Basilar artery.
  A. Normal anatomy (Figs. 6-1, 6-2).
    1. Origin: formed from union of right and left VAs ventral to inferior pons.
    2. Course: ventral to pons, terminates in interpeduncular cistern by bifurcating into right and left PCAs. Its course may be tortuous and is not a reliable marker for the ventral surface of the pons.
    3. Branches.
      a. Perforating branches.
        (1) Numerous small short and long segment circumflex branches arising along entire length of basilar artery. Three major groups.
          (a) Caudal group.
            i. Arise below origin of AICA. Occasionally may arise from AICA.
            ii. May give rise to pontomedullary artery, pyramidal vessels, hypoglossal nerve branches.
          (b) Middle group.
            i. Arise between AICA and superior cerebellar artery.
            ii. May give rise to pontomedullary artery, long pontine arteries, anterolateral or posterolateral branches.
          (c) Rostral group.
            i. Arise cephalad to superior cerebellar artery. May also originate from superior cerebellar or posterolateral arteries.
            ii. May give rise to anterolateral branches.
        (2) Supply: ventral pons, rostral brainstem.
      b. Anterior inferior cerebellar artery (paired).
        (1) Arises from the inferior basilar artery and courses posterolaterally around pons toward cerebellopontine angle and internal auditory canal (IAC) meatus. Near its origin, the AICA is usually crossed by CN VI. Near the

IAC meatus the AICA is typically anteroinferior to CNs VII and VIII, and may loop slightly into the meatus.

(2) Supplies: anterior margins of cerebellar hemispheres, inferolateral pons, middle cerebellar peduncle, flocculus, CNs VII and VIII.

c. Superior cerebellar artery (paired).

(1) Arises near apex of basilar artery and curve posterolaterally around pons and midbrain in pontomesencephalic groove, just below tentorial incisura. Courses below CNs III and IV; courses above CN V.

(2) Supplies: superior surface of vermis and cerebellar hemispheres as well as most of deep cerebellar white matter and dentate nuclei.

B. Variants.

1. Persistent embryonic carotid-vertebrobasilar anastomoses. (See Chapter 4.)

2. Posterior fossa arteries (SCA, AICA, PICA) can arise from ICA.

3. If PCA has "fetal origin" then distal basilar artery may be hypoplastic.

4. Occasionally may have fenestrated basilar artery (associated with increased incidence of aneurysms).

SUGGESTED READINGS

Ahuja A, Graves VB, Crosby DL, Strother CM: Anomalous origin of the posterior inferior cerebellar artery from the internal carotid artery, *AJNR* 13:1625-1626, 1992.

Akar ZC, Dujovny M, Gomez-Tortosa E, et al: Microvascular anatomy of the anterior surface of the medullar oblongata and olive, *J Neurosurg* 82:97-105, 1995.

Amarenco PA, Rosengart A, DeWitt D, et al: Anterior inferior cerebellar artery territory infarcts: mechanisms and clinical features, *Arch Neurol* 50:154-161, 1993.

Amarenco P, Roullet E, Goujon C, et al: Infarction in the anterior rostral cerebellum (the territory of the lateral branch of the superior cerebellar artery), *Neurology* 41:253-258, 1991.

Arnold V, Lehrmann R, Kursawe HK, Luckel W: Hypoplasia of vertebrobasilar arteries, *Neuroradiol* 33(suppl):426-427, 1991.

Cormier PJ, Long ER, Russell EJ: MR imaging of posterior fossa infarctions: vascular territories and clinical correlates, *Radiographics* 12:1079-1096, 1992.

Friedman DP: Abnormalities of the posterior inferior cerebellar artery: MR imaging findings, *AJR* 160:1259-1263, 1993.

Hardy DG, Peace DA, Rhoton AL: Microsurgical anatomy of the superior cerebellar artery, *Neurosurgery* 6:10-28, 1980.

Lister JR, Rhoton AL, Matsushima T, Peace DA: Microsurgical anatomy of the posterior inferior cerebellar artery, *Neurosurgery* 10:170-199, 1982.

Manabe H, Oda N, Ishii M, Ishii A: The posterior inferior cerebellar artery originating from the internal carotid artery, associated with multiple aneurysms, *Neuroradiol* 33:513-515, 1991.

Marinkovic SV, Gibo H: The surgical anatomy of the perforating branches of the basilar artery, *Neurosurgery* 33:80-87, 1993.

Naidich TP, Kricheff II, George AE, Lin JP: The normal anterior inferior cerebellar artery, *Radiol* 119:355-373, 1976.

Saeki N, Rhoton AL Jr: Microsurgical anatomy of the upper basilar artery and the posterior circle of Willis, *J Neurosurg* 46:563-578, 1977.

Savoiardo M, Bracchi M, Passerini A, Visciani A: The vascular territories in the cerebellum and brainstem: CT and MR study, *AJNR* 8:199-209, 1987.

Schrontz C, Dujoyny M, Ausman JI, et al: Surgical anatomy of the arteries of the posterior fossa, *J Neurosurg* 65:540-544, 1986.

Smoker WRK, Price MJ, Keyes WD, et al: High-resolution computed tomography of the basilar artery: I. Normal size and position, *AJNR* 7:55-60, 1986.

Takasato Y, Hayashi H, Kobayashi T, Hashimoto Y: Duplicated origin of right verteral artery with rudimentary and accessory left vertebral arteries, *Neuroradiol* 34:287-289, 1992.

Tanohata K, Maehara T, Noda M, et al: Anomalous origin of the posterior meningeal artery from the lateral medullary segment of the posterior inferior cerebellar artery, *Neuroradiol* 29:89-92, 1987.

Tran-Dinh HD, Soo YS, Jayasinghe LS: Duplication of the vertebrobasilar system, *Australian Radiol* 35:220-224, 1991.

7

Intracranial Venous System

Key Concepts

1. The cerebral venous system is composed of dural sinuses, superficial cortical and deep parenchymal veins. The venous vasculature is much more variable than the arterial system.
2. Dural sinuses are formed between dural reflections. They are endothelium-lined and contiguous with superficial cortical veins. No valves are present in dural sinuses.
3. The torcular Herophili (confluens sinuum) is the confluence of superior sagittal sinus (SSS) and straight sinus (SS).
4. The transverse sinuses (TS) are often asymmetric, with right TS being larger and showing preferential drainage toward the right jugular vein (50% to 80%).
5. The cavernous sinuses are complex multiseptated extradural venous spaces lateral to the sella. Important contents include the ICA and CNs III, IV, V_1, V_2, and VI. The right and left sides communicate via anterior and posterior intercavernous sinuses. In addition there are numerous connections to ECA branches as well as other dural sinuses.
6. Superficial cortical veins drain into dural sinuses.
7. Medullary veins drain the subcortical and deep white matter. They drain into subependymal veins, which then drain into internal cerebral veins, basal veins, and vein of Galen respectively.

I. Dural Sinuses: formed between dural reflections. Are endothelium-lined and contiguous with superficial cortical veins. No valves are present in dural sinuses. (Figs. 7-1, 7-2, 7-3, 7-4).
   A. Superior sagittal sinus (SSS).
      1. Unpaired midline structure situated between the inner table of the skull superiorly and the leaves of the falx cerebri laterally.
      2. SSS extends from origin near crista galli anteriorly to confluence with straight and lateral sinuses (torcular Herophili).
      3. SSS may end by becoming right transverse sinus.
      4. Occasionally rostral portion of SSS is hypoplastic or atretic (6% to 7%). In these cases substitute parasagittal intradural venous channels receive prominent tributaries from the cerebral cortex.
   B. Inferior sagittal sinus (ISS).
      1. Inconstant, unpaired midline channel in inferior (free) margin of falx cerebri.
      2. Joins with vein of Galen to form straight sinus.
   C. Straight sinus (SS).
      1. Unpaired midline channel that runs posteroinferiorly in dural confluence of the falx cerebri and tentorium cerebelli.
      2. Formed by union of vein of Galen and ISS.
      3. Ends by joining with SSS to form torcular Herophili.
      4. Occasionally SS ends by becoming left transverse sinus.
      5. SS may be hypoplastic or absent. In these cases an accessory falcine sinus is usually present.
   D. Torcular Herophili or confluens sinuum.
      1. Is the confluence of SSS and SS.
      2. Occurs at approximately the level of the internal occipital protruberance.
      3. Bifurcates into right and left transverse sinuses.
   E. Transverse sinuses (TS).
      1. Paired structures that extend from torcular along lateral tentorial attachments to the sigmoid sinuses.
      2. Often asymmetric with right TS being larger and showing preferential drainage toward the right jugular vein (50% to 80%).
      3. Agenesis of part or all of a TS may occur (1% to 5%) and should not be mistaken for dural sinus occlusion.
      4. Determination of dominant venous drainage patterns and potential collaterals is important in preoperative planning.
   F. Tentorial sinuses.
      1. Numerous additional tentorial sinuses drain into the dural sinuses near the torcular.

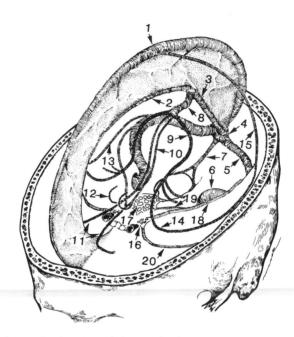

Fig. 7-1   Anatomic drawing of the cerebral venous and dural sinus system. Oblique overhead view.

1. Superior sagittal sinus
2. Inferior sagittal sinus
3. Straight sinus
4. Torcular Herophili (sinus confluence)
5. Transverse sinus
6. Sigmoid sinus
7. Occipital sinus
8. Vein of Galen
9. Basal vein of Rosenthal
10. Internal cerebral veins
11. Septal veins
12. Thalamostriate veins
13. Vein of Labbe
14. Superficial middle cerebral vein
15. Vein of Trolard
16. Cavernous sinus
17. Clival venous plexus
18. Superior petrosal sinus
19. Inferior petrosal sinus
20. Sphenoparietal sinus

(From Osborn A: *Diagnostic neuroradiology,* St Louis, 1994, Mosby.)

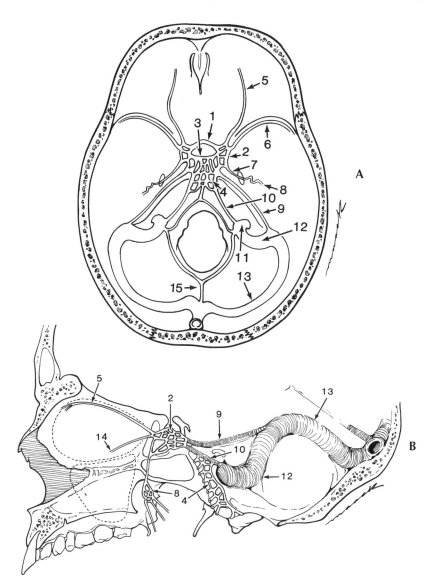

Fig. 7-2 Anatomic drawing of basal dural venous sinuses.
A. View from above; B. Lateral view
1. Anterior intercavernous sinus
2. Cavernous sinus
3. Posterior intercavernous sinus
4. Basilar or clival plexus
5. Superior ophthalmic vein
6. Sphenoparietal sinus
7. Foramen ovale plexus
8. Pterygoid plexus
9. Superior petrosal sinus
10. Inferior petrosal sinus
11. Internal jugular vein
12. Sigmoid sinus
13. Transverse sinus
14. Inferior opthalmic vein
15. Occipital sinus

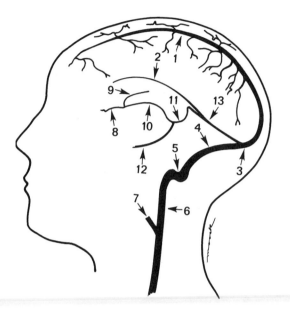

Fig. 7-3   Lateral anatomic drawing of cerebral venous system.
1. Superior sagittal sinus
2. Inferior sagittal sinus
3. Torcular Herophili
4. Transverse sinus
5. Sigmoid sinus, jugular bulb
6. Internal jugular vein
7. External jugular vein
8. Septal vein
9. Thalamostriate vein
10. Internal cerebral vein
11. Vein of Galen
12. Basal vein of Rosenthal
13. Straight sinus

     2. Provide significant drainage for adjacent cerebellar hemispheres.

     3. Can become significantly enlarged with SSS or SS occlusion.

G. Sigmoid sinuses.
     1. Paired S-shaped anteroinferior continuation of TS to jugular bulb.
     2. Joined by the inferior petrosal sinus and tributaries from the clival venous plexus.

H. Occipital sinus.
     1. Small midline or paramedian channel that courses from torcular

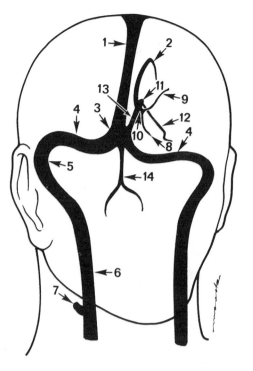

Fig. 7-4   Anatomic drawing of cerebral system. Oblique frontal view.

1. Superior sagittal sinus
2. Inferior sagittal sinus
3. Torcular Herophili
4. Transverse sinus
5. Sigmoid sinus, jugular bulb
6. Internal jugular bulb
7. External jugular bulb
8. Septal vein
9. Thalamostriate vein
10. Internal cerebral vein
11. Vein of Galen
12. Basal vein of Rosenthal
13. Straight sinus
14. Occipital sinus

and divides into right and left marginal branches that drain into the sigmoid sinuses or jugular bulbs.

2. May become prominent with agenesis or occlusion of transverse sinus.

I. Cavernous sinuses (Figs. 7-2, 7-5).

1. Complex multiseptated extradural venous spaces lateral to the

sella. Single cavity is uncommon. Right and left sides communicate via anterior and posterior intercavernous sinuses.
2. Important contents: internal carotid artery and CNs III, IV, V_1, V_2, and VI.
3. Receive superior and inferior ophthalmic veins.

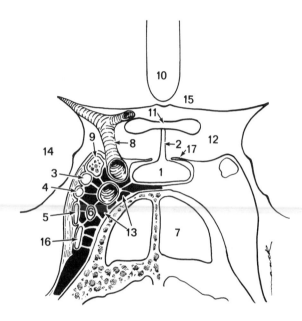

Fig. 7-5 Coronal anatomic drawing of sella turcica, cavernous sinus, and adjacent structures.

1. Pituitary gland
2. Infundibulum
3. Cranial nerve III
4. Cranial nerve IV
5. Cranial nerve V_1
6. Cranial nerve VI
7. Sphenoid sinus
8. Internal carotid artery
9. Anterior clinoid process
10. Third ventricle
11. Optic chiasm
12. Suprasellar cistern
13. Venous spaces of cavernous sinus
14. Temporal lobe
15. Hypothalamus
16. Cranial nerve V_2
17. Diaphragma sellae

4. Communicate posteriorly with clival (basilar) venous plexus.
5. Communicate superolaterally with sigmoid or transverse sinus via superior petrosal sinus.
6. Communicate inferiorly with jugular bulb via inferior petrosal sinuses.
7. Communicate anteriorly with deep facial veins via pterygoid venous plexus.
8. Communicate laterally with sphenoparietal sinuses along sphenoid wing.
  J. Sphenoparietal sinuses.
    1. Drain superficial middle cerebral vein into cavernous sinus.
    2. Course along greater sphenoid wings.
  K. Superior petrosal sinuses.
    1. Connect posterior part of cavernous sinus with transverse sinus.
    2. Course along the superior border of the petrous temporal bone.
  L. Inferior petrosal sinuses.
    1. Connect cavernous sinus with internal jugular vein.
    2. Course along the inferior border of the petrous temporal bone. Can join internal jugular vein within jugular foramen, at the exocranial opening of the foramen, or below the skull base.
    3. Usually course inferior to the glossopharyngeal nerve within the jugular foramen.
    4. Right and left sinuses can be assymmetric.
II. Cerebral veins (Figs. 7-1, 7-3, 7-4).
  A. Superficial (cortical) veins: highly variable, most unnamed.
    1. Superficial middle cerebral (sylvian) vein.
      a. Courses along sylvian fissure.
      b. Numerous anastomoses with deep cerebral veins, cavernous sinuses, facial veins via sphenoparietal sinus, pterygoid plexus, etc.
    2. Vein of Trolard.
      a. Large anastomotic cortical vein that courses cephalad from sylvian fissure to SSS.
    3. Vein of Labbe.
      a. Large anastomotic cortical vein that courses posterolaterally from sylvian fissure to TS.
    4. Vein of Rolando.
      a. Large anastomotic cortical vein from central sulcus to SSS.
  B. Deep veins.
    1. Medullary veins.
      a. Originate 1 to 2 cm below cortex and course centrally through white matter toward subependymal veins.
      b. Drain subcortical and deep white matter.

    2. Subependymal veins.
       a. Surround lateral ventricles and receive medullary veins of centrum semiovale.
       b. Two larger named subependymal veins unite to form internal cerebral veins.
         (1) Thalamostriate veins (paired): course over caudate nucleus.
         (2) Septal veins (paired): course posteriorly from frontal horn along septum pellucidum.
    3. Internal cerebral veins (ICV).
       a. Paired paramedian vessels. Formed by the union of thalamostriate and septal veins near the foramen of Monro.
       b. Course posteriorly from the foramen of Monro in the velum interpositum, just above the roof of the third ventricle.
       c. Join with basal veins to form vein of Galen.
    4. Basal veins.
       a. Paired vessels that course posterosuperiorly from deep sylvian fissure into the ambient cisterns around the midbrain.
       b. Drain the medial temporal lobes.
       c. Join with ICVs to form vein of Galen.
    5. Vein of Galen or great cerebral vein.
       a. Single midline U-shaped vein formed by the union of right and left ICVs and basal veins.
       b. Courses posteriorly under the splenium of the corpus callosum.
       c. Joins with the inferior sagittal sinus to form the straight sinus.
III. Posterior fossa veins (Fig. 7-6).
    A. Anterior pontomesencephalic vein.
       1. Not a single vein but a plexus of numerous small veins along the ventral surface of the pons and midbrain.
       2. Drains cephalad into vein of Galen.
       3. More accurately reflects the ventral margin of the pons than the basilar artery does.
    B. Precentral cerebellar vein (PCV).
       1. Anteriorly convex unpaired midline vein that lies in front of vermis just above and behind the roof of the fourth ventricle.
       2. Drains cephalad into vein of Galen, posterior to anterior pontomesencephalic vein.
    C. Superior vermian vein.
       1. Unpaired midline vein that courses behind superior vermis.
       2. Drains cephalad into vein of Galen, posterior to PCV.
    D. Inferior vermian vein.
       1. Unpaired midline vein that courses behind inferior vermis.

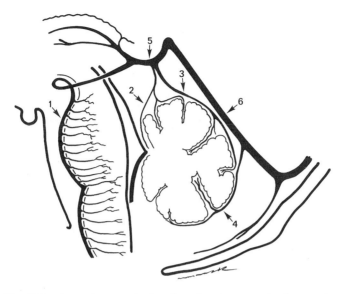

Fig. 7-6   Lateral anatomic drawing of major posterior fossa veins.
1. Anterior pontomesencephalic vein
2. Precentral cerebellar vein
3. Superior vermian vein
4. Inferior vermian vein
5. Vein of Galen
6. Straight sinus

2. Drains posterosuperiorly into straight sinus.
E. Hemispheric veins.
1. Drain the cerebellar hemispheres.

SUGGESTED READINGS

Andrews BT, Dujovny M, Mirchandani HG, Ausman JI: Microsurgical anatomy of the venous drainage into the superior sagittal sinus, *Neurosurgery* 24:514-520, 1989.

Bonneville JF, Cattin F, Racle A, et al: Dynamic CT of the laterosellar extradural venous spaces, *AJNR* 10:535-542, 1989.

Chakeres DW, Schmalbrock P, Brogan M, et al: Normal venous anatomy of the brain: demonstration with gadopentetate dimeglumine in enhanced 3-D MR angiography, *AJNR* 11:1107-1118, 1991.

Cure JK, van Tassel P, Smith MT: Normal and variant anatomy of the dural venous sinuses, *Semin US CT MR* 15:499-519, 1994.

Dean LM, Taylor GA: The intracranial venous system in infants: normal and abnormal findings on duplex and color doppler sonography, *AJR* 164:151-156, 1995.

Dora F, Zileli T: Common variations of the lateral and occipital sinuses at the confluens sinuum, *Neuroradiol* 20:23-27, 1980.

Gebarski SS, Gebarski KS: Inferior petrosal sinus: imaging-anatomic correlation, *Radiology* 194:239-247. 1995.

Goulao A, Alvarez H, Monaco RG, et al: Venous anomalies and abnormalities of the posterior fossa, *Neuroradiology* 31:476-482, 1990.

Hasegawa M, Yamasita J, Yamashima T: Anatomical variation of the straight sinus on magnetic resonance imaging: the infratentorial suprasellar approach to pineal region tumors, *Surg Neurol* 36:354-359, 1991.

Kaplan HA, Brosder J: Atresia of the rostral superior sagittal sinus: substitute parasagittal venous channels, *J Neurosurg* 38:602-607, 1973.

Lanzieri CF, Sacher M, Duchesneau PM, et al: The preoperative venogram in planning extended craniectomies, *Neuroradiology* 29:360-365, 1987.

Matsushima T, Suzuki SO, Fukui M, et al: Microsurgical anatomy of the tentorial sinuses, *J Neurosurg* 71:923-928, 1989.

Mattle HP, Wentz KU, Edelman RR, et al: Cerebral venography with MR, *Radiology* 178:453-458, 1991.

Okudera T, Huang YP, Ohta T, et al: Development of posterior fossa dural sinuses, emissary veins, and jugular bulb: morphological and radiological study, *AJNR* 15:1871-1883, 1994.

Osborn AG: *Introduction to cerebral angiography,* New York, 1980, Harper & Row, pp 327-377.

Rubenstein D, Burton BS, Walker AL: The anatomy of the inferior petrosal sinus, glossopharyngeal nerve, vagus nerve, and accessory nerve in the jugular foramen, *AJNR* 16:185-194, 1995.

8

Brain

Key Concepts

1. Knowledge of the anatomy and function of the different parts of the brain aids in the localization of pathology.
2. Identify the function(s) (e.g., motor, sensory, speech, vision, hearing, olfaction) involved and determine the pathway(s) involved.
3. If more than one function is involved, determine likely locations where multiple pathways could be affected by a single lesion (e.g., cortex, brainstem, spinal cord).
4. Determine the laterality of the affected lesion with relationship to possible decussation of pathway(s).

I. Prosencephalon (forebrain).
  A. Telencephalon: cerebrum.
    1. Lobes (named by the adjacent overlying bone) and major gyri
      (Figs. 8-1, 8-2).
      a. Frontal.
        (1) Superior frontal gyrus.
        (2) Middle frontal gyrus.
        (3) Inferior frontal gyrus.
        (4) Precentral gyrus.
        (5) Subcallosal gyrus.

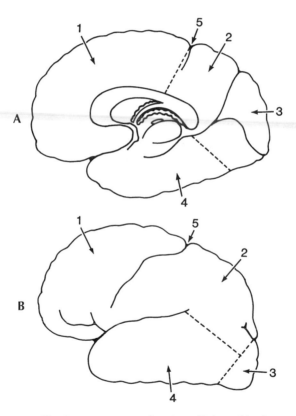

Fig. 8-1   Anatomic drawing of lobes of brain.
    A, Medial view. **B,** Lateral view.
    1. Frontal lobe
    2. Parietal lobe
    3. Occipital lobe
    4. Temporal lobe
    5. Central sulcus

b. Parietal.
  (1) Postcentral gyrus.
  (2) Superior parietal lobule.
  (3) Inferior parietal lobule.
  (4) Supramarginal gyrus.
  (5) Angular gyrus.
  (6) Pre-cuneate gyrus.
c. Occipital.
  (1) Cuneate gyrus.
  (2) Lingual gyrus.
d. Temporal.
  (1) Superior temporal gyrus.
  (2) Middle temporal gyrus.
  (3) Inferior temporal gyrus.
  (4) Hippocampal gyrus.
  (5) Parahippocampal gyrus.
2. Major fissures and sulci (Fig. 8-2).
  a. Interhemispheric fissure.
  b. Lateral sulcus or Sylvian fissure.
  c. Superior frontal sulcus.
  d. Inferior frontal sulcus.
  e. Cingulate sulcus.
  f. Precentral sulcus.
  g. Central sulcus (of Rolando).
  h. Postcentral sulcus.
  i. Intraparietal sulcus.
  j. Parieto-occipital sulcus.
  k. Calcarine sulcus.
  l. Superior temporal sulcus.
  m. Middle temporal sulcus.
  n. Inferior temporal sulcus.
  o. Hippocampal sulcus.
  p. Parahippocampal sulcus.
3. Functional localization of cerebral cortex (Fig. 8-3 on p. 88).
  a. Motor cortex.
    (1) Primary motor area.
      (a) Location: pre-central gyrus.
      (b) Function: gives rise to descending motor fibers of corticobulbar and corticospinal tracts that decussate in the medulla and subsequently control voluntary movement of the contralateral body; the motor homonculus has inverted representation of body (upper/medial corresponds to foot, lower/lateral corresponds to hand/face).

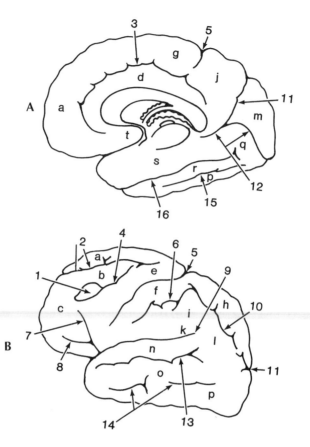

Fig. 8-2   For legend, see following page.

(2) Premotor area.
   (a) Location: posterior portions of superior, middle, and inferior frontal gyri.
   (b) Function: programs the activity of the primary motor area and controls coarse postural movements through connections to basal nuclei.
b. Sensory cortex.
   (1) Primary somesthetic area.
      (a) Location: post-central gyrus.
      (b) Function: receives major sensory pathways from contralateral body, after sensory decussation in inferior medulla.
   (2) Somesthetic association area.

Fig. 8-2—cont'd Anatomic drawing of major cerebral sulci and gyri.
A, Medial view. **B,** Lateral view.
Sulci.
  1. Inferior frontal sulcus
  2. Superior frontal sulcus
  3. Cingulate sulcus
  4. Precentral sulcus
  5. Central sulcus
  6. Postcentral sulcus
  7. Anterior ascending ramus of the lateral sulcus
  8. Anterior horizontal ramus of the lateral sulcus
  9. Posterior ramus of the lateral sulcus
 10. Intraparietal sulcus
 11. Parieto-occipital sulcus
 12. Calcarine sulcus
 13. Superior temporal sulcus
 14. Middle temporal sulcus
 15. Inferior temporal (occipitotemporal) sulcus
 16. Collateral sulcus
Gyri.
  a. Superior frontal gyrus
  b. Middle frontal gyrus
  c. Inferior frontal gyrus
  d. Cingulate gyrus
  e. Precentral gyrus
  f. Postcentral gyrus
  g. Paracentral lobule
  h. Superior parietal lobule
  i. Inferior parietal lobule
  j. Precuneate gyrus
  k. Supramarginal gyrus
  l. Angular gyrus
  m. Cuneate gyrus
  n. Superior temporal gyrus
  o. Middle temporal gyrus
  p. Inferior temporal gyrus
  q. Lingual gyrus
  r. Fusiform gyrus
  s. Parahippocampal gyrus
  t. Subcallosal gyrus

            (a) Location: superior and inferior parietal lobules.
            (b) Function: integrate and recognize different sensory
                modalities.
        c. Speech cortex.
            (1) Sensory ("receptive") speech area.

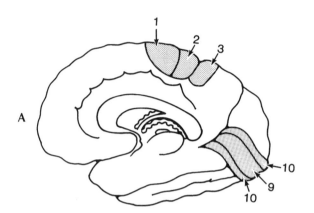

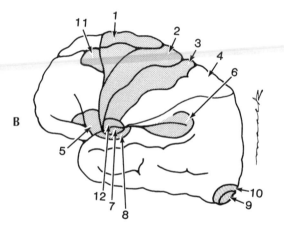

Fig. 8-3   Anatomic drawing of functional localization of the cerebral cortex.
A, Medial view. **B,** Lateral view.
1. Premotor area
2. Primary motor area
3. Primary sensory area
4. Sensory association area
5. Motor speech area
6. Sensory speech area
7. Primary auditory area
8. Secondary auditory area
9. Primary visual area
10. Secondary visual area
11. Frontal eye area
12. Taste area

    (a) Location: inferior parietal lobule (supramarginal and angular gyri) of dominant hemisphere.

    (b) Function: written and spoken language comprehension.

  (2) Broca's motor ("expressive") speech area.

    (a) Location: inferior frontal gyrus of dominant hemisphere.

    (b) Function: coordination of voluntary muscles involved in speech formation.

 d. Auditory cortex.

  (1) Primary auditory area.

    (a) Location: superior temporal gyrus, in floor of lateral sulcus, (Heschl's convolutions).

    (b) Function: receives major auditory sensory information from bilateral cochlea, although there is greater representation from the contralateral ear.

  (2) Secondary auditory area or auditory association cortex.

    (a) Location: superior temporal gyrus, lateral surface.

    (b) Function: auditory comprehension.

    Note: originally named Wernicke's area, but now term loosely refers to both secondary auditory area as well as sensory speech area.

 e. Visual cortex.

  (1) Primary visual area.

    (a) Location: adjacent to calcarine sulcus (cuneate and lingual gyri).

    (b) Function: receives major visual sensory information.

     i. Receives fibers from the temporal half (nasal field) of ipsilateral retina and from the nasal half (temporal field) of contralateral retina.

     ii. Fibers from the superior retinal quadrants (inferior field) pass to the superior wall of the calcarine sulcus while fibers from the inferior retinal quadrants (superior field) pass to the inferior wall of the calcarine sulcus.

  (2) Secondary visual area.

    (a) Location: pre-cuneate, cuneate, and lingual gyri.

    (b) Function: interpretation and recognition of visual information.

  (3) Occipital eye area.

    (a) Location: within secondary visual area.

    (b) Function: involuntary tracking.

      f. Eye motor cortex.
         (1) Frontal eye area.
           (a) Location: middle frontal gyrus.
           (b) Function: controls voluntary scanning eye movements independent of visual stimuli.
     g. Olfactory cortex.
         (1) Primary (lateral) olfactory area.
           (a) Location: uncal cortex, anterior hippocampal gyrus, amygdala (nonlimbic portion).
           (b) Function: receives major olfactory sensory information.
         (2) Secondary (medial) olfactory area.
           (a) Location: subcallosal gyrus.
           (b) Function: allows connection to limbic system.
     h. Taste cortex.
         (1) Location: lower end of post-central gyrus in the superior wall of the lateral sulcus.
         (2) Function: receives fibers from nucleus solitarius.
     i. Prefrontal cortex.
         (1) Location: superior, middle, and inferior frontal gyri, orbital gyrus, medial gyrus, and anterior portion of cingulate gyrus.
         (2) Function: involved in formation of personality, including emotion, initiative, and judgment.
  4. White matter tracts (major).
     a. Association (intrahemispheric) fibers: connect cortical areas in the ipsilateral hemisphere.
         (1) Short association fibers: U-shaped bands connecting adjacent gyri.
         (2) Long association fibers.
           (a) Fronto-occipital fasciculus: connects frontal lobe to parietal and occipital lobes.
           (b) Uncinate fasciculus: connects inferior frontal lobe with temporal pole.
           (c) Cingulum: connects frontal and parietal lobes with parahippocampal regions.
           (d) Superior longitudinal fasciculus: connects anterior frontal lobe to parietal and temporal lobes.
           (e) Inferior longitudinal fasciculus: connects occipital lobe to temporal lobe.
     b. Commissural (intrahemispheric) fibers: connect cortical areas with contralateral hemisphere.
         (1) Corpus callosum: largest commissure connecting hemispheres.

        (a) Rostrum: thin anteroinferior portion, continuous with lamina terminalis.

        (b) Genu: curved anterior portion.

        (c) Body: longitudinal portion beneath interhemispheric fissure.

        (d) Splenium: bulbous posterior portion.

    (2) Anterior commisure: small bundle of fibers crossing in lamina terminalis, connecting anterior perforated substance, olfactory tract, and temporal lobes.

    (3) Commissure of the fornix or hippocampal commisure: between columns of fornix, connect hippocampal formations.

    (4) Posterior commisure: small bundle of fibers crossing immediately above the cerebral aqueduct, carry fibers involved in pupillary light reflex.

    (5) Habenular commisure: small bundle of fibers that cross in the superior part of the pineal stalk, connect habenular nuclei.

  c. Projection fibers: connect cortical or limbic areas with corpus striatum or diencephalon.

    (1) Fornix: hippocampus to hypothalamus.

    (2) Corona radiata and internal capsule.

    (3) Optic radiations as well as terminal fibers of other sensory pathways.

 5. Basal nuclei (originally incorrectly designated as basal ganglia): deep grey matter.

  a. Amygdaloid body: located in the anterior temporal lobe, near uncus; olfactory and limbic functions.

  b. Claustrum: thin sheet of gray matter lateral to external capsule and medial to extreme capsule; function not well understood.

  c. Corpus striatum: involved in motor coordination.

    (1) Caudate nucleus: large C-shaped mass of gray matter closely related to lateral ventricle, lateral to thalamus and medial to internal capsule.

    (2) Lentiform nucleus: wedge-shaped mass of gray matter with apex directed medially, lateral to internal capsule and medial to external capsule.

        (a) Globus pallidus: medial portion of lentiform nucleus.

        (b) Putamen: lateral portion of lentiform nucleus.

B. Diencephalon: paired relay nuclei.

 1. Thalamus.

  a. Largest subdivision of diencephalon.

      b. Major relay station of general sensory and voluntary motor pathway, including connections to the cerebellum.

      c. Major nuclei.

        (1) Anterior thalamic nucleus: receives the mammillothalamic tract and has connections to cingulate gyrus and hypothalamus (part of Papez circuit).

        (2) Dorsomedial nucleus: large nucleus with connections to other thalamic nuclei, prefrontal cortex, hypothalamus; responsible for integration of sensory information.

        (3) Ventral anterior nucleus: connected to reticular formation, corpus striatum, premotor cortex, and other thalamic nuclei; influences activities of motor cortex.

        (4) Ventral lateral nucleus: connections to cerebellum and red nucleus; influences activities of motor cortex.

        (5) Ventral posterior nucleus: receives ascending sensory tracts from the body and conveys thalamocortical projections through posterior limb of internal capsule and corona radiata to reach primary sensory cortex.

        (6) Pulvinar: interconnections with other thalamic nuclei and association areas; responsible for integration of sensory information.

2. Hypothalamus.

      a. Most anteroinferior subdivision of diencephalon.

      b. Includes floor of infundibular recess of third ventricle, base of pituitary infundibulum, tuber cinereum, and mammillary bodies.

      c. Integration of autonomic and neuroendocrine pathways for maintaining body homeostasis.

      d. Nuclei.

        (1) Preoptic nucleus.

        (2) Paraventricular nucleus.

        (3) Dorsomedial nucleus.

        (4) Ventromedial nucleus.

        (5) Infundibular nucleus.

        (6) Posterior nucleus.

        (7) Supraoptic nucleus.

        (8) Lateral nucleus.

        (9) Tuberomammillary nucleus.

       (10) Lateral tuberal nucleus.

       (11) Suprachiasmatic nucleus.

3. Epithalamus.

      a. Smallest portion of diencephalon.

      b. Lies along roof of third ventricle.

      c. Includes pineal gland, habenular structures, and stria medullaris thalamus.

      d. Integration of olfactory, visceral, and somatic afferent pathways.

      e. Nuclei.

        (1) Habenular nucleus.

        (2) Pineal gland: does not actually possess nerve cells; instead contains pinealocytes and glial cells.

   4. Subthalamus.

      a. Located inferior to thalamus, posterior to hypothalamus, and above midbrain.

      b. Relay station for extrapyramidal motor pathways descending to striated muscles.

   5. Metathalamus.

      a. Posteroinferior to thalamus.

      b. Two nuclei.

        (1) Medial geniculate nucleus: relay station for auditory pathway (M for music).

        (2) Lateral geniculate nucleus: relay station for visual pathway (L for light).

II. Mesencephalon (midbrain).

  A. Geographic features.

   1. Dorsal surface.

      a. Quadragemina.

        i. Superior colliculi (paired): involved in visual reflexes.

        ii. Inferior colliculi (paired): relay station in auditory pathway.

      c. Superior cerebellar peduncles or brachium conjunctiva.

   2. Ventral surface.

      a. Cerebral peduncle or crus cerebri or basis pedunculi.

      b. Interpeduncular fossa.

   3. Internal.

      a. Cerebral peduncles: anterior portion of midbrain, ventral to substantia nigra.

      b. Tegmentum: posterior portion of midbrain, dorsal to substantia nigra but ventral to cerebral aqueduct.

      c. Decussation of superior cerebellar peduncles: occupy much of tegmentum.

      d. Tectum: small portion of midbrain dorsal to cerebral aqueduct.

      e. Cerebral aqueduct.

      f. Central gray or periaqueductal gray matter.

B. Major nuclei.
    1. Cranial nerves: III, IV, mesencephalic nucleus of V (see Chapter 9).
    2. Red nucleus: large round nucleus between substantia nigra and cerebral aqueduct; relay station between cerebellum and other parts of CNS.
    3. Substantia nigra: large nucleus between cerebral peduncle and tegentum; involved in extrapyramidal motor pathway.
    4. Superior colliculus: superior bulge of tectum; involved in control of involuntary tracking.
    5. Inferior colliculus: inferior bulge of tectum; relay station for auditory pathway.
    6. Reticular formation: throughout brainstem; but smallest in midbrain, located in tegmentum.
C. Major fiber tracts.
    1. Corticobulbar and corticospinal tracts: descending voluntary motor pathway, located in cerebral peduncle.
    2. Corticopontine tract: part of corticopontocerebellar pathway, in cerebral penduncle.
    3. Medial lemniscus: pathway for proprioception, vibration and touch discrimination.
    4. Lateral lemniscus: auditory pathway.
    5. Lateral spinothalamic tract: pathway for pain, temperature, and touch.
III. Rhombencephalon (hindbrain).
  A. Metencephalon: pons and cerebellum.
    1. Pons.
      a. Geographic features.
        (1) Dorsal surface.
          (a) Median sulcus: posterior midline groove.
          (b) Medial eminence: paramedian longitudinal bulge.
          (c) Sulcus limitans: groove lateral to medial eminence.
          (d) Facial colliculus: expanded inferior end of medial eminence, formed by root of CN VII looping around the nucleus of CN VI (see Chapter 9).
          (e) Floor of fourth ventricle.
          (f) Middle cerebellar peduncle or brachium pontis.
        (2) Ventral surface.
          (a) Basilar groove: shallow midline groove dorsal to basilar artery.
          (b) Basal portion of pons.
        (3) Lateral surface.
          (a) Root entry zone of CN V.

    (4) Pontomedullary junction.

        (a) Exit of CNs VI, VII, and VIII (see Fig. 9-2).

    (5) Internal.

        (a) Basal portion: large anterior part, ventral to trapezoid body and medial lemniscus.

        (b) Tegmentum: posterior part, dorsal to trapezoid body but ventral to fourth ventricle.

  b. Major nuclei.

    (1) Cranial nerves: V, VI, VII, VIII (cochlear nuclei and superior part of vesibular nuclear complex) (see Chapter 9).

    (2) Pontine nuclei (for corticobulbar/spinal tracts): basal pons.

    (3) Pontine paramedian reticular formation: lateral gaze center.

    (4) Reticular formation: distributed throughout brainstem.

  c. Major fiber tracts.

    (1) Corticobulbar and corticospinal tract, basal pons.

    (2) Medial lemniscus: see above.

    (3) Lateral lemniscus and trapezoid body: auditory pathway (see Chapter 9).

    (4) Lateral spinothalamic tract: (*Note*: decussation occurs in spinal cord within one or two vertebral segments from entry of spinal nerve root).

    (5) Rubrospinal, spinocerebellar, and pontocerebellar tracts: pathways for unconscious proprioception.

    (6) Medial longitudinal fasciculus: connects vestibulocochlear nuclei with nuclei controlling extraocular muscles.

2. Cerebellum.

  a. Lobules (Fig. 8-4).

    (1) Cerebellar hemispheres.

        (a) Anterior lobe.

            i. Ala of central lobule.

            ii. Quadrangular lobule.

        (b) Posterior lobe.

            i. Simple lobule.

            ii. Superior semilunar lobule.

            iii. Inferior seminlunar lobule.

            iv. Gracilis lobule.

            v. Biventral lobe.

            vi. Tonsil.

        (c) Flocculonodular lobe.

            i. Flocculus.

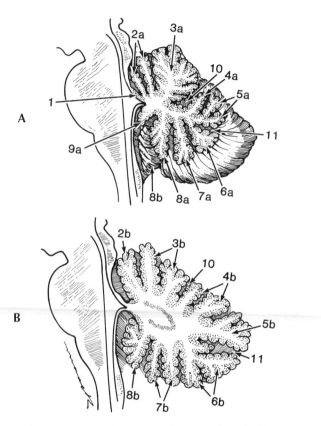

Fig. 8-4   Lateral anatomic drawing of cerebellum.
A, Midline sagittal view. **B,** Parasagittal view, 1 cm from midline.
 1. Lingula
2a. Central lobule
2b. Ala of central lobule
3a. Culmen
3b. Quadrangular lobule
4a. Declive
4b. Simple lobule
5a. Folium
5b. Superior semilunar lobule
6a. Tuber
6b. Inferior semilunar lobule
7a. Pyramis
7b. Biventral lobule
8a. Uvula
8b. Tonsil
9a. Nodule
10. Primary fissure
11. Horizontal fissure

    (2) Vermis.

        (a) Anterior lobe.

            i. Lingula (lacks hemispheric counterpart).

            ii. Central lobule.

            iii. Culmen.

        (b) Posterior lobe.

            i. Declive.

            ii. Folium.

            iii. Tuber (attached to inferior semilunar and gracilis lobules).

            iv. Pyramis.

            v. Uvula.

        (c) Flocculonodular lobe.

            i. Nodule.

  b. Major fissures.

    (1) Primary fissure: between anterior and posterior lobes.

    (2) Horizontal fissure: between the superior and inferior semilunar lobules.

    (3) Uvulonodular fissure: between the posterior and flocculonodular lobes.

  c. Nuclei (Fig. 8-5).

    (1) Dentate nucleus: largest, situated in white matter of cerebellar hemisphere.

    (2) Globose nucleus: one or more rounded cell groups antero-medial to emboliform nucleus.

    (3) Emboliform nucleus: ovoid nucleus medial to dentate nucleus and posterior to globose nucleus.

    (4) Fastigial nucleus: most anterior and paramedian, near roof of fourth ventricle.

  d. Peduncles.

    (1) Superior cerebellar peduncle or brachium conjunctivum.

        (a) Connects lower midbrain to cerebellum.

        (b) Efferent fibers: from the dentate, emboliform, and globose nuclei.

        (c) Afferent fibers: anterior spinocerebellar, rubrocerebellar, tectocerebellar tracts.

    (2) Middle cerebellar peduncle or brachium pontis.

        (a) Largest peduncle, formed by transverse pontine fibers.

        (b) Part of extensive corticopontocerebellar pathway.

    (3) Inferior cerebellar peduncle or restiform body or restibrachium.

        (a) Connects posterolateral medulla to cerebellum.

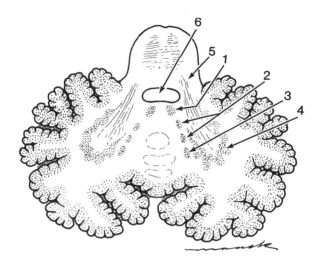

Fig. 8-5   Cross-sectional anatomic drawing of cerebellum.
1. Fastigial nucleus
2. Globose nucleus
3. Emboliform nucleus
4. Dentate nucleus
5. Superior cerebellar peduncle
6. Fourth ventricle

      (b) Afferent fibers: posterior spinocerebellar, cuneocerebellar, olivocerebellar, reticulocerebellar, vestibulocerebellar tracts.

      (c) Efferent fibers: from the fastigial nucleus; cerebellovestibular, cerebelloreticular tracts.

B. Myelencephalon: medulla.
   1. Geographic features.
      a. Dorsal surface.
         (1) Posterior median sulcus: continuous with that of spinal cord.
         (2) Gracile tubercle or clava: longitudinal paramedian bulge formed by nucleus gracilis.
         (3) Cuneate tubercle: longitudinal bulge formed by nucleus cuneatus; lateral to clava.
         (4) Tuberculum cinereum: longitudinal ridge formed by the spinal tract of trigeminal nerve; anterior to fasciculus cuneatus.
         (5) Floor of fourth ventricle.

    b. Ventral surface.

        (1) Anterior median fissure: continuous with that of spinal cord.

        (2) Pyramid: paramedian longitudinal ridge formed by corticospinal tract.

    c. Lateral surface.

        (1) Pre-olivary sulcus: rootlets of CN XII emerge.

        (2) Olive: bulge formed by inferior olivary nucleus.

        (3) Post-olivary sulcus: roots of CNs IX, X and XI emerge.

        (4) Inferior cerebellar peduncle or restiform body or restibrachium.

    d. Internal.

        (1) Pyramidal decussation: crossing of corticospinal tracts, occurs in caudal medulla, slightly below sensory decussation.

        (2) Sensory (proprioception) decussation: from posterior column to medial lemniscus.

        (3) Inferior fourth ventricle.

        (4) Obex: junction between inferior fourth ventricle and central canal of spinal cord.

2. Major nuclei.

    a. Cranial nerves: VIII (inferior part of vestibular nuclear complex), IX, X, XI, XII (see Chapter 9).

    b. Nucleus of spinal tract of CN V (see Chapter 9).

    c. Nucleus ambiguus (see Chapter 9).

    d. Nucleus solitarius (see Chapter 9).

    e. Superior and inferior salivatory nuclei (see Chapter 9).

    f. Nucleus gracilis: sensory information from posterior columns corresponding to lower part of body.

    g. Nucleus cuneatus: sensory information from posterior columns corresponding to upper part of body.

    h. Olivary nuclei: relay between cerebellum and other CNS areas.

    i. Reticular formation (see above).

3. Major fiber tracts.

    a. Corticospinal tract (see above).

    b. Lateral spinothalamic tract.

    c. Rubrospinal, vestibulospinal, spinocerebellar, and olivocerebellar tracts.

    d. Medial lemniscus: sensory fibers from posterior columns after decussation.

    e. Fasciculus gracilis: before decussation.

    f. Fasciculus cuneatus: before decussation.

    g. Medial longitudinal fasciculus (see above).

SUGGESTED READINGS

Bindman L: *The neurophysiology of the cerebral cortex,* Austin, 1981, University of Texas Press.

Brazis PW, Masdeu JC, Biller J: *Localization in clinical neurology,* ed 2, Boston, 1990, Little, Brown and Company.

Ito, M: *The cerebellum and neural control,* New York, 1984, Raven Press.

Snell RS: *Clinical neuroanatomy for medical students,* ed 3, Boston, 1992, Little, Brown and Company.

Schnitzlein HN, Murtagh FR: *Imaging anatomy of the head and spine,* ed 2, Baltimore, 1990, Urban and Schwarzenberg.

Sobotta, J: *Atlas of human anatomy,* ed 10, Baltimore, 1983, Urban and Schwarzenberg.

9

Cranial Nerves

Key Concepts

1. Knowledge of the anatomy and function of each of the cranial nerves provides a means of localizing a suspected lesion and aids tailoring an imaging study appropriately. (See Figs. 9-1, 9-2.)
2. Identify the cranial nerve(s) involved. If more than one cranial nerve is involved, identify location(s) where multiple cranial nerves are adjacent. For example, multiple nerves can be injured by a lesion in the orbit, cavernous sinus, interpeduncular cistern, brainstem, or jugular foramen.
3. Are the symptoms unilateral or bilateral? If bilateral, could this represent a more "central" lesion above the level of the nucleus?
4. Do the deficits encompass all or only part of the cranial nerve functions? If only some of the functions are involved, where in the cranial nerve pathway would a lesion be likely?
5. Are parasympathetic functions involved? If so, remember that parasympathetic fibers can travel along segments of more than one cranial nerve. (For more detailed discussion of cranial nerves, particularly regarding pathology and imaging issues, please refer to H. Ric Harnsberger's *Handbook of head and neck imaging,* ed 2, St Louis, 1985, Mosby.)

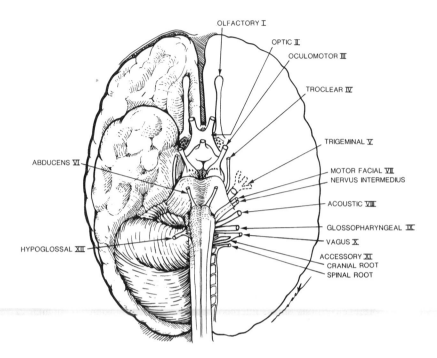

Fig. 9-1   Axial global cranial nerve anatomic drawing. Cranial nerves are labeled with Roman numerals.

I. ICN I: Olfactory nerve.
   A. Anatomy.
      1. Olfactory epithelium in roof of nasal cavity, superior nasal conchae, and nasal septum.
      2. Nerve fibers pierce cribriform plate to synapse in olfactory bulb (enlarged tip of olfactory tract).
      3. Right and left olfactory tracts run along undersurface of inferior frontal lobes to olfactory areas. Traditionally the bulb and tract have been incorrectly referred to as the olfactory "nerve."
      4. Rhinencephalon.
         a. Medial olfactory area: subcallosal gyrus.
         b. Lateral olfactory area: cortex of the uncus, anterior hippocampus, amygdala.
   B. Function.
      1. Sensory: olfaction.
      2. Motor: none.

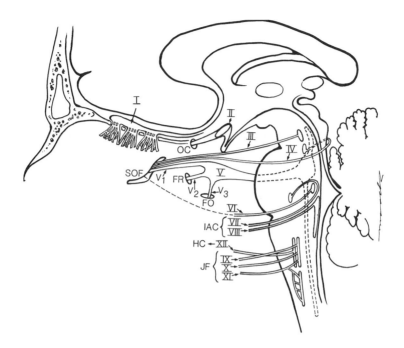

Fig. 9-2   Sagittal global cranial nerve anatomic drawing. Cranial nerves are labeled with Roman numerals. Divisions of CN V labeled V_1, V_2, V_3. Also:

OC: Optic canal
SOF: Superior orbital fissure
FR: Foramen rotundum
FO: Foramen ovale
IAC: Internal auditory canal
JF: Jugular foramen
HC: Hypoglossal canal

   C. Clinical importance.
      1. Unilateral or bilateral anosmia may be caused by anterior cranial fossa masses or skull base fractures traversing the cribriform plate.
      2. Olfactory hallucinations may be caused by temporal lobe lesions or temporal seizures.
 II. CN II: Optic nerve and visual pathway.
   A. Anatomy.
      1. Optic nerve.
         a. Ganglion cells in retina synapse with fibers that form optic nerve.

  b. Is not truly a nerve but a fiber tract (developmentally part of the brain).

  c. Travels through orbital apex and optic canal.

  d. Visual information at this level pertains to ipsilateral eye.

 2. Optic chiasm.

  a. Right and left optic nerves unite to form optic chiasm, located above sella and below third ventricle.

  b. Fibers carrying visual information from the medial retina (i.e., temporal visual fields) decussate at this level.

  c. Fibers carrying visual information from the lateral retina (i.e., nasal visual fields) do not decussate.

 3. Retrochiasmal pathway.

  a. Optic tract is continuation of both crossed and uncrossed fibers that course posteriorly to synapse in the lateral geniculate nucleus.

  b. Lateral geniculate nucleus is located in the posteroinferior thalamus.

  c. Most axons from the lateral geniculate body pass posteriorly as the optic radiation or geniculocalcarine tract. Superior (parietal) fibers carry information from the lower visual field while inferior (temporal) fibers carry information from the upper field.

  d. The optic radiation terminates in the visual cortex of the occipital lobe. The superior wall of the calcarine fissure represents the lower visual field while the inferior wall represents the upper field.

  e. A few fibers pass to the pretectal area and superior colliculus of midbrain, subsequently synapsing in Edinger-Westphal nucleus. These are involved in the afferent pathway for pupillary and accomodation reflexes, which are subsequently effected through CN III.

B. Function.

 1. Sensory.

  a. Vision.

  b. Afferent limb of pupillary light reflex and accomodation reflex.

 2. Motor: none.

C. Clinical importance.

 1. Monocular visual loss suggests a lesion in the globe, orbit, or optic nerve. Additional involvement of CNs III, IV, VI, and V_1 suggests an orbital apex lesion.

 2. Bitemporal hemianopsia suggests a median chiasmal lesion.

3. Unilateral nasal field defect suggests a unilateral marginal (lateral) chiasmal lesion.
4. Homonymous hemianopsia suggests a retrochiasmal lesion.
5. Upper quadrantonopia suggests a lesion in the temporal optic radiations or inferior calcarine fissure.
6. Lower quadrantonopia suggests a lesion in the parietal optic radiations or superior calcarine fissure.

III. CN III: Oculomotor nerve.
  A. Anatomy.
    1. Nuclei.
      a. Oculomotor nucleus (motor): paramedian tegmentum of midbrain ventral to superior colliculi.
      b. Edinger-Westphal nucleus (parasympathetic): dorsal to oculomotor nucleus.
    2. Course.
      a. Intraaxial segment: anteriorly through red nucleus, substantia nigra, and medial cerebral peduncle.
      b. Cisternal segment.
        (1) Exits from anterior midbrain in the interpeduncular cistern.
        (2) Passes between posterior cerebral artery and superior cerebellar artery.
        (3) Courses below posterior communicating artery and medial to uncus.
      c. Cavernous segment (see Fig. 7-5).
        (1) Enters roof of cavernous sinus and travels in lateral wall, superolateral to internal carotid artery.
        (2) Is the most cephalad structure in the cavernous sinus.
      d. Orbital segment.
        (1) Exits skull through superior orbital fissure (SOF) to orbit, passing through tendinous ring.
        (2) Within orbit innervates the superior, medial, and inferior recti, inferior oblique and levator palpebrae muscles.
        (3) Parasympathetic fibers synapse at ciliary ganglion and then travel on short ciliary nerve (V_1) to innervate constrictor pupillae muscle of the iris and ciliary muscles.
  B. Function.
    1. Sensory: none.
    2. Motor.
      a. All oculomotor movements except lateral gaze and inferolateral rotation.

          b. Elevation of upper eyelid.
    3. Parasympathetic.
          a. Pupillary constriction and accommodation.
  C. Clinical importance.
    1. Ipsilateral ophthalmoplegia and contralateral hemiplegia or tremor suggests a midbrain lesion.
    2. Oculomotor palsy, ptosis, and loss of pupillary reflex suggest mass effect along the course of CN III (e.g., PCoA aneurysm, uncal herniation).
    3. Oculomotor palsy and ptosis with intact pupilary reflex suggests diabetic ischemia.
    4. Partial ptosis is unrelated to CN III injury, as in Horner's syndrome (sympathetic innervation to superior tarsal muscle affected).
    5. Additional involvement of CNs IV, VI, and V_1 suggests a SOF lesion (e.g., spheniod meningioma).
IV. CN IV: Trochlear nerve.
  A. Anatomy.
    1. Nucleus: paramedian tegmentum of midbrain, caudal to CN III nuclear complex and ventral to inferior colliculus.
    2. Course.
          a. Intraaxial segment: courses around the cerebral aqueduct and decussates just before exiting the dorsal midbrain, below inferior colliculus.
          b. Cisternal segment (perimesencephalic): courses around mid-brain.
          c. Cisternal segment (interpeduncular): in the interpeduncular cistern, nerve courses inferolateral to CN III and also passes between posterior cerebral artery and superior cerebellar artery.
          d. Tentorial segment: passes forward just inferior to free edge of the tentorium.
          e. Cavernous segment: enters cavernous sinus just below CN III (see Fig. 7-5).
          f. Orbital segment.
             (1) Exits skull via superior orbital fissure to enter orbit.
             (2) Innervates the superior oblique muscle.
  B. Function.
    1. Sensory: none.
    2. Motor: inward rotation and inferolateral movement of the ocular globe.
  C. Clinical importance.
    1. Because of its long intracranial course and its position adja-

cent to the tentorium, the nerve is at risk during midbrain surgery.

2. Trochlear nerve palsy may signal the presence of a posterior communicating aneurysm although isolated involvement is rare.

V. CN V: Trigeminal nerve.

   A. Anatomy.

      1. Nuclei.

         a. Mesencephalic nucleus (proprioception): projects cephalad from lateral tegmentum of pons to the level of the inferior colliculus.

         b. Main sensory nucleus (tactile sensation): lateral tegmentum of pons, along anterolateral aspect of the fourth ventricle, at the level of the root entry zone of the nerve.

         c. Motor nucleus: anteromedial to main sensory nucleus.

         d. Spinal nucleus (pain and temperature sensation): projects caudally from main sensory nucleus into the medulla and upper cervical spinal cord (to C2).

      2. Preganglionic segment.

         a. Root entry zone: nerve emerges from lateral pons as a large sensory root and a smaller motor root.

         b. Courses anterosuperiorly through prepontine cistern.

         c. Enters Meckel's cave via porus trigeminus.

         d. Nerve carries dural covering and leptomeninges into Meckel's cave, resulting in a CSF-filled subarachnoid space referred to as the trigeminal cistern.

         e. The gasserian or trigeminal or semilunar ganglion lies in Meckel's cave.

      3. The nerve trifurcates into three peripheral branches.

         a. Ophthalmic nerve (V_1).

            (1) Courses in lateral wall of cavernous sinus, then exits skull through superior orbital fissure, into orbit.

            (2) Main branches.

               (a) Lacrimal nerve.

               (b) Frontal nerve: supraorbital, supratrochlear branches.

               (c) Nasociliary nerve: ethmoidal, nasal, infratrochlear, ciliary branches.

         b. Maxillary nerve (V_2).

            (1) Courses in lateral wall of cavernous sinus as the most caudal structure, then exits skull through foramen rotundum, to reach pterygopalatine fossa.

            (2) Main branches.

       (a) Zygomatic nerve: zygomaticofacial, zygomatico-temporal branches.

       (b) Pterygopalatine nerve: pharyngeal, nasal, palatine, orbital branches.

       (c) Infraorbital nerve: main trunk of V_2, which continues into orbit through inferior orbital fissure, then courses in infraorbital groove to reach the midface through infraorbital foramen. Branches include anterior, middle, and posterior superior alveolar nerves.

   c. Mandibular nerve (V_3).

     (1) Course.

       (a) Does not traverse cavernous sinus.

       (b) Runs along skull base and exits via foramen ovale to enter masticator space.

       (c) Carries small motor root.

     (2) Main branches.

       (a) From proximal main trunk:

         i. Nerve to tensor tympani.

         ii. Nerve to tensor veli palatini.

       (b) From anterior division (mostly motor).

         i. Masticator nerve: innervates masseter, temporalis, medial, and lateral pterygoid muscles.

         ii. Buccal nerve (sensory).

       (c) From posterior division (mostly sensory).

         i. Auriculotemporal nerve.

         ii. Lingual nerve.

         iii. Inferior alveolar nerve.

            a. Mylohoid nerve (motor): branch arises from proximal inferior alveolar nerve just before the mandibular canal, innervates mylohyoid and anterior belly of digastric muscles.

            b. Inferior alveolar nerve: enters posterior mandibular ramus through mandibular foramen, travels in mandibular canal and emerges through paramedian mandibular body at mental foramen.

            c. Mental nerve: continuation of inferior alveolar nerve after exit from mental foramen, to supply skin of chin.

B. Function.

  1. Sensory.

    a. Sensory type.

     (1) Proprioception from face (mesencephalic nucleus).

        (2) Tactile sensation from face (main sensory nucleus).

        (3) Pain and temperature from face (spinal nucleus).

   b. Facial distribution.

        (V_1): anterior scalp, forehead, upper eyelid, globe, nose, sinuses (frontal, ethmoid, sphenoid).

        (V_2): midface, lower eyelid, lateral nose, upper lip, upper teeth, upper cheek, maxillary sinuses, nasopharynx.

        (V_3): lower face, tongue, floor of mouth, lower cheek, jaw.

   c. Comments.

        (1) Afferent sensory fibers synapse at the ipsilateral main sensory nucleus. However, most postsynaptic fibers decussate in trigeminal lemniscus (above the level of the nucleus) to reach contralateral sensory cortex.

        (2) V_1 provides afferent limb of corneal reflex.

        (3) Directly provides tactile sensation to tongue, not taste. However, chorda tympani nerve (branch of CN VII), which provides taste to anterior two thirds of tongue, joins lingual nerve (V_3) in infratemporal fossa.

 2. Motor.

   a. Dampening of tympanic membrane.

   b. Tenses soft palate and opens eustachian tube aperture.

   c. Controls muscles of mastication.

 3. Parasympathetic.

   a. Does not directly have autonomic function. However, parasympathetic fibers from CNs III, VII, and IX travel with branches of CN V.

        (1) Parasympathetic fibers originating from Edinger-Westphal nucleus (CN III) synapse at ciliary ganglion, then travel with short ciliary nerves.

        (2) Greater superficial petrosal nerve (CN VII) synapses in pterygopalatine ganglion. Parasympathetic fibers then ride with zygomaticotemporal branch of V_2 for short distance before traveling with lacrimal nerve branch of V_1 to innervate lacrimal gland.

        (3) Chorda tympani (CN VII) joins with lingual nerve of V_3 in infratemporal fossa to reach anterior two thirds of tongue.

        (4) Lesser petrosal nerve (arising from tympanic branch of CN IX) synapses in otic ganglion and then travels with auriculotemporal branch of V_3 to reach parotid gland.

C. Clinical importance.

 1. Involvement of V_1, V_2, and V_3 suggests a "central" or preganglionic nerve lesion. Remember that the "central" pathway decussates.

    2. Abnormal sensation in a specific facial distribution suggests the peripheral branch involved: upper face (V_1); midface (V_2); lower face (V_3).

    3. Loss of the corneal reflex also suggests a lesion of V_1.

    4. Serous otitis media and atrophy of the muscles of mastication suggest injury to V_3 proximally.

    5. Atrophy of the mylohyoid and anterior belly of digastric muscles alone suggest injury to V_3 distally.

    6. Loss of certain parasympathetic functions can also occur simultaneously with injury to portions of CN V (see above).

VI. CN VI: Abducens nerve.

  A. Anatomy.

    1. Nucleus: paramedian tegmentum of pons.

    Note: Axons of the facial nerve (CN VII) loop around the abducens nucleus, creating a bulge in the floor of the fourth ventricle, known as the facial colliculus.

    2. Course.

      a. Intraaxial segment: anteroinferiorly through pons to emerge from the brainstem at ventral aspect of pontomedullary junction.

      b. Cisternal segment: ascends through prepontine cistern.

      c. Intracavernous segment.

        (1) Pierces dura covering the posterior sphenoid bone, at Dorello's canal.

        (2) Travels within cavernous sinus as the most medial (i.e., most susceptible) of the intracavernous nerves.

      d. Orbital segment (see Fig. 7-5).

        (1) Exits skull through superior orbital fissure.

        (2) Innervates lateral rectus muscle.

  B. Function.

    1. Sensory: none.

    2. Motor: lateral gaze.

  C. Clinical importance.

    1. Isolated abducens nerve palsy can be caused by skull base fractures or petrous apicitis (Gradenigo's syndrome).

    2. Lateral gaze palsy and facial palsy suggests a lesion in the facial colliculus.

    3. Complete gaze palsy with or without loss of the corneal reflex and abnormal sensation to the upper face suggests a lesion in the cavernous sinus. However, because CN VI is the most susceptible intracavernous nerve, a lesion in the cavernous sinus may not yet affect the remaining nerves.

VII. CN VII: Facial nerve.
  A. Anatomy.
   1. Central connections.
     a. Presynaptic corticobulbar fibers from motor cortex mostly decussate above the level of the nucleus.
     b. A few fibers remain ipsilateral and represent supply to upper face.
   2. Nucleus.
     a. Motor nucleus: nuclear column in lateral pontine tegmentum.
     b. Superior salivatory nucleus (parasympathetic): pontomedullary junction, anterior to fourth ventricle.
     c. Nucleus, solitarius (sensory): posterior medulla.
   3. Course.
     a. Intraaxial segment.
       (1) Motor fibers loop dorsally (internal genu) around abducens nucleus in pontine tegmentum, forming bulge in floor of fourth ventricle, known as facial colliculus.
       (2) Fibers from additional nuclei join in anterolateral pons, forming the smaller nervus intermedius, which exits pontomedullary junction immediately lateral to motor fibers.
     b. Cerebellopontine angle segment: nerve exits pontomedullary junction at cerebellopontine angle (CPA) medial to CN VIII and crosses CPA cistern.
     c. Internal auditory canal segment: enters internal auditory canal (IAC) through porus acousticus, traveling in anterosuperior quadrant of the IAC.
     d. Labyrinthine segment: runs anterolaterally through facial canal of temporal bone, over the cochlea, to reach geniculate ganglion.
     e. Tympanic segment: turns backward from geniculate ganglion (i.e., anterior genu) to course posteroinferiorly under lateral semicircular canal in medial wall of the tympanic cavity.
     f. Mastoid segment.
       (1) Turns inferiorly (i.e., posterior genu) to reach stylomastoid foramen.
       (2) Exits skull base through stylomastoid foramen.
     g. Parotid segment: extracranial facial nerve travels between superficial and deep lobes of parotid gland, eventually terminating in the muscles of facial expression.

4. Branches.
   a. Greater superficial petrosal nerve.
      (1) Exits at geniculate ganglion and runs anteriorly to pterygopalatine ganglion.
      (2) Parasympathetic fibers then travel with branches of CN V to innervate lacrimal gland.
   b. Stapedius nerve.
      (1) Exits at proximal mastoid segment of facial nerve.
      (2) Innervates stapedius muscle.
   c. Chorda tympani nerve.
      (1) Exits from mastoid segment of facial nerve, proximal to stylomastoid foramen.
      (2) Joins lingual nerve of CN V to reach tongue.
   d. Nonfacial muscular branches.
      (1) Posterior auricular nerve.
      (2) Nerve to posterior belly of digastric.
      (3) Stylohyoid nerve.
   e. Terminal branches of muscles of facial expression.
      (1) Temporal.
      (2) Zygomatic.
      (3) Buccal.
      (4) Mandibular.
      (5) Cervical.
B. Function.
   1. Sensory.
      a. Taste to anterior two thirds of tongue.
   2. Motor.
      a. Sound dampening via stapedius reflex.
      b. Control of muscles of facial expression.
   3. Parasympathetic.
      a. Lacrimation.
      b. Salivation: sublingual and submandibular glands.
C. Clinical importance.
   1. Paresis of the lower facial muscles of one side suggests a lesion in the "central" pathway of the contralateral hemisphere, such as the sensory cortex or posterior internal capsule. Most of the supranuclear fibers decussate, but a few fibers supplying the upper face remain ipsilateral. Therefore the upper face receives bilateral "central" innervation and will be spared in an upper motor neuron lesion.
   2. Paresis of the entire face of one side suggests a lesion at the level of the ipsilateral nucleus or the CN VII nerve.
   3. Involvement of both CNs VI and VII suggests a lesion at the facial colliculus.

4. Involvement of both CN VII and VIII suggests a CPA or IAC lesion.
5. Loss of special functions (lacrimation, stapedius reflex, and taste to anterior two thirds of tongue) suggests a lesion in the temporal bone.
6. Sparing of only lacrimation suggests a lesion in the tympanic segment or beyond.
7. Sparing of lacrimation with normal stapedius reflex but loss of taste to anterior two thirds of tongue suggests a lesion in the mastoid segment or beyond.
8. Sparing of all three special functions suggests a lesion of the extracranial segment.
9. The extracranial segment can be injured during forceps delivery in an infant because the mastoid process is not yet fully developed.

VIII. CN VIII: Vestibulocochlear nerve.
  A. Anatomy.
    1. Cochlear portion.
      a. Sensory afferent fibers from spiral ganglion of cochlea.
      b. Cochlear fibers run in anteroinferior quadrant of IAC.
      c. After joining with vestibular fibers, the vestibulocochlear nerve courses across cerebellopontine angle cistern.
      d. Enters brainstem at lateral pontomedullary junction.
      e. Synapse at dorsal and ventral cochlear nuclei in lateral aspect of inferior cerebellar peduncle.
      f. Most postsynaptic fibers decussate in the trapezoid body, located in the pontine tegmentum.
      g. Fibers continue through lateral lemniscus to reach medial geniculate body. Some fibers remain in the ipsilateral lateral lemniscus.
      h. Subsequently terminate in contralateral superior temporal gyrus, although there is a small degree of representation in the ipsilateral superior temporal gyrus.
    2. Vestibular portion.
      a. Sensory afferent fibers from vestibular apparatus of inner ear.
      b. Vestibular fibers run in posterior half of IAC: superior and inferior portions.
      c. After joining with cochlear fibers, the vestibulocochlear nerve courses across cerebellopontine angle cistern.
      d. Enters brainstem at lateral pontomedullary junction.
      e. Synapse at vestibular nuclear column spanning caudal pons and rostral medulla, ventral to cochlear nuclei.
  B. Function.
    1. Sensory.

        a. Cochlear portion: hearing.

           (1) Sensory component (cochlear).

           (2) Neural component (retrocochlear acoustic pathway).

        b. Vestibular portion: balance, equilibrium.

    2. Motor: none.

  C. Clinical importance.

    1. Unilateral sensorineural hearing loss suggests a lesion between the cochlea and the cochlear nuclei.

    2. Bilateral sensorineural hearing loss suggests a lesion in the central auditory pathway. Such a lesion usually causes greater hearing loss in the contralateral side.

IX. CN IX: Glossopharyngeal nerve.

  A. Anatomy.

    1. Nuclei

        a. Nucleus ambiguus (motor): lateral medulla.

          Note: also shared by CN X and XI.

        b. Inferior salivatory nucleus (parasympathetic): rostral medulla, posterior aspect.

        c. Nucleus solitarius or solitary nucleus (sensory): posterior medulla, lateral to inferior salivatory nucleus.

          Note: also shared by CNs VII and X.

    2. Course.

        a. Exits lateral medulla at retroolivary sulcus.

        b. Courses across medullary cistern to jugular foramen.

        c. Exits skull through pars nervosa (anterior portion of jugular foramen).

        d. Runs in carotid space.

    3. Branches.

        a. Tympanic branch (Jacobsen's nerve): ascends in inferior tympanic canaliculus and innervates:

           (1) Tympanic membrane, middle ear, and bony eustachian tube.

           (2) Parotid gland: via lesser petrosal nerve, which synapses in otic ganglion, then travels with auriculotemporal branch of V_3.

        b. Stylopharyngeus branch.

        c. Sinus nerve: innervates the carotid sinus and carotid body (baroreceptors, chemoreceptors).

        d. Pharyngeal branches: innervate posterior oropharynx and soft palate. Constitute afferent limb of gag reflex.

        e. Lingual branch: innervate posterior third of tongue.

  B. Function.

    1. Sensory.

a. Tympanic membrane, middle ear, and bony eustachian tube.
b. Posterior oropharynx and soft palate. (Afferent limb of gag reflex.)
c. Taste and general sensation from posterior third of tongue.
2. Motor.
a. Stylopharyngeus muscle.
3. Parasympathetic.
a. Baroreceptor and chemoreceptor input from carotid sinus and body.
b. Salivation from Parotid gland.
C. Clinical importance.
1. Involvement of CN IX, X, and XI suggests a lesion in the jugular foramen.
2. Involvement of CN IX, X, XI, and XII suggests a lesion in the nasopharyngeal carotid space.
X. CN X: Vagus nerve.
A. Anatomy.
1. Nuclei: three nuclear columns located in the rostral and mid-medulla.
a. Nucleus ambiguus (motor): lateral medulla.
Note: also shared by CN IX and XI.
b. Nucleus solitarius or solitary nucleus (sensory): posterior medulla, lateral to dorsal motor nucleus.
Note: also shared by CNs VII and IX.
c. Dorsal motor nucleus (parasympathetic): posterior medulla, below inferior salivatory nucleus.
2. Course.
a. Exits lateral medulla at retroolivary sulcus.
b. Courses across medullary cistern to jugular foramen.
c. Exits skull through pars vascularis (posterior portion of jugular foramen).
d. Runs inferiorly in carotid space, along posterolateral aspect of carotid artery.
e. Continues through neck, thorax, and abdomen.
3. Branches.
a. Proximal vagus branches.
(1) Pharyngeal plexus (motor): Efferent limb of gag reflex.
(2) Superior laryngeal nerve: divides into:
(a) Internal laryngeal nerve (sensory): to hypopharynx and larynx above true cords.
(b) External laryngeal nerve (motor): to inferior constrictor and cricothyroid muscles.

b. Recurrent laryngeal nerves (motor).

(1) Right recurrent laryngeal nerve arises in clavicular region, loops around right subclavian artery, courses cephalad in tracheoesophageal groove, and innervates endolaryngeal muscles.

(2) Left recurrent laryngeal nerve arises in region of aorto-pulmonary window, loops around ligamentum arteriosum, courses cephalad in tracheoesophageal groove, and innervates endolaryngeal muscles.

Note: components of fibers from nucleus ambiguus are also provided by medullary component o CN XI.

c. Distal innervation of thoracic and abdominal viscera.

B. Function.

1. Sensory.

a. External ear.

b. Pharynx, larynx, trachea, esophagus, thoracic, and abdominal viscera.

c. Taste from epiglottis.

2. Motor.

a. Swallowing, gagging.

b. Phonation.

3. Parasympathetic.

a. Thoracic and abdominal viscera.

C. Clinical importance.

1. Involvement of CNs IX, X, and XI suggests a lesion in the jugular foramen.

2. Involvement of CNs IX, X, XI, and XII suggests a lesion in the nasopharyngeal carotid space.

3. Isolated involvement of CN X suggests a lesion in or below the infrahyoid carotid space.

4. Isolated vocal cord paralysis suggests a lesion along the course of the recurrent laryngeal nerve.

XI. CN XI: Spinal accessory nerve.

A. Anatomy.

1. Origin.

a. Nucleus ambiguus (motor to endolarynx): lateral medulla. *Note:* also shared by CN IX and X.

b. Upper spinal cord (motor to trapezius, sternocleidomastoid): anterior horn cells of C1 to C5 segments.

2. Course.

a. Spinal segment emerges from lateral cervical cord and ascends through foramen magnum to join fibers from medullary origin.

b. Medullary fibers exit at retroolivary sulcus.

c. Coalescing fibers form nerve, which courses across medullary cistern, adjacent to CNs IX and X, to jugular foramen.

d. Exits skull through pars vascularis.

e. Runs for short distance in nasopharyngeal carotid space.

f. Spinal fibers run inferiorly along steroncleidomastoid muscle to posterior cervical space of neck. Innervate trapezius and sternocleidomastoid muscles.

g. Medullary fibers run with vagus nerve to innervate endolaryngeal muscles via recurrent laryngeal nerve.

B. Function.

1. Sensory: none.

2. Motor.

a. Trapezius and sternocleidomastoid muscle function.

b. Control of endolaryngeal muscles.

C. Clinical importance.

1. Involvement of CNs IX, X, and XI suggests a lesion in the jugular foramen.

2. Involvement of CNs IX, X, XI, and XII suggests a lesion in the nasopharyngeal carotid space.

XII. CN XII: Hypoglossal nerve.

A. Anatomy.

1. Nucleus.

a. Paramedian location along posterior medulla, ventral to floor of fourth ventricle.

b. The bulge made by the nucleus into the fourth ventricle is known as the hypoglossal eminence.

2. Course.

a. Exits medulla in preolivary sulcus.

b. Multiple rootlets course in medullary cistern to exit skull via hypoglossal canal.

c. Nerve runs for short distance in nasopharyngeal carotid space to level of hyoid bone.

d. Ascends and runs forward in sublingual space of oral cavity.

e. Innervates tongue musculature.

Note: C1 nerve root rides on hypoglossal nerve to help supply motor innervation to geniohyoid and thyrohyoid muscles. C1 also combines with C2 and C3 roots to form ansa hypoglossus (innervates infrahyoid strap muscles).

B. Function.

1. Sensory: none.

2. Motor.

a. Intrinsic tongue musculature.

        (1) Longitudinal.
        (2) Vertical.
        (3) Transverse.
    b. Extrinsic tongue musculature.
        (1) Genioglossus.
        (2) Geniohyoid.
        (3) Hypoglossus.
        (4) Styloglossus.
  C. Clinical importance.
    1. Involvement of CNs IX, X, XI, and XII suggests a lesion in the nasopharyngeal carotid space.

SUGGESTED READINGS

Bradley WG Jr: MR of the brain stem: a practical approach, *Radiology* 179:319-332, 1991.

Flannigan BD, Bradley WG Jr, Mazziotta JC, et al: Magnetic resonance imaging of the brain stem: normal structure and basic functional anatomy, *Radiology* 154:375-383, 1985.

Harnsberger HR: *Handbook of head and neck imaging,* ed 2, St Louis, 1995, Mosby.

Harnsberger HR (guest ed): Cranial nerve imaging, *Semin US CT MR* September 1987 (entire monograph).

Hirsch WL, Kemp SS, Martinez AJ, et al: Anatomy of the brain stem: correlation of in vitro MR images with histologic sections, *AJNR* 10:923-928, 1989.

Lanzieri CF: MR imaging of the cranial nerves, *AJR* 154:1263-1267, 1990.

Lufkin R, Flannigan BD, Bentson JR, et al: Magnetic resonance imaging of the brain stem and cranial nerves, *Surg Radiol Anat* 8:49-66, 1986.

Samii M, Jannetta P: *The cranial nerves: anatomy, pathology, pathophysiology, diagnosis and treatment,* New York, 1981, Springer-Verlag.

Solberg MD, Fournier D, Potts DG: MR imaging of the excised human brainstem: a correlative neuroanatomic study, *AJNR* 11:1001-1013, 1990.

Wilson-Pauwels L, Akesson EJ, Stewart PA: *Cranial nerves: anatomy and clinical comments,* St Louis, 1988, Mosby.

SECTION II
Brain Development and Congenital Malformations

10

Normal Brain Development and Classification of Congenital Malformations

---

Key Concepts

1. Early events in brain development.
   a. Neurulation (formation of neural plate, folds).
   b. Neural tube closure.
   c. Formation of brain vesicles (primitive ventricles).
   d. Embryonic brain flexes and bends.
   e. Disjunction of cutaneous, neural ectoderm.
   f. Process of diverticulation and cleavage forms forebrain, midbrain, hindbrain.
2. Between 2 and 5 months.
   a. Germinal matrix forms.
   b. Migration of neurons from subependymal region to cortex occurs.
   c. Gyri, sulci form.
   d. Commissural fibers (e.g., corpus callosum) form.
3. Third trimester to adulthood.
   a. Myelination occurs (peak from 30 weeks' gestational age to 8 months postnatal but continues into adulthood).
   b. Brain generally myelinates from caudad to cephalad, dorsal to ventral, central to peripheral, sensory before motor.

Understanding the basics of how the central nervous system is formed is essential for understanding the congenital malformations of the brain, spine, and spinal cord that are encountered in clinical practice. In this chapter we briefly delineate the salient features of neuroembryology, then discuss the general classification of CNS malformations.

I. Normal brain development.
  A. Neurulation.
    1. Neural plate forms and invaginates, forming neural groove.
    2. Neural groove thickens laterally, forming neural folds.
    3. Neural folds appose in midline, forming neural tube.
  B. Neural tube closure.
    1. Neural tube closes like zipper.
    2. Neural tube closure starts in the middle (future hindbrain area) and progresses towards both ends of the embryo.
  C. Formation of brain vesicles, flexures.
    1. Three hollow, fluid-filled primary vesicles (rostral expansions of the neural tube) form.
      a. Forebrain (prosencephalon).
      b. Midbrain (mesencephalon).
      c. Hindbrain (rhombencephalon).
    2. Tubelike caudal end will form future spinal cord.
    3. Rostral end of neural tube then constricts to form five secondary vesicles.
      a. Telencephalon (future cerebral hemispheres).
      b. Diencephalon (thalamus, hypothalamus).
      c. Mesencephalon (tectum, midbrain).
      d. Metencephalon (pons, cerebellum).
      e. Myelencephalon (medulla).
    4. Three bends develop.
      a. Midbrain flexure (divides cerebrum from cerebellum).
      b. Pontine flexure.
      c. Cervical flexure (divides medulla from spinal cord).
  D. Disjunction of cutaneous, neural ectoderm.
    1. After neural tube closes, superficial ectoderm separates from underlying neural ectoderm and then closes over it.
    2. Mesenchyme migrates dorsally between neural tube and skin.
  E. Diverticulation and cleavage.
    1. Forebrain development.
      a. Telencephalon develops bilateral outpouchings or cerebral vesicles that will form the future lateral ventricles.
      b. Outpouchings expand in all directions, covering diencephalon.
    2. Midbrain (mesencephalon) formation.

      a. Neural canal narrows, forming cerebral aqueduct.

      b. Neuroblasts from midbrain alar plate form tectum, colliculi.

      c. Basal plate neuroblasts form tegmentum.

   3. Hindbrain (rhombencephalon) formation.

      a. Rostral segment (metencephalon) gives rise to pons, cerebellum.

      b. Caudal segment (myelencephalon) becomes medulla.

 F. Neuronal proliferation, differentiation, histogenesis (2 to 4 months).

   1. Cellular layers in walls of the developing cerebral vesicles form the germinal matrix (7 weeks' gestation).

   2. Neuronal, glial precursors proliferate in the germinal zones (process begins at approximately 7 weeks' gestation, involutes around 28 to 30 weeks).

   3. Choroid plexus is formed; CSF production begins.

 G. Cellular migration and sulcation (2 to 5 months).

   1. Peripheral migration of developing neurons along radial glial fibers forms cerebral cortex.

   2. Cortical layers form from "inside out" (deep to superficial).

   3. Gyri, sulci form.

   4. Commissural fibers (e.g., corpus callosum) develop between approximately 8 and 17 gestational weeks.

 H. Myelination, maturation (6 gestational months to adulthood).

   1. Oligodendrocytes produce myelin.

   2. Peak myelin formation occurs from 30 weeks' gestational age to 8 months postnatal.

   3. In general, myelination progresses from:

      a. Caudad to cephalad.

      b. Dorsal to ventral.

      c. Central to peripheral.

   4. In general, sensory tracts myelinate earlier than motor tracts.

II. Abnormal development.

 A. One third of all major fetal anomalies involve the CNS.

 B. Interaction between genetic, environmental factors.

   1. Inheritance (recessive or dominant) accounts for 20%.

   2. Spontaneous chromosomal mutations may account for up to 10% of CNS malformations.

   3. Intrauterine environmental factors (e.g., infection) cause approximately 10%.

   4. No causal factor is identified in 60%.

 C. Simplified classification of brain malformations corresponds to major developmental stages of neuroembryology.

   1. Disorders of organogenesis.

     a. Neural tube closure disorders.
     b. Disorders of diverticulation/cleavage.
     c. Disorders of sulcation/cellular migration.
  2. Disorders of histogenesis (i.e., the neurocutaneous syndromes).
  3. Disorders of cytogenesis (congenital neoplasms).

SUGGESTED READINGS

Barkovich AJ: Normal development of the neonatal and infant brain, skull, and spine. In *Pediatric neuroimaging,* ed 2, New York, 1995, Raven Press, pp 9-54.

Osborn AG: Normal brain development and general classification of congenital malformations. In *Diagnostic neuroradiology,* St Louis, 1994, Mosby, pp 3-14.

11

Neural Tube Disorders and the Chiari Malformations

Key Concepts

1. Neural tube closure disorders are early developmental abnormalities, occurring at 3 to 4 gestational weeks.
2. Chiari II malformation arises from a defect in neural tube closure.
3. Chiari II malformation and myelomeningocele almost invariably occur together.
4. Myelomeningocele, Chiari II malformation, and lacunar skull do not cause each other; they merely develop in concert.

Neural tube defects are among the most common congenital fetal anomalies, with a prevalence in the United States of approximately 0.5 to 2 per 1000 live births. If the neural tube fails to close properly, a spectrum of abnormalities may result. Anencephaly and spina bifida account for most of these defects. One of the most complex of these anomalies encountered in radiologic practice is the Chiari II malformation. Other CNS anomalies that may arise from defects in neural tube closure include the congenital cephaloceles (see Chapter 12).

Congenital hindbrain anomalies in which cerebellar tissue is displaced into the cervical canal are called the "Chiari malformations" (named after the German pathologist, Hans Chiari, who described three of these cases in 1891). They are grouped together, although they are embryologically unrelated (Table 11-1).

I. Chiari I Malformation. This malformation, also called congenital cerebellar tonsillar ectopia, has *no* relationship to the Chiari II malformation; it is *not* associated with myelomeningocele.
   A. Pathology (Fig. 11-1).
      1. Elongated, peglike tonsils displaced caudally through foramen magnum (≥5 mm).
         a. About two thirds are at C1 level.
         b. One quarter are at C2.
         c. Occasionally extend below C3.
         d. Tonsils may be asymmetric in position.
      2. Osseous anomalies in 25%.
         a. Craniovertebral junction malformations with basilar invagination (25% to 50%), atlantooccipital assimilation (1% to 5%).
         b. Klippel-Feil (5% to 10%).
         c. Cervical spina bifida occulta (5%).
         d. *No spinal dysraphism.*
      3. Hydromyelia (accumulation of CSF in enlarged central canal of spinal cord, usually the cervical segment) in 20% to 75%.
      4. Nonspecific hydrocephalus in 20% to 50% (fourth ventricle is normal in position).
      5. Other than tonsillar ectopia and mild/moderate hydrocephalus, *brain abnormalities are not a feature of Chiari I malformation.*
   B. Clinical presentation.
      1. May be asymptomatic (herniation usually <5 mm) or cause nonspecific symptoms (headache, cervical pain).
      2. Central cord syndrome (e.g., sensory loss) in 50% to 65% with syringohydromyelia.
      3. Foramen magnum compression (e.g., ataxia, corticospinal tract, and cranial nerve deficits) in 20% to 25%.
      4. Cerebellar syndrome (e.g., nystagmus, truncal ataxia) in 10%.

Table 11-1   Chiari Malformations Compared

Type	Pathology
Chiari I	**Brain**
	Cerebellar tonsillar ectopia ($\geq$5 mm below foramen magnum)
	No other major anomalies (20% to 50% mild hydrocephalus)
	Spine (associated anomalies in 25%)
	No myelomeningocele
	Craniovertebral malformations (25% to 50%)
	Klippel-Feil (5% to 10%)
	Spinal cord
	Hydromyelia (20% to 75%)
Chiari II	Skull and dura
	Lacunar skull
	Small posterior fossa
	Low-lying torcular, transverse sinuses
	Fenestrated falx
	Heart-shaped incisura
	Gaping foramen magnum
	Concave clivus, petrous temporal bones
	Brain
	Inferiorly displaced vermis (nodulus), choroid plexus
	Medullary spur, kink
	Tectal beaking
	"Creeping" cerebellum, "towering" vermis
	Gyral anomalies (stenogyria, interdigitating gyri)
	Callosal dysgenesis
	Ventricles
	Hydrocephalus (uncommon at birth but eventually develops in >90%)
	Elongated fourth ventricle
	Large massa intermedia in third ventricle
	Enlarged occipital horns of lateral ventricles ("colpocephaly")
	Spine, spinal cord
	Myelomeningocele (essentially 100%)
	Syringohydromyelia (50% to 90%)
	Diastematomyelia
Chiari III	Brain
	Variable features of Chiari II
	Hindbrain herniation into cephalocele
	Spine
	Low occipital/high cervical cephalocele
Chiari IV	Brain
	Severe cerebellar hypoplasia
	Small brainstem
	Large cisterna magna
	Spine
	No associated abnormalities

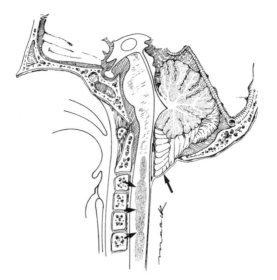

Fig. 11-1 Anatomic diagram depicts essential features of the Chiari I malformation. Pointed, low-lying tonsils are seen (large black arrow). Syringohydromyelia is indicated by the small black arrows. (From Osborn AG: *Diagnostic neuroradiology,* St Louis, 1994, Mosby.)

C. Imaging findings (best depicted on sagittal T1-weighted or high-resolution T2-weighted FSE MR scans).
1. Tonsils elongated, pointed ("peglike"), with folia and sulci angled inferiorly.
2. Tonsils >5 mm below foramen magnum. (Tonsillar herniation of 6 mm should not be considered pathologic in patients between 5 and 15 years of age.)
3. Osseous anomalies (see above).
4. Hydromyelia (intramedullary CSF collection that may be focal or involve entire cervical cord; may be collapsed, or cord may be grossly expanded).
5. Cine-mode phase-contrast velocity MRI may disclose abnormal CSF dynamics (e.g., absence of vallecula flow, decreased CSF velocity, shorter periods of caudal CSF flow at foramen magnum) or increased tonsillar velocities.
D. Miscellaneous: An "acquired" Chiari I malformation has been reported after multiple lumbar punctures and spinal shunting. Intracranial hypotension (spontaneous or iatrogenic) may cause descending tonsillar herniation; occasionally meningeal thickening and abnormal enhancement is identified on MR scans.

II. Chiari II malformation. This malformation is a complex anomaly that may affect the skull, dura, brain, spine, and spinal cord.
  A. Etiology (theoretic).
    1. Fetal neural tube fails to close.
    2. CSF leaks through dehiscent tube.
    3. Primitive ventricular system decompresses.
    4. Fourth ventricle is not adequately distended.
    5. Fourth ventricle collapse alters the normal inductive effect on surrounding mesenchyme.
    6. Enchondral bone formation is adversely affected.
    7. An abnormally small posterior fossa is formed.
    8. Development of the hindbrain within the abnormally small posterior fossa results in herniation of cerebellum, brainstem upwards through dysplastic tentorium, inferiorly through gaping foramen magnum into upper cervical canal.
  B. Clinical.
    1. Open spina bifida in nearly all cases.
    2. Obstetric sonography detects many cases.
    3. Amniocentesis with alpha-fetoprotein screening, karyotype analysis may be useful in some cases.
  C. Pathology and imaging (Fig. 11-2).
    1. Findings are variable; no single case manifests all potential abnormalities seen in Chiari II malformation.
    2. Skull and dura.
      a. Lacunar skull (craniolacunae or luckenschadel skull). Focal thinning causes "scooped-out" appearance of calvarium; changes diminish with age and are *not* caused by hydrocephalus.
      b. Small posterior fossa.
      c. Low-lying venous confluence, transverse sinuses.
      d. Fenestrated falx cerebri.
      e. Hypoplastic tentorium, heart-shaped incisura.
      f. "Gaping" foramen magnum.
      g. Concave clivus, petrous temporal bones.
    3. Cerebellum, hindbrain (some abnormalities of these structures are always present in Chiari II malformation).
      a. Medulla, vermis (usually nodulus, uvula) herniate inferiorly into upper cervical canal.
      b. "Cascade" of herniated tissue drapes inferiorly over cervical spinal cord.
      c. Cerebellum, vermis herniate superiorly, "towering" upwards through widened, gaping incisura.

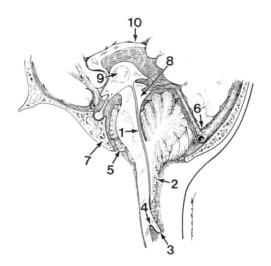

Fig. 11-2 Anatomic diagram depicts key features of the Chiari II malformation. (From Osborn AG: *Diagnostic neuroradiology,* St Louis, 1994, Mosby.)

1. Elongated, tubelike fourth ventricle
2. "Cascade" of inferiorly displaced vermis (nodulus), choroid plexus
3. Medullary "spur"
4. Medullary "kink"
5. Cerebellar hemispheres "creep" anteriorly around brainstem
6. Low-lying torcular herophili, transverse sinuses
7. Concave clivus
8. "Beaked" tectum
9. Large massa intermedia
10. Partial callosal agenesis

      d. Cerebellar hemispheres "creep" anteromedially around brainstem.

   4. Midbrain.

      a. "Beaked" or pointed tectum (deformity probably caused by mass effect from superiorly displaced cerebellum).

   5. Cerebral hemispheres.

      a. Callosal absence, dysgenesis common.

      b. Prominent, enlarged massa intermedia.

      c. Gyral abnormalities are common.

         (1) Stenogyria (short narrow gyri).

         (2) Interdigitated midline gyri.

         (3) Polymicrogyria.

      d. Sulcation, migration anomalies (e.g., heterotopic gray matter) common.

6. Cerebrospinal fluid spaces (abnormal in >90%).
    a. Hydrocephalus in >90%.
    b. Inferiorly displaced, elongated, tubelike fourth ventricle.
    c. If corpus callosum is absent, third ventricle may be high-riding.
    d. Enlarged occipital horns of lateral ventricles (colpocephaly).
    e. After shunting, walls of lateral ventricles often appear scalloped, pointed, and angulated.
    f. Hypoplastic/fenestrated falx, interdigitating gyri may cause "serrated" appearance of interhemispheric fissure.
    g. Small/inapparent cisterna magna.
7. Spine and spinal cord (abnormalities are a constant in Chiari II).
    a. Dorsally dysraphic spine (usually lumbar).
    b. Myelomeningocele (virtually 100% of cases).
    c. Syringohydromyelia (50% to 90%).
    d. Diastematomyelia (5% to 10%).
    e. Incomplete C1 ring (50%).
    f. Segmentation anomalies (<10%).

III. Chiari III malformation.
    A. Pathology and imaging.
        1. Variable features of Chiari II malformation.
        2. Low occipital or high cervical cephalocele.
        3. Herniation of dysplastic, gliotic brain, sometimes ventricles into cephalocele.

IV. Chiari IV malformation (etiologically unrelated to the other Chiari malformations).
    A. Pathology, imaging.
        1. Absent/severely hypoplastic cerebellum and vermis.
        2. Small brainstem.
        3. Large posterior fossa CSF spaces (posterior fossa is normal-sized).
        4. No hydrocephalus, other CNS anomalies.

SUGGESTED READINGS

Babcook CJ, Goldstein RB, Barth RA, et al: Prevalence of ventriculomegaly in association with myelomeningocele: correlation with gestational age and severity of posterior fossa deformity, *Radiol* 190:703-707, 1994.

Babcook CJ, Goldstein RB, Filly RA: Prenatally detected fetal myelomeningocele: is karyotype analysis warranted? *Radiol* 194:491-494, 1995.

Ball WS Jr, Crone KR: Chiari I malformation: from Dr. Chiari to MR imaging, *Radiol* 195:602-604, 1995.

Bhadelia RA, Bogdan AR, Wolpert SM, et al: Cerebrospinal fluid flow waveforms: analysis in patients with Chiari I malformation by means of gated phase-contrast

MR imaging velocity measurements, *Radiol* 196:195-202, 1995.

Castillo M, Quencer RM, Dominguez R: Chiari III malformation: imaging features, *AJNR* 13: 107-113, 1992.

Filly RA, Callen PW, Goldstein RB: Alpha-fetoprotein screening programs: what every obstetric sonologist should know, *Radiol* 188:1-9, 1993.

Huang PP, Constantini S: "Acquired" Chiari I malformation, *J Neurosurg* 80: 1099-1102, 1994.

McLone DG, Naidich TP: Developmental morphology of the subarachnoid space, brain vasculature, and contiguous structures, and the cause of the Chiari II malformation, *AJNR* 13:463-482, 1992.

Osborn AG: Disorders of neural tube closure. In *Diagnostic neuroradiology*, St Louis, 1994, Mosby-Year Book.

Wolpert SM, Bhadelia RA, Bogdan AR, Cohen AR: Chiari I malformations: assessment with phase-contrast velocity MR, *AJNR* 15:1299-1308, 1994.

12

Cephaloceles and Corpus Callosum Anomalies

Key Concepts

1. Cephaloceles are protrusions of intracranial structures through a skull defect. They may contain meninges, cerebrospinal fluid, brain, or a combination.
2. Corpus callosum anomalies occur between 8 and 20 weeks of gestational age.
3. Callosal anomalies are the most common malformation associated with other CNS anomalies.
4. Lipomas are brain malformations, not true neoplasms.
5. Nearly half of all intracranial lipomas occur in the midline and are commonly associated with callosal dysgenesis.

Cephaloceles are caused by defects in neural tube closure during early embryologic development. Congenital cephaloceles have a prevalence of approximately 1 to 3 per 10,000 live births. The type and location of cephaloceles vary with geographic region. For example, occipital cephaloceles are the most common cephaloceles in white North Americans and Europeans, whereas frontoethmoidal lesions are more common in Southeast Asians.

Anomalies of the corpus callosum are the most common anomalies that accompany other brain malformations.

I. Cephaloceles. By definition, a skull defect plus herniated intracranial contents is termed a *cephalocele*. A *meningocele* contains only meninges and CSF. If the defect contains leptomeninges, CSF, and brain, it is termed a *meningoencephalocele*.
   A. Occipital cephalocele.
      1. Pathology: Variable but cephalocele usually contains dysplastic, gliotic cerebellum.
      2. Clinical.
         a. Accounts for 80% to 90% of cephaloceles in white North Americans, Europeans.
         b. Female predominance.
      3. Imaging.
         a. Skull defect plus meninges, brain (may contain dural venous sinuses, distorted ventricles).
         b. Association with neural tube defects (Chiari II, III) and other anomalies such as Dandy-Walker malformation, cerebellar dysplasias, and neuronal migration anomalies.
   B. Parietal cephalocele.
      1. Pathology: variable.
      2. Clinical.
         a. Represents 10% to 15% of cephaloceles in white North Americans, Europeans.
         b. Male predominance.
      3. Imaging.
         a. Skull defect between lambda, bregma.
         b. Variable contents.
         c. Association with midline malformations (absent/dysplastic corpus callosum, Dandy-Walker malformation, holoprosencephalies).
         d. "Atretic cephalocele" is a small, hairless midline mass near the vertex; most atretic parietal cephaloceles are associated with other midline anomalies, whereas atretic occipital cephaloceles have a low incidence of associated malformations.

C. Anterior cephaloceles and other congenital midline nasal masses.
1. Embryology: Frontonasal diverticulum that normally connects ectoderm of developing nose with brain fails to regress.
2. Pathology: varies from dermal sinus tract to cephaloceles.
    a. Dermal sinus: skin dimple over dorsum of nose; occurs with or without hair-containing fistula and a cephalad sinus tract that extends a variable distance (may pass through foramen cecum into cranial vault).
    b. Dermoid/epidermoid tumors: may develop anywhere along the sinus tract.
    c. Anterior cephalocele: formed by herniation of intracranial tissues into the patent dural projection through the foramen cecum; can be located between frontal, nasal bones ("frontoethmoidal cephalocele"), between nasal bone and nasal cartilage ("nasoethmoidal cephalocele"), or between frontal process of the maxilla and the lacrimal bone, lamina papyracea of ethmoid bone ("naso-orbital cephalocele").
    d. Nasal glioma: not a true neoplasm; is an extracranial rest of glial tissue (dysplastic brain) in nasal cavity that is separated from intracranial contents.
3. Clinical.
    a. Frontoethmoidal cephaloceles are the most common type seen in Southeast Asians, aboriginal Australians.
    b. Dermal sinuses and anterior cephaloceles may cause nasal stuffiness, recurrent meningitis.
4. Imaging.
    a. Nasal dermoid/dermal sinus: Fusiform mass of fat density in nasal septum; may have enlarged foramen cecum, bifid crista galli, broadened nasal septum if sinus tract is present.
    b. Cephaloceles.
       (1) Hypertelorism, bone defect (crista galli absent/eroded).
       (2) Nasal mass with variable contents (CSF, brain).
       (3) Associated anomalies common (craniofacial anomalies common with frontoethmoidal cephaloceles; corpus callosum anomalies, lipomas, neuronal migration anomalies common with nasofrontal cephaloceles).
D. Nasopharyngeal cephaloceles. These are rare. A base of skull defect with well-defined sclerotic margins is typical. A nasopharyngeal mass of CSF, soft tissue that may contain hypothalamus, pituitary gland, optic chiasm, third ventricle is present.
II. Corpus callosum anomalies. Because the cerebral hemispheres, cerebellum, and corpus callosum all form at about the same time, callosal hypogenesis is the most common CNS anomaly that is

associated with other developmental disorders such as Chiari II and Dandy-Walker malformations. Callosal anomalies are also part of many syndrome complexes such as Aicardi syndrome (see below).

   The most common callosal anomalies are agenesis and hypogenesis. The corpus callosum may also be completely formed but hypoplastic. Lipoma is also often associated with developmental anomalies of the corpus callosum.

A. Normal development, anatomy of the corpus callosum.
   1. Forms between 8 and 17 weeks of gestation.
      a. Forms from front to back (exception: rostrum forms last).
   2. Four segments (Fig. 12-1, *A*).
      a. Rostrum.
      b. Genu.
      c. Body.
      d. Splenium.
   3. Shape, thickness of corpus callosum is quite variable. Commissural fibers normally course side-to-side (Fig. 12-1, *B*).
B. Corpus callosum agenesis.
   1. Pathology and imaging (Fig. 12-2).
      a. Absence of corpus callosum, cingulate gyri.
      b. Gyri oriented in a radiating pattern.
      c. Third ventricle is "high-riding" and open dorsally to the interhemispheric fissure.
      d. Lateral ventricles appear parallel, nonconverging.
      e. Longitudinal white matter tracts ("Probst bundles") indent superomedial aspect of lateral ventricles.
   2. Associated CNS anomalies (present in approximately 50% of all cases).
      a. Lipoma.
      b. Cephalocele.
      c. Chiari II, Dandy-Walker malformations.
      d. Holoprosencephalies.
      e. Azygous anterior cerebral artery.
      f. Migration disorders (heterotopic gray matter).
   3. Extracranial anomalies associated with callosal agenesis.
      a. Midline facial anomalies.
      b. Ocular colobomata.
      c. Skeletal anomalies.
      d. Aicardi syndrome (callosal agenesis plus ocular abnormalities and infantile spasms).
C. Corpus callosum hypogenesis.
   1. Embryology: Because corpus callosum forms from front to back (exception: rostrum, which forms last), hypogenesis is characterized by presence of earlier-formed parts (genu, body) and

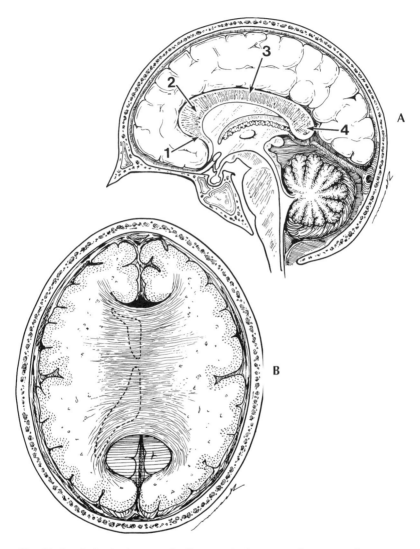

Fig. 12-1   **A,** Sagittal anatomic diagram depicts normal corpus callosum.
1. Rostrum
2. Genu
3. Body
4. Splenium

B, Axial anatomic drawing of the normal corpus callosum shows commissural fiber tracts as they course side-to-side between the white matter (centrum semiovale) of the cerebral hemispheres.

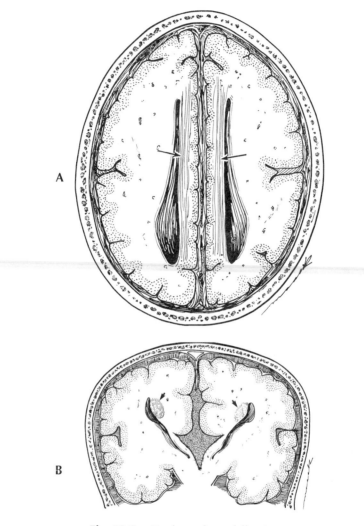

Fig. 12-2   For legend, see following page.

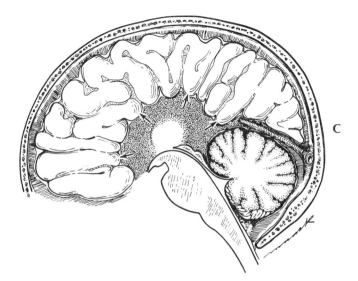

Fig. 12-2, cont'd   Axial **(A)**, coronal **(B)**, and sagittal **(C)** anatomic diagrams depict findings in complete callosal agenesis. Probst bundles (longitudinally oriented white matter tracts) are shown (A,B, arrows). Note "spoke-wheel" arrangement of gyri (C, arrows) around the high-riding third ventricle. The third ventricle is open dorsally and is contiguous with the interhemispheric fissure.

absence of later-formed segments (splenium, rostrum). Exception: holoprosencephaly (see Chapter 13).
2. Pathology and imaging: Genu and part of body are present; splenium and rostrum are absent.
3. Associated anomalies: usually none.
D. Corpus callosum lipoma.
1. Embryology: Brain malformation (not a true neoplasm), probably caused by persistence of meninx primitiva (mesenchymal neural crest derivative).
2. Pathology: nonneoplastic fatty tissue.
3. Imaging.
   a. Fat density/signal mass along interhemispheric fissure; may extend through choroidal fissure into lateral ventricles.
   b. Variable calcification (curvilinear, nodular).
   c. Two general types.
      (1) "Tubulonodular" lipoma: Bulky, lobulated mass usually seen with complete agenesis (Fig. 12-3).
      (2) "Curvilinear" lipoma: thin lesion that curves around splenium; callosal dysgenesis is mild or absent.
   d. Warning: Blood vessels may course directly through lipoma!

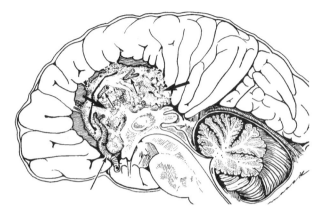

Fig. 12-3 Anatomic diagram, lateral view, shows interhemispheric lipoma (large arrows) with complete callosal agenesis. Note the anterior cerebral artery courses *through* the lipoma (small arrows).

SUGGESTED READINGS

Barkovich AJ: Congenital malformations of the brain and skull. In *Pediatric neuroimaging,* ed 2, New York, 1995, Raven Press, pp 177-275.

Bernardi B, Fonda C: Cefaloceli, *Riv di Neuroradiol* 7:171-186, 1994.

Castillo M: Congenital abnormalities of the nose: CT and MR findings, *AJR* 162:1211-1217, 1994.

Ferrario VF, Sforza C, Serrao G, et al: Shape of the human corpus callosum, *Invest Radiol* 29:677-681, 1994.

Fujii Y, Konishi Y, Kuriyama M, et al: Corpus callosum in developmentally retarded infants, *Pediatr Neurol* 11:219-223, 1994.

Gabrielli O, Salvolini U, Bonifazi V, et al: Morphological studies of the corpus callosum by MRI in children with malformative syndromes, *Neuroradiol* 35:109-112, 1993.

Menezes AV, Enzenauer RW, Buncic JR: Aicardi syndrome—the elusive mild case, *Br J Ophthalmol* 78:494-496, 1994.

Naidich TP, Altman NR, Braffman BH, et al: Cephaloceles and related malformations, *AJNR* 13:655-690, 1992.

Oba H, Barkovich AJ: Holoprosencephaly: an analysis of callosal formation and its relation to development of the interhemispheric fissure, *AJNR* 16:453-460, 1995.

Osborn AG: Disorders of neural tube closure. In *Diagnostic neuroradiology,* St Louis, 1994, Mosby.

Rubinstein D, Youngman V, Hise JH, Damiano TR: Partial development of the corpus callosum, *AJNR* 15:869-875, 1994.

13

Holoprosencephaly

Key Concepts

1. Holoprosencephalies form a spectrum from most (alobar) to least (lobar) severe.
2. Craniofacial anomalies such as cyclops and cleft palate are common in the more severe forms of holoprosencephaly.
3. The falx cerebri and interhemispheric fissure are absent in alobar holoprosencephaly.
4. Corpus callosum anomalies occur in holoprosencephaly but are atypical; the *posterior* portion of the corpus callosum is formed, whereas the *anterior* segment is absent.

If the prosencephalon (forebrain) fails to cleave and differentiate properly during early fetal development, the result is the congenital malformation termed holoprosencephaly. In holoprosencephaly there is failure of both lateral cleavage (into distinct cerebral hemispheres) and transverse cleavage (into diencephalon and telencephalon).

Holoprosencephaly occurs in 1 in 16,000 live births. It is associated with several chromosomal abnormalities, including trisomy 13 (Patau syndrome).

Holoprosencephaly affects the rostral basal regions of the brain most severely. Holoprosencephaly is classically divided into three types by the degree of brain cleavage, although these disorders actually form a continuum with no distinct division between the different types. From most to least severe these three types are:

1. Alobar holoprosencephaly.
2. Semilobar holoprosencephaly.
3. Lobar holoprosencephaly.

Some authors also include two less severe anomalies, septooptic dysplasia and arrhinencephaly, in the holoprosencephaly spectrum. (See Table 13-1.)

I. Holoprosencephaly.
  A. Alobar holoprosencephaly.
    1. Pathology and imaging (Fig. 13-1).
      a. Brain is a primitive-appearing unsegmented "holosphere" (no division into hemispheres or lobes).
      b. Single primitive horseshoe-shaped central monoventricle.
      c. Fused thalami, basal ganglia.
      d. No falx cerebri, interhemispheric fissure.
      e. Large dorsal cyst common.
    2. Associated anomalies ("the face predicts the brain").
      a. Severe midline craniofacial defects (e.g., cyclops, midline proboscis).
      b. Hypotelorism.

Table 13-1   Holoprosencephalies Compared

Pathology	Alobar	Semilobar	Lobar
Facial anomalies	Severe	Mild	None
Ventricles	Monoventricle	Rudimentary	Boxlike frontal horns
Septum pellucidum	Absent	Absent	Absent
Falx cerebri	None	Partial	Formed
Interhemispheric fissure	None	Partial	Present
Thalami	Fused	Partial separation	Separated

       c. Azygous anterior cerebral artery.

       d. Midline venous structures often absent.

       e. Trisomy 13, 18 syndromes.

  B. Semilobar holoprosencephaly.

    1. Pathology and imaging.

       a. Intermediate in severity.

       b. Brain is partially diverticulated with formation of rudimentary lobes.

       c. Minimal differentiation of ventricles with rudimentary occipital, temporal horns present; absent septum pellucidum.

       d. Incompletely formed interhemispheric fissure, rudimentary falx (usually posterior) are present.

       e. Thalami, basal ganglia may be partially separated.

    2. Associated anomalies.

       a. Less severe craniofacial defects (cleft lip, cleft palate).

       b. Hypotelorism.

       c. Semilobar holoprosencephaly may occur with middle interhemispheric fusion (here the corpus callosum genu, splenium are present but the body is absent).

       d. Corpus callosum spleniuim may be present and genu, anterior body, and rostrum absent (holoprosencephaly is the sole

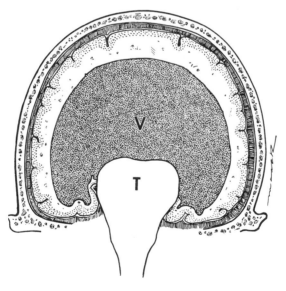

Fig. 13-1   Coronal anatomic diagram depicts alobar holoprosencephaly. There is virtually complete lack of cleavage. Note the undifferentiated central monoventricle (V) and the fused thalami (T). The interhemispheric fissure and falx are absent.

exception to the general rule that partial absence of the corpus callosum always involves the posterior structures such as splenium and body).

    e. Corpus callosum also may be absent or severely dysgenetic; in some cases, the hippocampal commissure is prominent, giving a "splenium-like" appearance.

    f. Azygous anterior cerebral artery.

C. Lobar holoprosencephaly.

  1. Pathology and imaging.

    a. Brain cleavage is nearly complete.

    b. Ventricles, lobes are well formed.

    c. Septum pellucidum is absent (giving the frontal horns of the lateral ventricles a "squared-off" appearance).

    d. Interhemispheric fissure, falx cerebri present.

    e. Some brain fusion, usually involving the inferior frontal lobes, is still present.

  2. Associated anomalies.

    a. Facies usually normal.

    b. Mild hypotelorism may be present.

    c. Hypoplastic optic vesicles, absence of olfactory bulbs common.

    d. Hypothalamic-pituitary axis dysfunction.

II. Related anomalies.

A. Septooptic dysplasia (also known as de Morsier syndrome).

  1. Pathology and imaging.

    a. Absence or dysgenesis of septum pellucidum gives undivided frontal horns a boxlike appearance.

    b. Hypoplastic optic nerves.

  2. Associated anomalies.

    a. Two subsets identified.

      (1) Schizencephaly, gray matter heterotopias, hypothalamic-pituitary dysfunction.

      (2) Hypoplastic white matter with ventriculomegaly, normal cortex.

    b. Septooptic dysplasia may occur with other brain anomalies such as Chiari II malformation, aqueductal stenosis.

B. Arrhinencephaly.

  1. Pathology and imaging.

    a. Absence of olfactory bulbs, tracts.

  2. Associated anomalies.

    a. Holoprosencephaly.

    b. Kallmann syndrome (anosmia, hypogonadism, mental retardation).

SUGGESTED READINGS

Barkovich AJ, Quint DJ: Middle interhemispheric fusion: An unusual variant of holoprosencephaly, *AJNR* 14:431-440, 1993.

Castillo M, Bouldin TW, Scatliff JH, Suzuki K: Alobar holoprosencephaly, *AJNR* 14:1151-1156, 1993.

Lehman CD, Nyberg DA, Winter TC III, et al: Trisomy 13 syndrome: prenatal US findings in a review of 33 cases, *Radiol* 194:217-222, 1995.

Oba H, Barkovich AJ: Holoprosencephaly: an analysis of callosal formation and its relation to development of the interhemispheric fissure, *AJNR* 16:453-460, 1995.

Triulzi F: Anomalie della linea mediana, *Riv di Neuroradiol* 7:187-198, 1994.

14

Sulcation and Cellular Migration Disorders

Key Concepts

1. Lissencephaly ("smooth brain") has a thick cortex with shallow sylvian fissures, few sulci, and broad, flat gyri.
2. Schizencephaly ("split brain") is a gray matter–lined cleft that extends from the ventriclar ependyma to the pia.
3. Gray matter heterotopias can be focal or diffuse with a nodular, laminar, or masslike appearance.

The subependymal germinal matrix appears during the seventh gestational week. Neurons are formed in the germinal zone, then subsequently migrate outwards along radial glial fibers to form the cerebral cortex. Disruption of normal neuronal migration or cortical organization causes a spectrum of disorders depending on timing and severity of the insult.

I. Sulcation disorders.
  A. Lissencephaly ("smooth brain").
    1. Pathology: Lissencephaly can be complete (agyria) or incomplete (pachygyria).
    2. Imaging.
      a. Smooth agyric brain (resembles normal fetal brain at 23 to 24 gestational weeks).
      b. Shallow sylvian fissures ("figure-of-eight" appearance).
      c. Thick cortex (in pachygyria, a few broad, flat gyri are present).
      d. Smooth gray-white matter interface.
    3. Associated abnormalities.
      a. Miller-Dieker syndrome (characteristic facies, spasticity).
      b. Walker-Warburg syndrome (ocular malformations, hypomyelination, cephaloceles, severe hypotonia).
      c. Fukuyama's syndrome (congenital muscular dystrophy with diffuse cortical dysplasia).
II. Migration abnormalities. If neuronal migration along the radial glial fibers is arrested, gray matter heterotopias are the result. Migration abnormalities thus represent ectopic collections of otherwise normal neurons in abnormal locations.
  A. Heterotopias.
    1. Laminar ("band") heterotopia (Fig. 14-1).
      a. Etiology and pathology.
        (1) Diffuse arrest of neuronal migration.
        (2) One or more layers of neurons are interposed between the ventricle and cortex.
      b. Clinical.
        (1) Clinical course can be related to severity of imaging findings.
        (2) Seizure onset correlated with severity of pachygyria, thickness of heterotopic band.
        (3) Development, intelligence correlate with ventricular enlargement.
      c. Imaging.
        (1) Layered, laminated appearance caused by alternating bands of gray, white matter ("double cortex" appearance).

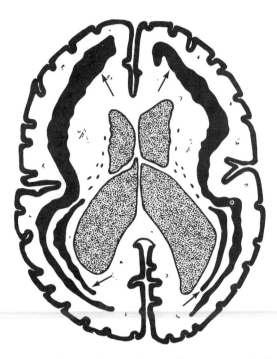

Fig. 14-1 Anatomic diagram depicts laminar heterotopia. The bandlike layers of heterotopic gray matter are shown here as dark areas (arrows) within the hemispheric white matter. Note thinning of the overlying cortical gray matter.

        (2) Gray, white matter are normal signal.
        (3) Overlying cortex is often thinned, may be dysplastic.
    d. Associated abnormalities.
        (1) Lissencephaly (may be a mild form of laminar hetero-
           topia).
  2. Nodular heterotopias.
    a. Pathology and imaging.
        (1) Subependymal (Fig. 14-2) or focal subcortical (Fig.
           14-3) collections of heterotopic gray matter.
        (2) Heterotopias are isointense with cortex, do not enhance
           following contrast administration.
    b. Differential diagnosis.
        (1) Subependymal nodules (SENs) in tuberous sclerosis
           (TS) (SENs often calcify, may enhance, and their signal
           does not precisely parallel gray matter).
        (2) Focal subcortical heterotopias may resemble tumor,
           especially on CT scans (heterotopic gray matter does not
           enhance, signal is the same as cortex).

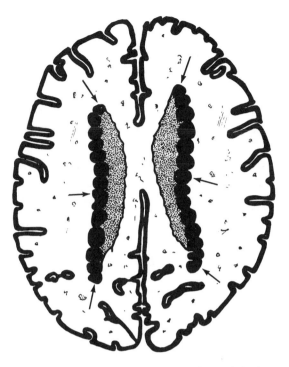

Fig. 14-2 Anatomic diagram depicts periventricular nodular heterotopia. Note the focal, rounded nodules of heterotopic gray matter, shown here as the subependymal dark areas (arrows).

  B. Schizencephaly ("split brain").
     1. Etiology: may represent arrest of a column of migrating neurons.
     2. Pathology (Fig. 14-4).
       a. Cerebrospinal fluid cleft extends from ventricular ependyma to pia.
       b. Cleft is lined by gray matter (usually dysplastic).
       c. Can be unilateral or bilateral, symmetric or asymmetric.
       d. Cleft can be open or closed.
     3. Imaging.
       a. CSF cleft ("pial-ependymal seam").
       b. Slight outpouching ("nipple") of CSF from ventricle.
       c. Dysplastic, heterotopic gray matter lines cleft.
       d. In "open-lip" schizencephaly, the cleft walls are separated, and the skull may be expanded over the opening (especially if the cleft is large).
     4. Associated abnormalities.

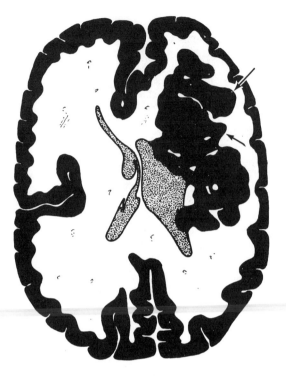

Fig. 14-3 Anatomic diagram depicts subcortical focal heterotopias (arrows). The mass of heterotopic gray matter may superficially resemble a neoplasm, but the signal intensity on MR scans is similar to cortex. Note adjacent malformed lateral ventricle.

        a. Septum pellucidum is absent in 80% to 90% of cases.
        b. Optic nerve hypoplasia occurs in up to one third of cases.
        c. Other foci of heterotopic or dysplastic gray matter are common.
   C. Unilateral megalencephaly ("hemimegalencephaly").
     1. Pathology.
        a. Hamartomatous overgrowth of part or all of one cerebral hemisphere.
        b. Localized neuronal migrational anomalies.
     2. Imaging.
        a. Affected hemisphere is enlarged.
        b. Ipsilateral ventricle often enlarged.
        c. White matter can be hypoplastic or hyperplastic, gliotic.
        d. Dysplastic cortex (may be thickened, calcified, abnormally sulcated).
        e. Heterotopic gray matter often present.

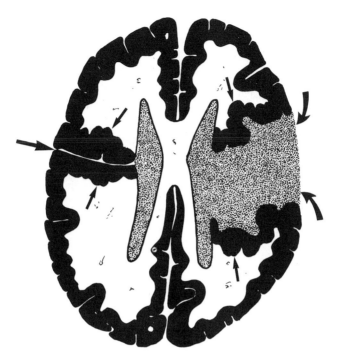

Fig. 14-4   Anatomic diagram depicts schizencephaly. On the left, a closed-lip schizencephaly is shown. Note the pial-ependymal "seam" (large arrow) is lined with heterotopic gray matter (small arrows). On the right, an open-lip schizencephaly (curved arrows) is depicted. Heterotopic gray matter (small arrows) lines the wide cleft.

   3. Associated abnormalities.
    a. Linear sebaceous nevus syndrome.
    b. Hypomelanosis of Ito.
 III. Abnormalities of neuronal organization. In this group of disorders, neurons migrate normally, but their cortical organization is deranged.
  A. Nonlissencephalic cortical dysplasias. These anomalies are also classified as "polymicrogyria/pachygyria complex."
   1. Pathology and imaging.
    a. Focal or diffusely thickened cortex.
    b. Irregular, "bumpy" gyral pattern.
    c. Relative paucity of underlying white matter (may be gliotic).
    d. Calcification may occur, can indicate intrauterine infection (e.g., cytomegalovirus).
    e. In utero ischemic injury may cause polymicrogyria.
   2. Associated abnormalities.
    a. Partial CSF cleft.
    b. Anomalous venous drainage.

SUGGESTED READINGS

Barkovich AJ: Congenital malformations. In *Pediatric Neuroradiology,* ed 2, New York, 1995, Raven Press.

Barkovich AJ, Chuang SH: Unilateral megalencephaly, *AJNR* 11:523-531,1990.

Barkovich AJ, Guerrini R, Battaglia G, et al: Band heterotopias: correlation of outcome with magnetic resonance imaging parameters, *Ann Neurol* 36:609-617, 1994.

Barkovich AJ, Kjos BO: Schizencephaly: Correlation of clinical findings with MR characteristics, *AJNR* 13:85-94, 1992.

Barkovich AJ, Rowley H, Bollen A: Correlation of prenatal events with the development of polymicrogyria, *AJNR* 16:822-827, 1995.

Canapicchi R, Guerrini R: Malformazioni della corteccia cerebrale, *Riv di Neuroradiol* 7:209-219, 1994.

Ferrie CD, Jackson GD, Giannakodimos S, Panayiotopoulos CP: Posterior agyria-pachygyria with polymicrogyria, *Neurol* 45:150-153, 1995.

Huttenlocher PR, Taravath S, Mojtahedi S: Periventricular heterotopia and epilepsy, *Neurol* 44:51-55, 1994.

Osborn AG: Disorders of diverticulation and cleavage, sulcation and cellular migration. In *Diagnostic neuroradiology,* St Louis, 1994, Mosby, pp 37-58.

Sébire G, Goutières F, Tardieu M, et al: Extensive macrogyri or no visible gyri: distinct clinical, electroencephalographic, and genetic features according to different imaging patterns, *Neurol* 45:1105-1111, 1995.

15

Dandy-Walker Complex and Miscellaneous Posterior Fossa Malformations

---

Key Concepts

1. Dandy-Walker complex represents a spectrum of posterior fossa cystic malformations.
2. Classic triad of findings in D-W malformation.
   a. Complete or partial vermian agenesis.
   b. Cystic dilatation of fourth ventricle.
   c. Enlarged posterior fossa with elevated torcular Herophili.
3. Findings in vermian-cerebellar hypoplasia ("Dandy-Walker variant") include:
   a. Varying degrees of vermian, cerebellar hypoplasia.
   b. Normal-sized posterior fossa.
   c. Prominent retrocerebellar CSF space that communicates freely with fourth ventricle.
   d. Fourth ventricle is normal or minimally dilated.
4. In mega cisterna magna, the cisterna magna is enlarged and communicates freely with the perimedullary subarachnoid space. The fourth ventricle, vermis, and cerebellar hemispheres are normally formed.
5. Midline posterior fossa arachnoid cysts are retrocerebellar CSF collections that do not communicate with the fourth ventricle and perimedullary subarachnoid spaces. They are not associated with cerebellar dysgenesis.

Posterior fossa malformations and cysts represent a spectrum of unrelated developmental anomalies (Table 15-1). The Chiari malformations were discussed in the chapter on neural tube closure abnormalities. In this chapter we discuss miscellaneous posterior fossa anomalies such as the Dandy-Walker (D-W) malformation as well as other entities (such as mega cisterna magna and posterior fossa arachnoid cyst) that can sometimes be confused with D-W. Finally, we also briefly delineate miscellaneous unrelated cerebellar malformations that are occasionally encountered in clinical practice. ·

I. Dandy-Walker complex. This spectrum of disorders includes the classic D-W malformation as well as the so-called Dandy-Walker "variant" and "mega cisterna magna." Because it is often difficult to distinguish these entities, some authors suggest using the term "Dandy Walker complex" (DWC) for all cases.

A. Dandy-Walker malformation (DWM).
   1. Etiology (unknown).
      a. May be caused by insult to both developing fourth ventricle, cerebellum.
      b. May be caused by delayed/absent opening of the foramen of Magendie.
   2. Prevalence and inheritance.
      a. One per 25,000 to 30,000 live births.
      b. Seems to occur as isolated malformation without definite evidence for inheritance.
   3. Clinical.
      a. Diagnosed by age 1 year in 80%.
      b. Most common presentation is hydrocephalus (>80%).
      c. Older children may have symptoms that mimic posterior fossa neoplasm (ataxia, nystagmus, cranial nerve palsies).
   4. Pathology and imaging (Fig. 15-1 on p. 157).
      a. Enlarged posterior fossa with upward displacement of torcular, transverse sinuses, tentorium (torcular-lambdoidal suture inversion).
      b. Cystic dilatation of fourth ventricle.
      c. Varying vermian, cerebellar hypoplasia.
      d. Vermian remnant is displaced anterosuperiorly over the cyst.
      e. Cerebellar hemispheres "winged" outwards.
   5. Associated abnormalities.
      a. Hydrocephalus develops in 75% to 90%.
      b. Corpus callosum dysgenesis in one third.
      c. Neuronal migration anomalies in 5% to 10%.
      d. Cephaloceles (usually occipital) in up to 16%.
      e. Brainstem may be hypoplastic.

Table 15-1   Differential Diagnosis of Posterior Cysts and Cystlike Masses*

Finding	Dandy-Walker Malformation	Dandy-Walker Variant	Mega Cisterna Magna	Posterior Fossa Arachnoid Cyst
Location	Occupies most of posterior fossa	Midline posterior	Midline, posterior; typically minimal/absent extension in front of cerebellopontine angle	Posterior midline; cerebellopontine angle
Fourth ventricle	Floor present; open dorsally to large cyst	"Keyhole" appearance	Normal	Normal but displaced
Vermis	Absent/hypoplastic; everted over cyst	Inferior lobules hypoplastic, otherwise normal	Normal	Normal but distorted
Obstructive hydrocephalus	Common	Absent	Absent	Variable
Enhancement after contrast	Absent	Absent	Absent	Absent
Calcification	Absent	Absent	Absent	Absent
Cyst density/signal	CSF	CSF	CSF	~CSF
Margins	Smooth	Smooth	Smooth	Smooth
Skull	Large posterior fossa; lambdoid-torcular inversion	Normal	Inner table may be scalloped	Usually normal

*From Osborn AG: *Diagnostic neuroradiology.* St Louis, 1994, Mosby.

Continued.

Table 15-1–Cont'd   Differential Diagnosis of Posterior Cysts and Cystlike Masses*

Finding	Inflammatory Cyst	Dermoid	Epidermoid Tumor	Cystic Neoplasm
Location	Any location	Midline, fourth ventricle	Cerebellopontine angle; fourth ventricle	Vermis, cerebellum
Fourth ventricle	Normally formed; may be distorted	Normal but distorted/ displaced	Normal but distorted/ displaced	Normal but displaced
Vermis	Normal	Normal but distorted	Normal but dis- torted	Normal but distorted
Obstructive hydro- cephalus	Variable	Variable	Variable	Common
Enhancement after contrast	Common	Uncommon	Unusual	Common
Calcification	Common	Common	Unusual	Common
Cyst density/signal	Often slightly hyper- dense/intense compared to CSF	Iso/hypodense on NECT; often like fat on MR	Equal or slightly higher than CSF	Often hyperdense/ hyperintense compared to CSF
Margins	Smooth	Smooth/lobulated	Irregular, frondlike	Smooth/lobulated
Skull	Normal	May have sinus tract	Normal	Normal

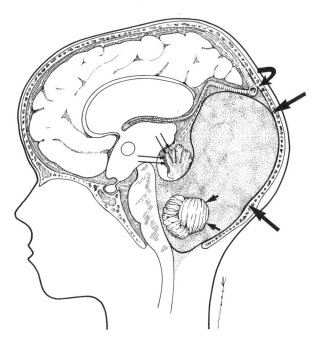

Fig. 15-1 Anatomic drawing depicting the key features of Dandy-Walker malformation is shown. A large posterior fossa cyst (large black arrows) is present. The cyst enlarges the posterior fossa, elevating the confluence of the sinuses ("torcular Herophili") (curved arrow). The vermis is hypoplastic (double arrows) and is displaced anterosuperiorly above the cyst. The cerebellar hemispheres (small black arrows) are hypoplastic. On sagittal T1-weighted MR scans they may appear to "float" within the large pool of CSF that forms the posterior fossa cyst.

    B. Dandy-Walker "variant" (also called vermian-cerebellar hypoplasia).

        1. Pathology, etiology.

           a. Milder form of D-W.

           b. May result from insult that primarily involves developing cerebral hemispheres.

           c. Variable hypoplasia of inferior vermis.

        2. Imaging.

           a. Normal-sized posterior fossa (no torcular-lambdoid inversion).

           b. Varying degrees of cerebellar, vermian hypoplasia (partial vermian hypoplasia always affects the inferior lobules).

           c. Prominent retrocerebellar CSF space communicates with normal or minimally dilated fourth ventricle through a prominent vallecula ("keyhole" appearance).

3. Associated anomalies.
   a. Hydrocephalus usually absent (hydrocephalus is present in approximately one third of cases).
   b. May have associated supratentorial abnormalities (e.g., callosal dysgenesis, heterotopias, gyral malformations).
   c. Syndromes associated with vermian-cerebellar hypoplasia include:
      (1) Joubert syndrome.
      (2) Walker-Warburg syndrome.
      (3) Cerebro-oculo-muscular syndrome.

C. Mega cisterna magna.
   1. Etiology.
      a. Now thought to represent the mildest form of D-W malformation.
      b. May result from insult primarily to developing fourth ventricle.
   2. Prevalence.
      a. Accounts for slightly more than half of cystlike posterior fossa malformations.
   3. Pathology.
      a. Cisterna magna enlarged, communicates freely with perimedullary subarachnoid space.
      b. Fourth ventricle, vermis, cerebellar hemispheres are morphologically intact.
   4. Imaging.
      a. Prominent cisterna magna (may extend laterally, superiorly, and posteriorly far beyond normal anatomic limits of cisterna magna; some cases even extend supratentorially through posterior dehiscence of the tentorium).
      b. Posterior fossa may appear either normal or enlarged with high tentorium (15%).
      c. Normal-appearing fourth ventricle, cerebellum; all vermian lobules present.
      d. Pulsatile CSF may cause prominent scalloping of occipital bone.
      e. Hydrocephalus is absent or mild (most cases are discovered incidentally at imaging).
      f. Can be asymmetric and manifest mild mass effect, mimic arachnoid cyst.

II. Miscellaneous congenital posterior fossa cysts.
   A. Posterior fossa arachnoid cyst (PFAC).
      1. Pathology.
         a. True intraarachnoid cyst.

    b. CSF-filled.
    c. Do not communicate with fourth ventricle and perimedullary subarachnoid space.
    d. Vermis, cerebellar hemispheres are morphologically intact.
  2. Prevalence.
    a. Arachnoid cysts account for 1% of all intracranial masses.
  3. Location: 20% of all intracranial arachnoid cysts are infratentorial.
    a. 10% cerebellopontine angle.
    b. 10% midline, retrovermian.
  4. Clinical.
    a. Variable hydrocephalus.
    b. Signs of mass effect (e.g., ataxia).
  5. Imaging.
    a. Parallels CSF in density or signal intensity (unless intracyst hemorrhage has occurred).
    b. Two thirds are large (>5 cm).
    c. Sharply, smoothly marginated.
    d. Nearly always unilocular; CSF density, signal intensity.
    e. No enhancement following contrast administration.
    f. Fourth ventricle and cerebellum are normally formed but may appear displaced, compressed.
  6. Differential diagnosis (Table 15-1).
    a. D-W cyst.
    b. Mega cisterna magna.
    c. Epidermoid cyst (diffusion-weighted MR may be helpful).
    d. Cystic neoplasm.
B. Enterogenous (neurenteric) cyst.
  1. Pathology, etiology.
    a. Notochord, foregut fail to separate during formation of alimentary canal.
    b. Cyst wall consists of single columnar or cuboidal epithelium, mucin-secreting goblet cells.
  2. Location.
    a. Usually intraspinal.
    b. 10% to 15% occur in posterior fossa.
    c. Cerebellopontine angle cistern, craniocervical junction (anterior to brainstem).
  3. Imaging.
    a. Well-delineated, noncalcified, nonenhancing round or lobulated mass.
    b. Attenuatation, signal vary with cyst contents (usually slightly hyperintense to CSF on MR).

III. Miscellaneous posterior fossa malformations.
  A. Chiari IV malformation.
    1. Etiology.
      a. Unknown.
      b. Related to Chiari II malformation in name only!
      c. Also termed median cerebellar hypoplasia; may be considered part of Dandy-Walker complex.
    2. Pathology, imaging.
      a. Normal-sized posterior fossa.
      b. Small brainstem.
      c. Cerebellar hemispheres, vermis absent or extremely hypoplastic.
      d. Large CSF cisterns.
  B. Joubert syndrome.
    1. Inheritance, gender.
      a. Autosomal recessive.
      b. Twice as common in males.
    2. Clinical presentation.
      a. Respiratory disturbances.
      b. Abnormal eye movements.
      c. Ataxia, facial asymmetry.
    3. Pathology, imaging.
      a. Vermis absent or hypoplastic; remnant appears disorganized (split or segmented).
      b. Superior cerebellar peduncle is horizontal.
      c. On sagittal views fourth ventricle appears upwardly convex, elongated; on axial studies has "bat-wing" shape.
      d. Cerebellar hemispheres appose in midline; if vermis is completely absent, hemispheres are separated by a narrow interhemispheric cleft that connects fourth ventricle with cisterna magna.
    4. Associated anomalies.
      a. Mental retardation.
      b. Callosal dysgenesis.
      c. Polydactyly, cystic kidney disease.
  C. Rhombencephalosynapsis.
    1. Pathology, imaging.
      a. Absent or hypoplastic vermis.
      b. Midline fusion of cerebellar hemispheres.
      c. Brainstem normal, but tectum may be fused.
    2. Associated anomalies.
      a. Absent septum pellucidum, ventriculomegaly.
      b. Thalami may be fused.
      c. Callosal dysgenesis.

D. Lhermitte-Duclos syndrome (dysplastic gangliocytoma of the cerebellum).
  1. Pathology.
    a. Focally enlarged, disorganized cerebellar cortex.
    b. Thickening, hypermyelination of molecular layer.
    c. Large pleomorphic cells replace the Purkinje, granular cell layers.
    d. No mitoses, necrosis, neovascularity.
    e. Biopsy may be called gangliocytoma.
  2. Imaging.
    a. CT shows hypodense, nonenhancing cerebellar mass.
    b. MR shows "striated cerebellum" (distinctive laminated-appearing mass caused by thickened, ribbon-like folia).
    c. Alternating linear bands of hypointense, isointense linear striations on T1WI that show hyperintensity and isointensity (relative to gray matter) on T2WI.
    d. Fourth ventricle may be displaced, compressed; causes hydrocephalus in 50%.
    e. Mass usually does not enhance following contrast administration (some heterogeneous pial enhancement may be present).
  3. Associated abnormalities.
    a. Cowden disease (multiple hamartoma syndrome).
      (1) Cutaneous lesions (facial papules, oral mucosal papillomatoses, sclerotic fibromas).
      (2) Breast carcinoma.
      (3) Uterine, cervical, renal pelvis, and urinary bladder carcinomas.
      (4) Skeletal, solid visceral tumors.
      (5) Gastrointestinal polyps.
      (6) CNS lesions (posterior fossa gangliocytoma).
    b. Megalencephaly, heterotopias.
    c. Local gigantism, polydactyly.

SUGGESTED READINGS

Altman NR, Naidich TP, Braffman BH: Posterior fossa malformations, *AJNR* 13:691-724, 1992.

Awad EE, Levy E, Martin DS, Merenda O: Atypical MR appearance of Lhermitte-Duclos disease with contrast enhancement, *AJNR* 16:1719-1720, 1995.

Demaerel P, Kendall BE, Wilms G, et al: Uncommon posterior cranial fossa anomalies: MRI with clinical correlation, *Neuroradiol* 37:72-76, 1995.

Harned RK, Buck JL, Sobin LH: The hamartomatous polyposis syndromes: clinical and radiologic features, *AJR* 164:565-571, 1995.

Kollias SS, Ball WS Jr, Prenger EC: Cystic malformations of the posterior fossa: Differential diagnosis clarified through embryologic analysis, *Radiographics* 13:1211-1231, 1993.

Meltzer CC, Smirniotopoulos JG, Jones RV: The striated cerebellum: an MR imaging sign in Lhermitte-Duclos disease (dysplastic gangliocytoma), *Radiol* 194:699-703, 1995.

Strand RD, Barnes PD, Poussaint TY, et al: Cystic retrocerebellar malformations: unification of the Dandy-Walker complex and the Blake's pouch cyst, *Pediatr Radiol* 23:258-260, 1993.

16

Neurofibromatosis

Key Concepts

1. Neurofibromatosis Type 1 (NF-1), also known as von Recklinghausen disease, is the most common neurocutaneous syndrome.
2. NF-1 is caused by chromosome 17 mutation.
3. Neoplasms reported in NF-1 are lesions of neurons and astrocytes.
4. Neurofibromatosis Type 2 (NF-2) is caused by a defect on chromosome 22.
5. Neoplasms in NF-2 are typically schwannomas, meningiomas, and spinal cord ependymomas.
6. NF-1 and NF-2 are considered as hereditary tumor syndromes of the nervous system.

The neurocutaneous syndromes, also known as "phakomatoses," are a heterogeneous group of disorders that mainly affect structures of ectodermal origin. With a few exceptions, these syndromes thus have both central nervous system and cutaneous manifestations. Visceral, osseous, and connective tissue lesions are additional features of some neurocutaneous syndromes.

In this chapter, we focus on the most common neurocutaneous syndrome, neurofibromatosis. Neurofibromatosis is actually a heterogeneous group of disorders with two distinct types that are recognized: Neurofibromatosis Type 1 (NF-1), also known as von Recklinghausen disease, and Neurofibromatosis Type 2 (NF-2) (Table 16-1).

   I. Neurofibromatosis Type 1 (NF-1).
     A. Prevalence, inheritance.
       1. Most common neurocutaneous syndrome (1 per 2000 to 3000 live births).
       2. Represents >90% of neurofibromatosis cases.
       3. Autosomal dominant (high penetrance, variable expressivity).

Table 16-1   NF-1 and NF-2 Compared

	NF-1	NF-2
Inheritance	Chromosome 17	Chromosome 22
Cutaneous lesions	Common	Rare
Brain lesions	Optic nerve glioma	Schwannomas (cranial nerves)
	Nonoptic astrocytomas	Meningiomas
	Hamartomas (white matter, basal ganglia)	Choroid plexus calcifications
Skull	Sphenoid wing hypoplasia, sutural defects	
Spine	Dural ectasia, meningoceles, kyphoscoliosis	Meningiomas
Spinal roots	Neurofibromas	Schwannomas
Spinal cord	Astrocytoma	Ependymoma
Miscellaneous	Plexiform neurofibroma (any location)	
	Lisch nodules (iris)	
	Buphthalmos	
	Retinal phakomas	
	Vascular stenoses, ectasias	
	Visceral, endocrine tumors	
	Ribbon ribs, pseudoarthroses	
	Tibial bowing	
	Focal limb overgrowth	

4. Tumor suppressor on chromosome 17 (encodes for protein "neurofibromin").
5. Approximately half of patients with NF-1 are new mutations.

B. Clinical.
1. Prominent skin manifestations (e.g., cafe-au-lait spots, axillary or inguinal freckling).
2. Diagnosis requires two or more criteria established by National Institutes of Health Consensus Development Conference in 1988.
   a. Six or more 5 mm (or larger) cafe-au-lait spots.
   b. One plexiform neurofibroma *or* two or more neurofibromas of any type.
   c. Two or more pigmented iris hamartomas (so-called "Lisch nodules").
   d. Axillary or inguinal freckling.
   e. Optic nerve glioma.
   f. First-degree relative with NF-1.
   g. Presence of a characteristic bone lesion (e.g., dysplasia of the greater sphenoid wing, pseudarthrosis).

C. Pathology, imaging.
1. Neoplasms (multiple neoplasms are a hallmark of NF-1, considered a hereditary tumor syndrome of nervous system).
   a. Optic pathway glioma.
      (1) Occurs in 5% to 15%.
      (2) Most are low-grade astrocytoma or hamartoma.
      (3) Between 10% and 20% more malignant and clinically aggressive.
      (4) Hypointense to isointense on T1WI, hyperintense on T2WI, variable enhancement.
   b. Nonoptic glioma.
      (1) Usually low-grade astrocytoma.
      (2) Midbrain, tectum, brainstem are common sites (may cause obstructive hydrocephalus).
   c. Plexiform neurofibroma.
      (1) Considered diagnostic of NF-1.
      (2) Found in one third of NF-1 cases.
      (3) Unencapsulated, infiltrating masses of neurons, Schwann cells, collagen.
      (4) Orbit, scalp (CN V_1 distribution), exiting spinal nerve roots are common sites.
      (5) Imaging studies show poorly delineated, variably enhancing wormlike infiltrating mass.

    d. Neurofibrosarcoma.
      (1) Sarcomatous degeneration of neurofibromas occurs in 5% to 15% of patients with NF-1.
      (2) Orbit and skull base, spinal nerve roots are common sites.
2. Nonneoplastic lesions (benign brain parenchymal abnormalities).
    a. Represent hamartomatous foci of glial proliferation, vacuolar or spongiotic change.
    b. Found in >75% of patients with NF-1.
    c. Basal ganglia and internal capsules, optic radiations, brainstem, cerebral peduncles, pons, and cerebellum are common sites.
    d. Age-related (uncommon before age 3 or after age 20).
    e. Often multiple, bilateral.
    f. Increase in size, number until age 10 or 12 years, then diminish.
    g. Usually isointense or slightly hyperintense on T1WI, hyperintense on T2WI.
    h. Typical lesions have little or no mass effect, do not enhance.
    i. Lesions with mass effect, enhancement should be followed as they may represent a nonoptic glioma.
    j. Proton MR spectroscopy is different from glioma, similar to that of normal brain.
3. Osseous, dural dysplasias.
    a. Hypoplastic sphenoid wing.
    b. Sutural defects.
    c. "Ribbon ribs."
    d. Tibial bowing.
    e. Pseudarthroses.
    f. Focal overgrowth (localized gigantism) of digit, ray, limb.
    g. Patulous dura (optic nerve sheath, internal auditory canal enlargement).
    h. Spine (see below).
4. Ocular/orbital manifestations.
    a. Optic nerve glioma.
    b. Pigmented iris hamartomas ("Lisch nodules").
    c. Enlarged globe ("buphthalmos").
    d. Retinal phakomas.
    e. Plexiform neurofibroma (cutaneous branches of ophthalmic division, trigeminal nerve).
    f. Dysplastic/absent sphenoid wing (temporal lobe herniation into orbit may cause pulsatile exophthalmos); often

but not invariably associated with plexiform neurofibroma of orbit.

5. Spine, spinal cord/nerve roots (abnormalities seen in 60% of NF-1 cases).
   a. Scoliosis (most common skeletal abnormality in NF-1, seen in one third of cases; thought to be secondary to vertebral body dysplasia).
   b. Dural ectasia (most common cause of posterior vertebral body scalloping in NF-1) and meningoceles (note: meningoceles, nerve root tumors can both enlarge neural foramina).
   c. Neurofibromas of exiting roots.
   d. Astrocytoma of spinal cord.
   e. Nonneoplastic white matter lesions (much less common than brain).
6. Vascular lesions/dysplasias.
   a. Most common (85%): Intimal proliferation with progressive cerebral arterial occlusive disease (may cause "Moya-moya" pattern).
   b. Aneurysms are second most common vascular lesion in NF-1.
   c. Nonaneurysmal vascular ectasias.
7. Miscellaneous.
   a. Visceral, endocrine tumors (4% of cases).

II. Neurofibromatosis Type 2 (NF-2) (neurofibromatosis with bilateral acoustic schwannomas) is a severe inherited disorder that is genetically and clinically distinct from the more common NF-1 (von Recklinghausen neurofibromatosis).
A. Prevalence, inheritance.
   1. Estimated incidence is one in 40,000 live births.
   2. Accounts for approximately 10% of neurofibromatosis cases.
   3. Autosomal dominant, high penetrance (children of an affected individual have a 50% risk of developing the disorder).
   4. Tumor suppressor gene on chromosome 22 (encodes for "merlin" protein).
   5. Approximately 50% of cases represent new mutations.
B. Clinical.
   1. Cutaneous manifestations much less common than in NF-1.
   2. Clinical manifestations (e.g., intracranial neoplasms) may not develop until adulthood.
   3. N.I.H. consensus panel diagnostic criteria.
      a. Bilateral acoustic schwannomas establish the diagnosis of NF-2.

   b. First-degree relative with NF-2 and either of the following:
      (1) Unilateral CN VIII tumor.
      (2) Two of the following: neurofibroma, meningioma, glioma, schwannoma, or juvenile posterior subcapsular lenticular opacity.
 C. Pathology, imaging (*Note:* CNS lesions develop in nearly all patients with NF-2).
   1. Brain (lesions of schwann cells, meninges).
      a. CN VIII ("acoustic") schwannomas.
      b. Schwannomas of other cranial nerves.
      c. Meningiomas (often multiple).
      d. Nonneoplastic intracranial calcifications (choroid plexus most commonly involved), glial hamartomas.
      e. Schwannomas, meningiomas both enhance intensely following contrast administration.
      f. Discovery of a schwannoma or meningioma in a pediatric-age patient should prompt intensive search for other lesions.
   2. Spinal cord and nerve roots.
      a. Spinal cord ependymomas.
      b. Nerve root schwannomas (often multiple).
      c. Meningiomas.
   3. Spinal column.
      a. Vertebral body scalloping (secondary to spinal cord neoplasm).
      b. Neural foramen enlargement (secondary to nerve root tumors).

SUGGESTED READINGS

Akeson P, Holtas S: Radiological investigation of neurofibromatosis type 2, *Neuroradiol* 36:107-110, 1994.

Barkovich AJ: The phakomatoses. In *Pediatric Neuroradiology,* ed 2, New York, 1995, Raven Press, pp 277-296.

Castillo M, Green C, Kwock L, et al: Proton MR spectroscopy in patients with neurofibromatosis type 1: evaluation of hamartomas and clinical correlation, *AJNR* 16:141-147, 1995.

DiPaolo DP, Zimmerman RA, Rorke LB, et al: Neurofibromatosis type 1: pathologic substrate of high-signal-intensity foci in the brain, *Radiol* 195:721-724, 1995.

Itoh T, Magnaldi S, White RM, et al: Neurofibromatosis type 1: the evolution of deep gray and white matter abnormalities, *AJNR* 15:1513-1519, 1994.

Louis DN, Ramesh V, Gusella JF: Neuropathology and molecular genetics of neurofibromatosis 2 and related tumors, *Brain Pathol* 5:163-172, 1995.

Rizzo J, Lessell S: Cerebrovascular abnormalities in neurofibromatosis type 1, *Neurol* 44:1000-1002, 1994.

von Deimling A, Krone W, Menon AG: Neurofibromatosis type 1: pathology, clinical features, and molecular genetics, *Brain Pathol* 5:153-162, 1995.

17

Major Neurocutaneous Syndromes Other Than Neurofibromatosis

Key Concepts

1. Tuberous sclerosis complex (TSC) causes hamartomatous growths in multiple organ systems including brain, kidneys, heart.
2. "Classic" clinical triad of cutaneous adenoma sebaceum, seizures, mental retardation is seen in less than 50% of patients with TSC.
3. Radiographic evidence of multiple calcified subependymal nodules that protrude into the ventricle indicates definite TSC; cortical tubers plus cerebral white matter lesions indicate probable TSC.
4. Benign subependymal nodules in TSC may enhance, but enlarging, enhancing nodule at foramen of Monro should be considered giant-cell astrocytoma until proved otherwise.
5. Sturge-Weber syndrome (SWS) consists of a facial angioma ("port wine" vascular nevus), paucity of normal cortical draining veins with overlying leptomeningeal angiomatosis.
6. Von Hippel-Lindau disease (VHL) is characterized by retinal angiomas, cerebellar and spinal cord hemangioblastomas, and visceral cysts or neoplasms.

After neurofibromatosis, the most important neurocutaneous syndromes encountered in clinical practice are tuberous sclerosis (TS), Sturge-Weber syndrome (SWS), and von Hippel-Lindau disease (VHL). In this chapter we summarize the clinical findings, pathology, and imaging spectrum of these disorders.

I. Tuberous sclerosis complex (TSC) (also known as Bourneville disease) is a multisystem disorder that primarily affects the brain, retina, kidneys, and skin.
   A. Prevalence, inheritance, gender.
      1. Approximately one in 10,000 to 20,000 live births (*forme fruste* probably more common).
      2. Autosomal dominant (variable expressivity, low penetrance).
      3. Genetically heterogeneous.
         a. Mapped to chromosomes 9 (TSC1) and 16 (TSC2).
         b. Two thirds of families map to chromosome 9q; slightly less than one third map to chromosome 16p; 5% do not map to any known region.
      4. No gender, racial predilection.
   B. Etiology.
      1. Germinal matrix abnormality affects neuronal-radial glial unit.
      2. Dysplastic, disorganized cells found in subependymal region, white matter, cortex.
   C. Clinical.
      1. "Triad" of adenoma sebaceum, seizures, mental retardation seen in <50% of patients with TSC.
      2. Papular facial rash consists of reddish-brown angiofibromas around nasolabial folds, cheeks.
      3. Diagnostic neuroimaging criteria include the following:
         a. Imaging evidence of multiple calcified subependymal nodules that project into ventricles establishes definite diagnosis of TSC.
         b. Imaging evidence of cortical tubers or noncalcified subependymal nodules plus cerebral white-matter "migration tracts" or heterotopias establishes diagnosis of probable TSC.
      4. Cerebral dysfunction correlates with lesions.
         a. More cortical tubers found in patients who have first seizure before 1 year, have infantile spasms or mental disability.
         b. Patients without seizures usually have no mental disability.
   D. Pathology, imaging.
      1. Subependymal hamartomas.
         a. Most common brain lesion in TSC (seen in 95% of patients).

    b. Typical location is lateral ventricles, along striothalamic groove.

    c. Calcifications increase with age (rare under 1 year of age).

    d. Variable signal on MR.

    e. Variable enhancement.

2. Cortical hamartomas ("tubers").

    a. Most characteristic lesion of TSC at pathologic examination.

    b. Found in 95% of patients with TSC.

    c. Grossly resemble distorted, expanded gyrus with poor gray-white matter definition.

    d. Microscopically consist of gliosis, disordered myelination, bizarre giant cells.

    e. On CT, pattern of expanded gyrus with hypodense underlying white matter is common; by age 10, calcified cortical tubers are present in half of all cases.

    f. MR signal varies with age (in infants and neonates, may appear quite hyperintense on T1WI, hypointense on T2WI; are usually hypointense on T1-, hyperintense on T2WI in older children and adults).

    g. Enhancement following contrast administration may occur in degenerated, calcified tubers but is uncommon.

    h. Cortical tubers do not undergo malignant degeneration.

3. White matter lesions.

    a. Disordered radial glial-neuronal unit with disordered, hypo-myelinated neurons and bizarre giant cells.

    b. Any part of white matter can be involved, from ependyma to cortex.

    c. CT shows lucent areas that may display focal or regional calcification.

    d. T2WI may disclose straight, curvilinear, wedge-shaped, or even "tumefactive" bands of increased signal intensity.

    e. Enhancement following contrast administration is uncommon.

    f. White matter lesions in TSC do not become malignant.

4. Subependymal giant-cell astrocytoma (SGCA).

    a. Seen in 5% to 15% of patients with TSC.

    b. Histologically benign, rarely invades brain; symptoms typically caused by obstructive hydrocephalus.

    c. Enlarging, enhancing subependymal nodule at foramen of Monro should be considered SGCA.

    d. MR spectroscopy may be helpful in distinguishing the hypometabolic subependymal nodules from SGCA.

5. Miscellaneous CNS lesions.

      a. Retinal hamartomas.

      b. Vascular dysplasias (aneurysm, progressive stenoses).

   6. Non-CNS lesions.

      a. Renal cysts, angiomyolipomas.

      b. Cardiac rhabdomyomas.

      c. Leiomyomas, adenomas of liver.

      d. Spleen, pancreas adenomas.

      e. Bone islands, cysts, periosteal new bone.

      f. Miscellaneous vascular ectasias, aneurysms, nonatheromatous stenoses.

II. Sturge-Weber syndrome (SWS).

  A. Etiology and pathology.

    1. Precise etiology unknown, but may be due to persistence of primordial sinusoidal vascular channels.

    2. Angiomatosis involves:

      a. Face ("port wine stain," most often in the distribution of CN V_1).

      b. Ocular choroid.

      c. Leptomeninges (plexus of thin-walled vessels between pia, arachnoid).

    3. Paucity of normal cortical draining veins.

    4. Dystrophic changes in brain underlying the leptomeningeal angioma.

      a. Atrophy (secondary to reduced perfusion or chronic ischemia caused by impaired venous drainage).

      b. Calcification (middle layers of cortex and subjacent white matter); may have "tram-track" appearance caused by calcification in apposing gyri.

    5. Calvarial thickening, paranasal and mastoid enlargement secondary to ipsilateral hemispheric atrophy.

  B. Imaging.

    1. Plain films may show "tram-track" calcification, thick calvarium, enlarged frontal sinus and mastoid.

    2. NECT.

      a. Cortical calcification.

        (1) Most common CT finding in SWS.

        (2) Unusual before 2 years of age.

        (3) Often gyriform, curvilinear.

        (4) Parietal, occipital lobes most common sites.

      b. Atrophy.

    3. CECT.

      a. Variable enhancement of pial angioma, underlying gyri (secondary to ischemia).

  b. Ipsilateral choroid plexus may be enlarged, show intense enhancement.
 4. MR.
  a. Dystrophic cortical, subcortical calcification seen as curvilinear areas of decreased signal on T2WI.
  b. Gliosis may prolong T1, T2 relaxation.
  c. Contrast enhancement shows:
   (1) Pial angioma enhances strongly.
   (2) Enlarged, intensely enhancing choroid plexus.
   (3) Prominent medullary, subependymal veins provide collateral deep venous drainage when superficial cortical venous system is deficient.
 5. Associated abnormalities.
  a. Ocular abnormalities seen in one third of SWS cases.
   (1) Scleral, choroidal angiomas.
   (2) Congenital glaucoma with buphthalmos.
  b. Angio-osteo-hypertrophy (Klippel-Trenaunay syndrome).
 6. Differential diagnosis: occipital calcifications at gray-white junction in celiac disease with folate deficiency may resemble SWS.
III. von Hippel-Lindau syndrome (VHL).
 A. Prevalence, inheritance.
  1. Estimated at one per 35,000 to 40,000.
  2. Autosomal dominant (incomplete penetrance, variable expressivity).
  3. Gene mapped to short arm of chromosome (3p 25-26), which has defective tumor suppressor gene.
  4. Occurs as new mutation in only 1% to 3% of cases.
 B. Clinical.
  1. Diagnostic criteria.
   a. Multiple CNS hemangioblastomas are diagnostic.
   b. One CNS hemangioblastoma plus a visceral manifestation (renal cell carcinoma, pheochromocytoma, cysts, and adenomas).
   c. First-order relative plus one central or visceral manifestation.
  2. Presentation.
   a. Rare before puberty.
   b. Typically become symptomatic in third or fourth decade.
    (1) 20s if retinal angioma present.
    (2) 30s with CNS hemangioblastoma.
    (3) 40s with renal cell carcinoma.
  3. Proposed National Cancer Institute classification of VHL.

   a. VHL without pheochromocytomas.
   b. VHL with pheochromocytomas.
      (1) Pheochromocytomas and retinal and CNS hemangio-blastomas.
      (2) Pheochromocytomas, retinal and CNS hemangioblasto-mas, renal cancers, and pancreatic involvement.
C. Pathology.
   1. CNS manifestations.
      a. Retinal angiomatosis.
         (1) Approximately 50% of patients with VHL.
         (2) Bilateral in half.
         (3) Multiple in one third.
         (4) Cause hemorrhage, subretinal exudates.
      b. Brain, spinal cord hemangioblastoma (>50% of patients with VHL).
         (1) 90% in posterior fossa (65% cerebellum, 20% brain-stem).
         (2) 10% to 15% spinal cord.
         (3) Rare above tentorium.
         (4) Multiple in 40% of patients with VHL.
   2. Non-CNS lesions.
      a. Renal cysts and carcinoma (25%).
      b. Pheochromocytoma (35%).
      c. Nonneoplastic visceral cysts.
      d. Adenomas (liver).
D. Imaging.
   1. Hemangioblastoma.
      a. 80% are cystic.
         (1) Well-delineated mass (usually hyperintense on both T1-, T2WI).
         (2) Small subpial mural nodule enhances strongly following contrast administration.
         (3) Cyst wall usually does not enhance.
         (4) Hemorrhage may cause complex signal.
      b. 20% to 40% solid.
      c. High-velocity signal loss ("flow voids") in afferent, efferent vessels that supply tumor can often be detected.
      d. Angiography shows intense, prolonged vascular stain in tu-mor nodule; cyst causes avascular surrounding mass effect.
      e. Spinal cord hemangioblastoma may have extensive syrinx-like cyst.
      f. Look for hemorrhage, retinal detachment caused by ocular hemangioma.

2. Non-CNS lesions (patients with VHL should have abdominal, pelvic imaging studies).
   a. Cysts occur in virtually all visceral organs.
   b. Renal cell carcinoma (often multicentric or bilateral) occurs in up to 40% to 50% of cases.
   c. Pheochromocytomas in 10% to 15%.
   d. Epidydimal cysts, cystadenomas in males (3%).

SUGGESTED READINGS

Barkovich AJ: The phakomatoses. In *Pediatric neuroradiology,* ed 2, New York, 1995, Raven Press, pp 296-312.

Benedikt RA, Brown DC, Walker R, et al: Sturge-Weber syndrome: cranial MR imaging with Gd-DTPA, *AJNR,* 14:409-415, 1993.

Choyke PL, Glenn GM, Walther MM, et al: von Hippel-Lindau disease: genetic, clinical, and imaging features, *Radiol* 194: 629-642, 1995.

Duncan DB, Herholz K, Pietrzyk U, Heiss W-D: Regional cerebral blood flow and metabolism in Sturge-Weber disease, *Clin Nuc Med* 20:522-523, 1995.

Groenendaal F, Meiners LC, Gooskens R, de Vries LS: Cerebral proton magnetic resonance spectroscopic imaging in a neonate with tuberous sclerosis, *Neuropediatr* 25:154-157, 1994.

Halley D, Janssen B, Hesseling-Janssen A, et al: Cloning and characterization of tuberous sclerosis determining genes on 9q and 16p, *Am J Hum Genetics* 55(3): A187, 1994.

Karsdorp N, Elderson A, Wittebol-Post D, et al: Von Hippel-Lindau disease: new strategies in early detection and treatment, *Am J Med* 97:158-168, 1994.

Lea ME, Sage MR: Bilateral occipital calcification associated with celiac disease, folate deficiency, and epilepsy, *AJNR* 16:1498-1500, 1995.

Linehan WM, Lerman MI, Zbar B: Identification of the von Hippel-Lindau (VHL) gene: its role in renal cancer, *JAMA* 273: 564-568, 1995.

Neumann HPH, Lips CJM, Hsia YE, Zbar B: Von Hippel-Lindau syndrome, *Brain Pathol* 5:181-193, 1995.

Pascual-Castroviejo I, Diaz-Gonzalea C, Garcia-Melian RM, et al: Sturge-Weber syndrome: study of 40 patients, *Pediatr Neurol* 9:283-288, 1993.

Pont MS, Elster AD: Lesions of skin and brain: modern imaging of the neurocutaneous syndromes, *AJR* 158:1193-1203, 1992.

Sheperd CW, Houser OW, Gomez MR: MR findings in tuberous sclerosis complex and correlation with seizure development and mental impairment, *AJNR* 16:149-155, 1995.

Short MP, Richardson EP Jr, Haines JL, Kwiatowski DJ: Clinical neuropathological and genetic aspects of the tuberous sclerosis complex, *Brain Pathol* 5:173-179, 1995.

Smirniotopoulos JG, Murphy FM: The phakomatoses, *AJNR* 13:725-746, 1992.

Vogl TJ, Stemmler J, Bergman C, et al: MR and MR angiography of Sturge-Weber syndrome, *AJNR* 14:417-425, 1993.

18

Other Neurocutaneous Syndromes

Key Concepts

1. Rendu-Osler-Weber disease has multiple mucocutaneous telangiectasias with arteriovenous malformations in the liver, lungs, and brain.
2. Wyburn-Mason syndrome has ocular, brain vascular malformations.
3. Ataxia-telangiectasia has oculocutaneous telangiectasias and cerebellar atrophy.
4. Neurocutaneous melanosis has congenital nevi with primary meningeal melanosis.

More than 30 different neurocutaneous syndromes have been described. NF-1, TSC, and NF-2 are by far the most common of these disorders. Neurofibromatosis and the other major neurocutaneous syndromes were discussed in the preceding chapters. In this chapter we close our discussion of congenital brain malformations by briefly summarizing some of the more interesting minor neurocutaneous syndromes.

I. Rendu-Osler-Weber disease (ROW) (also known as hereditary hemorrhagic telangiectasia or HHT).
  A. Inheritance.
    1. Autosomal dominant.
    2. Strong penetrance, variable expressivity.
  B. Pathology.
    1. Multiple mucocutaneous capillary telangiectasias.
    2. AVMs, AVFs.
      a. 30% in liver.
      b. 15% to 20% lungs.
      c. 8% to 30% brain, spine.
      d. Often multiple.
    3. Aneurysms.
  C. Clinical.
    1. 85% of patients with ROW have epistaxis.
    2. 50% of CNS complications are caused by pulmonary AVFs (septic emboli, thrombosis caused by polycythemia).
    3. 50% of neurologic symptoms caused by intracranial AVMs, hepatic encephalopathy, or cerebral abscess.
  D. Imaging.
    1. Mucocutaneous telangiectasias appear as multiple small nests of abnormal vessels on angiography.
    2. Brain imaging may show multiple AVMs, infarcts, cerebritis, abscess.
II. Wyburn-Mason syndrome (WMS).
  A. Clinical.
    1. Cutaneous vascular nevi.
  B. Pathology, imaging.
    1. Retinal, optic nerve vascular malformations.
    2. Ipsilateral cerebral AVM (typically involves visual pathways, midbrain).
III. Ataxia-telangiectasia (AT) (also known as Louis-Bar syndrome) is a multisystem disease that consists of progressive cerebellar ataxia, oculomucocutaneous telangiectasias, sinus and lung infections, and a propensity to develop lymphoreticular neoplasms.
  A. Prevalence, inheritance.
    1. Approximately one per 40,000 live births.

  2. Autosomal recessive.
  3. Localized to chromosome 11q.
B. Clinical.
  1. Conjunctival, cutaneous telangiectasias.
  2. Progressive cerebellar ataxia with onset in infancy or childhood.
  3. Immunodeficiency (both cell-mediated and humoral immunity are impaired).
    a. Thymus absent or rudimentary.
    b. Recurrent sinus, lung infections.
    c. Bronchiectasis, pulmonary failure are most common causes of death.
  4. 10% to 15% of patients with AT develop malignant neoplasms.
    a. Lymphoma, leukemia in younger patients.
    b. Epithelial malignancies in adults.
C. Pathology, imaging.
  1. Cerebellar atrophy.
  2. Embolic cerebral infarcts secondary to pulmonary emboli may occur.
  3. Usually no macroscopic telangiectases in brain.
  4. Sinusitis in 80%.
IV. Neurocutaneous melanosis (NCM).
  A. Prevalence, clinical.
    1. Rare.
    2. Giant pigmented cutaneous nevi.
    3. No evidence for cutaneous melanoma.
  B. Pathology, imaging.
    1. Meningeal, parenchymal accumulations of melanocytes.
    2. MR shows scattered foci of T1, T2 shortening.
    3. Some cases may show abnormal leptomeningeal enhancement.
V. Meningioangiomatosis (MA).
  A. Prevalence, inheritance.
    1. Rare.
    2. May represent a *forme fruste* of neurofibromatosis.
  B. Pathology, imaging.
    1. Hamartomatous proliferation of thickened, hyperplastic meninges; may infiltrate along Virchow-Robin spaces, involve underlying cortex.
    2. T1-weighted MR scans show isointense to slightly hypointense cortically based mass that enhances strongly following contrast administration.

VI. Epidermal nevus syndromes.
   A. Linear sebaceous nevus syndrome.
      1. Hemimegalencephaly.
      2. Nonlissencephalic cortical dysplasias.
      3. Facial hemihypertrophy.
   B. Epidermal nevus syndrome.
      1. Ocular anomalies (e.g., colobomas, Coats disease).
   C. Blue rubber bleb nevus syndrome.
      1. Multiple intracranial venous angiomas.
      2. Sinus pericranii.
VII. Basal cell nevus syndrome (BCNS or Gorlin-Goltz syndrome).
   A. Inheritance.
      1. Autosomal dominant.
      2. High penetrance, variable expressivity (chromosome 9q31).
   B. CNS manifestations.
      1. Thickened, lamellar dural calcification (plain skull radio-
         graphs show falcine calcification in approximately 100% with
         BCNS).
      2. Callosal dysgenesis.
      3. CNS neoplasms (most often medulloblastoma).
   C. Non-CNS manifestations.
      1. Basal cell carcinomas of the skin.
      2. Facial dysmorphism (large bulging forehead, hypertelorism,
         flat nasal bridge).
      3. Jaw cysts (multiple odontogenic keratocysts).
      4. Bifid ribs.
VIII. Cowden disease (multiple hamartoma syndrome).
   A. CNS manifestations.
      1. Neoplasms.
         a. Neuromas.
         b. Neurofibromas.
         c. Meningiomas.
      2. Lhermitte-Duclos disease.
   B. Non-CNS manifestations.
      1. Mucocutaneous lesions (facial papules, oral mucosal papil-
         lomatoses, acral keratoses, multiple sclerotic fibromas).
      2. Cysts, tumors of thyroid, breast, adnexae.
      3. Gastrointestinal polyps.

SUGGESTED READINGS

Albrecht S, Goodman J C, Rajagopolan S, et al: Malignant meningioma in Gorlin's
   syndrome: cytogenetic and p53 gene analysis, *J Neurosurg* 81:466-471, 1994.

Barkovich AJ: The phakomatoses. In *Pediatric Neuroradiology,* ed 2, New York, 1995, Raven Press, pp 312-319.

Barkovich AJ, Frieden IJ, Williams ML: MR of neurocutaneous melanosis, *AJNR* 15:859-867, 1994.

Garcia-Monaco R, Taylor W, Rodesch G, et al: Pial arteriovenous fistula in children as presenting manifestation of Rendu-Osler-Weber disease, *Neuroradiol* 37:60-64, 1995.

Harned RK, Buck JL, Sobin LH: The hamartomatous polyposis syndromes: clinical and radiologic features, *AJR* 164: 565-571, 1995.

Kikuchi K, Kowada M, Sasajima H: Vascular malformations of the brain in hereditary hemorrhagic telangiectasia (Rendu-Osler-Weber disease), *Surg Neurol* 41:374-380, 1994.

Lazzeri S, Mascalchi M, Cellerini M, et al: Epidermal nevus syndrome: MR of intracranial involvement, *AJNR* 14:1255-1257, 1993.

Louis DN, von Deimling A: Hereditary tumor syndromes of the nervous system: overview and rare syndromes, *Brain Pathol* 5:145-151, 1995.

Ratcliffe JF, Shanley S, Ferguson J, Chenevix-Trench G: The diagnostic implication of falcine calcification on plain skull radiographs of patients with basal cell haevus syndrome and the incidence of falcine calcification in their relatives and two control groups, *Br J Radiol* 68:361-368, 1995.

Sardanelli F, Parodi RC, Ottonello C, et al: Cranial MRI in ataxia-telangiectasia, *Neuroradiol* 37:77-82, 1995.

SECTION III
Trauma and Intracranial Hemorrhage

19

Understanding Intracranial Hemorrhage

Key Concepts

1. CT appearance of intracranial hemorrhage (ICH) depends on only one factor, namely, electron density of clot.
2. Acute ICH is hyperdense on CT scans (exceptions: rapid bleeding, coagulopathy, extreme anemia), whereas chronic hemorrhage is hypodense compared with brain.
3. Signal intensity of ICH on MR scans depends on many *intrinsic factors* including hemoglobin oxidation state, red blood cell morphology, and macroscopic clot structure.
4. *Extrinsic factors* such as pulse sequences, flip angle, and field strength also affect the signal intensity of ICH on MR scans.

Suspected intracranial hemorrhage (ICH) is one of the most frequent indications for emergent neuroimaging. Despite the superior sensitivity of MR, CT remains the screening procedure of choice in evaluating patients with head trauma and acute cerebral infarction. CT is also useful in the initial evaluation of patients with sudden unexplained neurologic deterioration.

In this chapter we review the general imaging appearance of hemorrhage and follow clot evolution as it is depicted on both CT (Fig. 19-1) and MR (Table 19-1). The primary and secondary effects of intracranial trauma as well as the major nontraumatic causes of ICH are discussed in subsequent chapters.

I. Acute intracranial hemorrhage (0-4 days).
  A. Hyperacute hemorrhage (<4 hours).
    1. Pathology.
       a. Inhomogeneous loose clot contains extravasated erythrocytes (RBCs), activated platelets, fibrin, watery serum.
       b. Biconvex RBCs contain oxyhemoglobin.
    2. CT appearance.
       a. Clot usually hyperdense (compared with brain) with:

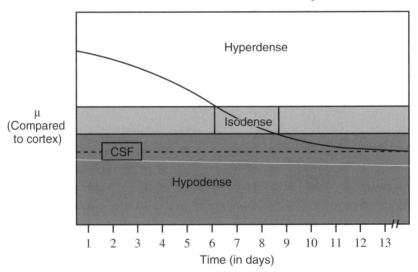

Fig. 19-1 Changing density of intracranial hemorrhage with time as shown on nonenhanced CT scan is depicted. Note that the attenuation of a typical acute hematoma is initially hyperdense compared to cortex. As clot density progressively diminishes over several days, the hematoma becomes isodense with brain. Late subacute or chronic hematomas are typically hypodense compared to brain and approach cerebrospinal fluid (CSF) in attenuation.

  (1) High hematocrit (90%).
  (2) High hemoglobin (>9 to 11 g/dl).
  b. Isodense with brain (rare).
  (1) Rapid hemorrhage with unretracted, semiliquid clot.
  (2) Coagulopathy.
  (3) Severe anemia.
  c. Fluid-blood levels.
  (1) Presence strongly suggests coagulopathy.
  3. MR appearance.
  a. T1WI: Isointense compared with brain.
  b. T2WI: Isointense to hyperintense (depends on amount of water in clot).
  c. Hypointense on gradient-refocussed (GRE or "GRASS") sequences.
B. Early acute hemorrhage (4 to 6 hours).
  1. Pathology.
  a. RBCs rapidly lose biconvex shape, become round.
  b. Clot retraction and hemoconcentration progresses.
  c. Peripheral edema surrounds clot.
  2. CT.
  a. Clot is typically hyperdense.
  b. Surrounding low-density area (edema, extruded serum).
  3. MR.
  a. T1WI: Isointense.
  b. T2WI: Hyperintense.
  c. GRE: Profoundly hypointense.
C. Late acute hemorrhage (7 to 72 hours).
  1. Pathology.
  a. RBC packing continues and further hemoconcentration occurs.
  b. RBCs shrink, assume spiculated configuration ("echino-cytes").

Table 19-1   CT and MR of Intracranial Hemorrhage (Density/Signal Intensity Compared to Cortex)

Time	NECT	CECT	T1WI	T2WI	GRE
4-6h	Hyperdense	—	Iso	Hyper	Hypo
7-72h	Hyperdense	—	Iso	Hypo	Very hypo
4-7d	Hyper/iso	—	Iso (center) Hyper (rim)	Hypo	Very hypo
1-4wks	Iso/hypo	Rim enh	Hyper	Hyper	Hypo
Chronic	Hypodense	—	Hypo	Hypo	Hypo

    c. Hemoglobin undergoes oxidation to deoxyhemoglobin,
       particularly in center of clot, which is profoundly hypoxic.
    d. Mass effect, edema surrounding clot increase.
  2. CT.
    a. Clot remains hyperdense.
    b. Edema, mass effect often continue to increase.
  3. MR.
    a. T1WI: Isointense.
    b. T2WI: Hypointense center, hyperintense periphery.
    c. GRE: Hypointense, "blooms."
II. Subacute hemorrhage (4 days to 4 weeks).
  A. Early subacute hemorrhage (4 to 7 days).
    1. Pathology.
      a. RBCs become microspherocytes.
      b. Hemoglobin undergoes further denaturation, with methemo-
         globin forming at edges of hematoma.
      c. Surrounding edema, mass effect persist.
    2. CT.
      a. Clot density decreases with time.
      b. Hematoma gradually becomes isodense compared with
         brain.
      c. Mass effect diminishes.
    3. MR.
      a. T1WI: Isointense center, hyperintense rim.
      b. T2WI: Hypointense.
      c. GRE: Hypointense, "blooms."
  B. Late subacute hemorrhage (1 to 4 weeks).
    1. Pathology.
      a. RBCs lyse, releasing methemoglobin.
      b. Clot density decreases as hematoma cavitates, forming pool
         of watery serum, dilute free methemoglobin.
      c. Sprouting capillaries with deficient blood-brain barrier begin
         to surround clot.
      d. Macrophages infiltrate clot periphery, ingest blood degrada-
         tion products.
    2. CT.
      a. Clot attenuation further decreases.
      b. Hematoma is typically hypodense compared with brain.
      c. Periphery enhances following contrast administration.
    3. MR.
      a. T1WI: Hyperintense.
      b. T2WI: Hyperintense.
      c. GRE: Hypointense, "blooms."

III. Chronic hemorrhage (months to years).
  A. Early chronic (months).
    1. Pathology.
      a. Hematoma cavity begins to shrink, and mass effect, edema diminish.
      b. Well-delineated vascularized clot wall surrounds cystic cavity.
      c. Hemosiderin, ferritin-laden macrophages are present in clot wall.
    2. CT.
      a. Cystic fluid collection is low density, resembles CSF.
      b. Rim enhancement diminishes.
    3. MR.
      a. T1WI: Hyperintense cavity, isointense to hypointense wall.
      b. T2WI: Hyperintense cavity, "blooming" of hypointense wall.
      c. GRE: Hypointense, prominent "blooming."
  B. Late chronic (months to years).
    1. Pathology.
      a. Slitlike gliotic scar.
      b. Iron storage products in macrophages.
    2. CT.
      a. May be difficult to discern.
      b. Contrast enhancement typically absent.
    3. MR.
      a. T1WI: Isointense to hypointense.
      b. T2WI: Hypointense (blooming).
      c. GRE: Hypointense (prominent blooming).

SUGGESTED READINGS

Chaney RK, Taber KH, Orrison WW Jr, Hayman LA: Magnetic resonance imaging of intracerebral hemorrhage at different field strengths, *Neuroimag Clin N Amer* 2:25-51, 1992.

Kirkpatrick JB, Hayman LA: Pathophysiology of intracranial hemorrhage, *Neuroimag Clin N Amer* 2:11-23, 1992.

Osborn AG: Intracranial hemorrhage. In *Diagnostic Neuroradiology,* St Louis, 1994, Mosby, pp 154-198.

Pfleger MJ, Hardee EP, Contant CF Jr, Hayman LA: Sensitivity and specificity of fluid-blood levels for coagulopathy in acute intracerebral hematomas, *AJNR* 15:217-223, 1994.

Pierce JN, Taber KH, Hayman LA: Acute intracranial hemorrhage secondary to thrombocytopenia: CT appearances unaffected by absence of clot retraction, *AJNR* 15:213-215, 1994.

20

Craniocerebral Trauma: Primary Manifestations

Key Concepts

1. Primary manifestations of head trauma include skull fractures, extracerebral hematomas, and intraaxial lesions (e.g., cortical contusions, white matter shearing injury).
2. CT scan with both soft tissue and bone detail is the imaging procedure of choice in evaluating patients with acute head injury.
3. Epidural hematomas are almost always unilateral and may cross dural attachments but only rarely cross sutures.
4. Subdural hematomas may be unilateral or bilateral, cross suture lines, but do not extend across dural attachments.
5. Cortical contusion and diffuse axonal injury are the most common primary causes of morbidity in patients with closed head injury.
6. Cranial manifestations of nonaccidental trauma (child abuse) include subdural hematomas of different ages, contusions, shearing injury, retinal hemorrhages, unexplained skull fractures, signs of inflicted skeletal injury.

Trauma is one of the most common causes of death in children and young adults worldwide. Head injury is the major contributor to mortality in at least 50% of these cases. In this chapter we consider the primary manifestations of craniocerebral trauma, including epidural and subdural hematomas, subarachnoid hemorrhage, diffuse axonal ("shearing") injury, and cortical contusions. Secondary effects of head trauma such as herniation syndromes, diffuse cerebral edema, and ischemia are delineated in Chapter 21.

  I. Clinical/imaging considerations in trauma.

    A. Background.

      1. Numerous studies have attempted both to predict outcome based on clinical assessment and determine so-called "high-yield" criteria that are associated with abnormal CT findings.

      2. Optimizing patient selection for emergency neuroimaging procedures remains a controversial topic.

      3. Some authors have shown that variables such as intoxication, antegrade amnesia, and prolonged loss of consciousness helped predict a CT abnormality.

      4. Other investigators report a roughly 10% incidence of intracranial abnormality in patients with only mild head trauma (brief loss of consciousness or amnesia with normal clinical assessment, i.e., Glasgow Coma Scale score of 15).

    B. General recommendation: Because CT is widely available and highly efficacious in depicting treatable lesions such as acute epidural and subdural hematomas, unenhanced cranial CT studies (*not* plain skull films) should be used relatively liberally.

    C. Suggested indications for emergency CT.

      1. Loss of consciousness or amnesia.

      2. Glasgow Coma Scale score <15.

      3. Focal neurologic abnormality.

      4. Intoxication.

      5. Depressed skull fracture/penetrating injury.

      6. Patient age <2 or >60 years (because very young and elderly patients with head trauma have a greater prevalence of abnormal CT findings than patients of other ages).

      7. Bleeding diathesis/anticoagulation.

    D. Suggested standard CT protocol.

      1. Scout view (look for skull/cervical spine fracture).

      2. 5 mm contiguous unenhanced axial scans (foramen magnum to vertex).

      3. Bone and soft tissue reconstruction algorithms.

      4. Photograph both bone, brain level/window settings (some authors also recommend a third or "subdural" setting; if not photographed, the radiologist should examine the images on

the monitor using several intermediate windows and levels).
   E. Optional/additional studies.
      1. Spiral CT of the neck (C1 or C2 fractures present in 5% of cases with substantial head trauma).
      2. Coronal CT scans (if patient's condition permits, cervical spine is normal, and facial/basal skull fractures are suspected).
      3. Contrast-enhanced CT scan (subacute hematoma or unexplained mass effect).
      4. MR scan (especially useful in defining/excluding contusion, axonal shearing injury, small extraaxial fluid collections).
II. Extraaxial traumatic lesions.
   A. Skull fracture.
      1. Types.
         a. Linear.
         b. Depressed.
         c. Diastatic.
      2. Frequency.
         a. Identified on CT scans in approximately two thirds of patients with severe head injury.
         b. Between 25% and 35% of severely traumatized patients have no skull fracture.
      3. Associated lesions.
         a. Fracture crossing middle meningeal artery or dural venous sinus occurs in 85% to 95% of patients with epidural hematoma (see below).
         b. Cervical spine fracture-dislocations are common in patients with severe craniocerebral trauma.
   B. Extraaxial hemorrhage.
      1. Types.
         a. Epidural hematoma.
         b. Subdural hematoma.
         c. Subarachnoid hemorrhage.
   C. Epidural hematoma (EDH) (Fig. 20-1).
      1. Etiology (most common).
         a. Forceful impact to calvarium fractures skull.
         b. Transient depression of skull fragment lacerates dural artery (usually middle meningeal artery).
         c. Blood extravasates from torn vessel, collecting between inner table of skull and outer layer of dura.
         d. As hematoma expands, dura is stripped away from inner table in focal fashion, forming biconvex mass.
      2. Clinical.
         a. Classic "lucid interval" seen in 50%.
         b. May have delayed onset.

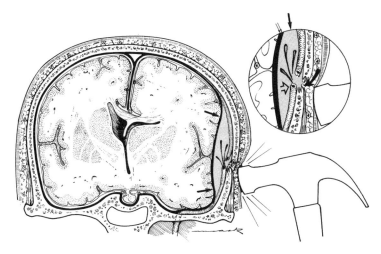

Fig. 20-1   Coronal anatomic diagram depicts formation of epidural hematoma (EDH). Impact typically causes skull fracture (insert, curved black arrow) that lacerates the middle meningeal artery (outlined black arrow). Blood extravasates from the torn artery, stripping the dura (heavy black line, indicated by the double black arrows) away from the inner table of the skull. Blood collects in the epidural space, forming the classic biconvex-shaped EDH (shown as the dotted area indicated by the small black arrows).

3. Incidence.
   a. Identified in <5% of patients imaged for craniocerebral trauma.
   b. Found in 10% of fatal injuries at autopsy.
4. Location.
   a. Between skull, dura.
   b. >95% unilateral.
   c. >95% supratentorial (temporoparietal is most common site).
   d. Crosses dural attachments but rarely crosses sutural lines.
5. CT.
   a. Displays imaging characteristics of extraaxial mass (gray-white matter interface displaced).
   b. Biconvex ("lentiform") shape.
   c. Two thirds hyperdense.
   d. One third may have hypodense foci within hyperdense collection. This represents rapid bleeding with unclotted blood.
6. MR.
   a. Biconvex shape.
   b. Displaced dura well visualized as thin, low-signal line between hematoma and brain.

        c. Signal intensity usually relatively isointense to brain on T1WI; mixed isointense, hyperintense on T2WI.

D. Subdural hematoma (SDH) (Fig. 20-2).

  1. Etiology.

      a. Sudden deceleration, rotation of head causes stretching, tearing of cortical veins as they cross the potential subdural space.

      b. Subacute, chronic SDHs may rebleed from vascularized neomembrane that surrounds the fluid collection.

  2. Incidence, clinical presentation.

      a. Found in 10% to 20% of patients with head injury.

      b. Impaired consciousness, neurologic deficits common.

  3. Location.

      a. Between dura, arachnoid.

      b. Often extensive.

      c. 95% supratentorial, 15% bilateral.

      d. Frontoparietal most common site.

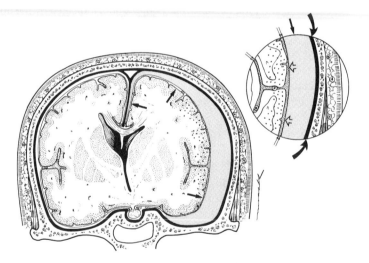

Fig. 20-2 Coronal anatomic diagram depicts acute subdural hematoma (SDH, shown as the crescentic-shaped dotted area and indicated by the small black arrows). An SDH collects between the dura (heavy black line, indicated by the curved arrows) and the arachnoid (outlined arrows). Note that the SDH extends over the convexity into the interhemispheric fissure but does not cross the dural attachment of the falx cerebri. Other lesions that commonly accompany SDH include traumatic subarachnoid hemorrhage (double arrows), cortical contusions (shown as large dots overlying the cortex), and mass effect with subfalcine herniation.

4. CT.
   a. Acute SDH.
      (1) Crescent-shaped.
      (2) 60% hyperdense, 40% mixed hyperdense, hypodense.
   b. Subacute SDH.
      (1) May be isodense with underlying cortex.
      (2) Look for cortical veins, sulci displaced away from inner table of calvarium.
      (3) Neomembrane may enhance with contrast administration.
   c. Chronic SDH.
      (1) May be biconvex, crescentic, multiloculated.
      (2) Low-density but repeated hemorrhage can cause complex pattern.
      (3) Calcification may occur in old, untreated SDHs.
5. MR (variable findings, especially if hemorrhages of differing ages are present).
   a. Hyperacute SDH (<6 hrs).
      (1) T1WI: Isointense compared to cortex.
      (2) T2WI: Isointense/hyperintense.
   b. Acute SDH (1-3 days).
      (1) T1WI: Isointense to hypointense.
      (2) T2WI: Hypointense.
   c. Early subacute SDH (4-7 days).
      (1) T1WI: Hyperintense.
      (2) T2WI: Hypointense.
   d. Late subacute SDH (1-4 weeks).
      (1) T1WI: Hyperintense.
      (2) T2WI: Hyperintense.
   e. Chronic SDH (>1 month).
      (1) T1WI: Variable; usually isointense.
      (2) T2WI: Hyperintense.
      (3) May enhance with contrast.
E. Subarachnoid hemorrhage (SAH).
   1. Prevalence.
      a. Traumatic SAH occurs in most patients with moderate to severe head injury (Fig. 20-2).
   2. Significance.
      a. Outcome worse than that of patients whose initial CT does not show traumatic SAH.
   3. Imaging.
      a. Similar to aneurysmal SAH (high density in cisterns, sulci on NECT scan).

   b. "Pseudodelta" sign (acute subdural or subarachnoid hemorrhage surrounding flowing blood in superior sagittal sinus).
  4. Associated lesions.
   a. Cortical contusion, diffuse axonal injury are often present (see below).
III. Intraaxial traumatic lesions.
 A. Diffuse axonal injury (DAI, also called "shearing" injury) (Fig. 20-3).
  1. Etiology, pathology.
   a. Acceleration/deceleration/rotation forces deform, tear axons and penetrating blood vessels.
   b. Microscopic "retraction balls" form at ends of severed axons.

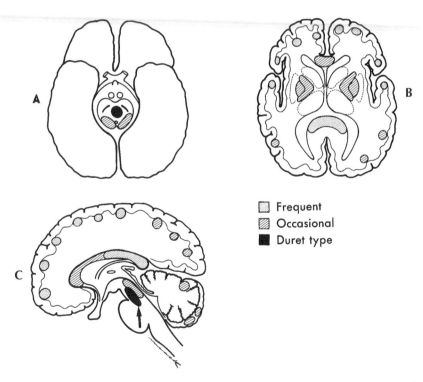

Fig. 20-3 **A** to **C**, Anatomic diagrams depict typical locations of diffuse axonal injury (DAI, or "shearing," injury). Secondary midbrain (Duret) hemorrhage is indicated (black area) in the mesencephalon (**C**, arrow). (From Osborn AG: *Diagnostic neuroradiology,* St Louis, 1994, Mosby.)

2. Incidence, clinical manifestations.
   a. 50% of intraaxial primary traumatic lesions.
   b. Patients typically lose consciousness immediately on impact.
   c. DAI uncommon in absence of severe closed head injury.
3. Location.
   a. Subcortical white matter (especially frontotemporal).
   b. Corpus callosum (splenium most often affected).
   c. Upper brainstem.
   d. Basal ganglia, internal capsule.
4. CT.
   a. Often initially normal.
   b. Petechial hemorrhages in typical locations.
5. MR.
   a. T1WI: Often normal.
   b. T2WI: Multifocal hyperintensities at typical locations.
   c. GRE: May demonstrate hypointense foci.
B. Cortical contusions (Fig. 20-4).
   1. Etiology, pathology.

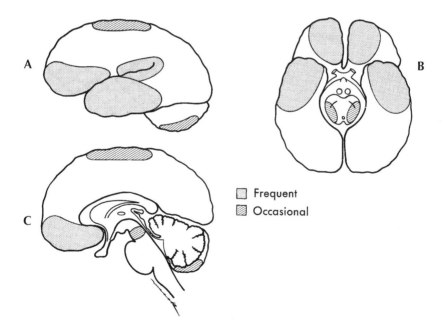

Fig. 20-4   **A** to **C,** Anatomic diagram depicts typical locations of contusional traumatic brain injuries. (From Osborn AG: *Diagnostic neuroradiology,* St Louis, 1994, Mosby.)

        a. Gyral crests impact osseous ridge or dural fold during trauma.

        b. Superficial (cortical) petechial hemorrhages, edema.

    2. Incidence, clinical.

        a. Second most common intraaxial traumatic lesion.

        b. Neurologic impairment varies with extent, association with other lesions (e.g., DAI, SDH).

    3. Location.

        a. Anteroinferior temporal lobes.

        b. Anteroinferior frontal lobes.

        c. Dorsolateral midbrain.

    4. CT.

        a. Often initially normal or subtly abnormal.

        b. Lesions, mass effect evolve with time.

        c. Mixed hyperdense, hypodense patchy foci represent petechial hemorrhage, edema, pulped brain.

        d. Focal SAH in sulci adjacent to contusion is very common.

    5. MR.

        a. T1WI: Mixed isointense, hypointense.

        b. T2WI: Hyperintense (edema); acute hemorrhage is seen as focal hypointense areas along cortical surfaces.

  C. Miscellaneous intraaxial lesions.

    1. Brainstem, deep gray nuclei injuries.

        a. 5% to 10% of primary traumatic lesions.

        b. Causes.

           (1) Shearing injury.

           (2) Impact against tentorial edge causes contusions.

           (3) Sudden craniocaudal brain displacement at time of injury.

    2. Intraventricular, choroid plexus hemorrhage.

        a. IVH in 1% to 5% of closed head injuries.

        b. Usually associated with other severe injuries.

        c. Poor prognosis.

IV. Nonaccidental trauma (child abuse).

  A. Suspect if:

    1. Multiple/complex/bilateral/depressed or unexplained skull fractures.

    2. Subdural hematomas (different ages).

    3. Cortical contusions/shearing injury.

    4. Retinal hemorrhages.

    5. Cerebral ischemia/infarction.

    6. Inflicted skeletal injury.

SUGGESTED READINGS

Dietrich AM, Bowman MJ, Ginn-Pease ME, et al: Pediatric head injuries: Can clinical factors reliably predict an abnormality on computed tomography? *Ann Emerg Med* 22:1535-1540, 1993.

Gean AD: *Imaging of Head Trauma,* New York, 1994, Raven Press.

Kakarieka A, Braakman R, Schakel EH: Clinical significance of the finding of subarachnoid blood on CT scan after head injury, *Acta Neurochir (Wien):* 129:1-5, 1994.

Kleinman PK, Marks SC Jr, Richmond JM, Blackbourne BD: Inflicted skeletal injury: a postmortem radiologic-histopathologic study in 31 infants, *AJR* 165:647-650, 1995.

Link TM, Schuierer G, Hufendiek A, et al: Substantial head trauma: value of routine examination of the cervicocranium, *Radiol* 196:741-745, 1995.

Numerow LM, Fong TC, Wallace CJ: Pseudodelta sign on computed tomography: an indication of bilateral interhemispheric hemorrhage, *Can Assoc Radiol J:* 45:23-27, 1994.

Orrison WW, Gentry LR, Stimac GK, et al: Blinded comparison of cranial CT and MR in closed head injury evaluation, *AJNR* 15:351-356, 1994.

Osborn AG: Craniocerebral trauma. In *Diagnostic Neuroradiology,* St Louis, 1994, Mosby, pp 199-247.

Schynoll W, Overton D, Krome R, et al: A prospective study to identify high-yield criteria associated with acute intracranial computed tomography findings in head-injured patients, *Am J Emerg Med* 11:321-326, 1993.

21

Secondary Effects of Craniocerebral Trauma

Key Concepts

1. Secondary effects of trauma may be more devastating than the primary injuries.
2. Major secondary effects of trauma.
   a. Cerebral herniations.
   b. Traumatic ischemia/infarctions.
   c. Diffuse cerebral edema.
   d. Hypoxia.
3. "Brain death" is a medicolegal concept; imaging studies complement clinical assessment.

Primary cerebral trauma may cause secondary effects that are significant causes of morbidity and mortality. Cerebral herniation syndromes, hypoxic/ischemic injury, and diffuse cerebral edema are discussed in this chapter. The vascular manifestations and complications of craniocerebral trauma are delineated in Chapter 22.

I. Cerebral herniations (Fig. 21-1).
   A. Anatomy, pathology.
      1. After sutures close, skull is a closed space.
      2. Dural folds and bony ridges functionally divide intracranial cavity into compartments.
         a. Supratentorial (two halves).
         b. Infratentorial.
      3. Accumulation of blood, edema causes mass effect that is initially focal (gyral swelling, sulcal effacement).
      4. Further volume increase of affected lobe or hemisphere causes displacement of brain, CSF spaces, blood vessels from one compartment into another.
   B. Classification (see box).
      1. Subfalcine herniation (also known as cingulate, supracallosal, transfalcial herniation).
         a. Most common type.
         b. Pathology.
            (1) Caused by unilateral frontal, parietal, or temporal mass (e.g., epidural or subdural hematoma).
            (2) Brain, accompanying vessels are displaced away from mass below the inferior (free) margin of falx cerebri.
            (3) Contralateral lateral ventricle enlarges (secondary to foramen of Monro obstruction).
         c. Imaging.
            (1) Cingulate gyrus, lateral and third ventricles, anterior cerebral artery (pericallosal branches), internal cerebral veins shifted across midline.
            (2) Rarely, severe herniation may occlude distal ACA (see below).
      2. Descending transtentorial herniation.
         a. Second most common type.
         b. Pathology.
            (1) Early.
               (a) Uncus, parahippocampal gyrus displaced medially over tentorial incisura.
               (b) May cause oculomotor nerve (CN III) compression with loss of light response followed by pupillary

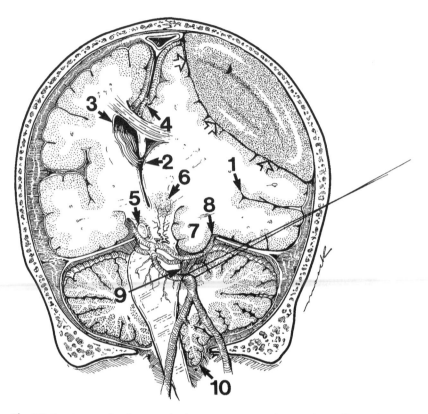

Fig. 21-1   Anatomic diagram depicts some potential secondary effects of a large epidural hematoma (open arrows). 1, Inferior displacement of sylvian fissure, middle cerebral artery branches. 2, Subfalcine herniation of lateral ventricles with compression of ipsilateral ventricle. 3, Contralateral lateral ventricle dilates secondary to functional obstruction at the foramen of Monro. 4, Anterior cerebral arteries (cut across), shifted across the midline by the mass effect, return to midline under the falx cerebri (may cause secondary ACA infarct). 5, Midbrain contusion (Kernohan notch) produced by displacement from the mass effect causing the cerebral peduncle to strike the opposite edge of the tentorial incisura. 6, Midbrain hemorrhage (Duret hemorrhage) caused by downward displacement. 7, Medial temporal lobe herniates over the tentorial incisura (descending transtentorial herniation). 8, Ipsilateral posterior cerebral artery (PCA) is compressed against the tentorial incisura (may cause secondary PCA infarct). 9, Ipsilateral cerebellopontine angle cistern is widened as the brainstem is displaced by the herniating temporal lobe. 10, Descending tonsillar herniation. (From Osborn AG: *Diagnostic neuroradiology,* St Louis, 1994, Mosby.)

Cerebral Herniations

Subfalcine
Transtentorial
  Descending
  Ascending
Transalar (transsphenoidal)
  Descending
  Ascending
Tonsillar
Miscellaneous (e.g., transdural/transcranial)

---

            dilatation (pupilloconstrictor fibers course in superior aspect of nerve).

     (2) Late.

        (a) Herniated brain completely fills suprasellar cistern.

        (b) Midbrain, pons displaced inferiorly.

  c. Imaging.

     (1) Early: lateral aspect of suprasellar, perimesencephalic cisterns subtly effaced.

     (2) Late.

        (a) Suprasellar CSF space obliterated as herniating brain completely plugs incisura.

        (b) Herniating brain displaces midbrain, compresses it against opposite edge of tentorium (may cause "Kernohan notch").

        (c) Sagittal MR shows midbrain, tectum, pons compressed and displaced inferiorly.

        (d) Ipsilateral cerebellopontine angle cistern initially widened.

        (e) Severe herniation may occlude posterior cerebral artery, cause occipital lobe infarct (see below).

  3. Ascending transtentorial herniation.

    a. Much less common than descending type.

    b. Pathology, imaging.

     (1) Posterior fossa mass forces vermis, cerebellar hemispheres superiorly through incisura.

     (2) Quadrigeminal cistern, tectal plate are displaced, deformed.

     (3) Severe herniation may occlude aqueduct, cause obstructive hydrocephalus.

  4. Transalar herniation.

a. Rare.
b. Pathology.
  (1) Large middle fossa mass displaces temporal lobe, middle cerebral artery (MCA) anterosuperiorly over sphenoid wing (ascending transalar herniation).
  (2) Large anterior fossa mass displaces frontal lobe posteroinferiorly over sphenoid wing (descending transalar herniation).
c. Imaging.
  (1) Ascending: temporal lobe, MCA, sylvian fissure displaced up and over sphenoid wing.
  (2) Descending: gyrus rectus displaced inferiorly, MCA displaced posteriorly.

5. Tonsillar herniation.
  a. Common with both severe descending transtentorial herniation and intrinsic posterior fossa masses.
    (1) Two thirds of patients with upward transtentorial herniation have concurrent tonsillar herniation.
    (2) One half of patients with downward transtentorial herniation have concurrent tonsillar herniation.
  b. Pathology: Tonsils forced inferiorly through foramen magnum, obliterating cisterna magna.
  c. Imaging: best demonstrated on sagittal MR.
    (1) Foramen magnum is measured by line extending from basion to opisthion.
    (2) Normal tonsil position relative to foramen magnum (FM) varies with age.
      (a) Approximately 5 mm below FM in first decade.
      (b) Between 3 and 4 mm in older adults.
    (3) Tonsillar herniation.
      (a) 6 mm or more below FM in children.
      (b) 5 mm or more second, third decades.
      (c) 4 mm fourth through eighth decades.
      (d) 3 mm in ninth decade.

II. Cerebral hyperemia, ischemia, infarction.
  A. Cerebral blood flow and metabolism.
    1. Hyperemia occurs in 7% of children with severe head injury.
    2. Inverse correlation exists between cerebral blood flow, intracranial pressure.
    3. Cerebrovascular reactivity may be impaired in most severely injured children.
    4. Focal or regional hyperemia is common adjacent to edematous, pericontusional zones (SPECT).
  B. Cerebral ischemia (often accompanied by cerebral edema).

1. One of the most common sequelae of severe head trauma.
2. Can be focal or global, may cause:
   a. Local vasogenic edema.
   b. Severe anoxia and diffuse cerebral edema (see below).
3. Early changes can be demonstrated by MRS, SPECT, functional MR.
C. Cerebral infarction.
   1. Usually occurs as complication of brain herniations.
   2. Most common site is occipital lobe (with severe descending transtentorial herniation, PCA is compressed against tentorial incisura).
   3. Miscellaneous sites.
      a. Cingulate gyrus (distal ACA is compressed against free edge of falx cerebri).
      b. Basal ganglia (perforating arteries are compressed against skull base with severe descending herniation).
      c. Border zone (watershed), basal ganglionic infarctions may also occur with systemic hypotension.
III. Secondary hemorrhage.
   A. Midbrain ("Duret") hemorrhage.
      1. Central tegmental hemorrhages may occur with severe descending transtentorial herniation.
      2. Caudal brainstem displacement compresses thalamoperforating arteries, causing ischemia, hemorrhage, or both.
      3. Differential diagnosis is brainstem contusion (these are typically dorsolateral, not central).
   B. Peduncular hemorrhage.
      1. Can occur as direct result of brainstem impacting against tentorium during trauma.
      2. May also occur secondary to descending transtentorial herniation.
         a. Herniating temporal lobe displaces midbrain.
         b. Contralateral cerebral peduncle is compressed against tentorial incisura ("Kernohan notch" is term used to describe the indentation on the peduncle caused by the dural edge of the tentorium).
         c. Compression may result in focal ischemia or hemorrhagic necrosis of peduncle.
IV. Cerebral edema.
   A. Some focal edema is common with parenchymal injury (DAI, contusion).
   B. Diffuse cerebral edema with elevated intracranial pressures is life-threatening (50% mortality).
      1. Occurs in 10% to 20% of severe head trauma cases.

2. Occurs at all ages (especially children).
3. Often accompanied by other lesions (subdural or epidural hematoma, contusion) but may occur as isolated event.
C. Imaging.
1. Early.
a. Gyral swelling.
b. Sulcal effacement.
c. Loss of gray matter-white matter interface.
2. Late.
a. Diffuse low attenuation of brain.
b. Generalized effacement of subarachnoid cisterns.
c. Lateral ventricles appear compressed, small.
d. Dural structures (falx, tentorium) and cerebral arteries may appear abnormally prominent (caused by low density brain and should not be mistaken for subarachnoid hemorrhage).
e. Severe edema of hemispheres may cause posterior fossa structures to appear comparatively hyperdense ("cerebellar reversal sign" or "white cerebellum sign").
V. Brain death.
A. Medicolegal term.
1. Irreversible cessation of higher brain function.
2. Definition, documentation varies with jurisdiction.
B. Pathology.
1. Intracranial pressure exceeds intraarterial pressure.
2. Hemispheric blood flow ceases.
C. Imaging.
1. MR and CT show diffuse cerebral edema, severe descending transtentorial herniation.
2. Vascular studies (conventional cerebral angiography, dynamic CECT, transcranial doppler U/S, scintigraphic perfusion studies, MRA) show no flow distal to cavernous internal carotid artery.
3. 99mTc-HMPAO has high specificity, demonstrates no uptake in brain parenchyma.

SUGGESTED READINGS

Gean AD: Brain herniation. In *Imaging of head trauma,* New York, 1994, Raven Press, pp 249-297.

Itoyama Y, Fujioka S, Ushio Y: Kernohan's notch in chronic subdural hematoma: findings on magnetic resonance imaging, *J Neurosurg* 82:645-646, 1995.

Lemmon GW, Franz RW, Roy N, et al: Determination of brain death with use of color duplex scannings in the intensive care unit settings, *Arch Surg* 130:517-520, 1995.

Osborn AG: Secondary effects of craniocerebral trauma. In *Diagnostic neurora-diology,* St Louis, 1994, Mosby, pp 222-247.

Reich JB, Sierra J, Camp W, et al: Magnetic resonance imaging measurements and clinical changes accompanying transtentorial and foramen magnum brain herniation, *Ann Neurol* 33:159-170, 1993.

Sakas, DE, Bullock MR, Patterson J, et al: Focal cerebral hyperemia after focal head trauma in humans: a benign phenomenon? *J Neursurg* 83:277-284, 1995.

Sharples PM, Matthews DSF, Eyre JA: Cerebral blood flow and metabolism in children with severe head injuries. Part 2: cerebrovascular resistance and its determinants, *J Neurol Neurosurg Psychiatr* 58:153-159, 1995.

Sharples PM, Stuart AG, Matthews DSF: Cerebral blood flow and metabolism in children with severe head injury. Part 1: relation to age, Glasgow coma score, outcome, intracranial pressure, and time after injury, *J Neurol Neurosurg Psychiatr* 58:145-152, 1995.

Wijdicks EFM: Determining brain death in adults, *Neurol* 45:1003-1011, 1995.

22

Vascular Effects of Trauma

Key Concepts

1. Primary vascular injuries.
   a. Laceration, intimal tear.
   b. Dissection, transection.
   c. Pseudoaneurysm.
   d. Thrombosis and occlusion.
   e. Arteriovenous fistula.
   f. Dural sinus/cortical vein laceration, occlusion.
2. Secondary vascular effects.
   a. Occlusion caused by cerebral herniations (ACA, PCA, lenticulostriate arteries).
   b. Flow reduction caused by markedly increased intracranial pressure.

Craniocerebral trauma may injure the cerebral arteries as well as damage the dural sinuses and cortical veins (see box). These injuries can be direct or indirect, primary or secondary. Direct causes include both blunt trauma and penetrating injury. In this chapter we focus on the most important primary vascular injuries: arterial dissection, traumatic aneurysm, and arteriovenous fistula. Secondary vascular effects such as vascular occlusion induced by cerebral herniation syndromes and flow reduction caused by markedly increased intracranial pressure are considered in Chapter 21.

I. Arterial dissections.
   A. Pathology (Fig. 22-1).
      1. Arterial wall continuity is disrupted.
      2. Hematoma forms in or around vessel.
      3. Dissection occurs as blood splits vessel layers and creates a false lumen.
   B. Etiology.
      1. Penetrating injury (gunshot wound, knife, other sharp objects such as pencil or sticks).

Vascular Manifestations and Complications of Craniocerebral Trauma

Primary Injuries
   Arterial
      Transection
      Laceration
      Subintimal tear
      Dissection
      Pseudoaneurysm
      Thrombosis
      Arteriovenous fistula
   Venous
      Cortical vein rupture/thrombosis
      Dural sinus laceration/thrombosis
Secondary Injuries
   Arterial
      Occlusion, infarction secondary to herniation
      Vasospasm
      "Brain death" secondary to massively elevated ICP
   Venous
      Thrombosis
      Venous infarction

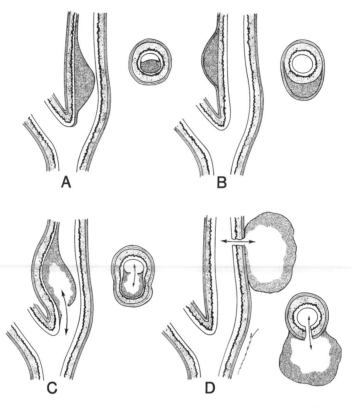

Fig. 22-1 Anatomic diagrams compare carotid artery dissection, dissecting aneurysm, and pseudoaneurysm. Both lateral and cross-sectional views are illustrated. **(A),** Typical *subintimal dissection* is shown. The subintimal hematoma is indicated by the heavily dotted area. **(B),** A *subadventitial dissection* is less common. Note the paravascular hematoma is external to the media and under the intima. Vessel lumen may be normal in such cases, and conventional angiography can appear unremarkable. **(C),** If the intima overlying a typical dissection ruptures, a communication between the hematoma and the vessel lumen is created. This produces a true *dissecting aneurysm*. Angiography typically discloses an outpouching that communicates with the narrowed lumen. **(D),** A complete vessel wall laceration may cause a paravascular hematoma to develop. The hematoma contains no layers of the parent vessel wall. If the paravascular hematoma then cavitates and a connection is created between the hematoma cavity and vessel lumen, a *pseudoaneurysm* is formed.

2. Nonpenetrating injury.
   a. Spine fracture.
      (1) Cervical fracture may injure vertebral artery (24% on MR angiography).
3. Blunt trauma (hyperextension, lateral flexion).
   a. Athletic activity (e.g., wrestling).
   b. Chiropractic manipulation.
   c. Deceleration injury.
   d. Violent sneezing.
4. Miscellaneous causes of arterial dissection.
   a. Spontaneous (no underlying abnormality).
   b. Underlying vasculopathy (fibromuscular dysplasia, Marfan syndrome).
   c. Pharyngeal infection.
   d. Drug abuse.
   e. Trivial trauma (coughing, sneezing, nose blowing, head turning).
C. Clinical presentation.
   1. Penetrating injury.
      a. Physical examination can exclude injury in over 99% of patients with penetrating neck wounds.
      b. Arteriography is sensitive but has very low yield (1% to 2%).
   2. Blunt trauma.
      a. May be asymptomatic.
      b. Symptom onset may be delayed (typically a few days up to 2 or 3 weeks).
      c. Symptoms.
         (1) Neck pain.
         (2) Stroke (usually caused by distal cerebral emboli).
         (3) Postganglionic Horner's syndrome.
D. Location.
   1. Internal carotid artery.
      a. Bulb usually spared.
      b. Mid to distal extracranial ICA is most common site with blunt trauma, deceleration injury.
      c. Cavernous ICA can be injured with skull base fracture.
      d. Supraclinoid ICA is a rare site but can occur, especially in children with closed head injury.
   2. Vertebral artery.
      a. Most common site is between C2, skull base.
      b. Midsegment VA injury may occur with cervical spine fractures that involve foramen transversarium.
      c. Proximal segment (aortic arch to C6) is uncommon.

E. Imaging.
   1. Angiography (conventional, CTA, MRA) shows smooth or irregularly narrowed, tapered lumen.
   2. MR shows blood in false lumen, paravascular hematoma.

II. Traumatic aneurysm.
   A. Pathology (Fig. 22-1).
      1. Dissecting intramural hematoma extends towards adventitia with focal aneurysmal dilatation (*Note:* The term "dissecting aneurysm" should be applied only to a dissection with a projection from the lumen that extends beyond the normal vessel boundaries. If no projection is present, the simple term "dissection" should be used).
      2. Most traumatic aneurysms are actually pseudoaneurysms, that is, they are formed when cavitation of a paravascular hematoma communicates with the parent vessel lumen.
      3. Pseudoaneurysms are not contained by normal components of the vessel wall.
   B. Incidence.
      1. Trauma accounts for less than 1% of all intracranial aneurysms.
      2. Extracranial traumatic aneurysms are common.
   C. Etiology.
      1. Penetrating trauma.
         a. Gunshot wound (50% prevalence of major vascular injury).
         b. Knife, pencil, other sharp objects.
      2. Nonpenetrating trauma.
         a. Skull fracture (>50% of traumatic aneurysms have associated skull fracture).
         b. Blunt trauma.
         c. Closed head injury (e.g., artery impacts against dura).
   D. Location.
      1. Extracranial.
         a. Skull base (at exocranial opening of carotid canal) is most common site.
      2. Intracranial.
         a. Cavernous sinus (skull fracture, residuum from carotid-cavernous fistula).
         b. Distal ACA (artery is lacerated by impaction against falx cerebri).
         c. Cortical arteries adjacent to skull fracture (approximately 50% of cases involve distal middle cerebral artery branches).
   E. Imaging.
      1. Delayed traumatic intracranial hemorrhage suggests presence of traumatic aneurysm.

      2. Conventional angiography shows aneurysm.

      3. Subacute hematoma may obscure lesion on MR, 3D TOF MRA.

III. Arteriovenous fistulae.

  A. Etiology.

      1. Arterial dissection or laceration.

      2. Spontaneous communication between injured artery, adjacent dural sinus or vein develops.

  B. Location.

      1. Cavernous sinus (carotid-cavernous fistula).

      2. Below petrous temporal bone (internal carotid artery-jugular vein).

      3. Foramen magnum (skull base-C1, C1-C2 vertebral artery-occipital veins).

      4. Squamous temporal bone (middle meningeal artery-vein AVF).

IV. Venous injuries.

  A. Thrombosis.

      1. Etiology, pathology.

         a. Depressed skull fracture.

         b. Laceration with compression from venous epidural hematoma.

         c. May have associated cortical vein thrombosis, venous infarct.

      2. Imaging.

         a. NECT: high density in affected sinus, vein; may have associated cortical/subcortical hemorrhage (caution: flowing blood in patent vascular structures is normally somewhat hyperdense compared with adjacent brain).

         b. CECT: "Empty delta sign" (enhancing dural wall surrounds nonenhancing thrombus).

         c. "Pseudo empty delta sign": NECT scan with high-density subarachnoid or subdural blood outlines dural sinus.

         d. MR/MR venography demonstrates clot.

  B. Laceration.

      1. Etiology.

         a. Depressed or linear skull fracture that crosses major venous sinus.

         b. Tearing of meningeal or diploic veins.

         c. Penetrating injury.

      2. Imaging.

         a. Adjacent epidural hematoma near.

            (1) Torcular Herophili.

            (2) Transverse sinus.

         b. MR, MR venography, conventional angiography may demonstrate laceration.

SUGGESTED READINGS

Beitsch P, Weigelt JA, Flynn E, Easley S: Physical examination and arteriography in patients with penetrating zone II neck wounds, *Arch Surg* 129:577-581, 1994.

Freidman D, Flanders A, Thomas C, Millar W: Vertebral artery injury after acute cervical spine trauma: rate of occurrence as detected by MR angiography and assessment of clinical consequences, *AJR* 164:443-447, 1995.

Gean AD: Vascular injury. In *Imaging of head trauma,* pp 299-366, 1994.

Holmes B, Harbaugh RE: Traumatic intracranial aneurysms: a contemporary review, *J Trauma* 35:855-860, 1993.

Jinkins JR, Dadsetan MR, Sener RN, et al: Value of acute-phase angiography in the detection of vascular injuries caused by gunshot wounds to the head, *AJR* 159:365-368, 1992.

Osborn AG: Vascular manifestations and complications of craniocerebral trauma. In *Diagnostic neuroradiology,* St Louis, 1994, Mosby, pp 232-247.

Pretre R, Reverdin A, Kalonji T, Faidutti B: Blunt carotid artery injury: difficult therapeutic approaches for an underrecognized entity, *Surgery* 115:375-381, 1994.

Tulyapronchote R, Selhorst JB, Malkoff MD, Gomez CR: Delayed sequelae of vertebral artery dissection and occult cervical fractures, *Neurol* 44:1397-1399, 1994.

23

Nontraumatic Intracranial Hemorrhage

Key Concepts

1. Primary intracranial hemorrhage (ICH) causes 10% to 13% of "strokes."
2. Hypertension causes between 70% and 90% of all nontraumatic intracerebral hematomas.
3. Important causes of ICH by age group.
   a. Premature neonate: germinal matrix hemorrhage.
   b. Term neonate: traumatic delivery.
   c. Young, middle-aged adults: Aneurysm, vascular malformation, drug abuse, pregnancy complication.
   d. Elderly adult: hypertensive ICH, amyloid angiopathy, hemorrhagic infarction.
4. Dural sinus or venous occlusion is rare but underdiagnosed, important cause of nontraumatic ICH.

Craniocerebral trauma is the most common overall cause of intracranial hemorrhage (ICH). However, there are numerous nontraumatic lesions that may produce ICH as either their primary or secondary imaging manifestation (see box below). Spontaneous ICH is relatively common, accounting for between 10% and 13% of all "strokes." In this chapter we briefly summarize and discuss the nontraumatic causes of intracerebral hemorrhage.

I. Perinatal hemorrhage.
   A. Premature infants.
      1. Periventricular-intraventricular hemorrhage (PVH-IVH).
         a. Incidence.
            (1) 25% to 40% in infants <1500g, <32 weeks' gestation.
         b. Pathogenesis.
            (1) Germinal matrix contains fragile arteries and capillaries, thin-walled veins, proliferating neuronal precursors.
            (2) Germinal matrix involutes between 34 and 36 gestational weeks.
            (3) Hypoxia may cause hypertension and subsequent rupture of vessels (arteries or veins) within the germinal matrix.

Etiology of Nontraumatic Intracranial Hemorrhage

Most common
   Hypertension (especially older adults)
   Aneurysm
   Vascular malformation (especially AVM, cavernous angioma)
   Premature infants
Common
   Embolic stroke with reperfusion
   Amyloid angiopathy
   Coagulopathies/blood dyscrasias
   Drug abuse
   Tumor (primary or metastatic)
Uncommon
   Venous infarct
   Eclampsia
   Herpes encephalitis
   Vasculitis (especially fungal)
   Sepsis, emboli
Rare
   Abscess (unless immunocompromised)
   Vasculitis (nonfungal)

   c. Timing: The germinal matrix involutes between 34 and 36
      gestational weeks. Therefore:
      (1) Germinal matrix hemorrhages are characteristic of im-
          mature brain.
      (2) Germinal matrix hemorrhages are very uncommon in
          term infants.
      (3) Germinal matrix hemorrhages almost never occur
          beyond the first 4 weeks of life (90% occur by day 6).
   d. Imaging.
      (1) Transcranial ultrasound shows subependymal, intraven-
          tricular hyperechoic foci.
      (2) Germinal matrix hemorrhages are graded from I (con-
          fined to one or both germinal matrices) to IV (large
          parenchymal hemorrhages; may be secondary to ische-
          mia).
2. Periventricular leukomalacia (PVL).
   a. Incidence.
      (1) 7% to 22% of premature infants at autopsy.
      (2) 29% to 58% of premature infants with PVH-IVH.
   b. Etiology and pathogenesis.
      (1) Vascular watershed zone of developing fetus is in the
          periventricular white matter.
      (2) Ischemic infarct causes coagulation necrosis of deep
          periventricular white matter.
      (3) Subsequent cavitation occurs; hemorrhage is found in up
          to 20% of cases.
   c. Imaging.
      (1) Early: U/S shows increased echogenecity along lateral
          ventricles from frontal horns to trigone.
      (2) Late: cystic changes.
B. Term infants.
   1. Incidence: ICH less common compared with premature infants.
   2. Location: usually extraaxial or cortical.
   3. Etiology.
      a. Traumatic delivery.
         (1) Scalp edema, subgaleal hemorrhage.
         (2) Cephalohematoma.
         (3) Subdural hematoma.
      b. Hypoxic-ischemic injury.
         (1) Can be prenatal, perinatal, or postnatal.
         (2) Deep gray nuclei may show T1 shortening on MR scans.
         (3) Perirolandic hemorrhage may cause T2 shortening.

II. Young, middle-aged adults.
   A. Aneurysm (see Chapter 35).
      1. Acute SAH.
         a. Incidence: Between 80% and 90% of acute nontraumatic subarachnoid hemorrhage (SAH) is caused by aneurysm rupture.
         b. Imaging.
            (1) Acute SAH appears as high density in CSF spaces (especially suprasellar cistern, interhemispheric fissure) on NECT scans.
            (2) Hydrocephalus (extraventricular) may occur relatively quickly.
            (3) Acute SAH is isointense with brain on T1-weighted MR scans and appears slightly hyperintense on long TR/short TE ("proton density-weighted") sequences.
            (4) Visualization of SAH may be improved by using special MR pulse sequences such as fluid attenuated inversion recovery ("FLAIR").
      2. Chronic SAH (superficial siderosis).
         a. Pathology: leptomeningeal, subpial hemosiderin deposition.
         b. Etiology: bleeding source found in only 50% of autopsies (may be trauma, tumor, vascular malformation, aneurysm).
         c. Imaging: very hypointense lines along brain, spinal cord, cranial nerves.
   B. Vascular malformations (see Chapter 36).
      1. Pathology.
         a. Arteriovenous malformation (pial).
            (1) Usually solitary.
            (2) Hemorrhage rate 2% to 3% per year, cumulative.
            (3) Usually causes parenchymal hemorrhage.
         b. Cavernous angioma.
            (1) Often multiple.
            (2) Hemorrhage rate estimated 0.5% to 1.0% per year.
            (3) Most common vascular malformation associated with other types of vascular malformations (e.g., venous angioma).
            (4) MR typically shows mixed-signal foci within low signal rim.
         c. Venous "angioma."
            (1) Developmental anomaly of white matter veins, not true vascular malformation.
            (2) Usually solitary.

(3) Rarely hemorrhage unless associated with other malformation (e.g., cavernous angioma).

C. Hemorrhagic infarction (HI) (see Chapter 37).

1. Arterial.
   a. HI typically occurs as hemorrhagic transformation of initially ischemic ("bland") infarct (see Chapter 37).
   b. Basal ganglia, cortical gray matter most common sites.
   c. May occur as complication of pregnancy, contraceptives, drug abuse.

2. Venous infarction (see Chapter 40).
   a. Cortical vein thrombosis causes patchy hemorrhagic infarction.
   b. Subcortical white matter most common site.
   c. Often (but not always) occurs with dural sinus occlusion.
   d. May occur as complication of pregnancy, contraceptives, drug abuse.

D. Hypertension.

1. Hypertensive intracranial hemorrhage (see below).

2. Hypertensive encephalopathies.
   a. Preeclampsia/eclampsia.
   b. Renal failure.
   c. Systemic lupus erythematosus.
   d. Hemolytic-uremic syndrome.
   e. Some neurotoxins (e.g., cyclosporine).

E. Hemorrhagic neoplasms, cysts (see below).

III. Elderly adults.

A. Hypertensive intracerebral hemorrhage.

1. Prevalence.
   a. Most common cause of nontraumatic ICH in adults.
   b. Accounts for 70% to 90% of nontraumatic ICH.

2. Etiology.
   a. May be caused by rupture of lenticulostriate artery microaneurysm (Charcot-Bouchard aneurysm).
   b. Caution.
      (1) Only one third to one half of patients with lobar ICHs have hypertension (look for other etiologies such as neoplasm, vascular malformation).
      (2) Aneurysm or AVM is cause of deep (basal ganglionic) hemorrhage in 13% of hypertensive patients.

3. Location.
   a. Putamen/external capsule most common site (60% to 65%).
   b. Thalamus (15% to 20%).

  c. Pons (5% to 10%).
  d. Cerebellum (2% to 5%).
  e. Hemispheric white matter (1% to 2%).
4. Imaging.
  a. NECT.
    (1) High-density mass in basal ganglia.
    (2) May rupture into adjacent lateral ventricle, cause hydro-cephalus.
  b. MR.
    (1) Depends on age of clot (see Chapter 19).
    (2) Old hemorrhages appear as slitlike low-signal cavities.
B. Cerebral amyloid angiopathy (CAA).
  1. Incidence.
    a. Common cause of nontraumatic ICH in normotensive elderly.
    b. May account for up to 10% to 15% of nontraumatic ICHs in patients over 60.
    c. May cause 20% of lobar ICHs in patients >70 years.
  2. Pathology.
    a. Amyloid protein deposited in cortical, leptomeningeal vessel walls.
    b. Thickened vessels stain with Congo red.
    c. Increased vascular fragility may cause lobar parenchymal hemorrhages.
  3. Imaging.
    a. Corticomedullary junction, lobar hemorrhages.
    b. Often multiple, different ages.
    c. Spares basal ganglia, brainstem.
C. Hemorrhagic infarction (see above).
D. Coagulopathies.
  1. Etiology.
    a. Complication of medication (anticoagulation or chemo-therapy).
    b. Blood dyscrasias.
    c. Systemic malignancy.
  2. Imaging.
    a. Intracerebral hematoma with fluid-blood level.
      (1) 60% sensitive to presence of coagulopathy.
      (2) 98% specific for coagulopathy.
E. Neoplasms.
  1. Incidence.
    a. 1% to 11% of nontraumatic parenchymal ICHs caused by neoplasm.

    b. <0.5% of nontraumatic SAH caused by neoplasm.

    c. Hemorrhage occurs in 10% of neoplasms.

    d. Primary and metastatic tumors bleed with approximately equal frequency.

  2. Pathology.

    a. Primary brain tumors that commonly hemorrhage.

      (1) Anaplastic astrocytoma.

      (2) Glioblastoma multiforme.

      (3) Pituitary adenoma.

    b. Primary tumors that less commonly hemorrhage.

      (1) Meningioma.

    c. Primary brain tumors that rarely hemorrhage.

      (1) Low-grade astrocytoma.

      (2) Schwannoma.

    d. Metastatic tumors that commonly hemorrhage.

      (1) Melanoma.

      (2) Choriocarcinoma.

      (3) Renal cell carcinoma.

      (4) Lung, breast metastases may also cause hemorrhage.

    e. Metastatic tumors that uncommonly hemorrhage.

      (1) Gastrointestinal malignancy.

  3. Imaging of benign versus neoplastic hemorrhage.

    a. Benign hemorrhage typically undergoes orderly evolution (see Chapter 19), has well-defined complete hemosiderin rim; often multiple.

    b. Neoplastic hemorrhage often more bizarre appearance, incomplete rim, may show nonhemorrhagic areas that enhance after contrast administration; usually solitary (unless caused by hemorrhagic metastases).

SUGGESTED READINGS

Brady AP, Stack JP: Case report: magnetic resonance demonstration of haemorrhagic acoustic neuroma, *Clin Radiol* 49:61-63, 1994.

Halpin SFS, Britton JA, Byrne JV et al: Prospective evaluation of cerebral angiography and computed tomography in cerebral haematoma, *J Neurol Neurosurg Psychiatr* 57:1180-1186, 1994.

Komiyama M, Yasui T, Tamura K, et al: Simultaneous bleeding from multiple lenticulostriate arteries in hypertensive intracerebral haemorrhage, *Neuroradiol* 37:129-130, 1995.

Lazaro CM, Guo WY, Sami M et al: Haemorrhagic pituitary tumors, *Neuroradiol* 36:111-114, 1994.

Noguchi K, Ogawa T, Inugami A, et al: Acute subarachnoid hemorrhage: MR imaging with fluid-attenuated inversion recovery pulse sequences, *Radiol* 196:773-777, 1995.

Osborn AG: Intracranial hemorrhage. In *Diagnostic neuroradiology,* St Louis, 1994, Mosby, pp 154-198.

Pfleger MJ, Hardee EP, Contant CF Jr, Hayman LA: Sensitivity and specificity of fluid-blood levels for coagulopathy in acute intracerebral hematomas, *AJNR* 15:217-223, 1994.

Phytinen J, Paakko E, Ilkko E: Superficial siderosis in the central nervous system, *Neuroradiol* 37:127-128, 1995.

Schwartz RB, Bravo SM, Klufas RA, et al: Cyclosporine neurotoxicity and its relationship to hypertensive encephalopathy, *AJR* 165:627-631, 1995.

Vinters HV, Duckwiler GR: Intracranial hemorrhage in the normotensive elderly patient, *Neuroimag Clin N Amer* 2:153-169, 1992.

SECTION IV

Intracranial Neoplasms and Tumor-like Lesions

24

Classification

Key Concepts

1. Intracranial neoplasms are classified according to histology.
2. Current most widely used scheme is the World Health Organization (WHO) classification.
3. Brain tumors can be grouped by prevalence: approximately two thirds are primary and one third are metastatic.
4. Primary CNS neoplasms are divided into two general groups: glial and nonglial tumors.
5. Neoplasms can also be grouped into adult and pediatric tumors, as well as by location.

I. Classification by histology.
  A. Neuronal tumors.
    1. Olfactory neuroblastoma or esthesioneuroblastoma.
  B. Glial tumors (gliomas).
    1. Astrocytoma.
    2. Oligodendroglioma.
    3. Ependymoma.
    4. Choroid plexus tumors.
    5. Mixed gliomas.
  C. Mixed neuronal-glial tumors.
    1. Ganglioglioma, gangliocytoma.
    2. Central neurocytoma.
    3. Dysembryoplastic neuroepithelial tumor.
    4. Desmoplastic infantile ganglioglioma.
  D. Primitive neurectodermal tumors (PNET).
    1. Primary cerebral neuroblastoma (cerebral PNET).
    2. Medulloblastoma (posterior fossa PNET).
    3. Pineoblastoma.
    4. Retinoblastoma.
    5. Olfactory neuroblastoma or esthesioneuroblastoma.
    6. Ependymoblastoma.
    7. Medulloepithelioma.
  E. Tumors of embryonal remnants (developmental or malformative tumors).
    1. Epidermoid, dermoid.
    2. Craniopharyngioma, Rathke's cleft cyst.
    3. Colloid cyst.
    4. Lipoma.
    5. Hamartoma.
  F. Germ cell tumors.
    1. Germinoma.
    2. Teratoma.
    3. Embryonal carcinoma.
    4. Yolk sac tumor (endodermal sinus tumor).
    5. Choriocarcinoma.
    6. Mixed germ cell tumors.
  G. Pineal parenchymal tumors.
    1. Pineoblastoma.
    2. Pineocytoma.
  H. Pituitary neuroendocrine tumors.
    1. Pituitary adenoma.
    2. Pituitary adenocarcinoma.
  I. Nerve sheath tumors.

      1. Schwannoma.

      2. Neurofibroma.

  J. Meningothelial tumors.

      1. Meningioma.

  K. Reticuloendothelial tumors.

      1. Lymphoma.

      2. Leukemia.

      3. Plasmacytoma, multiple myeloma.

      4. Langerhans cell histiocytosis.

  L. Mesenchymal tumors.

      1. Hemangiopericytoma.

      2. Hemangioblastoma.

      3. Miscellaneous benign mesenchymal tumors.

      4. Sarcomas.

  M. Metastatic tumors.

II. Classification by prevalence (Fig. 24-1).

  A. Primary brain tumors: two thirds of intracranial neoplasms.

      1. Gliomas: most common group of primary neoplasms: 45% to 50%.

         a. Astrocytoma: 35% to 40% (75% of gliomas).

         b. Oligodendroglioma: 2% (5% of gliomas).

         c. Ependymoma: 3% (7% of gliomas).

         d. Choroid plexus tumors: <1% (3% of pediatric brain neoplasms).

      2. Meningioma: 15%.

      3. Pituitary adenoma: 10%.

      4. Medulloblastoma: 6%.

      5. Schwannoma: 6%.

      6. Craniopharyngioma: 3%.

      7. Pineal tumors: 1%.

      8. Primary CNS lymphoma: 1%.

      9. Hemangioblastoma: 1%.

    10. Other: 5% to 10%.

  B. Metastatic tumors: one third of intracranial neoplasms.

      1. Location.

         a. Parenchyma: most common, tend to occur at gray-white junction.

         b. Leptomeninges: more common with CNS dissemination of primary CNS tumors, usually diffuse or multifocal.

         c. Dura: less common, usually associated with calvarial metastasis.

         d. Calvarium: common.

      2. Etiology (in descending order of frequency).

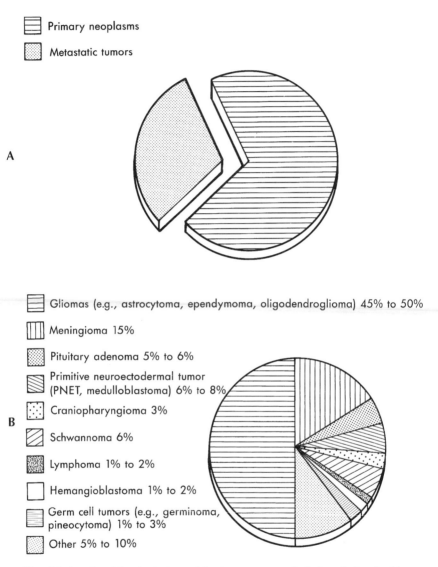

Primary neoplasms

Metastatic tumors

A

Gliomas (e.g., astrocytoma, ependymoma, oligodendroglioma) 45% to 50%

Meningioma 15%

Pituitary adenoma 5% to 6%

Primitive neuroectodermal tumor
(PNET, medulloblastoma) 6% to 8%

Craniopharyngioma 3%

B

Schwannoma 6%

Lymphoma 1% to 2%

Hemangioblastoma 1% to 2%

Germ cell tumors (e.g., germinoma,
pineocytoma) 1% to 3%

Other 5% to 10%

Fig. 24-1   Graphic depiction of brain tumors and their relative incidence.
A, Primary neoplasms account for approximately two thirds of all brain tumors;
metastases from extracranial primary malignancies account for the remainder.
B, Incidence of common primary brain tumors. Gliomas are the largest single group
of primary brain tumors, and astrocytomas are the most frequently encountered
glioma. High-grade astrocytomas (anaplastic astrocytoma and glioblastoma multiforme) are the most common of all primary cerebral neoplasms. (From Osborn
AG: *Diagnostic neuroradiology,* St Louis, 1994, Mosby.)

a. Lung: 45%.

b. Breast: 15%.

c. Melanoma: 10% to 15%.

d. GI/GU: 10% to 15%.

III. Classification by age and general location.

A. Adult.

1. General.

a. 80% to 85% of all intracranial neoplasms occur in adults.

b. Primary (2/3) > metastatic (1/3).

c. Metastases more common in adults than children.

d. Increasing age correlates with increasing malignancy.

2. Location.

a. Supratentorial (3/4).

(1) Common.

(a) Astrocytoma (anaplastic, GBM).

(b) Meningioma.

(c) Pituitary adenoma.

(d) Oligodendroglioma.

(e) Metastases.

(2) Uncommon.

(a) Lymphoma.

(3) Rare.

(a) Ependymoma.

b. Infratentorial (1/4).

(1) Common.

(a) Schwannoma.

(b) Meningioma.

(c) Epidermoid.

(d) Metastases.

(2) Uncommon.

(a) Hemangioblastoma.

(b) Brainstem glioma.

(3) Rare.

(a) Choroid plexus papilloma.

B. Pediatric.

1. General.

a. 15% to 20% of all intracranial neoplasms occur in children.

b. 15% of all pediatric neoplasms are intracranial.

c. CNS tumors are the second most common pediatric neoplasm (after leukemia).

d. Most intracranial neoplasms are primary.

e. CNS metastases are rare.

(1) 6% from extracranial non-CNS neoplasms.

(2) CNS dissemination of primary intracranial neoplasm more common (medulloblastoma, ependymoma, choroid plexus tumors, germinoma, cerebral PNET, pineoblastoma or high-grade astrocytoma).

2. Less than 2 years of age: intracranial neoplasm rare (1% to 2%).

a. Etiology: most are probably congenital.

b. Histology: tumors tend to be large, highly malignant.

(1) Astrocytoma (usually anaplastic or GBM).

(2) PNETs.

(3) Teratoma.

(4) Choroid plexus tumors.

c. Location: supratentorial (⅔) > infratentorial (⅓).

3. Children over 2 years of age.

a. Histology.

(1) Astrocytomas (pilocytic or low grade fibrillary): 50%.

(2) PNETs: 15%.

(3) Ependymoma: 10%.

(4) Craniopharyngioma: 10%.

(5) Pineal region tumors: 3%.

b. Location.

(1) Supratentorial (50% to 70%).

(a) Astrocytomas (low-grade fibrillary, pilocytic): 45% to 50%.

(b) Craniopharyngioma: 12%.

(c) Opticochiasmatic-hypothalamic glioma: 12%.

(d) Choroid plexus papilloma: 12%.

(e) Ependymoma: 10%.

(f) Pineal region tumors: 5%.

(g) Others: rare.

(2) Infratentorial (30% to 50%).

(a) Cerebellar astrocytomas (pilocytic > fibrillary): 25% to 30%.

(b) Medulloblastoma: 25% to 30%.

(c) Brainstem glioma: 15% to 25%.

(d) Ependymoma: 12% to 15%.

SUGGESTED READINGS

Burger PC, Scheithauer BW: *Atlas of tumor pathology (third series, fascicle 10),* Washington, 1994, Armed Forces Institute of Pathology.

Kleihues P, Burger PC, Scheithauer BW: The new WHO classification of brain tumours, *Brain Pathol* 3:255-268, 1993.

Osborn AG: Brain tumors and tumor-like masses: classification and differential diagnosis. In *Diagnostic Radiology,* St Louis, 1994, Mosby, pp 399-528.

Russell DS, Rubinstein LJ: *Pathology of tumors of the nervous system,* ed 5, Baltimore, 1989, Williams and Wilkins.

25

Astrocytoma

Key Concepts

1. Glial tumors (gliomas) include:
   a. Astrocytomas.
   b. Oligodendrogliomas.
   c. Ependymomas.
   d. Choroid plexus tumors.
2. Gliomas constitute the most common primary intracranial neoplasms (45% to 50%); 75% are astrocytomas, of which half are glioblastoma multiforme (GBM) and one quarter are anaplastic.
3. Astrocytomas can be divided into two general groups: diffuse and circumscribed.
4. Diffusely infiltrating astrocytomas are most often fibrillary, less commonly protoplasmic or gemistocytic.
5. Fibrillary astrocytomas are classified as low-grade, anaplastic, or glioblastoma multiforme (GBM).
6. Diffuse fibrillary astrocytomas are generally tumors of adults and are situated in deep cerebral hemispheres or gray/white junction. Increasing age generally correlates with higher grade and worse prognosis.
7. Diffuse fibrillary astrocytomas in children usually involve the brainstem, particularly the pons.

I. Neuroglial tissue: general comments.
   A. Normal glia.
      1. Astrocytes.
         a. Types and location.
            (1) Fibrous or fibrillary: normal mature stellate astrocyte; mainly white matter.
            (2) Protoplasmic: normal mature stellate astrocyte; mainly gray matter.
            (3) Gemistocytic: large reactive astrocyte with abundant cytoplasm; normally at sites of injury.
            (4) Pilocytic: thin elongated reactive astrocyte; laid down along major white matter tracts.
         b. Function.
            (1) Developmental lattice, mechanical support.
            (2) Do not generate/propagate impulses; probably augment neuronal functions.
            (3) Formation of reactive scar tissue in response to injury.
      2. Oligodendrocytes.
         a. Location: white matter (WM) > gray matter (GM).
         b. Function: production, maintenance of CNS myelin.
      3. Ependymal cells.
         a. Location.
            (1) Line ventricles, central canal of cord.
            (2) Modified ependyma in choroid plexus.
         b. Function: secretion, transport of CSF.
      4. Microglial cells.
         a. Location: ubiquitous, migratory.
         b. Function: phagocytosis; activated in response to injury.
   B. Gliomas: most common group of primary intracranial neoplasms (45% to 50%).
         a. Astrocytomas: 75% of gliomas; 35% to 40% of primary neoplasms.
         b. Oligodendrogliomas: 6% of gliomas; 2% of primary neoplasms.
         c. Ependymomas: 8% of gliomas; 2% to 3% of primary neoplasms.
         d. Choroid plexus tumors: 1% to 3% of gliomas; <1% of primary neoplasms.
II. Astrocytic tumors: general comments.
   A. Histology.
      1. Types.
         a. Astrocytoma: (fibrillary, protoplasmic, gemistocytic).
         b. Pilocytic astrocytoma.

      c. Pleomorphic xanthoastrocytoma (PXA).

      d. Subependymal giant cell astrocytoma.

  2. Immunopositive for glial fibrillary acidic protein (GFAP) and S-100 protein.

B. Grading.

  1. Traditional: previously (Kernohan-Sayer) four-tiered, based on degree of "dedifferentiation" but no distinction between low-grade fibrillary and pilocytic astrocytomas under Grade I.

  2. Current.

    a. New WHO classification: still four categories but essentially three-tiered for fibrillary astrocytoma, sometimes designated by numerator/denominator system (e.g., anaplastic astrocytoma = grade 2/3 or II/III).

      (1) Grade I: reserved for specific circumscribed tumors (e.g., pilocytic astrocytoma).

      (2) Grade II (low grade): nuclear atypia.

      (3) Grade III (anaplastic): nuclear atypia, mitoses, and no necrosis.

      (4) Grade IV (GBM): nuclear atypia, mitoses, endothelial proliferation, and/or necrosis.

    b. Daumas-Daport (St. Anne/Mayo) classification: generally reserved for diffuse or fibrillary astrocytoma; based on presence of four variables (nuclear atypia, mitoses, endothelial proliferation, and necrosis).

      (1) Grade 1: absence of above features.

      (2) Grade 2: one variable.

      (3) Grade 3: two variables.

      (4) Grade 4: three or four variables.

III. Diffuse astrocytomas.

A. Histology.

  1. Types.

    a. Fibrillary astrocytoma.

      (1) Most common.

      (2) Location: proportional to white matter.

      (3) Diffuse (more common).

        (a) Adult: usually cerebral hemisphere (especially frontal, temporal).

        (b) Children: usually brainstem (pons > medulla, midbrain).

      (4) Focal (uncommon): usually cerebellum, diencephalon of children/young adults.

      (5) Gliomatosis cerebri (rare): extensive infiltration (see Chapter 26).

    b. Protoplasmic astrocytoma.

    (1) "Pure" form rare.
    (2) Age: children/young adults.
    (3) Location: cortical (temporal > frontal).
    (4) Generally lower grade.
  c. Gemistocytic astrocytomas.
    (1) "Pure" form rare.
    (2) Age: average 40 years.
    (3) Location: cerebral hemisphere.
    (4) Frequently aggressive, anaplastic.
  2. Cytogenetics: genetic alterations include mutation of p53 tumor suppressor gene; loss of heterozygosity (LOH) of chromosomes 9p, 10, 13q, 17p, 19q; and amplification of epidermal growth factor receptor (EGFR) gene.
IV. Low-grade astrocytomas (WHO grade II).
  A. Incidence: less common than high-grade; 15% to 25% of astrocytomas.
  B. Age: older children, young adults (25 to 45 years).
  C. Gender: slight male predilection.
  D. Location.
    1. Adult.
      a. Usually cerebral white matter (especially frontal, temporal).
      b. Less common in cerebellum.
      c. Rarely intraventricular.
    2. Children: brainstem (especially midbrain, cervicomedullary junction).
  E. Clinical features.
    1. Hemispheric tumors more likely to present with seizures than functional deficits (reverse is true for higher grade tumors).
    2. Surgical treatment unless brainstem location (especially pons). Adjuvant radiation beneficial for older patients, but may increase risk of malignant transformation in childhood tumors.
    3. Moderate prognosis: 30% 5-year survival; average survival 2 to 8 years.
    4. Prognosis improved with younger age, supratentorial tumors.
    5. Worse prognosis with diffuse pontine lesions (unresectable).
    6. CNS dissemination rare (5%).
    7. Death more commonly due to malignant transformation rather than progressive low-grade disease.
  F. Imaging.
    1. Angiography: avascular mass effect, no significant neovascularity or arteriovenous (AV) shunting.
    2. CT.
      a. Ill-defined hypodense white matter lesion with mild mass effect and minimal edema.

       b. Enhancement usually absent.

       c. Calcification uncommon (15% to 25%), although more likely than higher grades.

    3. MRI.

       a. Hypointense or isointense to GM on T1WI, hyperintense on T2WI. Microcalcifications may cause T1 hyperintensity.

       b. Margins ill-defined on T1WI, better delineated on T2WI.

       c. Brainstem tumors may be focal or diffusely infiltrating (more likely in higher grades).

       d. Hemorrhage rare (more likely in higher grades).

       e. Occasional intratumoral cysts.

       f. No necrosis unless postradiation.

  G. Differential diagnosis (hemispheric lesion).

    1. Oligodendroglioma (cortical, usually calcified).

    2. Gangliocytoma (rare, more likely in temporal lobe but may be indistinguishable).

    3. Demyelinating lesion of MS (usually multiple, typically at callososeptal interface).

    4. Infarct (typical vascular territory, involves gray and white matter, often gyral enhancement).

    5. Encephalitis (often bilateral, patchy enhancement, more likely to hemorrhage).

V. Anaplastic astrocytomas (WHO grade III).

  A. Incidence: second most common grade of astrocytoma (25% to 30%).

  B. Age: any age, peak at 40 to 60 years.

  C. Gender: slight male predilection.

  D. Location.

    1. Adult: usually cerebral white matter (especially frontal, temporal)

    2. Children: young adults; brainstem (especially pons, medulla).

  E. Clinical features.

    1. Symptoms nonspecific, location-dependent.

    2. Treatment: surgery, radiation therapy, chemotherapy.

    3. Poor prognosis: 20% 5-year survival; average survival 2 to 3 years.

    4. CNS dissemination frequent.

  F. Imaging.

    1. Angiography: mass effect with variable vascularity.

    2. CT.

       a. Heterogeneous mass with moderate to marked mass effect and edema.

       b. Often partially enhancing, although variable pattern. May have irregular ring enhancement (indistinguishable from GBM).

    c. Calcification uncommon, unless malignant transformation of preexisting low-grade astrocytoma.

    d. Intratumoral hemorrhage may occur.

    e. Brainstem tumors diffusely expansile, often difficult to detect on CT.

  3. MRI.

    a. Heterogeneous signal on both T1WI and T2WI. Surrounding T2 hyperintensity due to edema and/or tumor infiltration; latter may extend beyond T2 hyperintensity, especially for recurrent tumors.

    b. Tendency to spread through white matter tracts (see GBM).

    c. Diffuse pontine tumors may displace or encircle basilar artery anteriorly, compress fourth ventricle posteriorly (see Fig. 26-1, *D).*

 G. Differential diagnosis (brainstem lesion).

  1. Pilocytic astrocytoma (usually focal, with dorsal exophytic component).

  2. Infarct (less mass effect, less enhancement).

  3. Demyelinating lesion (smaller lesion, no mass effect, typically at root entry zone of CN V or cerebellar peduncles).

VI. Glioblastoma multiforme (WHO grade IV).

 A. Incidence.

  1. Most common primary intracranial neoplasm; most common grade of astrocytoma (50%).

  2. May arise spontaneously or from precursor lower grade tumor.

 B. Age: usually older patient >50 years; rarely <30.

 C. Gender: slight male predilection.

 D. Location (Fig. 25-1).

  1. Usually cerebral white matter (especially frontal, temporal); occasionally basal ganglia or posterior fossa.

  2. Multilobed and bihemispheric tumors that cross the corpus callosum common.

  3. Extension along white matter tracts most common (corpus callosum, anterior/posterior commissures, optic radiations, internal/external capsules, corticospinal and spinothalamic tracts).

  4. Meningeal ependymal, subpial, perivascular, and subarachnoid spread common.

  5. Synchronous or metachronous multiple tumor foci (up to 10%).

    a. Multifocal (more common): microscopic connections.

    b. Multicentric (occasional): no detectable microscopic connections.

 E. Clinical features.

  1. Rapidly progressive neurologic deficit.

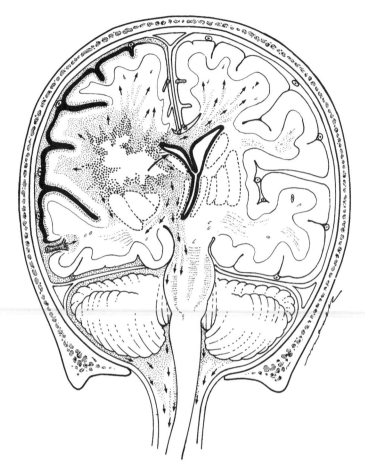

Fig. 25-1 Anatomic diagram illustrates common routes of spread of GBM. Tumor dissemination along white matter tracts, subpial space, and the subarachnoid space is indicated by the dots. Tumor also spreads along the ependyma and leptomeninges (heavy black lines). Note tumor spread along penetrating blood vessels and Virchow-Robin spaces, as shown in the right temporal lobe. Spread outside the CNS to sites such as bone and liver occurs but is rare. Dural (pachymeningeal) GBM spread is also uncommon. (From Osborn AG: *Diagnostic neuroradiology,* St Louis, 1994, Mosby.)

2. Treatment: surgery, radiation, chemotherapy.
3. Dismal prognosis: 5% 5-year survival; average survival <1 year.
4. CNS dissemination (10% to 25%) rapid, widespread.
5. Distant metastases (e.g., bone, liver, lung) rare.
   F. Imaging.

1. Angiography.
    a. Large mass with striking tumor blush, contrast stasis, neovascularity.
    b. AV shunting and early draining veins common.
    c. Occasionally mimics AVM or "luxury perfusion" of infarct.
2. CT.
    a. Infiltrative ill-defined heterogeneous mass with central low density, marked mass effect, and edema extending along white matter tracts.
    b. Extension across corpus callosum gives "butterfly" appearance.
    c. Irregular, thick rim enhancement typical, although rare tumors without hypervascularity and necrosis may have minimal enhancement.
    d. Hemorrhage common (> lower grade).
    e. Calcification rare (15%), unless GBM developed from malignant transformation of low grade astrocytoma.
    f. May have multiple tumor foci.
3. MRI.
    a. Mixed-signal, infiltrative mass with central necrosis. Surrounding T2 hyperintensity does not accurately reflect tumor extent (see anaplastic astrocytoma).
    b. May have hemorrhages of different ages.
    c. May have prominent vascular flow voids.
    d. May have ependymal, leptomeningeal or subarachnoid spread (grave prognosis).
4. Nuclear medicine.
    a. Lesions as small as 1 cm can be detected on radionuclide cerebral imaging; sensitivity improved with SPECT.
    b. Tumor grade may be predicted by degree of activity on PET, Thallium-201 SPECT, or Tc99m-MIBI.
G. Differential diagnosis.
    1. Ring-enhancing lesion.
        a. Lymphoma (usually homogeneously enhancing but ring enhancement in immunosuppressed patient may be indistinguishable).
        b. Metastasis (usually small and multiple but large solitary lesion may be indistinguishable).
        c. Abscess (often multiple, usually thin-walled, may see associated extraaxial/extracranial infection).
        d. Subacute infarction (conforms to vascular territory, involves gray and white matter, may have gyral enhancement).
        e. Resolving hematoma (milder more uniform edema).

      f. Radiation necrosis (may be indistinguishable on CT/MR, nuclear imaging may be helpful).

      g. Active giant MS plaque (usually minimal mass effect/ edema, usually multiple lesions in typical locations).

  2. Parenchymal hemorrhagic lesion (see Chapter 23).

      a. Other hemorrhagic primary or metastatic tumors (may be indistinguishable).

      b. AVM (hemosiderin rim suggests chronic duration, may see serpiginous vessels or flow voids).

      c. Cavernoma (heterogeneous mixed-density "popcorn" appearance, often multiple).

      d. Hypertensive hemorrhage (predilection for basal ganglia, pons).

      e. Amyloid angiopathy-related (often multiple, situated at corticomedullary junction).

      f. Hemorrhagic infarct (predilection for basal ganglia, cortex).

  3. "Butterfly" callosal lesions.

      a. Anaplastic astrocytoma vs. GBM (indistinguishable).

      b. Lymphoma (see above).

      c. Active giant MS plaque (see above).

      d. Deep falcine meningioma (usually homogeneously enhancing unless aggressive, coronal imaging demonstrates extraaxial location and dural attachment).

SUGGESTED READINGS

Alvord EC Jr: Commentary: patterns of growth of gliomas, *AJNR* 16:1013-1017, 1995.

Arita N, Taneda M, Hayakawa T: Leptomeningeal dissemination of malignant gliomas: Incidence, diagnosis and outcome, *Acta Neurochir* 126:84-92, 1994.

Aronen HJ, Gazit IE, Louis DN, et al: Cerebral blood volume maps of gliomas: comparison with tumor grade and histologic findings, *Radiol* 191:41-51, 1994.

Blankenberg FG, Teplitz RL, Ellis W, et al: The influence of volumetric tumor doubling time, DNA ploidy, and histologic grade on the survival of patients with intracranial astrocytomas, *AJNR* 16:1001-1012, 1995.

Bognar L, Turjman F, Vilanyi E, et al: Tectal plate gliomas, Part II: CT scans and MR imaging of tectal gliomas, *Acta Neurochir* 127:48-54, 1994.

Brunberg JA, Chenevert TL, McKeever PE, et al: In vivo MR determination of water diffusion coefficients and diffusion anisotropy: correlation with structural alteration in gliomas of the cerebral hemispheres, *AJNR* 16:361-371, 1995.

Burger PC, Scheithauer BW: Tumors of neuroglia and choroid plexus epithelium. In *Atlas of tumor pathology (third series, fascicle 10): tumors of the central nervous system,* Washington, 1994, Armed Forces Institute of Pathology, pp 25-162.

Delbeke D, Meyerowitz C, Lapidus RL, et al: Optimal cutoff levels of F-18 flurodeoxyglucose uptake in the differentiation of low-grade from high-grade brain tumors with PET, *Radiol* 195:47-52, 1995.

Dirks PB, Jay V, Becker JE, et al: Development of anaplastic changes in low-grade astrocytomas of childhood, *Neurosurg* 34:68-78, 1994.

Gajjar A, Bhargava R, Jenkins JJ, et al: Low grade astrocytoma with neuraxis dissemination at diagnosis, *J Neurosurg* 83:67-71, 1995.

Goraj B, Spiller M, Valsamis MP, Kasoff SS, Tenner MS: Determinants of signal intensity in MRI of human astrocytomas, *Eur Radiol* 7:74-92, 1995.

Kane AG, Robles HA, Smirniotopoulos JG, Heironimus JD, Fish MH: Radiologic-pathologic correlation: diffuse pontine astrocytoma, *AJNR* 14:941-945, 1993.

Kondziolka D, Lunsford LD, Martinez AJ: Unreliability of contemporary neurodiagnostic imaging in evaluating suspected adult supratentorial (low-grade) astrocytoma, *J Neurosurg* 79:533-536, 1993.

Kurki T, Lundbom N, Kalimo H, Valtonen S: MR classification of brain gliomas: value of magnetization transfer and conventional imaging, *Mag Resonance Imaging* 13:501-511, 1995.

Kuroiwa T, Numaguchi Y, Rothman MI, et al: Posterior fossa glioblastoma multiforme: MR findings, *AJNR* 16:583-589, 1995.

Lang FF, Miller DC, Koslow M, Newcomb EW: Pathways leading to glioblastoma multiforme: a molecular analysis of genetic alterations in 65 astrocytic tumors, *J Neurosurg* 81:427-436, 1994.

Mihara F, Ikeda M, Rothman MI, Numaguchi Y, Kristt D: Vertebral body metastasis of glioblastoma multiforme with epidural mass formation, *Clin Imaging* 18:286-289, 1994.

Mineura K, Sasajima T, Kowada M, et al: Perfusion and metabolism in predicting the survival of patients with cerebral gliomas, *Cancer* 73:2386-2394, 1994.

Oriuchi N, Tamura M, Shibazaki T, et al: Clinical evaluation of thallium-201 SPECT in supratentorial gliomas: relationship to histologic grade, prognosis and proliferative activities, *J Nucl Med* 34:2085-2089, 1993.

Osborn AG: Astrocytomas and other glial neoplasms. In *Diagnostic radiology,* St Louis, 1994, Mosby, pp 529-578.

Russell DS, Rubinstein LJ: Tumours of central neuroepithelial origin. In *Pathology of tumours of the nervous system,* ed 5, Baltimore, 1989, Williams and Wilkins, pp 83-350.

Rutherfoord GS, Hewlett RH, Truter R: Contrast enhanced imaging is critical to glioma nosology and grading, *International J Radiol* 1:28-38, 1995.

Tien RD, Felsberg GJ, Friedman H, Brown M, MacFall J: MR imaging of high-grade cerebral gliomas: value of diffusion-weighted echoplanar pulse sequences, *AJR* 162:671-677, 1994.

Yuh WTC, Nguyen HD, Tali ET, et al: Delineation of gliomas with various doses of MR contrast material, *AJNR* 15:983-989, 1994.

26

Astrocytoma Variants

Key Concepts

1. Circumscribed astrocytomas include:
   a. Pilocytic astrocytoma.
   b. Pleomorphic xantho astrocytoma (PXA).
   c. Subependymal giant cell astrocytoma.
2. Both diffuse fibrillary and pilocytic astrocytomas can involve brainstem and cerebellar hemispheres; however, diffuse fibrillary astrocytoma is more common in brainstem, whereas pilocytic astrocytoma is more common in cerebellar hemisphere.
3. Pilocytic astrocytoma and subependymal giant cell astrocytoma are generally pediatric neoplasms.
4. Subependymal giant cell astrocytoma is associated with tuberous sclerosis.
5. Differential diagnosis of cyst with mural nodule in a young patient includes:
   a. Pilocytic astrocytoma.
   b. PXA.
   c. Ganglioglioma.
6. Differential diagnosis of cyst with mural nodule in an older patient includes:
   a. Hemangioblastoma.
7. Unusual glial tumors include gliomatosis cerebri, gliosarcoma, and primary leptomeningeal gliomatosis.

I. Pilocytic astrocytoma.
  A. Histology.
    1. Types.
      a. Juvenile: elongated "hairlike" astrocytes.
      b. Adult: more uniform packing of pilocytic astrocytes than in juvenile type.
    2. Immunopositive for glial fibrillary acidic protein (GFAP), Rosenthal fibers.
  B. Incidence.
    1. Juvenile type more common.
      a. One of two most common pediatric intracranial neoplasms, along with medulloblastoma.
      b. 30% of pediatric gliomas.
      c. One of two most common pediatric posterior fossa neoplasms (25% to 30%) along with medulloblastoma (studies differ as to which is most common).
      d. Most common histology of cerebellar astrocytoma (80%).
      e. Optic pathway lesions often associated with NF-1 (5% to 15% of NF patients, whereas 25% of optic pathway astrocytomas associated with NF-1).
    2. Adult type rare, 2% to 10% of adult intracranial astrocytomas.
  C. Age and gender: children/young adults; no gender predilection.
    1. Opticochiasmatic-hypothalamic tumors: <12 years.
    2. Cerebellar tumors: peak at 10.
    3. Cerebral hemispheric tumors: peak at 20.
    4. Rare adult type: 40 to 50.
  D. Location (in descending order of frequency).
    1. Cerebellar hemispheres, vermis.
    2. Opticochiasmatic-hypothalamic.
    3. Cerebral hemispheres.
    4. Intraventricular.
    5. Brainstem (although less common than fibrillary astrocytoma).
  E. Clinical features.
    1. Symptoms location-dependent; often seizures.
    2. Generally benign, slow-growing.
    3. Clinically malignant tumors or malignant degeneration rare (latter is more likely in adult type or after radiation).
    4. Surgical treatment with adjuvant radiation for subtotal resection.
    5. Good prognosis: 85% 5-year survival and 70% 20-year survival for all surgeries; total resection cure rate approaches 100%.

6. Even unresectable chiasmatic-hypothalamic lesions can have 75% 10-year survival, although some have fatal outcome.
7. Brainstem pilocytic astrocytomas have better prognosis than fibrillary astrocytomas.
8. "Recurrence" often due to cyst reformation, can be drained with impressive clinical improvement.
9. CNS dissemination rare.

F. Imaging (Fig. 26-1, *A*).
   1. Angiography:
      a. Usually avascular mass effect.
      b. Occasionally mural nodule will show neovascularity.
   2. CT.
      a. Typically well-defined partly solid/cystic spheric mass with minimal edema. However, cyst uncommon in opticochiasmatic-hypothalamic and brainstem tumors.
      b. Cyst in supratentorial tumors (80%) usually small. Posterior fossa tumor cyst (50%) usually large.
      c. Calcification uncommon (<10%).
      d. Strong but variable enhancement of solid portion; cyst wall typically does not enhance. Occasional fluid/contrast level or enhancing fluid on delayed CECT.
      e. Brainstem tumors may be difficult to detect on CT.
      f. Obstructive hydrocephalus more common with tumors of fourth ventricle or vermis; relatively mild/late onset in brainstem tumors.
   3. MRI.
      a. Solid portion mildly hypointense or isointense to GM on T1WI; moderately hyperintense on T2WI. Cystic portion similar to or slightly greater than CSF-signal.
      b. Chiasmatic-hypothalamic tumors may be contiguous with optic nerve tumors or extend into retrochiasmatic optic pathway.
      c. Brainstem tumors often dorsally exophytic, compress fourth ventricle posteriorly.
      d. MRI is modality of choice for suspected brainstem tumors.

G. Differential diagnosis.
   1. Cerebellar lesions (Fig. 26-1).
      a. Medulloblastoma (usually midline and homogeneously enhancing, although atypical adult tumors may be indistinguishable).
      b. Ependymoma (usually fills/dilates fourth ventricle, may extrude into adjacent cisterns, more heterogeneous, frequent calcification).

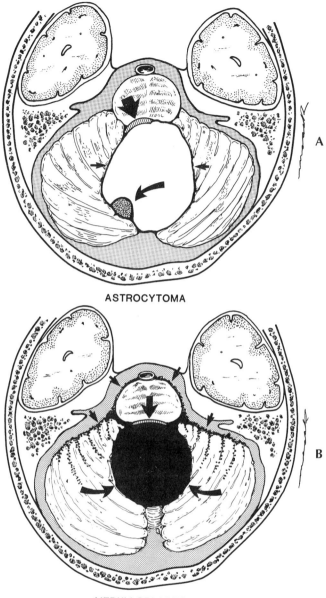

ASTROCYTOMA

MEDULLOBLASTOMA

Fig. 26-1 Axial anatomic drawings depict the four most common posterior fossa neoplasms in children.

A, A typical midline cerebellar astrocytoma is shown. The lesion consists of a mural nodule (curved black arrow) and a cyst (small black arrows). The cyst wall is usually benign and consists of compressed cerebellum. The fourth ventricle (large black arrow) is displaced anteriorly.

B, Medulloblastoma (posterior fossa primitive neuroectodermal tumor) is shown. The typical medulloblastoma (curved black arrows) is hyperdense on unenhanced CT scans and lies in the midline, displacing the fourth ventricle (large black arrow) anteriorly. At least 50% of medulloblastomas have cerebrospinal fluid dissemination (small black arrows) at the time of initial diagnosis.

Continued.

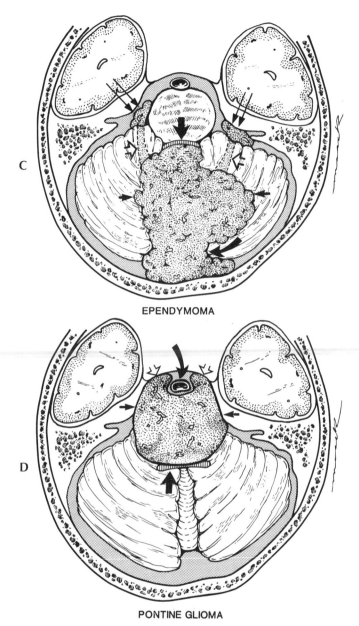

EPENDYMOMA

PONTINE GLIOMA

Fig. 26-1, cont'd   Axial anatomic drawings depict the four most common posterior fossa neoplasms in children.

C, The typical fourth ventricular ependymoma (small black arrows) has a "plastic" configuration, extending posteriorly through the foramen of Magendie (curved black arrow) into the cisterna magna, and anteriorly through the foramina of Luschka (outlined arrows) into the cerebellopontine angles (double arrows). The fourth ventricle (large black arrow) appears filled with tumor.

D, Diffuse pontine glioma (small black arrows) grossly expands the pons, displacing the fourth ventricle (large black arrow) posteriorly. Exophytic tumor extension (outlined arrows) may surround and engulf the basilar artery (curved arrow), displacing it posteriorly away from the clivus.

    c. Hemangioblastoma (extremely rare in <20 years of age, strongly enhancing mural nodule abuts pial surface).

    d. Intraventricular demoid (rare, no mural nodule, usually resembles fat density/signal).

    e. Intraventricular epidermoid (uncommon, no mural nodule, contents slightly heterogeneous, usually resembles CSF).

    f. Dandy-Walker cyst (no mural nodule, homogeneous midline cyst communicating with fourth ventricle, vermian hypoplasia, enlarged posterior fossa).

  2. Opticochiasmatic-hypothalamic lesions.

    a. Suprasellar germinoma (homogeneous enhancement, often associated CSF dissemination).

    b. Suprasellar teratoma (heterogeneous, may have calcification or fat).

    c. Pituitary adenoma (larger intrasellar component, sellar expansion, chiasm displaced superiorly).

    d. Craniopharyngioma (suprasellar/intrasellar, usually calcified, cysts more common, chiasm displaced superiorly).

    e. Langerhans cell histiocytosis (enhancing infundibulum or suprasellar mass).

    f. Hypothalamic hamartoma (nonenhancing mass between infundibulum and mammillary bodies).

  3. Cerebral hemispheric lesions.

    a. Pleomorphic xanthoastrocytoma (cortical, mural nodule usually abuts surface).

    b. Ganglioglioma (most common in temporal lobe, may be indistinguishable).

  4. Brainstem lesions.

    a. Fibrillary astrocytoma (more diffusely infiltrating and expansile without exophytic component).

II. Pleomorphic xanthoastrocytoma.

  A. Histology.

    1. Tumor of morphologically variable lipid-laden astrocytes.

    2. Immunopositive for GFAP and S-100 protein.

  B. Incidence: rare, <1% of astrocytomas.

  C. Age and gender: children, young adults (90% <30 years); occasionally 40 to 50; no gender predilection.

  D. Location.

    1. Cortical, commonly involving adjacent leptomeninges.

    2. Usually supratentorial (temporal > parietal, occipital, frontal); rarely cerebellum.

  E. Clinical features.

    1. Typically long seizure history.

2. Usually indolent.
3. Treatment primarily resection with postoperative survival up to 25 years.
4. Recurrence frequent.
5. Malignant transformation into anaplastic astrocytoma or GBM uncommon (10% to 25%).

F. Imaging.
   1. Angiography.
      a. Avascular or hypovascular mass effect.
      b. Tumor nodule may demonstrate neovascularity.
   2. CT.
      a. Typically discrete partly solid/cystic hypodense superficial mass with mild edema. Less commonly solid or infiltrating.
      b. Calcification rare.
      c. Mural nodule or solid component abuts leptomeninges, enhances strongly. Cyst wall usually does not enhance although infiltrating margins may enhance.
   3. MRI.
      a. Solid portion hypointense or isointense to GM on T1WI; hyperintense on T2WI. Cytic portion similar to or slightly greater than CSF signal.

G. Differential diagnosis.
   1. Pilocytic astrocytoma (deeper location, mural nodule not restricted to surface).
   2. Ganglioglioma (may be indistinguishable).
   3. Oligodendroglioma (usually calcified, large cyst uncommon).
   4. Meningioma (usually distinctly extraaxial, usually homogeneously solid, although cystic meningioma may have similar appearance).

III. Subependymal giant cell astrocytoma (Tuberous sclerosis).
   A. Histology.
      1. Tumor of giant multinucleated astrocytes probably resulting from enlargement, degeneration of subependymal tubers.
      2. Immunopositive for S-100 protein; GFAP weakly positive.
   B. Incidence: almost always occurs in tuberous sclerosis (TS), although only 10% to 15% of TS patients will be affected; "isolated" cases may represent forme fruste of TS.
   C. Age: usually <20 years.
   D. Location: almost exclusively at foramen of Monro.
   E. Clinical features.
      1. Symptoms usually due to obstructive hydrocephalus.
      2. Slow-growing.

3. Treatment primarily resection with good prognosis and long-term survival.
F. Imaging.
   1. Angiography.
      a. Variable vascularity.
      b. Subependymal veins stretched around dilated ventricles.
   2. CT.
      a. Well-defined rounded or lobulated heterogeneous lateral ventricular mass at foramen of Monro.
      b. Calcification and cyst formation common.
      c. Strong heterogeneous enhancement. (Because 30% to 80% of benign subependymal nodules (SEN) may enhance, enlarging size is more useful indicator of transformation than enhancement.)
      d. May cause obstructive hydrocephalus.
      e. Usually associated with subependymal or cortical tubers of TS, which are often calcified (see Chapter 17).
   3. MRI.
      a. Heterogeneous mixed signal: generally hypointense or isointense to GM on T1WI; isointense to hyperintense on T2WI.
      b. MRI more sensitive for detecting SENs, cortical tubers, and other white matter lesions (modality of choice for suspected TS), although CT is helpful for detection of calcification.
G. Differential diagnosis.
   1. Central neurocytoma (may be indistinguishable without other findings/history of TS).
   2. Ependymoma (supratentorial lesions usually extend into paraventricular parenchyma but occasionally can remain intraventricular and be difficult to distinguish).
   3. Subependymoma (rare, often pedunculated/attached to septum pellucidum, absent or variable enhancement).
   4. Colloid cyst (smoothly spheric, midline, nonenhancing, homogeneously hyperdense).
IV. Gliomatosis cerebri.
A. Histology: extensive infiltration of brain by neoplastic glial cells (usually fibrillary astrocytes) with destruction of myelin sheaths. Controversy whether distinct neoplasm or extremely diffuse glioma.
B. Incidence: rare.
C. Age and gender: any age, usually 20 to 40 years; no gender predilection.

D. Location.
  1. White matter tracts (optic chiasm, corpus callosum, fornices, cerebral/cerebellar peduncles) > gray matter (basal ganglia, thalami). May be hemispheric or bilateral.
  2. Infiltration is perineuronal, perivascular, and subpial.
E. Clinical features.
  1. Symptoms disproportionately mild compared with extent of brain involvement.
  2. Slowly progressive.
  3. Unresectable due to infiltration. Steroids useful in short term. Radiation and chemotherapy of questionable benefit. Poor prognosis.
F. Imaging.
  1. Angiography: normal or avascular mass effect.
  2. CT.
    a. Diffuse ill-defined isodense mass with loss of gray/white differentiation. Occasionally multifocal hypodense areas.
    b. Usually no enhancement, although small enhancing foci may be seen as late manifestation.
    c. CT may appear normal; full extent of tumor difficult to determine on CT.
  3. MRI.
    a. Usually hypointense to GM on T1WI; hyperintense on T2WI (tumor infiltration and demyelination). Underlying cerebral structures relatively preserved.
    b. May see multiple enhancing foci.
    c. MRI more sensitive than CT, better delineates extent of tumor.
G. Differential diagnosis.
  1. Herpes HSV-1 encephalitis (may initially be unilateral but typically becomes bilateral, often hemorrhagic).
  2. White matter disorders (variable characteristic patterns, depending on etiology [see Chapters 49 to 54]).
  3. Pachygyria (enlargement of cortex without abnormal signal).
  4. Hemimegalencephaly (unilateral hemispheric/ventricular/calvarial enlargement without abnormal signal, may have associated migrational anomalies).
V. Gliosarcoma.
  A. Histology.
    1. Neoplastic gliomatous (GBM > oligodendroglial) and sarcomatous (fibrosarcoma, MFH) elements. Typically glial component surrounds sarcomatous center.

2. May arise spontaneously or sarcoma may arise in preexisting glioma.

B. Incidence: rare, <5% of astrocytomas.

C. Age and gender: usually 40 to 70 years; no gender predilection.

D. Location.
   1. Tendency to peripheral location with dural invasion.
   2. Favors similar locations as GBM, temporal lobe common.

E. Clinical features.
   1. Symptoms nonspecific.
   2. Survival similar to GBM.
   3. Extracranial metastases frequent (15% to 30%).
   4. Death usually due to intracerebral neoplasm rather than metastases.

F. Imaging.
   1. Angiography.
      a. Prominent vascular stain with well-defined margins, neovascularity, early cortical draining veins.
      b. Blood supply pial or mixed pial-dural.
   2. CT.
      a. Discrete slightly hyperdense (densely cellular, vascular) peripheral mass with mild to moderate edema.
      b. May contact skull or falx but lacks broad dural attachment of meningioma. Occasionally erodes through skull.
      c. Strong homogeneous or irregular ringlike enhancement.
   3. MRI.
      a. Variable inhomogeneous appearance, with mixed hypointensity and hyperintensity on T1- and T2WI.
      b. Hemorrhage and necrosis common.
      c. Heterogeneous strong enhancement.

G. Differential diagnosis.
   1. GBM (deeper location, no dural/calvarial involvement).
   2. Meningioma (more homogeneously hyperdense, broad dural attachment, less edema).
   3. Hemangiopericytoma (may be indistinguishable).
   4. Other sarcomas (may be indistinguishable).

VI. Primary leptomeningeal gliomatosis.
   A. Histology: glioma (astrocytic > oligodendroglial) restricted to leptomeninges without identifiable parenchymal source.
   B. Incidence: rare.
   C. Age and gender: all ages; no gender predilection.
   D. Location: intracranial or intraspinal leptomeninges.

E. Clinical features.
   1. Symptoms nonspecific.
   2. Poor operability. Prognosis poor, depends on degree of histologic malignancy.
F. Imaging: not well described; generally diffuse leptomeningeal thickening or enhancement expected.
G. Differential diagnosis: all causes of diffuse leptomeningeal infiltrative process (see Chapter 56).

SUGGESTED READINGS

Burger PC, Scheithauer BW: Tumors of neuroglia and choroid plexus epithelium. In *Atlas of tumor pathology (third series, fascicle 10): tumors of the central nervous system,* Washington, 1994, Armed Forces Institute of Pathology, pp 25-162.

Felsberg GJ, Silver SA, Brown MT, Tien RD: Radiologic-pathologic correlation: gliomatosis cerebri, *AJNR* 15:1745-1753, 1994.

Fulham MJ, Melisi JW, Nishimiya J, Dwyer AJ, Di Chiro G: Neuroimaging of juvenile pilocytic astrocytomas: an enigma, *Radiol* 189:221-225, 1993.

Hayostek CJ, Shaw EG, Scheithauer B, et al: Astrocytomas of the cerebellum: a comparative clinicopathologic study of pilocytic and diffuse astrocytomas, *Cancer* 72:856-869, 1993.

Kepes JJ: Pleomorphic xanthoastrocytoma: the birth of a diagnosis and a concept, *Brain Pathol* 3:269-274, 1993.

Lipper MH, Eberhard DA, Phillips CD, Vezina L-G, Cail WS: Pleomorphic xanthoastrocytoma, a distinctive astroglial tumor: neuroradiologic and pathologic features, *AJNR* 14:1397-1404, 1993.

Mamelak AN, Prados MD, Obana WG, Cogen PH, Edwards MSB: Treatment options and prognosis for multicentric juvenile pilocytic astrocytoma, *J Neurosurg* 81:24-30, 1994.

Osborn AG: Astrocytomas and other glial neoplasms. In *Diagnostic radiology,* St Louis, 1994, Mosby, pp 529-578.

Preul MC, Espinosa JA, Tampieri D, Carpenter S: Unusual evolution and computerized tomographic appearance of a gliosarcoma, *Can J Neurol Sci* 21:141-145, 1994.

Robertson PL, Allen JC, Abbott IR, et al: Cervicomedullary tumors in children: a distinct subset of brainstem gliomas, *Neurol* 44:1798-1803, 1994.

Russell DS, Rubinstein LJ: Tumours of central neuroepithelial origin. In *Pathology of tumours of the nervous system,* ed 5, Baltimore, 1989, Williams and Wilkins, pp 83-350.

Shin YM, Chang KH, Myung NH, et al: Gliomatosis cerebri: comparison of MR and CT features, *AJR* 161:859-862, 1993.

Strong JA, Hatten HP Jr, Brown MT, et al: Pilocytic astrocytoma: correlation between the initial imaging features and clinical aggressiveness, *AJR* 161:369-372, 1993.

Tien RD, Cardenas CA, Rajagopalan S: Pleomorphic xanthoastrocytoma of the brain: MR findings in six patients, *AJR* 159:1287-1290, 1992.

Vandertop WP, Hoffman HJ, Drake JM, et al: Focal midbrain tumors in children, *Neurosurg* 31:186-194, 1992.

Wasdahl DA, Scheithauer BW, Andrews BT, Jeffrey RA Jr: Cerebellar pleomorphic xanthoastrocytoma: case report, *Neurosurg* 35:947-950, 1994.

27

Nonastrocytic Glial Tumors

Key Concepts

1. Nonastrocytic glial neoplasms include:
   a. Oligodendroglioma.
   b. Ependymoma.
   c. Subependymoma.
   d. Choroid plexus tumors.
2. Oligodendroglioma is the most likely brain neoplasm to calcify; however, because astrocytoma is much more common, a calcified tumor is still more likely to be astrocytoma.
3. Ependymoma is more commonly infratentorial (fourth ventricle); supratentorial tumors are usually extraventricular due to periventricular parenchymal extension.
4. Ependymoma and choroid plexus papilloma are generally pediatric neoplasms.

I. Oligodendroglial tumors.
  A. Histology.
    1. Types.
        a. Oligodendroglioma.
        b. Mixed oligo-astrocytoma.
        c. Anaplastic oligodendroglioma.
        d. Anaplastic mixed oligo-astrocytoma.
    2. Cytology: "fried-egg" appearance (perinuclear halo) occurs when specimen fixation delayed, not seen on frozen section.
    3. Immunonegative for glial fibrillary acidic protein (GFAP).
  B. Incidence.
    1. Oligodendroglial tumors uncommon; 2% to 5% of primary intracranial neoplasms, 5% to 10% of gliomas.
    2. >50% mixed (astrocytoma or anaplastic astrocytoma).
    3. "Pure" oligodendroglioma uncommon.
    4. Actual incidence of anaplastic oligodendroglial tumors uncertain; likely previously diagnosed as GBM due to presence of necrosis.
  C. Age: any age, adults > children (8:1), peak at 35 to 45 years.
  D. Gender: slight male predilection.
  E. Location.
    1. Cortical/subcortical; originates in white matter but infiltrative and often involves cortex.
    2. 85% supratentorial (frontal > parietal, temporal).
    3. Can invade ventricles; rarely purely intraventricular. (Most previous cases of intraventricular oligodendroglioma probably central neurocytoma.)
    4. Posterior fossa uncommon (although more likely in children).
  F. Clinical features.
    1. Symptoms frequently seizures, headache.
    2. Due to infiltrative nature, not completely resectable. Adjuvant radiation and/or chemotherapy especially for anaplastic tumors.
    3. Prognosis for "pure oligodendroglioma" most dependent on tumor grade.
        a. Moderate prognosis with low-grade: 75% 5-year survival; 45% 10-year survival, median survival 10 years.
        b. Poor prognosis with high-grade: 40% 5-year survival; 20% 10-year survival, median survival 4 years.
        c. Prognosis improved with younger age, absence of neurologic deficits, gross total resection.
    4. Mixed oligodendroglioma has intermediate prognosis.
    5. Propensity for tumor progression, malignant degeneration, although slower than astrocytoma.

G. Imaging.
  1. Angiography.
     a. Low-grade tumors typically avascular or faintly vascular mass effect.
     b. Anaplastic tumors may have neovascularity.
  2. CT.
     a. Infiltrative heterogeneous hypodense or isodense superficial mass with mild edema.
     b. Dense, coarse calcification common: up to 90%. (Note: calcified neoplasm still more likely to be astrocytoma because astrocytomas >> oligodendrogliomas.)
     c. Cystic degeneration common, although lack large cysts.
     d. Mild-moderate enhancement (more likely with higher grade or mixed tumors).
     e. Hemorrhage uncommon.
     f. Overlying skull may show scalloped erosion.
  3. MRI.
     a. Typically mixed hypointensity and isointensity on T1WI; hyperintense with hypointense calcific foci on T2WI. Variable signal if hemorrhage occurs.
H. Differential diagnosis.
     a. Astrocytoma (deeper in parenchyma, less frequent/smaller calcifications).
     b. Ganglioglioma (more commonly involves temporal lobes, often prominent cystic component, calcification less common).
     c. PXA (typical mural nodule/cyst configuration without calcification).
II. Ependymal tumors.
  A. Ependymoma (see Figs. 26-1,*C,* 27-1).
     1. Histology.
        a. Types: cellular, papillary, clear cell; anaplastic (malignant).
        b. Cytology: GFAP and S-100 positive; cells form perivascular pseudorosettes.
        c. Cytogenetics: some cases associated with chromosome 22 deletion.
     2. Incidence.
        a. 2% to 6% of all primary intracranial neoplasms.
        b. Third most common pediatric intracranial neoplasm (8% to 10%), after PNET and pilocytic astrocytoma.
        c. Fourth most common pediatric posterior fossa tumor (15%).
        d. Some association with NF-2.
     3. Age: children > adults (5:1); peak at 1 to 5 years, second smaller peak mid-30s.

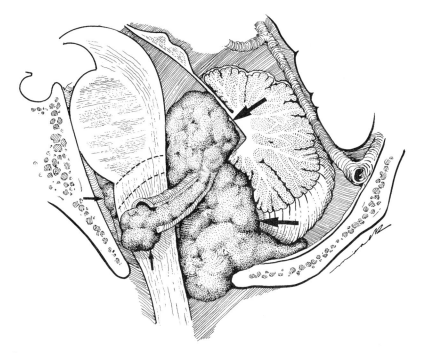

Fig. 27-1 Anatomic drawing shows a typical fourth ventricular ependymoma. The tumor (large arrows) expands the fourth ventricle and extends out the foramen of Magendie into the cisterna magna and through the foramina of Luschka into the cerebellopontine angle cisterns (small arrows). The tendency of this tumor to squeeze out these foramina gives rise to the appellation "plastic" ependymoma. (From Osborn AG: *Diagnostic neuroradiology,* St Louis, 1994, Mosby.)

4. Gender: slight male predilection.
5. Location.
   a. 60% infratentorial; >90% in fourth ventricle, occasionally foramen of Luschka/CPA.
   b. 40% supratentorial; extraventricular > intraventricular (tendency to extend into periventricular parenchyma).
   c. Spine: myxopapillary ependymoma is unique tumor of filum/conus.
6. Clinical features.
   a. Symptoms location-dependent.
      (1) Supratentorial: nonspecific.
      (2) Infratentorial: symptoms related to hydrocephalus.
      (3) Spine: pain, paresthesias, neurologic deficits.
   b. Moderately radiosensitive, often receive prophylactic spinal axis radiation in addition to surgery and chemotherapy.

    c. Moderate prognosis: 45% 5-year survival.

    d. CNS dissemination frequent (10% to 30%); extraneural metastases rare (lymph nodes, lung, liver, bone).

    e. Death usually due to tumor progression or recurrence.

7. Imaging.

    a. Angiography: varies from hypovascular to extremely hypervascular.

    b. CT.

        (1) Infratentorial tumors are typically lobulated isodense mass that fills/dilates fourth ventricle; may extrude into CPA cisterns, cisterna magna, or foramen magnum.

        (2) Supratentorial tumors usually extend into periventricular parenchyma.

        (3) Punctate calcification fairly common (50%).

        (4) Mild to moderate heterogeneous enhancement.

        (5) Cyst formation common.

        (6) Hemorrhage uncommon.

        (7) Associated hydrocephalus (obstruction of fourth ventricle vs. impaired resorption due to tumor cells or protein).

    c. MRI.

        (1) Heterogeneous mixed-signal mass. Solid portions generally hypointense or isointense to GM on T1WI; hyperintense on T2WI. Cystic portions similar to CSF signal.

        (2) Supratentorial tumors may mimic astrocytoma.

        (3) May see subarachnoid seeding.

8. Differential diagnosis.

    a. Fourth ventricular lesion (see Fig. 26-1).

        (1) Medulloblastoma (usually homogeneous, displaces fourth ventricle anteriorly).

        (2) Cerebellar astrocytoma (off-midline hemispheric location, typically cyst/mural nodule configuration).

        (3) Pontine astrocytoma (diffuse brainstem infiltration, displaces fourth ventricle posteriorly).

        (4) Choroid plexus papilloma (rarely in fourth ventricle unless in adult, more homogeneous enhancement).

    b. Supratentorial extraventricular lesion.

        (1) Pilocytic astrocytoma (usually cyst/mural nodule configuration).

        (2) Anaplastic astrocytoma or GBM (may be indistinguishable).

        (3) Cerebral PNETs (may be indistinguishable).

        (4) Choroid plexus papilloma/carcinoma (large tumors with

parenchymal extension may be indistinguishable).

  c. Supratentorial intraventricular lesion.

    (1) Choroid plexus papilloma (more homogeneous marked enhancement).

    (2) Meningioma (usually located in trigone, more homogeneous enhancement).

    (3) Subependymal giant cell astrocytoma (foramen of Monro, usually other findings of TS).

    (4) Central neurocytoma (near foramen of Monro, may be indistinguishable).

    (5) Colloid cyst (midline, near foramen of Monro, homogenous nonenhancing hyperdense mass).

B. Subependymoma.

  1. Histology: prominent fibrillary background.

  2. Incidence: rare (<1%).

  3. Age: middle-aged, elderly adults.

  4. Location: along ventricular walls (especially floor of inferior fourth ventricle and septum pellucidum between frontal horns).

  5. Clinical features.

    a. Usually asymptomatic, discovered incidentally.

    b. Fourth ventricular tumors may present with symptoms related to obstructive hydrocephalus.

    c. Benign.

    d. Treatment primarily resection; occasionally adjunctive radiation for subtotal resection or recurrent tumor.

  6. Imaging.

    a. Angiography: usually avascular mass effect, rarely vascular.

    b. CT.

      (1) Well-circumscribed rounded hypodense or isodense subependymal or intraventricular mass. Fourth ventricular tumors may extend through foramina of Luschka or Magendie.

      (2) Calcification infrequent (more likely in fourth ventricle).

      (3) Variable enhancement: from absent to striking.

      (4) Hemorrhage uncommon.

    c. MRI.

      (1) Usually hypointense or isointense to GM on T1WI, mildly hyperintense on T2WI. May be pedunculated.

      (2) Mild signal heterogeneity may be due to cystic change, subclinical hemorrhage, or calcification.

      (3) Variable enhancement: from absent to striking.

  7. Differential diagnosis.

    a. Fourth ventricular lesions.

   (1) Intraventricular ependymoma (heterogeneous, moderately enhancing, frequently calcified).
   (2) Intraventricular meningioma (strongly enhancing).
   (3) Choroid plexus papilloma (strongly enhancing).
   (4) Metastasis (most common posterior fossa tumor in adults and may be indistinguishable).
  b. Septum pellucidum lesions.
   (1) Subependymal giant cell astrocytoma (heterogeneous, strongly enhancing, frequently calcified).
   (2) Central neurocytoma (moderately enhancing).
   (3) Ependymoma (heterogeneous, moderately enhancing, usually has parenchymal extension).
   (4) Colloid cyst (midline anterior third ventricle, smoothly rounded nonenhancing hyperdense mass).
III. Choroid plexus tumors.
 A. Histology.
  1. Types.
   a. Choroid plexus papilloma.
   b. Choroid plexus carcinoma.
  2. Arise from secretory epithelial cells (modified ependyma) lining choroid with glial component.
  3. Immunopositive for S-100 protein, cytokeratin and GFAP.
 B. Incidence.
  1. Choroid plexus papilloma:
   a. 0.5% of adult primary intracranial neoplasms.
   b. 2% to 5% of pediatric primary intracranial neoplasms.
   c. One of most common brain tumors in <2 years age.
  2. Choroid plexus carcinoma: uncommon; 10% to 20% of all choroid plexus neoplasms.
 C. Age.
  1. Choroid plexus papilloma: usually young children; 75% <2 years, 85% <5 years, rarely congenital; uncommon in adults.
  2. Choroid plexus carcinoma: 2 to 4 years.
 D. Gender: slight male predilection.
 E. Location: proportional to normal choroid plexus.
  1. Choroid plexus papilloma.
   a. Children: trigone >> third ventricle.
   b. Adult: fourth ventricle or lateral recess.
   c. Rarely extends into contiguous cistern or seeds subarachnoid space.
  2. Choroid plexus carcinoma: lateral ventricles.
 F. Clinical features.
  1. Symptoms usually secondary to hydrocephalus (cause of hydro-

cephalus uncertain: CSF overproduction vs. impaired resorption due to tumor cells, protein, or hemorrhage).
2. Treatment primarily resection. Adjuvant radiation for subtotal resection, dissemination, recurrence.
3. Good long-term survival for papilloma, even though recurrence is common. Malignant transformation rare (more likely in children).
4. Prognosis for carcinoma depends on extent of resection (favorable if complete, poor if incomplete).
5. CSF dissemination can occur with both papilloma and carcinoma (although more likely with carcinoma).

G. Imaging.
1. Angiography.
   a. Highly vascular with prominent, prolonged stain.
   b. Enlarged choroidal arteries and early draining veins may be seen.
2. U/S.
   a. Echogenic lobulated intraventricular mass.
3. CT.
   a. Large well-defined lobulated homogeneously isodense or hyperdense intraventricular mass. Less commonly hypodense or mixed density.
   b. Calcification uncommon (25%); slightly more common in fourth ventricular tumors and adults.
   c. Intense enhancement.
   d. Papillomas tend to be homogeneous (heterogeneity suggests carcinoma). However, papillomas in adults tend to be heterogeneous.
   e. Focal parenchymal infiltration occurs in both papilloma and carcinoma, although extent greater with carcinoma.
   f. Associated hydrocephalus.
4. MRI.
   a. Well-defined markedly enhancing frequently pedunculated intraventricular mass.
   b. Hypointense or isointense to GM on T1WI; isointense or slightly hyperintense on T2WI.
   c. More heterogeneous on MRI than CT with mottled appearance (trapped CSF, calcification, vascular flow voids).
   d. Choroid plexus carcinoma more likely to be heterogeneous and invasive with associated edema.
   e. May see subarachnoid seeding.

H. Differential diagnosis.
1. Lateral ventricular lesion.

   a. Ependymoma (usually more heterogeneous but may be indistinguishable).
   b. Astrocytoma with intraventricular extension (more likely heterogeneous, less marked enhancement).
   c. Cerebral PNETs (usually heterogeneous, largely parenchymal with possible secondary intraventricular extension).
   d. Subependymal giant cell astrocytoma (usually heterogeneous, frequently calcified, associated TS lesions).
   e. Central neurocytoma (heterogeneous, less marked enhancement).
2. Third ventricular lesion.
   a. Intraventricular ependymoma (rarely in third ventricle, may be indistinguishable).
   b. Hypothalamic pilocytic astrocytoma (closely related to floor of third ventricle and may be difficult to distinguish).
   c. Craniopharyngioma (usually suprasellar/intrasellar but may protrude into inferior third ventricle and mimic primary intraventricular lesion).
3. Fourth ventricular region lesion (rare, more likely in adults).
   a. Medulloblastoma (rare adult tumors tend to be more lateral).
   b. Ependymoma (heterogeneous, less marked enhancement, frequently calcified).
   c. Subependymoma (variable enhancement).
   d. Hemangioblastoma (typical mural nodule/cyst configuration).
   e. Solitary metastasis (most common adult posterior fossa tumor and may be indistinguishable).

SUGGESTED READINGS

Burger PC, Scheithauer BW: Tumors of neuroglia and choroid plexus epithelium. In *Atlas of tumor pathology (third series, fascicle 10): tumors of the central nervous system,* Washington, 1994, Armed Forces Institute of Pathology, pp 25-162.

Celli P, Norfrone I, Palma L, Cantore G, Fortuna A: Cerebral oligodendroglioma: prognostic factors and life history, *Neurosurg* 35:1018-1035, 1994.

Greene KA, Dickman CA, Marciano FF, Coons SW, Rekate HL: Pathology and management of choroid plexus tumors, *BNI Quarterly* 10:13-20, 1994.

Kyritsis AP, Yung WKA, Bruner J, Gleason MJ, Levin VA: The treatment of oligodendrogliomas and mixed gliomas, *Neurosurg* 34:365-371, 1993.

Lindboe CF, Stolt-Nielsen A, Dale LG: Hemorrhage in a highly vascularized subependymoma of the septum pellucidum: a case report, *Neurosurg* 31:741-745, 1992.

Nijssen PCG, Lekanne Deprez RH, Tijssen CC, et al: Familial anaplastic ependymoma: evidence of loss of chromosome 22 in tumour cells, *J Neurol, Neurosurg, Psychiatry* 57:1245-1248, 1994.

Oppenheim JS, Strauss RC, Mormino J, Sachdev VP, Rothman AS: Ependymomas of the third ventricle, *Neurosurg* 34:350-353, 1994.

Osborn AG: Astrocytomas and other glial neoplasms. In *Diagnostic radiology,* St Louis, 1994, Mosby, pp 529-578.

Russell DS, Rubinstein LJ: Tumours of central neuroepithelial origin. In *Pathology of tumours of the nervous system,* ed 5, Baltimore, 1989, Williams and Wilkins, pp 83-350.

Shaw EG, Scheithauer BW, O'Fallon JR, Davis DH: Mixed oligoastrocytomas: A survival and prognostic factor analysis, *Neurosurg* 34:577-582, 1994.

Shaw EG, Scheithauer BW, O'Fallon JR, Tazelaar HD, Davis DH: Oligodendrogliomas: the Mayo clinic experience, *J Neurosurg* 76:428-434, 1992.

Silverstein JE, Lenchik L, Stanciu MG, Shimkin PM: MRI of intracranial subependymomas, *J Comp Asst Tomogr* 19:264-267, 1995.

Tekkok IH, Ayberk G, Saglam S, Onol B: Primary intraventricular oligodendroglioma, *Neurochirurgia* 35:63-66, 1992.

Tice H, Barnes PD, Goumnerova L, Scott RM, Tarbell NJ: Pediatric and adolescent oligodendrogliomas, *AJNR* 14:1293-1300, 1993.

Tortori-Donati P, Fondelli MP, Cama A, et al: Ependymomas of the posterior cranial fossa: CT and MRI findings, *Neuroradiol* 37:238-243, 1995.

28

Neuronal, Mixed Neuronal-Glial, and Pineal Parenchymal Tumors

---

Key Concepts

1. Neuronal and mixed neuronal-glial tumors are uncommon and include:
   a. Ganglioglioma.
   b. Gangliocytoma (may not be true neoplasm but rather a hamartomatous process).
   c. Desmoplastic infantile ganglioglioma.
   d. Dysembryoplastic neuroepithelial tumor.
   e. Central neurocytoma.
2. Dysplastic cerebellar gangliocytoma or Lhermitte-Duclos disease is probably not a true neoplasm but rather a hamartoma or cortical dysplasia of cerebellar folia.
3. Pineal parenchymal tumors include:
   a. Pineocytoma.
   b. Pineoblastoma.
4. Pineoblastoma comprises immature neuronal cells and resembles other primitive neuroepithelial tumors, particularly medulloblastoma.

I. Ganglion cell tumors.
   A. Histology.
      1. Types.
         a. Ganglioglioma: mature, enlarged neuronal cells ("ganglion cells") mixed with neoplastic glial tissue (usually astrocytic).
         b. Gangliocytoma: mature, enlarged neuronal cells without glial component. Controversy whether true neoplasm or malformation/dysplasia.
         c. Desmoplastic infantile ganglioglioma (DIG): atypical, immature neuronal and astroglial cells with marked desmoplastic stroma (may have been previously diagnosed as cerebral neuroblastoma/PNET).
      2. Neuronal markers: neurofilaments, synapses, neuron-specific enolase (NSE), synaptophysin.
   B. Incidence.
      1. Ganglioglioma: uncommon; <1% of all primary CNS neoplasms; 8% to 10% of pediatric CNS neoplasms.
      2. Gangliocytoma: rare, 0.1%.
      3. Desmoplastic infantile ganglioglioma: rare, 0.3%.
   C. Age.
      1. Children and young adults more common; 60% to 80% <30 years.
      2. Desmoplastic infantile ganglioglioma: infants only; average 6 months.
   D. Gender: slight male predilection.
   E. Location.
      1. Ganglioglioma and gangliocytoma:
         a. Superficial location.
         b. Supratentorial (temporal > frontal, parietal) >> posterior fossa.
         c. Intracranial > spinal cord.
      2. Desmoplastic infantile ganglioglioma: superficial cerebral hemisphere (parietal > frontal >> occipital).
   F. Clinical features.
      1. Presentation.
         a. Gangliocytoma/ganglioglioma: usually seizures, headaches.
         b. DIG: increasing head size, seizures.
      2. Gangliocytomas and gangliogliomas: slow-growing. Surgery generally curative. Long postoperative survival, even if incompletely resected.
      3. Gangliogliomas: almost never fatal, malignant transformation rare (10% to 30%); graded according to neoplastic astrocytic

component, although prognosis may not correlate with traditional grading.

4. Desmoplastic infantile ganglioglioma: favorable prognosis with long postoperative survival if totally resected. However, due to large size and hypervascularity, resection often difficult. Unknown prognosis for partial resection. Usually do not receive radiation or chemotherapy due to age.

G. Imaging.
  1. Ganglioglioma.
     a. CT.
        (1) Variable appearance. Typically large, partly cystic/solid mass with isodense or hypodense mural nodule and mass effect. May also be homogeneously solid.
        (2) Mural nodule often calcified: 30%.
        (3) Variable enhancement; cyst margins can enhance.
        (4) May have scalloped erosion of adjacent skull.
     b. MRI.
        (1) Solid portion variable (hypointense or hyperintense to GM) on T1WI; hyperintense on T2WI. Cystic portion similar to CSF-signal.
        (2) Variable enhancement.
     c. Differential diagnosis.
        (1) Pleomorphic xanthoastrocytoma (mural nodule abuts leptomeninges).
        (2) Pilocytic astrocytoma (may be indistinguishable).
        (3) Oligodendroglioma (cortical/subcortical, more common in frontal lobes, usually calcified, less likely cystic).
        (4) Dysembryoplastic neuroepithelial tumor (lacks mural nodule/cyst configuration but may be indistinguishable from solid ganglioglioma).
  2. Gangliocytoma.
     a. CT.
        (1) Slightly hyperdense lesion with minimal mass effect.
        (2) Absent or minimal enhancement.
     b. MRI.
        (1) May be difficult to identify on T1WI.
        (2) Isointense to hyperintense to GM on PD; isointense to hypointense on T2WI.
     c. Differential diagnosis.
        (1) Low-grade astrocytoma (may be indistinguishable).
  3. Desmoplastic infantile ganglioglioma.
     a. CT.
        (1) Typically massive, heterogeneous, partly solid/cystic mass.

(2) Solid portion hyperdense, usually adjacent to meninges.
(3) Marked enhancement of solid portion extending to meninges.
(4) May have associated obstructive hydrocephalus.
  b. MRI.
(1) Heterogeneous mixed intermediate tissue and fluid signal.
  c. Differential diagnosis.
(1) Teratoma (usually midline, deeper location).
(2) Cerebral PNETs (usually deeper location, neuroblastomas commonly calcified, otherwise may be indistinguishable).
(3) Supratentorial ependymoma (usually deeper location, often calcification).
(4) Anaplastic astrocytoma or GBM (usually deeper location).
(5) Sarcomas (usually more peripheral, related to meninges).
(6) Desmoplastic cerebral astrocytoma (indistinguishable by imaging; pathologically determined by lack of neuronal elements).

II. Dysplastic cerebellar gangliocytoma (Lhermitte-Duclos disease) (see also Chapter 15).
  A. Histology: focal progressive expansion of cerebellar folia with disorganized progressive hypertrophic neurons. Probable hamartoma or cortical dysplasia rather than neoplasm.
  B. Incidence: rare; some association with congenital anomalies (megalencephaly, heterotopia and polydactyly), Cowden syndrome.
  C. Age: presents in adults.
  D. Location: cerebellar cortex.
  E. Clinical features.
    1. Symptoms of increased intracranial pressure rather than cerebellar dysfunction (uncommon).
    2. Slow-growing (hypertrophy rather than proliferation).
    3. Surgery relieves increased intracranial pressure.
  F. Imaging.
    1. CT: thickened, enlarged cerebellar folia.
    2. MRI: expansile mass with irregularly laminated or striated appearance with rare enhancement.
  G. Differential diagnosis.
    1. Infarct (typical vascular territory, less mass effect, may have gyral enhancement).

III. Dysembryoplastic neuroepithelial tumor (DNT).
  A. Histology.

       1. Diagnostic criteria include: columnar glioneuronal element, cellular polymorphism, multinodular glial architecture, and associated foci of cortical dysplasia (some prior controversy over hamartomatous origin).

       2. Immunopositive for neuronal markers (neurofilament, synaptophysin, NSE).

  B. Incidence: rare, although probably underestimated (only recently reported).

  C. Age: children, young adults.

  D. Gender: slight male predilection.

  E. Location.

       1. Predominantly cortical, can involve adjacent white matter.

       2. Temporal > frontal >> parietal, occipital lobes.

  F. Clinical features.

       1. Characteristic chronic intractable partial seizures with normal intelligence.

       2. Slow-growing, indolent course with favorable prognosis.

       3. Surgical resection performed for seizures.

  G. Imaging.

       1. CT.

          a. Typically rounded hypodense mass. However, may not be detectable on CT (10%).

          b. Absent to minimal enhancement.

          c. Calcification rare.

          d. May have adjacent scalloped skull erosion.

       2. MRI.

          a. Hypointense or isointense to GM on T1WI; hyperintense on T2WI. No edema.

          b. Occasionally may see multiple tiny cysts ("blister-like" nodules on pathology) on high-resolution T2WI.

          c. Absent to minimal enhancement.

  H. Differential diagnosis.

       1. Low-grade astrocytoma (temporal lobe tumors may be indistinguishable).

       2. Ganglioglioma (typically cyst/mural nodule configuration, although solid tumors may be indistinguishable).

       3. Gangliocytoma (may be indistinguishable).

       4. Oligodendroglioma (usually calcified, older presentation).

       5. Mesial temporal sclerosis (no mass effect or enhancement, older presentation).

       6. Choroidal fissure cyst (ovoid or spindle-shaped cyst related to choroidal fissure best distinguished on sagittal/coronal MRI).

       7. Unfused hippocampal fissure (small cysts related to fissure best distinguished on high-resolution T2WI).

IV. Central neurocytoma.
  A. Histology: small mature neuronal cells; resembles oligodendroglioma on light microscopy but neuronal characteristics confirmed by electron microscopy (synapses, neurosecretory granules, microtubules) and immunohistochemical studies (synaptophysin, NSE).
  B. Incidence: rare, 0.5% of primary brain tumors. (Probably underestimated; probably previously diagnosed as intraventricular oligodendroglioma, clear cell ependymoma, cerebral neuroblastoma.)
  C. Age: any age, usually young adults; peak at 20 to 30 years.
  D. Location: anterior portion of lateral ventricles near foramen of Monro > third ventricle.
  E. Clinical features.
    1. Presentation nonspecific, symptoms due to hydrocephalus.
    2. Benign. Good long-term survival.
    3. Total resection curative; radiation for subtotal resection.
  F. Imaging.
    1. Angiography.
      a. Varies from avascular mass effect to moderate homogenous tumor stain.
      b. May have vessel displacement due to hydrocephalus.
    2. CT.
      a. Well-defined rounded or lobulated heterogeneous isodense or slightly hyperdense intraventricular mass.
      b. Mild to moderate enhancement.
      c. Small cysts common: 70% to 85%.
      d. Punctate, scattered calcification common: 50% to 70%.
      e. Hemorrhage uncommon.
      f. May have associated obstructive hydrocephalus.
    3. MRI.
      a. Heterogeneous ("soap bubble" appearance) isointense or hyperintense to GM on T1WI; isointense or hyperintense on T2WI.
      b. Low or absent signal areas due to calcification or vessels.
      c. Mild to moderate enhancement.
  G. Differential diagnosis (foramen of Monro/septum pellucidum lesion).
    1. Subependymal giant cell astrocytoma (may be indistinguishable without associated findings of TS).
    2. Ependymoma (more commonly extraventricular, however, may be indistinguishable if purely intraventricular).
    3. Subependymoma (absent or variable enhancement, calcification uncommon).
    4. Colloid cyst (midline anterior third ventricle, homogeneously hyperdense, no calcification, nonenhancing).

V. Pineal parenchymal tumors.
  A. Pineocytoma.
    1. Histology: mature neuronal-type pineal cells; pineocytomatous rosettes.
    2. Incidence.
        a. Rare, <1% of primary CNS tumors.
        b. <15% of pineal region tumors.
    3. Age: any age, average 35 years.
    4. Gender: slight female or no gender predilection.
    5. Location: pineal gland.
    6. Prognosis: benign, slow-growing.
    7. Imaging.
        a. CT.
            (1) Small tumors usually solid but may be cystic and indistinguishable from benign pineal cysts.
            (2) Large tumors appear more aggressive.
            (3) Isodense or slightly hyperdense.
            (4) Dense calcification common.
            (5) Moderate to marked homogeneous enhancement.
        b. MRI.
            (1) Usually homogeneously enhancing, but cystic tumors may be indistinguishable from benign pineal cysts.
    8. Differential diagnosis.
        a. Solid tumors.
            (1) Germinoma (may have additional suprasellar lesion or subependymal involvement).
            (2) Meningioma (may be indistinguishable).
            (3) Glioma (usually located in tectum but occasionally from glial tissue in pineal gland, heterogeneous).
            (4) Solitary metastasis (rare, may be indistinguishable).
        b. Cystic tumors.
            (1) Benign pineal cyst (may be indistinguishable).
            (2) Arachnoid cyst (located in quadrigeminal cistern or velum interpositum, identical to CSF, may compress pineal gland inferiorly.
            (3) Epidermoid cyst (located in quadrigeminal cistern, mildly lobulated, often slightly heterogeneous, similar to or slightly greater than CSF density/signal).
            (4) Cavum velum interpositum (triangular shape, contiguous with quadrigeminal cistern).
  B. Pineoblastoma.

1. Histology.
   a. Tumor of malignant undifferentiated, immature neuronal-type pineal cells, resembles other PNETs especially medulloblastoma.
   b. Immunopositive for synaptophysin, NSE. No pineocytomatous rosettes.
2. Incidence.
   a. Uncommon.
   b. May be "third tumor" in trilateral retinoblastoma.
3. Age: young children.
4. Gender: slight female or no gender predilection.
5. Location: pineal gland.
6. Prognosis.
   a. Aggressive behavior, poor prognosis.
   b. CSF dissemination common.
7. Imaging.
   a. CT.
      (1) Large lobulated, heterogeneous isodense or hyperdense mass in pineal region with possible adjacent parenchymal invasion.
      (2) Dense calcification, hemorrhage, necrosis common.
      (3) Moderate to marked enhancement.
      (4) Associated obstructive hydrocephalus common.
   b. MRI.
      (1) Variable mixed signal: usually hypointense or isointense to GM on T1WI; isointense or hyperintense on T2WI.
      (2) May see ependymal spread or CNS dissemination.
      (3) MRI is modality of choice for craniospinal axis screening.
8. Differential diagnosis (pediatric).
   a. Germinoma (usually homogeneously enhancing, male predominance).
   b. Teratoma (may have fat density/signal).
   c. Choroid plexus papilloma in posterior third ventricle (large tumors may be indistinguishable).
   d. Tectal or pineal glioma (may be indistinguishable).
   e. Aneurysmal dilatation of vein of Galen (smoothly spheric with strong uniform intraluminal enhancement and flow void, relationship to internal cerebral veins/straight sinus best seen on MRI).

C. Mixed pineocytoma/pineoblastoma: intermediate prognosis, capacity for CNS dissemination.

SUGGESTED READINGS

Abe M, Tabuchi K, Tsuji T, et al: Dysembroplastic neuroepithelial tumor: report of three cases, *Surg Neurol* 43:240-245, 1995.

Awwad EE, Levy E, Martin DS, Merenda OO: Atypical MR appearance of Lhermitte-Duclos disease with contrast enhancement, *AJNR* 16:1719-1720, 1995.

Blatt GL, Ahuja A, Miller LL, Ostrow PT, Soloniuk DS: Cerebellomedullary ganglioglioma: CT and MR findings, *AJNR* 16:790-792, 1995.

Burger PC, Scheithauer BW: *Atlas of tumor pathology (third series, fascicle 10): tumors of the central nervous system,* Washington, 1994, Armed Forces Institute of Pathology.

Chang KH, Han MH, Kim DG, et al: MR appearance of central neurocytoma, *Acta Radiol* 34:520-526, 1993.

Daumas-Duport C: Dysembryoplastic neuroepithelial tumours, *Brain Pathol* 3:283-295, 1993.

Duffner PK, Burger PC, Cohen ME, et al: Desmoplastic infantile gangliogliomas: an approach to therapy, *Neurosurg* 34:583-589, 1994.

Hashimoto M, Fujimoto K, Shinoda S, Masuzawa T: Magnetic resonance imaging of ganglion cell tumours, *Neuroradiol* 35:181-184, 1993.

Hassoun J, Soylemezoglu F, Gambarelli D, et al: Central neurocytoma: a synopsis of clinical and histological features, *Brain Pathol* 3:297-306, 1993.

Koeller KK, Dillon WP: Dysembryoplastic neuroepithelial tumors: MR appearance, *AJNR* 13:1319-1325, 1992.

Lang FF, Epstein FJ, Ransohoff J, et al: Central nervous system gangliogliomas, Part 2: clinical outcome, *J Neurosurg* 79:867-873, 1993.

Meltzer CC, Smirniotopoulos JG, Jones RV: The striated cerebellum: an MR imaging sign in Lhermitte-Duclos disease (dysplastic gangliocytoma), *Radiol* 194:699-703, 1995.

Miller DC, Lang FF, Epstein FJ: Central nervous system gangliogliomas; Part 1: pathology, *J Neurosurg* 79:859-866, 1993.

Okamura A, Goto S, Sato K, Ushio Y: Central neurocytoma with hemorrhagic onset, *Surg Neurol* 43:252-255, 1995.

Osborn AG: Meningiomas and other nonglial neoplasms. In *Diagnostic radiology,* St Louis, 1994, Mosby, pp 579-625.

Raymond AA, Halpin SFS, Alsanjari N, et al: Dysembryoplastic neuroepithelial tumour: features in 16 patients, *Brain* 117:461-475, 1994.

Russell DS, Rubinstein LJ: *Pathology of tumours of the nervous system,* ed 5, Baltimore, 1989, Williams and Wilkins.

Smirniotopoulos JG, Rushing EJ, Mena H: From the archives of the AFIP: Pineal region masses: differential diagnosis, *Radiographics* 12:577-596, 1992.

VandenBerg SR: Desmoplastic infantile ganglioglioma and desmoplastic cerebral astrocytoma of infancy, *Brain Pathol* 3:275-281, 1993.

29

Primitive Neuroepithelial Tumors and Germ Cell Tumors

Key Concepts

1. PNETs are a diverse group of embryonal, largely undifferentiated tumors that generally occur in pediatric population, and include:
   a. Medulloblastoma.
   b. Cerebral neuroblastoma.
   c. Retinoblastoma.
   d. Pineoblastoma.
   e. Ependymoblastoma.
   f. Medulloepithelioma.
2. Medulloblastoma is prototypic infratentorial PNET, whereas cerebral neuroblastoma is prototypic supratentorial PNET.
3. Medulloblastoma is one of two most common pediatric posterior fossa tumors, along with cerebellar astrocytoma (studies differ as to which is most common).
4. Germ cell tumors include:
   a. Germinoma.
   b. Teratoma.
   c. Choriocarcinoma.
   d. Endodermal sinus (yolk sac) tumor.
   e. Embryonal carcinoma.
5. Germinoma is the most common intracranial germ cell tumor and the most common pineal region neoplasm.

I. Primitive neuroepithelial or embryonal tumors.
   A. Medulloblastoma (prototype infratentorial PNET).
      1. Histology.
         a. Spectrum of densely cellular undifferentiated tumors with areas of neuronal/neuroblastic or glial differentiation. Probably arise from bipotential embryologic cells in roof of fourth ventricle. Types are:
            (1) Classic: undifferentiated.
            (2) With neuroblastic or neuronal differentiation: may have neuroblastic Homer Wright rosettes, ganglion cells, synaptophysin, neuron-specific enolase (NSE).
            (3) With glial differentiation: glial fibrillary acidic protein (GFAP) positive.
            (4) With mixed glial-neuronal differentiation.
         b. Lateral cerebellar tumors tend to have desmoplastic response.
      2. Incidence.
         a. 6% of all primary brain tumors; 1% of adult intracranial neoplasms.
         b. One of two most common pediatric brain tumors (15% to 25%) along with astrocytoma.
         c. One of two most common pediatric posterior fossa tumors (25% to 30%) along with astrocytoma (studies differ as to which is most common).
         d. May be associated with basal cell nevus (Gorlin) syndrome.
      3. Age: children; 75% <15 years, rarely congenital; 15% in adults, second peak 25 to 30 years.
      4. Gender: slight male predominance (4:3 to 2:1).
      5. Location.
         a. Midline posterior fossa most common (75%).
         b. Lateral cerebellum uncommon (25%); more likely in young adults (50%).
         c. Occasionally extends through foramina of Luschka or Magendie. Rarely CPA mass.
         d. CNS dissemination common (50% to 60%).
         e. Non-CNS metastases rare (6%).
            (1) Bone (usually blastic) most common: pelvis, long bones, spine > ribs, skull.
            (2) Less commonly nodes, abdominal viscera, lungs.
      6. Clinical features.
         a. Symptoms due to obstructive hydrocephalus.
         b. Overall 5-year survival >50%.

    c. With total resection 5-year survival of 75%; 10-year survival of 25%.

    d. Early, widespread CNS dissemination frequent (20% to 50%), often receive adjuvant or prophylactic craniospinal radiation.

7. Imaging (see Fig. 26-1, *B*).

    a. Angiography.

        (1) Avascular or hypovascular mass effect; inferior displacement of PICA, anterior displacement of precentral cerebellar vein.

    b. CT.

        (1) Typically rounded or lobulated well-defined homogeneously hyperdense midline posterior fossa mass, although classic findings seen in only 30%.

        (2) Heterogeneity with cystic areas common (65%) although more likely in lateral tumors.

        (3) Fourth ventricle displaced anteriorly.

        (4) Calcification uncommon: 15% to 50%.

        (5) Moderate homogeneous enhancement. (Lateral tumors tend to have less intense and heterogeneous enhancement.)

        (6) Hemorrhage rare.

        (7) Associated obstructive hydrocephalus common: 95%.

    c. MRI.

        (1) Mildly heterogeneous fourth ventricular region mass that may extend into cisterna magna.

        (2) Hypointense to isointense on T1WI; hyperintense on T2WI. Occasionally hypointense on T2WI (may correlate with desmoplasia in adult tumors).

        (3) Cysts common: 75% to 80%.

        (4) Moderate to marked enhancement; occasionally patchy or absent.

        (5) Subarachnoid spread common.

        (6) MRI is modality of choice for craniospinal axis screening.

8. Differential diagnosis (see Fig. 26-1).

    a. Midline lesions (more common, usually children):

        (1) Ependymoma (more heterogeneous, dilates/fills fourth ventricle, may extrude into CPA cistern).

        (2) Vermian pilocytic astrocytoma (typical mural nodule/ cyst configuration).

    b. Lateral posterior fossa lesions (uncommon, usually adults, often heterogeneous, less intensely enhancing).

       (1) Pilocytic astrocytoma (also uncommon in adults but may be indistinguishable).

       (2) Ependymoma (usually fills/dilates fourth ventricle with extrusion into CPA).

       (3) Hemangioblastoma (typical mural nodule/cyst configuration).

       (4) Choroid plexus papilloma (rare in fourth ventricle or CPA, marked enhancement).

       (5) Metastasis (most common adult posterior fossa tumor, may be indistinguishable).

B. Primary cerebral neuroblastoma (prototype supratentorial PNET).

  1. Histology.

    a. Tumor of small, undifferentiated cells with focal areas of ganglionic (neuronal) differentiation, neuroblastic Homer Wright rosettes, immunopositive for synaptophysin, NSE.

    b. Types:

      (1) Classic (most common).

      (2) Ganglioneuroblastoma (rare): neuronal differentiation intermediate between neuroblasts and mature ganglion cells.

  2. Incidence.

    a. Rare, <1% of primary CNS tumors.

    b. One of most common congenital brain tumors, 20% <2 months age.

  3. Age and gender: infants, young children, 80% <10 years, occasionally young adults; no gender predilection.

  4. Location.

    a. Usually originates in deep white matter.

    b. Cerebral hemispheres (frontal, parietal lobes) > occipital lobes, basal ganglia, thalami, pineal, and intraventricular.

  5. Clinical features.

    a. Presentation nonspecific, usually due to increased intracranial pressure.

    b. Poor prognosis, 5-year survival 30%.

    c. Postsurgical recurrence common. CSF dissemination frequent.

  6. Imaging.

    a. Angiography: variable vascularity; usually avascular mass effect.

    b. CT.

      (1) Large, discrete, heterogeneous, hemispheric mass with absent or minimal peripheral edema.

      (2) Calcification common (60%).

        (3) Mild to moderate heterogeneous enhancement.
        (4) Cyst formation or necrosis common.
        (5) Hemorrhage uncommon (10%).
        (6) Associated macrocephaly common.
    c. MRI.
        (1) Variable signal on T1WI depending on presence of hemorrhage; hyperintense to GM on T2WI.
        (2) Minimal peripheral edema.
        (3) Modality of choice for screening craniospinal axis.
    d. Differential diagnosis.
        (1) Supratentorial extraventricular ependymoma (may be indistinguishable).
        (2) Teratoma (usually midline, may have fat density/signal components).
        (3) High-grade astrocytoma (calcification uncommon).
        (4) Sarcomas (usually more peripheral and related to meninges).

C. Medulloepithelioma.
  1. Histology: extremely undifferentiated PNET, composed of epithelium resembling embryonic neural tube in addition to varying glial, neuronal, or even mesenchymal differentiation.
  2. Incidence: rare.
  3. Age and gender: usually <5 years, occasionally congenital; no gender predilection.
  4. Location: supratentorial (deep, periventricular) > infratentorial.
  5. Clinical features.
    a. Usually increasing head size.
    b. Prognosis poor; average survival <1 year.
    c. CNS dissemination frequent; systemic metastases rare.
  6. Imaging.
    a. Large, bulky, lobulated, heterogeneous enhancing mass.
    b. May have cysts, calcification, hemorrhage.

D. Ependymoblastoma.
  1. Histology: ependymoblastic rosettes within undifferentiated cells, no similarity to conventional ependymoma.
  2. Incidence: rare.
  3. Age and gender: most <5 years, occasionally congenital, rare in adults; no gender predilection.
  4. Location: any portion of neuraxis; cerebrum most common.
  5. Clinical features.
    a. Usually increasing head size.
    b. Aggressive tumor, prognosis poor, average survival <1 year.
    c. Tendency to CNS dissemination.

6. Imaging: not well described; large discrete enhancing tumors similar to other cerebral PNETs.

II. Germ cell tumors.
  A. Histology.
    1. Primordial germ cells thought to persist in extragonadal sites including thymus, pineal gland, and hypothalamus. Subsequent neoplastic transformation of residual germ cells may be related to hormonal changes during puberty.
    2. Classification.
      a. Germinoma: histology identical to testicular seminoma, ovarian dysgerminoma.
      b. Teratoma: embryonal differentiation, more than one germ cell layer. Types are:
        (1) Immature or "malignant."
        (2) Mature or "benign."
      c. Choriocarcinoma: trophoblastic differentiation; may detect elevated HCG in CSF or serum.
      d. Endodermal sinus (yolk sac) tumor: yolk sac differentiation, may detect elevated α-fetoprotein in CSF or serum.
      e. Embryonal carcinoma: yolk sac differentiation; may detect elevated α-fetoprotein and HCG in CSF or serum.
      f. Mixed germ cell tumors.
  B. Incidence.
    1. 0.5% to 2% of primary brain tumors overall; 2% to 4% of pediatric primary brain tumors.
    2. Germinoma: most common intracranial germ cell tumor (60%); most common pineal tumor (40%).
    3. Teratoma: second most common intracranial germ cell tumor (20%), second most common pineal tumor (15%).
    4. Pure embryonal carcinoma, endodermal sinus tumor and choriocarcinoma are rare.
    5. Mixed forms 20%.
  C. Age: childhood, peak 10 to 20 years; rarely adult.
  D. Gender.
    1. Male predominance for germinomas of pineal region (10:1) and basal ganglia.
    2. No gender predilection for suprasellar germinomas.
  E. Epidemiology: slightly increased incidence in Japan.
  F. Location.
    1. Germinoma:
      a. Pineal 60% to 80%.
      b. Suprasellar (hypothalamus, infundibulum) 20% to 30%.
      c. Basal ganglia, thalamus 5% to 10%.

      d. Multiple sites (e.g., pineal and suprasellar) 10% to 40%.

      e. Subependymal and subarachnoid spread frequent.

G. Clinical features.

  1. Symptoms location-dependent:

      a. Pineal tumors may present with Parinaud's syndrome or symptoms related to obstructive hydrocephalus.

      b. Suprasellar tumors may present with diabetes insipidus or precocious puberty. Larger lesions present with visual field defects secondary to chiasmal compression.

      c. Basal ganglia/thalamic tumors may present with slowly progressive hemiparesis or dystonia.

  2. Germinoma.

      a. Pure germinoma highly radiosensitive, potentially curable. Treatment includes resection and radiation. Long postoperative survival typical.

      b. Infiltration of basal ganglia, white matter tracts may lead to hemiatrophy of the cerebrum or brainstem.

  3. Teratoma: treatment primarily resection; mature tumors have better prognosis than immature tumors.

  4. Embryonal carcinoma and endodermal sinus tumor: poorly radiosensitive, resistant to treatment, dismal prognosis. Widespread CNS dissemination common. Average survival <1 year.

  5. Choriocarcinoma: prognosis improving with new chemotherapy regimens.

  6. Rare cases of somatic "malignant transformation" (e.g., sarcoma, adenocarcinoma) with dismal prognosis.

H. Imaging.

  1. Germinoma.

      a. CT.

         (1) Typically discrete mildly hyperdense pineal or suprasellar mass.

         (2) Pineal tumor often engulfs pineal calcification.

         (3) Typically strong homogeneous enhancement.

         (4) Hemorrhage, cysts uncommon (more likely with basal ganglia and thalamic lesions).

         (5) Pineal tumor may have associated obstructive hydrocephalus secondary to aqueductal compression.

      b. MRI.

         (1) Often isointense to GM on all sequences, occasionally hyperintense on T1WI and mixed intensity on T2WI.

         (2) Strong enhancement.

         (3) Basal ganglia and thalamic involvement may be associated with cerebral or brainstem hemiatrophy.

(4) Suprasellar lesions may invade sella with anterior compression/displacement of pituitary gland.

(5) MRI more sensitive for detecting subarachnoid and subependymal spread.

2. Teratoma.

   a. CT.

      (1) Lobulated heterogeneous mixed-density midline mass.

      (2) May have calcification, fat, or cystic areas.

      (3) Mild to moderate heterogeneous enhancement of solid areas or cyst walls.

   b. MRI.

      (1) Heterogeneous mixed-signal intensity; solid portions generally hypointense to GM on T1WI; hyperintense on T2WI. Signal varies with calcification, fat, cystic areas.

      (2) Malignant teratomas prone to parenchymal invasion (e.g., tectum, thalamus) and subarachnoid spread.

3. Other germ cell tumors: imaging findings nonspecific; choriocarcinoma prone to hemorrhage, embryonal carcinoma prone to necrosis and hemorrhage.

I. Differential diagnosis.

1. Pediatric pineal region lesions.

   a. Germinoma (homogeneously enhancing, may have associated suprasellar lesion or subependymal involvement).

   b. Teratoma (heterogeneous, may have calcification or fat).

   c. Pineoblastoma (heterogeneous).

   d. Choroid plexus papilloma of posterior third ventricle (uncommon).

   e. Glioma (usually arises from tectum or rarely from pineal gland glial tissue).

2. Pediatric suprasellar lesions.

   a. Germinoma (homogeneously enhancing, may have associated pineal lesion or subependymal involvement).

   b. Teratoma (heterogeneous, may have calcification or fat).

   c. Craniopharyngioma (usually suprasellar/intrasellar, partly solid/cystic, usually calcified).

   d. Chiasmatic-hypothalamic glioma (usually homogeneously enhancing, involves chiasm, may extend posteriorly into retrochiasmatic optic pathway).

   e. Hypothalamic hamartoma (nonenhancing mass between infundibulum and mammillary bodies).

   f. Granulocytic sarcoma or chloroma of AML (rare, infundibular thickening or mass).

g. Lymphoma (rarely suprasellar, homogeneous enhancement of suprasellar mass or infundibular thickening, uncommon in children).

h. Sarcoidosis (rarely suprasellar, homogeneously enhancing hypothalamic mass or infundibular thickening, uncommon in children).

SUGGESTED READINGS

Becker RL, Becker AD, Sobel DF: Adult medulloblastoma: review of 13 cases with emphasis on MRI, *Neuroradiol* 37:104-108, 1995.

Bourgouin PM, Tampieri D, Grahovac SZ, et al: CT and MR imaging findings in adults with cerebellar medulloblastoma: comparison with findings in children, *AJR* 159:609-612, 1992.

Burger PC, Scheithauer BW: *Atlas of tumor pathology (third series, fascicle 10): tumors of the central nervous system,* Washington, 1994, Armed Forces Institute of Pathology.

Freilich RJ, Thompson SJ, Walker RW: Adenocarcinomatous transformation of intracranial germ cell tumors, *Am J Surg Pathol* 19:537-544, 1995.

Higano S, Takahashi S, Ishii K, et al: Germinoma originating in the basal ganglia and thalamus: MR and CT evaluation, *AJNR* 15:1435-1441, 1994.

Itoyama Y, Kochi M, Kuratsu J-I: Treatment of intracranial nongerminomatous malignant germ cell tumors producing alpha-fetoprotein, *Neurosurg* 36:459-466, 1995.

Meyers SP, Kemp SS, Tarr RW: MR imaging features of medulloblastomas, *AJR* 158:859-865, 1992.

Moon WK, Chang KH, Kim I-O, et al: Germinomas of the basal ganglia and thalamus: MR findings and a comparison between MR and CT, *AJR* 162:1413-1417, 1994.

Mueller DP, Moore SA, Sato Y, Yuh WTC: MRI spectrum of medulloblastoma, *Clinical imaging* 16:250-255, 1992.

Osborn AG: *Diagnostic radiology,* St Louis, 1994, Mosby.

Robles HA, Smirniotopoulos JG, Figueroa RE: Understanding the radiology of intracranial primitive neuroectodermal tumors from a pathological perspective: a review, *Semin Ultrasound CT MRI:* 13:170-181, 1992.

Russell DS, Rubinstein LJ: *Pathology of tumours of the nervous system,* ed 5, Baltimore, 1989, Williams and Wilkins.

Smirniotopoulos JG, Rushing EJ, Mena H: From the archives of the AFIP: Pineal region masses: differential diagnosis, *Radiographics* 12:577-596, 1992.

Sugiyama K, Uozumi T, Kiya K, et al: Intracranial germ-cell tumor with synchronous lesions in the pineal and suprasellar regions: report of six cases and review of the literature, *Surg Neurol* 38:114-120, 1992.

Sumida M, Uozumi T, Kiya K, et al: MRI of intracranial germ cell tumours, *Neuroradiol* 37:32-37, 1995.

30
Pituitary Adenoma and Tumors of Rathke's Pouch Origin

Key Concepts

1. Pituitary adenomas are the most common sellar/juxtasellar mass.
2. Microadenomas (<1 cm) usually present with endocrinopathy, macroadenomas (>1 cm) are usually nonfunctioning and symptoms are due to hypopituitarism, chiasm compression, or cranial nerve involvement in cavernous sinus.
3. Lesions of Rathke's pouch origin include:
   a. Craniopharyngioma.
   b. Rathke cleft cyst.
4. Craniopharyngioma is heterogeneous and largely suprasellar, whereas Rathke cleft cyst is unilocular and largely intrasellar.

I. Pituitary adenoma.
  A. Histology.
    1. Embryology.
      a. Neurohypophysis (posterior lobe) originates from downward extension of hypothalamus.
      b. Adenohypophysis (anterior lobe) traditionally thought to develop from Rathke's pouch (diverticulum of primitive buccal cavity), although recent studies suggest possible origin from ventral neural ridge (i.e., neuroectoderm).
    2. Adenohypophysis.
      a. Three parts: pars tuberalis, pars distalis, pars intermedia.
      b. Histologic origin of tumors (in descending order of frequency).
        (1) Prolactinoma (27%).
        (2) Null cell/nonfunctioning/chromophobic adenoma (26%).
        (3) Growth hormone (GH) cell adenoma (13%).
        (4) Corticotroph adenoma (10%).
        (5) Gonadotroph adenoma (9%).
        (6) Mixed GH/prolactin-cell adenoma (8%).
        (7) "Silent" corticotroph adenoma (5%).
        (8) Thyrotroph adenoma (1%).
        (9) Plurihormonal adenoma (1%).
    3. Neurohypophysis.
      a. Three parts: median eminence, infundibular stalk, neural lobe.
      b. Hormones produced in hypothalamus transported through infundibular stalk, released by neural lobe.
  B. Incidence.
    1. 10% of primary brain tumors.
    2. Most common sellar/juxtasellar mass (30% to 50%).
    3. Microadenoma >> macroadenoma (by autopsy), although macroadenoma more likely to present clinically.
  C. Age and gender.
    1. Usually adults; <10% in children; <2% of pediatric intracranial neoplasms.
    2. Prolactinoma: young adults, female predilection (5:1).
    3. Growth hormone-cell adenoma: male predilection (2:1).
    4. Corticotroph adenoma: usually young adults, 20% child/adolescent; female predilection.
    5. Plurihormonal: usually children.
  D. Location.
    1. Microadenoma (<1 cm) usually located in pars distalis of adenohypophysis in proportion to normal cell distribution.

a. Prolactinoma, growth hormone-cell adenomas are located laterally.

b. Thyrotroph, gonadotroph and corticotroph adenomas are located centrally (latter towards posterior portion of adeno-hypophysis).

2. Macroadenoma may have suprasellar extension.

E. Clinical features.

   1. Microadenoma.

      a. May be incidental, asymptomatic, 10% to 30% of autopsies.

      b. Endocrinopathy (75%).

         (1) Prolactinoma: amenorrhea, galactorrhea in young women; impotence in men (less likely to present in men until large with visual symptoms).

         (2) Growth hormone adenoma: gigantism in children, acromegaly in adults.

         (3) Corticotroph adenoma: Cushing disease or Nelson syndrome.

         (4) Gonadotroph adenoma: menstrual disturbance or infertility in women.

   2. Macroadenoma usually nonfunctioning; may present with hypopituitarism, visual impairment (chiasm compression), or cranial nerve palsy (cavernous sinus involvement).

   3. Generally benign, slow-growing.

   4. Treatment for prolactinoma primarily bromocriptine. Macroadenoma generally treated surgically.

   5. Surgical recurrence up to 15% at 8 years, 35% at 20 years.

   6. Malignant adenomas, metastases (subarachnoid, liver, lung, nodes) rare (<1%).

F. Imaging.

   1. Plain film: macroadenomas usually cause sellar expansion and erosion.

   2. CT.

      a. Microadenoma (<1 cm).

         (1) Small hypodense or isodense mass on NECT (may be invisible without contrast). Less enhancement compared with normal gland, particularly with rapid CECT.

         (2) May have focal superior convexity of gland.

         (3) May have focal sellar floor erosion or destruction.

         (4) Hemorrhage rare in microadenoma unless treated with bromocriptine.

      b. Macroadenoma (>1 cm).

         (1) Lobulated isodense sellar and suprasellar mass. "Snowman" or "figure-of-eight" configuration due to

constriction at diaphragma sella. Optic chiasm displaced superiorly.

   (2) Necrosis, hemorrhage, cyst formation common.
   (3) Calcification rare (1% to 8%).
   (4) Moderate enhancement.
   (5) May have associated hydrocephalus.

3. MRI.
   a. Generally procedure of choice for initial screening.
   b. Microadenoma.
      (1) Generally hypointense (80% to 90%) to gland on T1WI; isointense or hyperintense (30% to 50%) on T2WI.
      (2) Cavernous sinus invasion suggested by tumor encasement of cavernous internal carotid artery. Lack of invasion suggested by rimlike enhancing tissue interposed between microadenoma and cavernous sinus.
      (3) Enhances less rapidly than normal pituitary gland; hypointense on dynamic T1WI contrast study. Usually also hypointense on routine postcontrast study, but adenoma may enhance to degree of adjacent gland on more delayed imaging.
      (4) Pituitary stalk may be displaced (although finding is nonspecific).
   c. Macroadenoma.
      (1) Heterogeneity common (necrosis, hemorrhage, cyst formation).
      (2) Heterogeneous intense enhancement.
      (3) Normal pituitary gland usually displaced superiorly, although often difficult to distinguish.
      (4) Postoperative studies demonstrate lowering of normal gland into sella and reexpansion.

G. Differential diagnosis.
   1. Microadenoma.
      a. Pars intermedia or Rathke cleft cyst (purely cystic).
      b. Empty sella (intrasellar subarachnoid extension, flattening of pituitary gland, normal midline infundibulum).
      c. Pituitary hyperplasia (homogenous enlargement of gland without focal lesion).
   2. Macroadenoma.
      a. Craniopharyngioma (larger suprasellar component, partly cystic/solid, usually calcified, strong enhancement of solid portion, displacement/compression of normal pituitary inferiorly).

   b. Meningioma (homogeneously enhancing, usually suprasellar, may have "dural tail").
   c. Germinoma (usually suprasellar but if extends intrasellar usually displaces pituitary anteriorly).
   d. Chiasmatic-hypothalamic glioma (usually suprasellar solid mass involving chiasm, may extend into retrochiasmatic optic pathway).
   e. Metastasis, especially lung, breast, prostate (rare, no distinguishing features).
   f. Large Rathke cleft cyst (cystic, grows upward into suprasellar region without sellar expansion or erosion, absent or minimal peripheral enhancement).
   g. Juxtasellar aneurysm (round, frequent peripheral calcification, strong uniform luminal enhancement and flow void if patent).
   h. Lymphocytic hypophysitis: lymphocytic infiltration of adenohypophysis usually in peripartum females with hypopituitarism (enhancing intrasellar mass with possible suprasellar extension may be indistinguishable from macroadenoma).
II. Lesions of Rathke's pouch origin.
   A. Craniopharyngioma.
      1. Histology.
         a. Origin uncertain; thought to arise from squamous epithelial rests of Rathke's pouch origin at junction of pituitary stalk and adenohypophysis.
         b. Composed of nests of epithelial cells and cysts lined by squamous epithelium. Cyst contents include desquamated cells, keratin, cholesterol, protein, hemorrhage. Appearance ranges from straw-colored to turbid brown (classic "motor oil" appearance) due to old hemorrhage.
         c. Cell types.
            (1) Adamantinomatous (more common): partly solid/cystic with keratin and calcification.
            (2) Squamous papillary (less common, usually adults): predominantly solid, tend to lack keratin and calcification. Immunopositive for epithelial membrane antigen (EMA).
            (3) Mixed.
      2. Incidence.
         a. 3% to 5% of primary intracranial tumors.
         b. Most common pediatric nonglial intracranial neoplasm.
         c. 10% to 15% of pediatric supratentorial tumors.
         d. 50% of pediatric suprasellar tumors.

3. Age.
   a. Usually childhood <20 years, peak 10 to 15.
   b. Almost half occur in adults; second smaller peak in middle-aged adults (30 to 60).
4. Location.
   a. Suprasellar with smaller intrasellar component (75%).
   b. Predominantly suprasellar less common (20%).
   c. Purely intrasellar uncommon (5%).
   d. Rarely third ventricle (<1%).
5. Clinical features.
   a. Presentation.
      (1) Suprasellar lesions may present with endocrinopathy (e.g., diabetes insipidus or short stature) or visual impairment (e.g., field defects).
      (2) Third ventricle lesions may present with symptoms due to obstructive hydrocephalus.
      (3) Rupture can result in chemical meningitis, ventriculitis.
   b. Although histologically benign, can demonstrate aggressive infiltration.
   c. Treatment includes surgery with possible adjuvant radiation. Complete resection often impossible.
   d. Recurrence: 20% with complete resection and 75% with incomplete resection.
   e. Controversial whether recurrence rates lower with squamous papillary type (probably due to higher likelihood of complete resection).
6. Imaging.
   a. Plain film: large lesions usually cause sellar enlargement or destruction. Calcification common.
   b. CT.
      (1) Typically lobulated heterogeneous cystic and solid suprasellar mass. Rarely purely solid (15%), more likely in adults.
      (2) Nodular or eggshell calcification common: 90% in pediatric tumors, 30% to 40% in adult tumors.
      (3) Strong enhancement of solid portions and periphery.
   c. MRI.
      (1) Solid portions generally hypointense to GM on T1WI and hyperintense on T2WI.
      (2) Cystic portions usually resemble CSF signal, but can be hyperintense on T1WI with hemorrhage, cholesterol, or protein content.
7. Differential diagnosis.

  a. Pituitary macroadenoma (larger intrasellar component, usually solid, less enhancing, older presentation).

  b. Chiasmatic-hypothalamic glioma (usually homogenous solid mass involving chiasm, although cyst/mural nodule may be seen, may extend into retrochiasmatic optic pathway).

  c. Hypothalamic hamartoma (homogeneous solid mass between infundibulum and mammillary bodies without enhancement).

  d. Germinoma (homogeneous enhancement).

  e. Teratoma (heterogeneous, may have calcification or fat).

B. Rathke's cleft cyst, pars intermedia cyst.

 1. Histology: Rathke's pouch is an epithelial-lined diverticulum of the embryonic buccal cavity ectoderm (primitive stomatodeum) giving rise to adenohypophysis. Normally closes during embryologic development; otherwise epithelium-lined cleft persists between anterior and posterior lobes (pars intermedia). Cyst formed by accumulation of serous or mucinous fluid.

 2. Incidence: uncommon, <1% of primary intracranial tumors; however, may be incidental in 30% of autopsies.

 3. Age: any age, usually middle-aged adults.

 4. Location.

  a. Usually intrasellar with smaller suprasellar component (70%).

  b. Less commonly purely intrasellar (25%).

  c. Rarely purely suprasellar (<5%).

 5. Clinical features.

  a. Small intrasellar lesions (i.e., pars intermedia cyst) often asymptomatic, found incidentally at autopsy.

  b. Larger lesions (i.e., Rathke's cleft cyst) present with endocrinopathy or visual impairment.

  c. Large lesions requiring resection or aspiration rarely recur.

 6. Imaging.

  a. Plain film: unlike pituitary adenoma, no sellar enlargement.

  b. CT.

   (1) Typically small (<5 mm, but can be as large as 4 cm) homogeneous hypodense cystic mass predominantly in intrasellar region. Rather than expand sella, growth is upward into suprasellar region (probably due to soft consistency).

   (2) Hemorrhage uncommon but can result in increased density.

   (3) Calcification rare.

   (4) Minimal peripheral enhancement in 50% of cases.

  c. MRI.

(1) Variable homogeneous signal: two thirds hyperintense to GM (high protein, cholesterol, hemorrhage), one third hypointense on T1WI; variable on T2WI.

(2) Typically does not enhance, although may see strong enhancement of displaced, compressed pituitary gland around cyst.

7. Differential diagnosis.

a. Craniopharyngioma (predominantly suprasellar, partly solid/cystic, calcification, marked enhancement, younger presentation).

b. Necrotic or cystic pituitary adenoma (expands sella, partly solid/cystic).

c. Arachnoid cyst (predominantly suprasellar, identical to CSF).

d. Epidermoid cyst (predominantly suprasellar, slightly heterogeneous, similar to or slightly hyperintense to CSF).

e. Dermoid cyst (predominantly suprasellar, usually resembles fat density/signal).

f. Empty sella (intrasellar subarachnoid extension with flattening of pituitary gland, normal midline infundibulum).

g. Cysticercosis cyst (may see enhancing scolex or parenchymal calcifications, additional lesions).

SUGGESTED READINGS

Burger PC, Scheithauer BW: *Atlas of tumor pathology (third series, fascicle 10): tumors of the central nervous system,* Washington, 1994, Armed Forces Institute of Pathology.

Colombo N, Loli P, Vignati F, Scialfa G: MR of corticotropin-secreting pituitary microadenomas, *AJNR* 15:1591-1595, 1994.

Crotty TR, Scheithauer BW, Young WF Jr, et al: Papillary craniopharyngioma: a clinicopathological study of 48 cases, *J Neurosurg* 83:206-214, 1995.

Elster AD: Modern imaging of the pituitary, *Radiol* 187:1-14, 1993.

Epstein FJ, Handler MH (guest ed): Craniopharyngioma: the answer, *Ped Neurosurg* 21(suppl 1): entire monograph, 1994.

Girard N, Brue T, Chabert-Orsini V, et al: 3D-FT thin sections MRI of prolactin-secreting pituitary microadenomas, *Neuroradiol* 36:376-379, 1994.

Hald JK, Eldevik OP, Brunberg JA, Chandler WF: Craniopharyngiomas—the utility of contrast medium enhancement for MR imaging at 1.5 T, *Acta Radiol* 35:520-525, 1994.

Harrison MJ, Morgello S, Post KD: Epithelial cystic lesions of the sellar and parasellar region: a continuum of ectodermal derivatives? *J Neurosurg* 80:1018-1025, 1994.

Inoue Y, Saiwai S, Miyamoto T, Katsuyama J: Enhanced high-resolution sagittal MRI of normal pineal glands, *J Comp Assist Tomog* 18:182-186, 1994.

Knosp E, Steiner E, Kitz K, Matula C: Pituitary adenomas with invasion of the cavernous sinus space: a magnetic resonance imaging classification compared with surgical findings, *Neurosurg* 33:610-618, 1993.

Kobayashi S, Ikeda H, Yoshimoto T: A clinical and histopathological study of factors affecting MRI signal intensities of pituitary adenomas, *Neuroradiol* 36:298-302, 1994.

Kollias SS, Ball WS, Prenger EC: Review of the embryologic development of the pituitary gland and report of a case of hypophyseal duplication detected by MRI, *Neuroradiol* 37:3-12, 1995.

Kucharczyk W, Bishop JE, Plewes DB, Keller MA, George S: Detection of pituitary microadenomas: comparison of dynamic keyhole fast spin-echo, unenhanced, and conventional contrast-enhanced MR imaging, *AJR* 163:671-679, 1994.

Mindermann T, Wilson CB: Pediatric pituitary adenomas, *Neurosurg* 36:259-269, 1995.

Oka H, Kawano N, Suwa T, et al: Radiological study of symptomatic Rathke's cleft cysts, *Neurosurg* 35:632-637, 1994.

Osborn AG: *Diagnostic radiology,* St Louis, 1994, Mosby.

Partington M, Davis DH, Laws ER, Scheithauer BW: Pituitary adenomas in childhood and adolescence: results of transsphenoidal surgery, *J Neurosurg* 80:209-216, 1994.

Russell DS, Rubinstein LJ: *Pathology of tumours of the nervous system,* ed 5, Baltimore, 1989, Williams and Wilkins.

Steiner E, Math G, Knosp E, et al: MR-appearance of the pituitary gland before and after resection of pituitary macroadenomas, *Clin Radiol* 49:524-530, 1994.

Sumida M, Uozumi T, Yamanaka M, et al: Displacement of the normal pituitary gland by sellar and juxtasellar tumours: surgical-MRI correlation and use in differential diagnosis, *Neuroradiol* 36:372-375, 1994.

Teramoto A, Hirakawa K, Sanno N, Osamura Y: Incidental pituitary lesions in 1,000 unselected autopsy specimens, *Neuroradiol* 193:161-164, 1994.

Weiner HL, Wisoff JH, Rosenberg ME, et al: Craniopharyngiomas: a clinicopathological analysis of factors predictive of recurrence and functional outcome, *Neurosurg* 35:1001-1011, 1994.

Whyte AM, Sage MR, Brophy BP: Imaging of large Rathke's cleft cysts by CT and MRI: report of two cases, *Neuroradiol* 35:258-260, 1993.

31

Meningeal Tumors

Key Concepts

1. Meningioma is the second most common primary intracranial neoplasm, after astrocytoma.
2. Current World Health Organization (WHO) classification and grading:
   a. Typical meningioma: benign.
   b. Atypical meningioma: intermediate grade.
   c. Anaplastic (malignant) meningioma: necrosis or brain invasion.
3. Prior classification of meningioma.
   a. Syncytial.
   b. Fibroblastic.
   c. Transitional meningioma.
   d. "Angioblastic meningiomas" (subtypes hemangiopericytic and hemangioblastic) do not arise from meningothelial cells and are no longer grouped with meningiomas in WHO classification. Small group of remaining extremely vascular meningiomas more appropriately designated "angiomatous."
4. Imaging finding of "dural tail" now known to be nonspecific (reported in various tumors in addition to meningioma) and does not necessarily reflect tumor infiltration (may simply be benign reactive process).
5. Hemangioblastoma, although mostly sporadic (80% to 90%) is frequently associated with von Hippel-Lindau (VHL) disease (45% of patients). Discovery should prompt consideration of VHL and search for additional important lesions (e.g., renal cell carcinoma). Ten to 40% of hemangioblastomas secrete erythropoietin, resulting in polycythemia.
6. Differential diagnosis of solid extraaxial dural-based mass includes meningioma, hemangiopericytoma, sarcomas, plasmacytoma/multiple myeloma, dural metastasis, and nonneoplastic processes such as sarcoid.

I. Meningioma.
  A. Histology.
   1. Meningothelial origin; arachnoid cap cell. Immunopositive for epithelial membrane antigen (EMA).
   2. Cytogenetics: deletion on chromosome 22; others may contribute to expression of aggressiveness.
   3. Types.
      a. Classic meningioma:
        (1) Meningotheliomatous or syncytial.
        (2) Fibroblastic or fibrous.
        (3) Transitional (mixed).
      b. Less common histological variants include: psammomatous, microcystic, myxomatous, xanthomatous, lipomatous, granular, secretory, chondroblastic, osteoblastic, papillary and clear cell meningioma.
      c. *Note:* previously described "angioblastic meningiomas" (subtypes hemangiopericytic and hemangioblastic) do not originate from meningothelial cells, are no longer grouped with meningothelial tumors in WHO classification (see below). Small group of remaining extremely vascular meningiomas more appropriately designated "angiomatous."
   4. Grading: "all histologic varieties may display malignant characteristics."
      a. WHO.
        (1) Typical meningioma: benign; 90% to 95%.
        (2) Atypical meningioma: intermediate hypercellularity and mitotic activity; 5%.
        (3) Anaplastic (malignant) meningioma: necrosis, abundant mitosis, brain invasion; 1% to 2%.
      b. Helsinki group.
        (1) Grade I: benign.
        (2) Grade II: atypical.
        (3) Grade III: anaplastic.
        (4) Grade IV: sarcomatous.
   5. Morphologic types.
      a. Globose or globular: most common.
      b. Meningioma en-plaque: less common.
      c. Multicentric: uncommon (1% to 10%), present slightly earlier, favors single hemicranium. Note: not to be confused with meningiomatosis (NF-2), a reactive angiodysplasia with intracortical meningovascular and fibroblastic proliferation.
  B. Incidence.

1. Second most common primary brain tumor after astrocytoma (15% to 20%).
2. Most common intracranial extraaxial tumor.
3. 25% to 30% of spinal tumors.
4. Genetics: chromosome 22 aberrations often associated.
5. Associated with NF-2 (also have chromosome 22 mutation); 50% of multicentric meningiomas occur in NF-2.
6. Increased incidence with prior radiation; more aggressive.

C. Age.
1. Adults, peak incidence at 40 to 60 years.
2. Rare in children; more likely associated with NF-2 or multicentric tumors.

D. Gender.
1. Females > males (2:1 to 4:1); relationship to sex hormones suggested by association with breast cancer, pregnancy, and progesterone receptors.
2. Slight male predilection in children.

E. Location (Fig. 31-1).
1. Supratentorial > infratentorial:
   a. Parasagittal 25% (middle third > frontal third > posterior third).
   b. Convexity 20%.
   c. Sphenoid ridge 15% to 20%.
   d. Olfactory groove 5% to 10%.
   e. Parasellar 5% to 10%.
2. Posterior fossa (CPA, clival) 10%.
3. Other intracranial (intraventricular, pineal, optic nerve sheath) 2%.
4. Intraspinal common.
5. Extracranial (nasal cavity, paranasal sinuses, neck, skin, lungs, mediastinum, peripheral nerves) 1%.
6. Multiple 5% to 15%.
7. Pediatric meningiomas slightly more frequent in atypical locations (posterior fossa, lateral ventricles).

F. Clinical features.
1. Up to 3% of patients >60 years of age have incidental meningioma at autopsy.
2. Symptoms nonspecific, dependent on location and size.
3. Prognosis depends on location, resectability: 10-year recurrence is 10% to 20% with complete resection, 20% to 50% with subtotal resection.
4. 5-year recurrence: 5% for typical benign; 30% for atypical; 75% for anaplastic tumors.

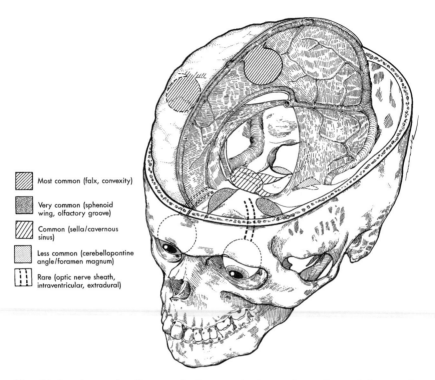

Most common (falx, convexity)

Very common (sphenoid wing, olfactory groove)

Common (sella/cavernous sinus)

Less common (cerebellopontine angle/foramen magnum)

Rare (optic nerve sheath, intraventricular, extradural)

Fig. 31-1 Anatomic diagram depicts meningioma sites. (From Osborn AG: *Diagnostic neuroradiology,* St Louis, 1994, Mosby.)

    5. Metastases rare (0.1%) but occurs with both benign and malignant tumors. Most common locations lung, abdominal viscera, bones, and nodes.

    6. Sarcomatous transformation rare (not to be confused with primary sarcomas or leptomeningeal sarcomatosis, which diffusely infiltrates meninges without focal mass).

    7. Pediatric and recurrent meningiomas more aggressive, may be multifocal.

    8. Treatment primarily surgical. Often preoperative embolization and adjunctive radiation. Recent developments include radiosurgery and hormonal therapy.

  G. Imaging (Fig. 31-2).

    1. Plain film.

      a. Calcified mass or hyperostosis.

      b. Secondary findings of bone erosion, enlarged vascular channels, or expanded paranasal sinus (pneumosinus dilatans) may be seen.

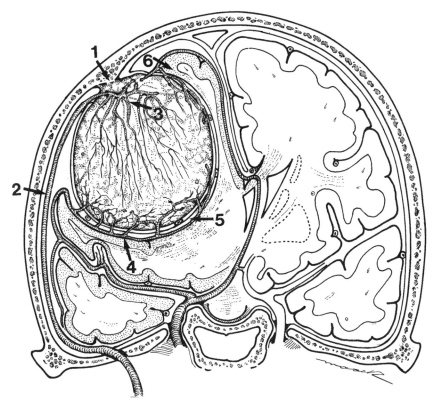

Fig. 31-2   Anatomic diagram, coronal plane, demonstrates the typical dual vascular supply of a large convexity meningioma: 1, Enostotic "spur" with vascular pedicle. 2, Enlarged middle meningeal artery. 3, Dural-derived vessels supply center of the meningioma. 4, Enlarged pial vessels supply the periphery. 5, CSF/vascular cleft between the tumor and adjacent brain. 6, Cortex displaced around the tumor confirms extraaxial location of the mass. (From Osborn AG: *Diagnostic neuroradiology,* St Louis, 1994, Mosby.)

2. Angiography.
    a. Usually vascular.
    b. Mostly supplied by meningeal and falcine arteries. Large tumor may have dual supply; additional pial branches of cerebral arteries supply periphery.
    c. Typical prolonged "sunburst" blush.
    d. Occasional AV shunting, early draining veins.
    e. May cause dural venous sinus occlusion.
    f. Preoperative embolization often performed to reduce vascularity.

3. CT.
   a. Discrete homogenous hyperdense extraaxial mass. Less commonly isodense (25%) or hypodense (1% to 5%).
   b. Usually rounded but often en-plaque (e.g., sphenoid wing), latter may be difficult to see on NECT.
   c. Typically abuts dural surface. Occasionally lacks dural attachment (more likely in children).
   d. Gross calcification uncommon (20% to 25%).
   e. Bone changes include variable hyperostosis or less commonly bone destruction (10% to 15%).
   f. Strong homogeneous enhancement (95%).
   g. Gross hemorrhage uncommon.
   h. Necrosis or cystic areas uncommon (5% to 10%), although more likely in children.
   i. Edema common (60%) but variable.
4. MRI.
   a. Globose tumors are typically well-defined extraaxial mass with CSF cleft adjacent to brain and "buckling" or displacement of gray/white interface.
   b. En-plaque tumors may be difficult to see on noncontrast study.
   c. Frequently isointense to GM on all sequences, but signal can be variable. (Some studies have shown correlation between histology and signal, although not confirmed by other studies.)
   d. May see flow voids with enlarged feeding/draining vessels.
   e. Cystic areas may be intratumoral or peritumoral (latter can be large, possibly due to arachnoid cysts or peripheral parenchymal degeneration).
   f. Extent of edema may correlate with invasiveness and difficulty in resection.
   g. "Dural tail sign" often associated, although nonspecific and found in many other lesions. Controversy whether this represents tumor infiltration or benign meningeal reaction.
H. Differential diagnosis.
   1. Intraosseous calvarial lesions.
      a. Osteoma (hyperostosis usually confined to outer table, no diploic involvement).
      b. Fibrous dysplasia (usually "ground-glass" appearance on plain film and CT, hypointense on T1- and T2WI).
      c. Blastic metastasis (uncommon).
   2. Intracranial convexity lesions.
      a. Hemangiopericytoma.

        b. Sarcomas.

        c. Plasmacytoma/solitary multiple myeloma.

        d. Osseus/dural metastasis.

    3. CPA lesions.

        a. Solid lesions.

           (1) Schwannoma ("ice-cream cone" appearance, enlargement of IAC, acute angle with petrous bone).

           (2) Choroid plexus papilloma (rarely isolated CPA lesion).

           (3) Ependymoma (rarely isolated CPA lesion).

           (4) Metastasis (may be indistinguishable).

           (5) Vascular ectasia, aneurysm (strong uniform intraluminal enhancement and flow void if patent).

        b. Cystic lesions.

           (1) Cystic schwannoma (extends into IAC along nerve, acute angle with petrous bone).

           (2) Epidermoid (lacks solid portion, no enhancement).

           (3) Arachnoid cyst (lacks solid portion, no enhancement).

II. Mesenchymal, nonmeningothelial tumors.

  A. Hemangiopericytoma (Meningeal hemangiopericytoma).

    1. Histology.

        a. Origin controversial, probably arise from pericytes (mesenchymal) around capillaries rather than meningothelial cells. A histologically identical neoplasm occurs in soft tissues.

        b. Not immunoreactive for EMA. (No longer grouped with meningothelial tumors in WHO classification.)

    2. Incidence: rare, <1% of primary CNS tumors; 2% of meningeal tumors.

    3. Age: peak at 30 to 60 years.

    4. Gender: equal gender or slight male predilection.

    5. Location: parallels conventional meningioma.

    6. Clinical features.

        a. Symptoms nonspecific.

        b. Highly aggressive, although deceptively easy to enucleate; almost always recur, prone to metastasis.

        c. 5-year survival of 65%, 10-year survival of 40%, 15-year survival of 25%.

        d. Treatment primarily resection with possible adjuvant therapy, although poor response to radiation and chemotherapy.

        e. Local recurrence within 5 to 20 years common (75% to 80%).

        f. Distant metastases (e.g., lung, bone) uncommon (15%).

7. Imaging.
   a. Angiography.
      (1) Extremely vascular with prolonged, dense heterogeneous stain.
      (2) Mixed dural-pial supply.
      (3) AV shunting, early draining veins common.
   b. CT.
      (1) Discrete heterogeneous (not hyperdense) extraaxial mass, often with dural attachment.
      (2) Cystic areas, necrosis common (latter especially with larger tumors).
      (3) Strong, heterogeneous enhancement.
      (4) Calcification uncommon.
      (5) Can invade/destroy adjacent calvarium, extend into scalp. Unlike meningioma, no hyperostosis.
   c. MRI.
      (1) Typically extradural mass.
      (2) Generally isointense to GM on T1WI; slightly hyperintense on PD; heterogeneous on T2WI. Minimal edema.
      (3) Prominent vascular flow voids may be seen.
8. Differential diagnosis.
   a. Meningioma (usually adjacent hyperostosis rather than calvarial destruction).
   b. Sarcomas (may be indistinguishable).
   c. Plasmacytoma/solitary multiple myeloma (originates in calvarium with secondary extension to epidural/dural region).
   d. Calvarial/dural metastasis (originates in calvarium with secondary invasion of epidural/dural region).
B. Hemangioblastoma (Capillary hemangioblastoma).
   1. Histology: nonmeningothelial capillary-rich neoplasm interspersed with lipidized stromal cells. Supratentorial hemangioblastoma previously designated "angioblastic meningioma" is histologically identical to cerebellar hemangioblastoma.
   2. Incidence.
      a. Uncommon, 1% to 2% of primary intracranial neoplasms; 10% of posterior fossa tumors.
      b. Most sporadic; 10% to 20% associated with von Hippel-Lindau (VHL) disease (often multiple tumors), whereas 45% of VHL patients develop hemangioblastoma.
   3. Age: Young, middle-aged adults, 30 to 65 years; rare in children.
   4. Gender: overall slight male predilection; slight female predilection in VHL.

5. Location.
   a. Cerebellar hemisphere most common (80% to 85%).
   b. Occasionally medulla: 2%.
   c. Spinal cord: 5% to 15%.
   d. Supratentorial: rare, controversy over designation as "angioblastic meningioma" or supratentorial hemangioblastoma.
   e. Multiple lesions: 10% overall; 40% of VHL associated tumors.
6. Clinical features.
   a. Presenting symptoms nonspecific, location-dependent.
   b. 10% to 40% may be associated with polycythemia (secrete erythropoietin).
   c. If associated with VHL, may present with other lesions (see Chapter 17).
   d. Benign, treatment primarily resection with possible adjuvant radiation.
   e. 25% recur, especially in younger patients with multicentric tumors or VHL disease.
7. Imaging.
   a. Angiography.
      (1) Vascular nodule has intense, prolonged stain.
      (2) Cystic component has avascular mass effect.
   b. CT.
      (1) 60% well-circumscribed low-density cystic intraparenchymal mass with mural nodule; 40% solid. Mural nodule tends to abut pial surface.
      (2) Strong enhancement of mural nodule. Typically no enhancement of cyst wall (not usually neoplastic), although occasional minimal enhancement reported.
      (3) Calcification, necrosis, hemorrhage rare.
      (4) May have associated hydrocephalus.
   c. MRI.
      (1) Solid portion isointense to GM on T1WI; slightly hyperintense on T2WI. Cystic portion often slightly greater than CSF on both T1 and T2WI due to protein. Mixed signal if hemorrhage present.
      (2) May have vessel flow voids.
      (3) May have associated syrinx in medulla or spinal cord lesions.
8. Differential diagnosis.
   a. Pilocytic astrocytoma (mural nodule not confined to periphery, usually in children).
   b. Pleomorphic xanthoastrocytoma (rare in cerebellum).

      c. Ganglioglioma (rare in cerebellum).

      d. Metastasis (most common adult posterior fossa tumor although rarely cystic).

C. Other mesenchymal tumors.

  1. Histology.

      a. Benign: lipoma, chondroma, osteochondroma, fibroma, fibrous histiocytoma/fibroxanthoma, leiomyoma, rhabdomyoma. ⁓

      b. Malignant: angiosarcoma, chondrosarcoma, osteosarcoma, rhabdomyosarcoma, fibrosarcoma, malignant fibrous histiocytoma (MFH), meningeal sarcomatosis.

  2. Incidence: uncommon; 1% to 2% of primary intracranial tumors.

      a. Chondroma associated with Ollier, Mafucci syndrome.

      b. Fibrosarcoma, MFH may arise in GBM (gliosarcoma), site of prior radiation, or pagetoid bone.

      c. Angiosarcoma usually systemic, rarely primary in CNS.

  3. Age and gender.

      a. Any age.

      b. Rhabdomyosarcoma, primary meningeal sarcomatosis: children > adult.

      c. No gender predilection.

  4. Location.

      a. Meninges >> brain parenchyma.

      b. Osteocartilagenous tumors predominantly involve bone (skull base or calvarium); rarely primary in meninges or brain.

      c. Rhabdomyosarcoma occurs predominantly in head/neck; if intracranial, more likely in posterior fossa.

      d. Primary leptomeningeal sarcomatosis: diffuse infiltration of meninges without large mass.

  5. Clinical features.

      a. Symptoms nonspecific, location-dependent.

      b. Malignant tumors (sarcomas) are aggressive, often difficult to resect; poor prognosis. Local recurrence common.

  6. Imaging.

      a. Due to rarity of lesions, imaging characteristics not well described.

      b. Generally sarcomas will show discrete contrast-enhancing meningeal-based mass with edema, mass effect.

      c. Primary meningeal sarcomatosis: diffuse meningeal involvement without large mass.

  7. Differential diagnosis of sarcomas.

       a. Meningioma.

       b. Hemangiopericytoma.

       c. Plasmacytoma/solitary multiple myeloma.

       d. Calvarial/dural metastasis (including lymphoma/leukemia).

III. Primary melanocytic neoplasms.

  A. Histology.

     1. Arise from normally occurring leptomeningeal melanocytes (more common at base of brain, upper cervical region). Not to be confused with intracranial metastases of cutaneous malignant melanoma.

     2. Types.

       a. Diffuse melanosis.

       b. Melanocytoma (benign).

       c. Primary meningeal malignant melanoma.

  B. Incidence: rare.

  C. Age.

     1. Diffuse melanosis more common in children.

     2. Melanocytoma more common in adults.

  D. Location: posterior fossa, cervical spinal canal, Meckel's cave.

  E. Clinical features.

     1. Diffuse melanosis may be associated with pigmented skin lesions: neurocutaneous melanosis.

     2. Melanocytoma prone to multiple local recurrences; rare transformation to malignant melanoma.

  F. Imaging: not well described.

     1. Melanocytoma: focal or en-plaque extraaxial isodense mass with homogeneous enhancement.

     2. Primary meningeal malignant melanoma: diffuse meningeal enhancement, may have associated hydrocephalus.

SUGGESTED READINGS

Black PM: Meningiomas, *Neurosurg* 32:643-657, 1993.

Bourekas EC, Wildenhain P, Lewis JS, et al: The dural tail sign revisited, *AJNR* 16:1514-1516, 1995.

Burger PC, Scheithauer BW: *Atlas of tumor pathology (third series, fascicle 10): tumors of the central nervous system,* Washington, 1994, Armed Forces Institute of Pathology.

Carpeggiani P, Crisi G, Trevisan C: MRI of intracranial meningiomas: correlations with histology and physical consistency, *Neuroradiol* 35:532-536, 1993.

Chiocca EA, Boviatsis EJ, Westmark RM, et al: Deep sylvian fissure meningioma without dural attachment in an adult: case report, *Neurosurg* 35:944-946, 1994.

Cosentino CM, Poulton TB, Esguerra JV, Sands SF: Giant cranial hemangiopericytoma: MR and angiographic findings, *AJNR* 14:253-256, 1993.

Croutch KL, Wong WHM, Coufal F, Georgy B, Hesselink JR: En plaque meningioma of the basilar meninges and Meckel's cave: MR appearance, *AJNR* 16:949-951, 1995.

Darling CF, Byrd SE, Reyes-Mugica M, et al: MR of pediatric intracranial meningiomas, *AJNR* 15:435-444, 1994.

De Jesus O, Rifkinson N, Negron B: Cystic meningiomas: a review, *Neurosurg* 36:489-492, 1995.

DeVries J, Wakhloo AK: Repeated multifocal recurrence of grade I, grade II, and grade III meningiomas: regional multicentricity (primary new growth) or metastases? *Surg Neurol* 41:299-305, 1994.

Florian CL, Preece NE, Bhakoo KK, et al: Cell type-specific fingerprinting of meningioma and meningeal cells by proton nuclear magnetic resonance spectroscopy, *Cancer Res* 55:420-427, 1995

Germano IM, Edwards MSB, Davis RL, Schiffer D: Intracranial meningiomas of the first two decades of life, *J Neurosurg* 80:447-453, 1994.

Gokalp HZ, Arasil E, Erdogan A, et al: Tentorial meningiomas, *Neurosurg* 36:46-51, 1995.

Goldmann A, Kunz U, Bader C, et al: MR imaging and MR angiography in preoperative evaluation of intracranial meningiomas, *Eur Radiol* 4:538-544, 1994.

Kasoff SS, Spiller M, Valsamis MP, et al: Relaxometry of noncalcified human meningiomas: correlation with histology and solids content, *Invest Radiol* 30:49-55, 1995.

Lunsford LD: Contemporary management of meningiomas: radiation therapy as an adjunct and radiosurgery as an alternative to surgical removal? *J Neurosurg* 80:187-190, 1994.

Maeda M, Itoh S, Kimura H, et al: Vascularity of meningiomas and neuromas: assessment with dynamic susceptibility-contrast MR imaging, *AJR* 163:181-186, 1994.

Nagele T, Petersen D, Klose U, et al: The "dural tail" adjacent to meningiomas studied by dynamic contrast-enhanced MRI: a comparison with histopathology, *Neuroradiol* 36:303-307, 1994.

Newman SA: Meningiomas: a quest for the optimum therapy, *J Neurosurg* 80: 191-194, 1994.

Olivero WC, Lister JR, Elwood PW: The natural history and growth rate of asymptomatic meningiomas: a review of 60 patients, *J Neurosurg* 83:222-224, 1995.

Osborn AG: *Diagnostic radiology,* St Louis, 1994, Mosby.

Prabhu SS, Lynch PG, Keogh AJ, Parekh HC: Intracranial meningeal melanocytoma: a report of two cases and a review of the literature, *Surg Neurol* 40:516-21, 1993.

Rawat B, Franchetto AA, Elavathil J: Extracranial metastases of meningioma, *Neuroradiol* 37:38-41, 1995.

Ruscalleda J, Feliciani M, Avila A, et al: Neuroradiological features of intracranial and intraorbital meningial hemangiopericytomas, *Neuroradiol* 36:440-445, 1994.

Russell DS, Rubinstein LJ: *Pathology of tumours of the nervous system,* ed 5, Baltimore, 1989, Williams and Wilkins.

Salpietro FM, Alafaci C, Lucerna S, et al: Peritumoral edema in meningiomas: microsurgical observations of different brain tumor interfaces related to computed tomography, *Neurosurg* 35:639-642, 1994.

Sridhark K, Ravi R, Ramamurthi B, Vasudevan MC: Cystic meningiomas, *Surg Neurol* 43:235-239, 1995.

Standard SC, Ahuja A, Livingston K, Guterman LR, Hopkins LN: Endovascular embolization and surgical excision for the treatment of cerebellar and brain stem hemangioblastomas, *Surg Neurol* 41:405-410, 1994.

Terstegge K, Schorner W, Henkes H, et al: Hyperostosis in meningiomas: MR findings in patients with recurrent meningioma of the sphenoid wings, *AJNR* 15:555-560, 1994.

Toye R, Jeffree MA: Metastatic bronchial adenocarcinoma showing the "meningeal sign": case note, *Neuroradiol* 35:272-273, 1993.

Wasenko JJ, Hochhauser L, Stopa EG, Winfield JA: Cystic meningiomas: MR characteristics and surgical correlations, *AJNR* 15:1959-1965, 1994.

Wellenreuther R, Kraus JA, Lenartz D, et al: Analysis of the neurofibromatosis 2 gene reveals molecular variants of meningioma, *Am J Pathol* 146:827-832, 1995.

Wilson CB: Meningiomas: genetics, malignancy, and the role of radiation in induction and treatment, *J Neurosurg* 81:666-675, 1994.

Younis GA, Saway R, DeMonte F, et al: Aggressive meningeal tumors: review of a series, *J Neurosurg* 82:17-27, 1995.

Zorludemir S, Scheithauer BW, Hirose T, et al: Clear cell meningioma: a clinicopathologic study of a potentially aggressive variant of meningioma, *Am J Surg Pathol* 19:493-505, 1995.

32

Reticuloendothelial Tumors and Intracranial Metastasis

Key Concepts

1. Intracranial lymphomas may be primary or secondary (usually NHL, B-cell).
2. Incidence of primary CNS lymphoma is rising in both immunocompetent and immunosuppressed (AIDS, congenital immunodeficiency, organ transplants) populations.
3. Leukemia and multiple myeloma usually involve CNS secondarily.
4. Cranial metastases are commonly parenchymal (lung, breast, melanoma, GI) or calvarial (prostate, breast, lung).
5. Parenchymal metastases are usually multiple, situated at gray/white matter junction and vascular watershed areas.
6. Leptomeningeal metastasis most commonly occurs from dissemination of primary CNS neoplasms (medulloblastoma, ependymoma, germinoma, cerebral neuroblastoma, pineoblastoma, choroid plexus tumors, high-grade astrocytoma, and primary CNS lymphoma).

I. Hematopoetic and reticuloendothelial neoplasms.
  A. Lymphoma.
    1. Primary CNS lymphoma.
      a. Histology: usually NHL, B-cell (rarely T-cell). In immuno-compromised populations probably arises from T-cell suppressor impairment and subsequent proliferation of B cells (may be associated with EBV infection).
      b. Incidence.
        (1) Rare, 1% to 2% of primary CNS tumors; immuno-suppressed > immunocompetent (however, increasing in both AIDS and non-AIDS populations).
        (2) 1% of primary NHL.
        (3) 2% of AIDS cases.
        (4) Possible associations: immunosuppression (e.g., congenital, AIDS, organ transplants), EBV, SLE, sarcoid, Sjogren's syndrome, rheumatoid arthritis, idiopathic thrombocytopenic purpura, leukemia.
      c. Age and gender: any age; slight male predilection.
        (1) Usually older adult if immunocompetent: peak 50 to 60 years.
        (2) Usually childhood or young adult if immunocompromised (e.g., congenital immunodeficiency, AIDS).
      d. Location.
        (1) Parenchymal.
          (a) Usually supratentorial (periventricular deep white matter, basal ganglia, thalami, corpus callosum).
          (b) Less commonly infratentorial (cerebellum, brainstem).
          (c) Solitary more likely in immunosuppressed, multiple more likely in AIDS.
        (2) Leptomeningeal and subependymal (frequent).
        (3) Uveal or vitreous deposits (common).
        (4) Spinal intramedullary masses (less frequent).
      e. Clinical features.
        (1) Presenting symptoms nonspecific.
        (2) Treatment includes corticosteroids, radiation, and/or chemotherapy.
        (3) Prognosis improved with solitary lesions and immunocompetence.
        (4) Although responds dramatically to steroids and highly radiosensitive, overall prognosis poor with frequent progression or recurrence within 1 year, average survival <1 or 2 years.

f. Imaging.
  (1) CT.
    (a) Usually ill-defined, isodense to moderately hyper-dense lesion(s). Can cross corpus callosum, giving "butterfly" appearance.
    (b) Minimal mass effect but marked peripheral edema.
    (c) Calcification uncommon.
    (d) Hemorrhage, necrosis uncommon (more likely in immunosuppressed).
    (e) Strong homogeneous enhancement usually in immunocompetent patients; may have irregular ring enhancement in immunosuppressed patients.
  (2) MRI.
    (a) Usually infiltrative, ill-defined lesion(s) involving deep gray nuclei and white matter.
    (b) Usually isointense to slightly hypointense to GM on T1WI; isointense to slightly hyperintense on T2WI.
    (c) May detect leptomeningeal seeding.
  (3) Nuclear imaging.
    (a) Relatively greater uptake than toxoplasmosis abscess demonstrated with PET and Thallium-201 SPECT imaging.
g. Differential diagnosis.
  (1) Solid lesion.
    (a) Low-grade astrocytoma (usually lacks enhancement).
  (2) Ring-enhancing lesion.
    (a) High-grade astrocytoma (may be indistinguishable).
    (b) Metastasis (usually multiple but solitary lesion may be indistinguishable).
    (c) Abscess, particularly toxoplasmosis (may be indistinguishable, diagnosis made by positive response to antibiotics).
    (d) Radiation necrosis (may be indistinguishable on CT/MR; nuclear imaging may be helpful).
  (3) Butterfly callosal lesions.
    (a) Astrocytoma, GBM.
    (b) Giant MS plaque.
2. Secondary CNS lymphoma.
  a. Histology: NHL >> Hodgkin's.
  b. Incidence.
    (1) Less common than primary CNS lymphoma; 1% of all CNS tumors; 5% to 30% of NHL.

        (2) Leptomeningeal >> dural or parenchymal.

        (3) Spinal >> cerebral.

    c. Age: any age.

    d. Location.

        (1) Leptomeningeal: subarachnoid, perivascular, and subependymal infiltration.

        (2) Dural/epidural.

        (3) Calvarium/spine.

        (4) Parenchymal (rare).

    e. Clinical features.

        (1) Symptoms nonspecific.

        (2) Prognosis dependent on NHL histology.

    f. Imaging: not well described.

B. Leukemia.

  1. Histology: secondary CNS involvement, usually acute leukemia (ALL > AML).

  2. Incidence.

    a. Rarely involves CNS at onset (10%), although is frequent site of recurrence.

    b. Leptomeningeal infiltration more common in lymphocytic leukemia.

    c. Focal masses (chloroma or granulocytic sarcoma) more common in myelocytic leukemia.

  3. Age and gender: childhood and adult leukemia; no gender predilection.

  4. Location.

    a. Meningeal: diffuse or focal infiltration; leptomeninges >> dura.

    b. Cerebrovascular: perivascular/intravascular invasion with impaction of leukemic cells in blood vessels, resulting in infarct, necrosis, and hemorrhage.

    c. Focal: solid masses (chloroma or granulocytic sarcoma): parenchymal, dural, epidural, or within bone.

    d. Spine: diffuse marrow infiltration; rarely focal mass.

  5. Clinical features: CNS symptoms nonspecific; treatment/prognosis dependent on underlying disease type.

  6. Imaging: generally homogeneously enhancing lesions, isointense to GM on T1 and T2WI.

C. Multiple myeloma and plasmacytoma.

  1. Multiple myeloma.

    a. Histology: disseminated malignant plasma cells arising from bone marrow.

    b. Incidence.

(1) Most common primary malignancy in adults.

(2) Axial skeleton most commonly involved.

(3) CNS involvement uncommon (<1%).

c. Age: usually older adults >40 years.

d. Location.

(1) Skeletal involvement correlates with sites of red marrow.

(2) Extension from involved calvarium or spine results in epidural mass or dural infiltration.

(3) Rarely metastatic leptomeningeal involvement.

e. Prognosis: poor, 5-year survival of 20%; death usually from renal failure or infection.

f. Imaging.

(1) Plain film.

(a) Skull: typically "punched out" multiple lytic lesions; occasionally sclerotic.

(b) Spine: typically expansile lytic vertebral body lesion(s) sparing pedicles; less commonly diffuse osteopenia.

(2) CT.

(a) Cranial: typically enhancing mass with calvarial destruction and possible epidural/dural involvement.

(b) Spinal: typically vertebral body destruction with epidural mass.

(3) MRI: similar characteristics as described for CT.

(4) Nuclear imaging.

(a) Bone scan: focal increased uptake in 75% of patients and 50% of sites.

(b) Gallium scan: focal increased uptake in 55% of patients and 40% of sites.

2. Plasmacytoma.

a. Histology: focal medullary or extramedullary proliferation of malignant plasma cells.

b. Incidence: much rarer than multiple myeloma; actual incidence uncertain because of possible later progression to disseminated form.

c. Age: middle-aged adults; average 50.

d. Location.

(1) Osseous.

(a) Axial skeleton more common. Vertebral lesion may extend into epidural space.

(b) Calvarial or skull base involvement rare, often involve adjacent dura, resembles meningioma.

(2) Extraosseous (rare).

(a) Typically nasal/oral cavity, lymph nodes.
(b) Primary intracranial lesions rare; usually attached to dura, rarely diffuse parenchymal lesion.
(c) Spinal epidural plasmacytoma without vertebral involvement reported.
  e. Prognosis: uncertain; some cases may actually represent initial presentation of multiple myeloma.
  f. Imaging: see multiple myeloma.
  g. Differential diagnosis.
(1) Solitary multiple myeloma lesion.
(2) Meningioma.
(3) Hemangiopericytoma.
(4) Sarcomas.
(5) Solitary osseus/dural metastasis.
  D. Langerhans cell histiocytosis.
  a. Histology: spectrum of proliferative lesions involving macrophages and histiocytes.
  b. Incidence: CNS involvement uncommon.
  c. Age: childhood.
  d. Location.
(1) Systemic locations include axial and peripheral skeleton, calvarium, lung, liver, spleen, lymphatics, skin.
(2) CNS involvement includes:
(a) Calvarium or skull base extension.
(b) Hypothalamic-pituitary (particularly in "Hand-Schuller-Christian" form).
(c) Leptomeningeal (particularly in "Letterer-Siwe" form).
(d) Periventricular parenchyma (rare).
  e. Prognosis: dependent on type of histiocytosis.
  f. Imaging.
(1) CT.
(a) Focal isodense to mildly hyperdense mass in region of hypothalamus and neurohypophysis.
(b) Strong homogeneous enhancement.
(2) MRI: typically isointense to GM on T1WI and T2WI with strong homogeneous enhancement.
II. Cranial metastases.
  A. Histology and patterns of spread.
    1. Histology.
    a. Bronchial carcinoma: 45% to 50%.
    b. Breast: 15%.
    c. Melanoma: 10% to 15%.
    d. GI/GU: 10% to 15%.

   e. Others: prostate, thyroid, sarcoma, lymphoma/leukemia.
   f. Primary site unknown: 10% to 15%.
2. Routes of spread.
   a. Hematogenous.
   b. CSF.
   c. Contiguous spread: through foramina (e.g., perineural), along surfaces, along white matter tracts.

B. Incidence.
   1. 25% of cancer patients.
   2. 25% to 40% of intracranial neoplasms.

C. Age.
   1. Older adults (>40 years).
   2. Rare in children; leptomeningeal metastasis more likely from primary CNS neoplasm (especially medulloblastoma, ependymoma, or germinoma).

D. Location.
   1. Parenchymal (common):
      a. Usually gray-white junction and vascular watershed areas, 80% supratentorial; 80% multiple.
      b. Uncommon sites include choroid plexus, pineal body, pituitary gland, orbit.
   2. Leptomeningeal infiltration (less common).
      a. Rarely from non-CNS primary, more likely in lymphoma/leukemia, breast, lung.
      b. Subarachnoid seeding more common with primary CNS neoplasms including medulloblastoma, ependymoma, germinoma, cerebral PNET, pineoblastoma, choroid plexus papilloma or carcinoma, high-grade astrocytoma, and primary CNS lymphoma.
      c. Cranial > spinal.
   3. Dural (rare).
      a. More likely due to extension from adjacent calvarial lesion with epidural mass.
      b. Rarely direct involvement without associated bony lesion.
   4. Skull and vertebral (common): more likely from prostate, breast, lung.

E. Clinical features.
   1. Symptoms nonspecific.
   2. 15% to 60% of patients with leptomeningeal metastases have positive CSF cytology.
   3. Poor prognosis; average survival <3 months. Longer survival (>1 year) may be seen with leptomeningeal involvement

in breast cancer or lymphoma.
4. Solitary metastasis may be resected with adjuvant radiation and/or chemotherapy with improved survival. Recently multiple metastatectomies have been reported.
F. Imaging.
  1. Parenchymal metastases.
    a. CT.
      (1) Multiple discrete masses of variable density centered at gray-white junction of cerebral hemisphere.
      (2) Moderate to marked enhancement. Can be homogeneous in smaller lesions or irregularly ring-enhancing in larger lesions with central necrosis. Rarely, smooth thin-walled ring-enhancement can mimic abscess.
      (3) Marked peripheral edema with larger lesions.
      (4) Hemorrhage may occur with melanoma, renal cell carcinoma, choriocarcinoma.
      (5) Calcification may occur with colon (carcinoid, mucinous adenocarcinoma), pancreas, osteosarcoma. Also reported with lung, breast, cervix, ovarian, NHL.
      (6) Small lesions may not be detectable, even with contrast (higher dose or delayed postcontrast scanning improves sensitivity).
    b. MRI.
      (1) Contrast-enhanced MRI is more sensitive than CT, particularly for small lesions.
      (2) Variable signal; isointense or hypointense on T1WI, isointense or hyperintense on T2WI. Mixed signal with hemorrhage. T2 hypointensity reported with colon carcinoma (probably due to mucus).
      (3) Lesions >10 mm detectable on noncontrast MRI. Lesions <10 mm may be missed unless contrast-enhanced; sensitivity further improved with delayed postcontrast imaging or higher dose (e.g., 0.3 mmol/kg).
      (4) Nonenhancing white matter lesions unlikely to represent metastases.
  2. Leptomeningeal (Meningeal carcinomatosis or carcinomatous meningitis).
    a. CT.
      (1) Obliteration of basal cisterns or sulci on noncontrast CT; with moderate to marked diffuse or linear enhancement.
      (2) May see ependymal enhancement.
      (3) Hydrocephalus is indirect sign.

b. MRI.
 (1) Contrast-enhanced MRI more sensitive than CT, especially in spine. Difficult to detect without contrast. Negative study does not exclude (up to 30% of cytology-confirmed leptomeningeal metastases will have negative MRI).
 (2) Typically moderate to markedly enhancing basilar cisterns or sulci.
 (3) Focal subarachnoid masses less common.
 (4) Carcinomatous encephalitis: rare phenomenon producing innumerable tiny subpial nodules.
3. Dural.
 a. CT.
 (1) More commonly due to extension from calvarial lesion. Typically diffusely thickened or nodular enhancing dura.
 (2) May be difficult to detect on CT due to adjacent calvarium.
 (3) Rarely focal dural mass may mimic meningioma.
 b. MRI.
 (1) Contrast-enhanced MRI more sensitive than CT.
 (2) Similar characteristics as described for CT.
4. Skull and vertebral.
 a. CT.
 (1) Destructive lytic lesion, which may be associated with epidural mass or dural thickening.
 b. MRI.
 (1) Typically hypointense patchy replacement of fatty marrow best seen on T1WI.
 (2) Larger lesions may be associated with paraspinal/epidural mass or dural involvement.
 (3) Typically infiltrated marrow enhances, as does epidural lesion or involved dura.

SUGGESTED READINGS

Bindal RK, Sawaya R, Leavens ME, Lee JJ: Surgical treatment of multiple brain metastases, *J Neurosurg* 79:210-216, 1993.

Boorstein JM, Wong KT, Grossman RI, Bolinger L, McGowan JC: Metastatic lesions of the brain: imaging with magnetization transfer, *Radiol* 191:799-803, 1994.

Burger PC, Scheithauer BW: *Atlas of tumor pathology (third series, fascicle 10):*

tumors of the central nervous system, Washington, 1994, Armed Forces Institute of Pathology.

Elster AD, Chen MYM: Can nonenhancing white matter lesions in cancer patients be disregarded? *AJNR* 13:1309-1315, 1992.

Ginsberg LE, Leeds NE: Neuroradiology of leukemia, *AJR* 165:525-534, 1995.

Gutmann J, Kendall B: Unusual appearances of primary central nervous system non-Hodgkin's lymphoma, *Clin Radiol* 49:696-702, 1994.

Hawighorst H, Schad LR, Gademann G, et al: A 3D T1-weighted gradient-echo sequence for routine use in 3D radiosurgical treatment planning of brain metastases: first clinical results, *Eur Radiol* 5:19-25, 1995.

Herman MD, Gordon LI, Kaul K, et al: Systemic T-cell lymphoma presenting with isolated neurological dysfunction and intraparenchymal brain lesions: case report, *J Neurosurg* 78:997-1001, 1993.

Hwang T-L, Valdivieso JG, Yang C-H, Wolin MJ: Calcified brain metastasis, *Neurosurg* 32:451-454, 1993.

Mayr NA, Yuh WTC, Muhonen MG, et al: Cost-effectiveness of high-dose MR contrast studies in the evaluation of brain metastases, *AJNR* 15:1053-1061, 1994.

Moots PL, Harrison MB, Vandenberg SR: Prolonged survival in carcinomatous meningitis associated with breast cancer, *South Med J* 88:357-362, 1995.

Morgan-Parkes JH: Metastases: mechanisms, pathways, and cascades, *AJR* 164:1075-1082, 1995.

Moulopoulos LA, Granfield CAJ, Dimopoulos MA, et al: Extraosseous multiple myeloma: imaging features, *AJR* 161:1083-1087, 1993.

Nakagawa H, Miyawaki Y, Fujita T, et al: Surgical treatment of brain metastases of lung cancer: retrospective analysis of 89 cases, *J Neurol Neurosurg Psychiatry* 57:950-956, 1994.

O'Malley JP, Ziessman HA, Kumar PN, et al: Diagnosis of intracranial lymphoma in patients with AIDS: value of ^{201}Tl single-photon emission computed tomography, *AJR* 163:417-421, 1994.

Osborn AG: *Diagnostic radiology,* St Louis, 1994, Mosby.

Oschmann P, Bauer T, Kaps M, Trittmacher S, Dorndorf W: Leptomeningeal metastasis: a CT and MRI study, *Eur Radiol* 4:337-340, 1994.

Pilkington GJ: Tumour cell migration in the central nervous system, *Brain Pathol* 4:157-166, 1994.

Pui MH, Fletcher BD, Langston JW: Granulocytic sarcoma in childhood leukemia: imaging features, *Radiol* 190:698-702, 1994.

Russell DS, Rubinstein LJ: *Pathology of tumours of the nervous system,* ed 5, Baltimore, 1989, Williams and Wilkins.

Suzuki M, Takashima T, Kadoya T, et al: Signal intensity of brain metastases on T2-weighted images: specificity for metastases from colonic cancers, *Neurochir* 36:151-155, 1993.

Torenbeek R, Scheltens PH, Strack van Schijndel RJM, et al: Angiotropic intravascular large-cell lymphoma with massive cerebral extension, *J Neurol Neurosurg Psychiatry* 56:914-916, 1993.

Watanabe M, Tanaka R, Takeda N: Correlation of MRI and clinical features in meningeal carcinomatosis, *Neuroradiol* 35:512-515, 1993.

Yuh WTC, Fisher DJ, Runge VM, et al: Phase III multicenter trial of high-dose Gadoteridol in MR evaluation of brain metastases, *AJNR* 15:1037-1051, 1994.

Yuh WTC, Tali ET, Nguyen HD, et al: The effect of contrast dose, imaging time, and lesion size in the MR detection of intracerebral metastasis, *AJNR* 16:373-380, 1995.

33

Regional Head and Neck Tumors with Intracranial Extension

Key Concepts

1. Nerve sheath tumors include:
   a. Schwannomas: composed of Schwann cells, commonly involve cranial nerves.
   b. Neurofibromas: composed of Schwann cells and fibroblasts, rarely intracranial.
2. Schwannomas are more common than neurofibromas; usually occur sporadically but can be associated with NF-2.
3. Neurofibromas are less common and are usually associated with NF-1.
4. Paragangliomas encompass adrenal pheochromocytoma, sympathetic paragangliomas (paratracheal, paraaortic), and parasympathetic paragangliomas (head/neck, spinal). Intratemporal tumors can extend intracranially and mimic other cerebellopontine angle tumors. Distinguishing feature is "salt and pepper" appearance on MRI due to hypervascularity.
5. Chordomas and nasopharyngeal carcinomas can extend through skull base and cause intracranial compression or infiltration.

I. Tumors of cranial and spinal nerves (Table 33-1).
   A. Schwannoma (neurilemoma, neurinoma).
      1. Histology.
         a. Benign tumor of Schwann cells (neural crest derivative) usually at transition between central and peripheral segments of nerve. Occasionally melanin-pigmented.
         b. Well-encapsulated, compresses but does not invade nerve.
         c. Like glial tumors, immunopositive for S-100 protein.
         d. Associated with deletion on chromosome 22, whether sporadic or associated with NF-2.
      2. Incidence.
         a. 6% to 8% of primary intracranial neoplasms; 75% to 80% of CPA tumors.
         b. More common than neurofibroma.
         c. Sporadic (95%) > inherited (5%).
         d. Inherited associated with NF-2.
            (1) 20% of solitary tumors occur in NF-2.

Table 33-1   Comparison Between Schwannoma and Neurofibroma

	Schwannoma	Neurofibroma (Plexiform Type)
Pathology	Schwann cells	Schwann cells + fibroblasts
	Encapsulated	Unencapsulated
	Focal	Infiltrating
	Round	Fusiform
	Cysts, necrosis, hemorrhage common	Cysts, necrosis, hemorrhage rare
	Don't undergo malignant degeneration	Malignant degeneration in 5% to 13%
	NF-2	NF-1
Incidence	Common (6% to 8% of primary brain tumors)	Uncommon (except in NF-1)
Age	40s to 60s	Any age
Location	Cranial nerves (especially CN VIII)	Cutaneous and spinal nerves (especially CN V_1 peripheral branches, exiting spinal nerves)
Imaging	Sharply delineated	Poorly delineated, infiltrating
	Heterogeneous (large lesions)	Homogeneous
	T1WI: 67% hypointense, 33% isointense	T1WI: mostly isointense with muscle
	T2WI: hyperintense	T2WI: hyperintense
	Enhance strongly	Enhance moderately/intensely

From Osborn AG: *Diagnostic neuroradiology*, St Louis, 1994, Mosby.

       (2) Bilateral "acoustic" neuromas pathognomonic for NF-2.

       (3) Multiple tumors (5%) more likely in NF-2.

3. Age.

  a. Usually adults, peak at 40 to 60 years.

  b. Slightly younger with NF-2 (20 to 30).

  c. Rare in children (0.1% pediatric intracranial tumors).

4. Gender: female predilection (2:1).

5. Location.

  a. Intracranial.

       (1) Cranial nerves III to XII, especially sensory nerves (VIII[vestibular] >> V). Cranial nerves I and II are actually brain tracts; no Schwann cells in sheath. Note: "acoustic" neuroma incorrect, as most actually arise from vestibular nerve; although acoustic symptoms > vestibular symptoms.

       (2) Rarely intraventricular or within brain parenchyma.

  b. Intraspinal: usually lumbosacral, cauda equina; dorsal (sensory) roots >> ventral (motor) roots; rarely intramedullary.

  c. Peripheral nerve (rare): intercostal nerves, major nerves near elbow, wrist, knee.

6. Clinical features.

  a. Symptoms location-dependent.

       (1) CN VIII (vestibular N.): gradual high-frequency sensorineural hearing loss, tinnitus (vestibular symptoms uncommon).

       (2) CN V: facial pain, numbness, masticator muscle weakness.

       (3) CN VII: gradual facial paralysis, occasionally hemifacial spasm.

       (4) Large tumors associated with additional cranial nerve palsies, symptoms of brainstem compression or hydrocephalus.

  b. Benign, slow-growing; unlikely to undergo malignant degeneration.

  c. Treatment primarily surgical resection. Occasionally treated with radiation or radiosurgery.

7. Imaging.

  a. Plain film: enlargement of bony canals (IAC or neural foramina) late manifestation.

  b. Angiography: variable vascularity; tumor blush and early draining veins uncommon.

  c. CT.

(1) Well-defined round hypodense or isodense extraaxial mass.
(2) Occasional calcification.
(3) Large tumors may be heterogeneous due to cystic degeneration, hemorrhage, or peripheral cysts.
(4) Strongly enhancing.
(5) May enlarge bony canals (e.g., IAC, intratemporal facial nerve canal, or other neural foramina). Partly intra-canalicular/extracanalicular tumors may have "dumb-bell" configuration.

d. MRI.

(1) Typically hypointense or isointense on T1WI; hyperin-tense on T2WI. Signal heterogeneous and varies with hemorrhage, necrosis, or intratumoral/peripheral cysts.
(2) Peripheral cysts may be due to arachnoid adhesions, may resemble CSF or be hyperintense to GM on both T1WI and T2WI (protein or hemorrhagic products).
(3) CPA tumors have "ice-cream cone" appearance due to larger round cisternal portion with small pointed exten-sion into IAC; acute angle with petrous bone. Usually distinct CSF/vascular "cleft" between tumor and brain.

8. Differential diagnosis.

a. Solid CPA lesions.

(1) Meningioma (only rarely extends into IAC, no IAC enlargement, obtuse angle with petrous bone, usually "dural tail").
(2) Choroid plexus papilloma (rarely isolated CPA lesion).
(3) Ependymoma (rarely isolated CPA lesion, usually heterogeneous).
(4) Metastasis (usually partly parenchymal with extension into adjacent cistern, more likely heterogeneous).
(5) Paraganglioma (origin in temporal bone or jugular fossa with uncommon extension into CPA, typical "salt and pepper" MRI appearance).
(6) Cavernous angioma (parenchymal, hemorrhagic com-ponents).
(7) Vascular ectasia, aneurysm (may have peripheral calci-fication, strong uniform intraluminal enhancement and flow void if patent).
(8) Pseudotumor (e.g., flocculus).

b. Cystic CPA lesions.

(1) Cystic meningioma (usually no IAC extension, obtuse angle with petrous bone, "dural tail").

       (2) Epidermoid (usually resembles CSF signal, often slightly heterogeneous, insinuates along CSF cisterns, non-enhancing).

       (3) Arachnoid cyst (CSF-signal intensity, homogeneous cyst).

       (4) Exophytic pilocytic astrocytoma (origin in cerebellar hemisphere).

       (5) Cholesterol granuloma (origin in petrous temporal bone with secondary invasion of IAC, hyperintense on T1WI).

B. Neurofibroma.

  1. Histology.

    a. Composed of Schwann cells as well as fibroblasts; are unencapsulated, diffusely infiltrate affected nerve or tissue.

    b. Two morphologic types.

       (1) Solitary or circumscribed: discrete fusiform or globular mass.

       (2) Plexiform: involve multiple fascicles within a nerve, occur only in NF-1.

    c. Immunopositive for S-100 protein.

  2. Incidence: uncommon, more likely with NF-1.

  3. Age and gender: any age; no gender predilection.

  4. Location.

    a. Cranial: rare involvement of peripheral (orbital segment) CN V_1 associated with NF-1.

    b. Intraspinal: rarely sporadic, more likely in NF-1.

    c. Peripheral nerve: plexiform > solitary.

    d. Cutaneous or dermal: cutaneous nodule, may be isolated or associated with NF-1 (30% to 50%).

  5. Clinical features.

    a. Symptoms due to nerve impingement.

    b. Generally benign, treatment primarily resection.

    c. Malignant degeneration uncommon (5% to 15%), although more likely than schwannoma.

  6. Imaging.

    a. CT.

       (1) Fusiform hypodense or isodense mass associated with nerve root. Plexiform tumors diffuse, multicompartmental.

       (2) Unlike schwannoma, no cystic component.

       (3) Variable enhancement.

    b. MRI: isointense or slightly hyperintense on T1WI; mixed hypointensity/hyperintensity on T2WI.

C. Malignant peripheral nerve sheath tumors.
  1. Histology: malignant neoplasm of peripheral nerve supportive tissue; may arise de novo or from malignant transformation (neurofibroma > schwannoma).
  2. Incidence.
      a. 50% arise from neurofibromas (5% to 15% of plexiform neurofibromas undergo malignant transformation), virtually always associated with NF-1.
      b. Occasionally secondary to prior radiation.
  3. Age and gender: adults; no gender predilection.
  4. Location: usually large nerves in extremities; rarely intracranial (CN V > CN VIII).
  5. Clinical: often unresectable, average survival <1 year.
  6. Imaging: no distinguishing features from benign tumors.
II. Parasympathetic paraganglioma (chemodectoma, glomus tumor).
  A. Histology.
      1. Neuroendocrine tumor arising in paraganglionic tissue in body; histologically similar to adrenal pheochromocytoma and para-aortic sympathetic paraganglioma.
      2. Immunopositive for neuron-specific enolase (NSE).
  B. Incidence.
      1. Fourth or fifth most common CPA mass (2% to 10%).
      2. Carotid body tumor may be familial, may be associated with pheochromocytoma, often bilateral.
      3. Unlike pheochromocytoma no known association with NF or MEN syndromes.
  C. Age: usually 40 to 60 years.
  D. Gender.
      1. Female predilection (2:1 to 4:1) for temporal bone and carotid body tumors.
      2. No gender predilection for intraspinal tumors.
  E. Location.
      1. Glomus tympanicum: middle ear, on cochlear promontory.
      2. Glomus jugulare: jugular fossa.
      3. Glomus jugulotympanicum: extends from jugular fossa to middle ear.
      4. Glomus vagale: skull base near jugular fossa.
      5. Carotid body tumor: nestles in CCA bifurcation.
      6. Intraspinal: usually filum terminale, cauda equina.
  F. Clinical features.
      1. Symptoms location-dependent.
          a. Temporal bone tumors: lower cranial neuropathies, pulsatile tinnitus.

       b. Intraspinal tumors: back pain, motor/sensory deficits, incontinence.
2. Glomus tympanicum appears as vascular retrotympanic mass.
3. Unlike pheochromocytoma, endocrine symptoms uncommon, although various hormones and neurotransmitters may be secreted (e.g., somatostatin, serotonin).
4. Majority benign, favorable postoperative course.
5. Local recurrence frequent: 50% for jugulare, 15% for vagale, 10% for carotid body tumors.
6. Malignant transformation, metastasis rare.

  G. Imaging.
    1. Angiography.
      a. Well-delineated dense persistent vascular stain with possible A-V shunting.
      b. Glomus jugulotympanicum supplied by various vessels including tympanic branch of ascending pharyngeal artery.
      c. Glomus vagale displaces vessels in carotid sheath anteriorly.
      d. Carotid body tumor usually supplied by ascending pharyngeal artery, splays ICA and ECA.
    2. CT.
      a. Well-circumscribed, isodense, strongly enhancing mass.
      b. Tympanicum tumors may erode ossicles.
      c. Jugulare tumors may destroy jugular foramen, erode jugular spine.
      d. Jugulotympanicum tumors may also destroy floor of middle ear.
      e. Large intratemporal tumors may extend into CPA.
      f. Intraspinal tumors attached to filum or cauda equina.
    3. MRI.
      a. Heterogeneous signal, hypointense or isointense to GM on T1WI(hyperintense if hemorrhage); hyperintense on T2WI.
      b. Speckled, "salt and pepper" appearance due to vascular flow voids.
      c. Strong enhancement.
      d. Glomus vagale may be partly intracranial/extracranial with "dumbbell" configuration.

III. Chordoma.
  A. Histology: arise from notochordal remnants in skull base and spine; distinctive markedly vacuolated physaliphorous cells.
  B. Incidence: uncommon (1% to 5% of primary bone neoplasms).
  C. Age: 30 to 70 years.
  D. Gender: male predilection (2:1).

    E. Location: usually at ends of neuraxis.
      1. Sacral: (50%).
      2. Cranial: spheno-occipital region (30%), rarely petrous apex, Meckel's cave.
      3. Vertebral: cervical > thoracic > lumbar.
    F. Clinical features.
      1. Intracranial tumors may present with headache, cranial nerve palsies, diplopia.
      2. Sacral tumors may present with pain, weakness, incontinence.
      3. Histologically benign but locally invasive.
      4. Treatment includes resection, radiation.
      5. Prognosis improved with younger age, wide resection.
      6. Prone to late recurrence. Occasional metastasis (lung, nodes, skin). Malignant degeneration to chondrosarcoma, fibrosarcoma, MFH rare.
    G. Imaging (cranial).
      1. CT.
        a. Destructive mass involving clivus.
        b. Calcification common (20% to 70%).
        c. Variable enhancement.
      2. MRI: heterogeneous enhancing mass centered in clivus.
IV. Carcinoma.
    A. Histology: regional squamous cell carcinomas (SCC), salivary gland tumors, or less commonly, basal cell carcinoma may extend intracranially by direct spread or perineural invasion.
    B. Incidence: intracranial involvement rare.
    C. Age and gender: usually adult; gender predilection dependent on underlying tumor type.
    D. Location.
      1. Nasopharyngeal (SCC): may enter skull base (usually "through" foramen lacerum) to involve meninges, cranial nerves.
      2. Paranasal sinus (SCC): maxillary > ethmoid, may erode through cribriform plate into anterior cranial fossa or extend perineurally along branches of CN V.
      3. Ear, mastoid antrum (SCC): may erode through bone and infiltrate adjacent dura, occasionally extend into CPA.
      4. Salivary gland tumors: may extend perineurally along branches of CN V or VII.
      5. Scalp (basal cell carcinoma): may extend through calvarium, infiltrate dura. Rarely transgresses leptomeninges to involve superficial cortex.

SUGGESTED READINGS

Asari S, Katayama S, Itoh T, Tsuchida S, Ohmoto T: CT and MRI of haemorrhage into intracranial neuromas, *Neuroradiol* 35:247-250, 1993.

Burger PC, Scheithauer BW: *Atlas of tumor pathology (third series, fascicle 10): tumors of the central nervous system,* Washington, 1994, Armed Forces Institute of Pathology.

Casadei GP, Komori T, Scheithauer BW, et al: Intracranial parenchymal schwannoma: a clinicopathological and neuroimaging study of nine cases, *J Neurosurg* 79:217-222, 1993.

Charabi S, Mantoni M, Tos M, Thomsen J: Cystic vestibular schwannomas: neuroimaging and growth rate, *J Laryng Otolog* 108:375-379, 1994.

Di Biasi C, Trasimeni G, Iannilli M, Polettini E, Gualdi G: Intracerebral schwannoma: CT and MR findings, *AJNR* 15:1956-1958, 1994.

Ezura M, Ikeda H, Ogawa A, Yoshimoto T: Intracerebral schwannoma: case report, *Neurosurg* 30:97-100, 1992.

Hall WH: National institutes of health consensus development conference statement on acoustic neuroma, December 11-13, 1991, *Arch Neurol* 51:201-207, 1994.

Jung J-M, Shin H-J, Chi JG, et al: Malignant intraventricular schwannoma: case report, *J Neurosurg* 82:121-124, 1995.

Lessin BD, Alenghat JP: Magnetic resonance imaging of hemorrhagic acoustic neuroma, *Clin Imaging* 17:142-145, 1993.

Lhuillier FM, Doyon DL, Halimi PhM, Sigal RC, Sterkers JM: Magnetic resonance imaging of acoustic neuromas: pitfalls and differential diagnosis, *Neuroradiol* 34:144-149, 1992.

Martin N, Sterkers O, Mompoint D, Nahum H: Facial nerve neuromas: MR imaging, *Neuroradiol* 34:62-67, 1992.

Mizerny BR, Kost KM: Chordoma of the cranial base: the McGill experience, *J Otolaryngol* 24:14-19, 1995.

Osborn AG: *Diagnostic radiology,* St Louis, 1994, Mosby.

Russell DS, Rubinstein LJ: *Pathology of tumours of the nervous system,* ed 5, Baltimore, 1989, Williams and Wilkins.

Tali ET, Yuh WTC, Nguyen HD, et al: Cystic acoustic schwannomas: MR characteristics, *AJNR* 14:1241-1247, 1993.

Wallace CJ, Fong CF, Auer RN: Cystic intracranial schwannoma, *Can Assoc Radiol J* 44:453-459, 1993.

34

Nonneoplastic Cysts and Tumor-Like Lesions

Key Concepts

1. Congenital dermoid and epidermoid cysts are formed from inclusion of ectodermal elements during neural tube closure. Epidermoids can also occur as acquired lesions from implantation.
2. Dermoids may be formed earlier than epidermoids, resulting in more midline location.
3. Dermoid contents usually resemble fat on CT and MRI, whereas epidermoids usually resemble CSF.
4. Congenital arachnoid cyst probably arises from arachnoid splitting or diverticulum. Cyst contents are identical to CSF on CT and MRI.
5. Colloid cyst grows by slow accumulation of cells, debris and has characteristic location at foramen of Monro. Sudden ventricular obstruction may cause "drop attack," coma, or sudden death.
6. Benign nonneoplastic pineal cyst may be difficult to distinguish from small cystic pineocytoma.
7. Intracranial lipoma is not a true neoplasm but results from malformation of meninx primitiva and is often associated with other congenital malformations (e.g., callosal dysgenesis).
8. Hypothalamic hamartoma is a focal malformation of neural and glial tissue situated between the infundibulum and mammillary bodies. Unusual symptoms include precocious puberty and gelastic (laughing) seizures.

I. Congenital inclusion cysts: dermoid and epidermoid (Table 34-1).
   A. Dermoid (inclusion) cyst.
      1. Histology.

Table 34-1   Comparison Between Epidermoid and Dermoid Tumors

	Epidermoid	Dermoid
Pathology	Ectodermal inclusion cyst	Ectodermal inclusion cyst (no mesoderm)
	Squamous epithelium	Squamous epithelium
	Keratinaceous debris	Keratinaceous debris
	Solid crystalline cholesterol	Liquid cholesterol
	No dermal appendages	Dermal appendages (hair, sebaceous glands)
	Grow by epithelial desquamation	Grow by epithelial desquamation + glandular secretion
	Rarely rupture	Commonly rupture
Incidence	0.2% to 1% of primary brain tumors	Uncommon (0.04% to 0.6% of primary brain tumors)
	4-9× more common than dermoid	
Age	20 to 60 years	30 to 50 years
	M = F	Slight male predominance
Location	Off-midline	Midline
	40% to 50% in cerebellopontine angle cistern; 10% to 15% parasellar, middle fossa space; 10% diploic space	Parasellar, frontobasal most common intracranial sites
		Vermis, fourth ventricle most common infratentorial sites
	Insinuates along CSF spaces	Subarachnoid spread from ruptured cyst
Imaging **CT**	NECT: low density (like CSF); calcification uncommon	NECT: very low density (like fat); calcification common; ± dermal sinus tract
	CECT: periphery occasionally enhances	CECT: no enhancement
MR	T1-, T2WI: often like CSF	Hyperintense on T1-, hypointense on T2WI

(From Osborn AG: *Diagnostic neuroradiology,* St Louis, 1994, Mosby.

a. Inclusion of ectodermal elements at time of neural groove closure (possibly earlier than for epidermoid cysts and therefore more midline). Contains epithelium, dermal appendages, occasional dental elements (ectodermal origin).
   b. Immunopositive for epithelial membrane antigen (EMA), cytokeratins.
   c. Arises from one germ cell layer, not two (common misconception probably originating from misnomer of ovarian "dermoid cyst," which is not an inclusion cyst but a teratoma of more than one germ cell layer with prominent dermal elements).
   d. Although both dermoid and epidermoid contain cholesterol crystals, dermoids (sweat/sebaceous glands) more often contain liquid cholesterol and lipid metabolites responsible for fat density/signal.
2. Incidence.
   a. Inclusion cysts common in subcutaneous tissues. Also occur in skull or orbit. Dermoids and epidermoid are most common pediatric scalp masses.
   b. Rare in the CNS, 0.5% of primary brain tumors.
   c. Less common than CNS epidermoids.
3. Age.
   a. Spinal lesions usually <20 years.
   b. Cranial lesions usually <10.
4. Gender: slight male predilection.
5. Location: CNS lesions tend to be near midline, in subarachnoid spaces.
   a. Skull: near anterior fontanelle.
   b. Intracranial: posterior fossa (adjacent to vermis, fourth ventricle), parasellar, pineal region.
   c. Spine: lumbosacral.
   d. Slightly more common in spine than cranium (reverse is true for epidermoid).
   e. May be associated with sinus tract, particularly in spine or skull base.
6. Clinical features.
   a. Symptoms nonspecific, location-dependent.
   b. Slow-growing; treatment primarily resection; late recurrence common due to incomplete resection; malignant transformation to squamous carcinoma very rare.
   c. Ruptured lesions may result in chemical meningitis or ventriculitis.
7. Imaging.

a. Plain film: skull lesions typically well-defined, lytic with sclerotic rim.
b. Angiography.
 (1) Avascular mass effect.
 (2) Chemical meningitis may induce vasospasm.
c. CT.
 (1) Typically discrete fat-density midline mass.
 (2) Mural or central coarse calcification can occur.
 (3) Enhancement usually absent.
 (4) Ruptured dermoids may show fat-density droplets in subarachnoid space or fat-CSF levels in ventricles.
 (5) Sinus tract may be seen, particularly with spine or skull base lesions.
 (6) Skull lesions typically fat-density intradiploic mass without cortical destruction, although erosion (outer > inner table) can occur.
d. MRI.
 (1) Typically hyperintense to GM on T1WI and hypointense on T2WI. Occasionally dermoids with less lipid content are hypointense on T1WI and hyperintense on T2WI, resembling epidermoid.
 (2) May see intracystic fluid/fluid level.
 (3) Ruptured dermoids may show T1 hyperintense droplets in CSF.
8. Differential diagnosis.
 a. Epidermoid (usually off-midline, mildly lobulated, often slightly heterogeneous, usually resembles CSF signal).
 b. Arachnoid cyst (identical to CSF).
 c. Lipoma (frequently associated with callosal dysgenesis, engulfs vessels).
B. Epidermoid tumor.
 1. Histology.
  a. Inclusion or implantation of ectodermal elements.
   (1) Congenital: CNS lesions probably from inclusion at time of neural closure (possibly later than dermoid cysts, thereby resulting in more variable sites).
   (2) Acquired: traumatic implantation of skin can occur from lumbar puncture or surgery.
  b. Composed of squamous epithelial lined capsule and contains desquamated epithelium, keratin, and cholesterol crystals.
 2. Incidence.
  a. Epidermoid tumors common in subcutaneous tissues,

middle ear (cholesteotoma). Also occur in skull and orbit. Epidermoids and dermoids are most common pediatric scalp mass.

 b. CNS lesions rare (1% of primary brain tumors), although 5 to 10 times more common than CNS dermoids.

 c. Third most common CPA mass (7% to 9%), after acoustic schwannoma and meningioma.

3. Age and gender: any age, usually 20 to 60 years; no gender predilection.

4. Location: CNS lesions not restricted to midline.

 a. Cerebellopontine angle most common (40% to 50%).

 b. Parasellar, middle cranial fossa 10% to 15%.

 c. Skull 10%.

 d. Intraventricular (fourth ventricle) 5% to 10%.

 e. Spine: any location; less common than cranial lesions.

5. Clinical features.

 a. Symptoms nonspecific, location-dependent.

 b. Slow-growing; treatment primarily resection, although asymptomatic lesions may be observed.

 c. Late recurrence common due to incomplete resection; malignant transformation to squamous carcinoma rare.

 d. Rupture of cystic components less common than with dermoids.

6. Imaging.

 a. Plain film: skull lesions typically well defined, lytic with sclerotic rim.

 b. Angiography: avascular mass effect.

 c. CT.

  (1) Typically discrete, midly lobulated, homogeneous CSF-density mass. Margins may be imperceptible. Occasionally may be hyperdense due to hemorrhage or protein content.

  (2) Calcification uncommon (10% to 25%).

  (3) Usually enhancement absent, although occasional peripheral enhancement.

  (4) CT cisternography: intrathecal contrast surrounds mass and delineates lobulated "cauliflower-like" margins.

  (5) Skull lesion has low density with margins similar to dermoid.

 d. MRI.

  (1) Usually resembles CSF-signal intensity. However, frequently mildly heterogeneous and slightly hyper-

intense to CSF on all sequences. Occasionally epidermoids with high lipid content are hyperintense on T1WI and hypointense on T2WI, resembling dermoid.
(2) Tend to insinuate along CSF spaces.
(3) Margins often imperceptible, often difficult to differentiate from adjacent CSF. Diffusion weighting, magnetization transfer, or heavily T1-weighted imaging may improve conspicuity.
  7. Differential diagnosis (CPA lesion).
   a. Arachnoid cyst (identical to CSF density/signal, smooth margins).
   b. Cystic acoustic neuroma (strong enhancement of solid portion, "ice-cream cone" extension into IAC).
   c. Cystic meningioma (rare, strong enhancement of solid portion, "dural tail").
   d. Neurenteric cyst (rare, may be associated with anterior dysraphism or cleft).
   e. Cysticercosis cyst (usually multiple lesions, may see enhancing scolex or calcifications).
II. Congenital arachnoid cyst (not to be confused with extra-arachnoid leptomeningeal cyst due to dural tear or meningitis).
 A. Origin.
   1. Probable congenital maldevelopment of arachnoid membrane resulting in splitting of arachnoid or arachnoidal diverticulum.
   2. May be associated with partial agenesis of temporal lobe.
   3. Controversy over whether antecedent temporal lobe maldevelopment favors secondary formation of cyst.
 B. Incidence: 1% of intracranial masses.
 C. Age: any age, usually children (75%).
 D. Gender: male predilection (3:1).
 E. Location.
   1. Middle cranial fossa most common: 50% to 65%.
   2. Suprasellar cistern 5% to 10%.
   3. Quadrigeminal cistern 5% to 10%.
   4. Cerebral convexities 5%.
   5. Posterior fossa (CPA, cisterna magna) 5% to 10%.
 F. Clinical features.
   1. Usually asymptomatic, occasional symptoms location-dependent.
    a. Middle cranial fossa lesions may cause temporal epilepsy.
    b. Posterior fossa lesions may cause hydrocephalus.
    c. Suprasellar lesions may cause endocrinopathies or visual defects.

2. Benign, usually stable.
3. Small percentage may slowly enlarge and cause increased head size in infants or compressive effects such as hydrocephalus.
4. Need for treatment controversial, evacuation may or may not relieve symptoms.
G. Imaging.
1. Plain film: may cause scalloped erosion of adjacent calvarium.
2. CT.
   a. Typically well-defined cystic CSF-density extraaxial mass. Often spheric indentation of adjacent brain.
   b. No enhancement.
   c. May have associated scalloped erosion of adjacent calvarium.
3. MRI.
   a. Homogeneous CSF-signal intensity mass.
   b. Rarely, signal may be complicated by hemorrhage or protein content.
H. Differential diagnosis.
1. Epidermoid (mildly lobulated, usually resembles CSF, and may be indistinguishable, although frequently slightly hyperintense to CSF on T1- and T2WI).
2. Dermoid (located in midline, resembles fat density/signal).
III. Colloid cyst.
A. Histology: origin controversial, probably congenital.
1. Thought to be of neuroepithelial origin, although histologic similarity to Rathke cleft and neuroenteric cysts also suggests endodermal origin.
2. Slow expansion by accumulation of contents: including mucin, lipid, protein, desquamated cells, hemorrhage, CSF.
B. Incidence: uncommon, <1% of primary brain tumors; 15% to 20% of intraventricular masses.
C. Age: usually young, middle-aged adults; peak at 20 to 50 years.
D. Gender: slight male predilection.
E. Location: anterior third ventricle at foramen of Monro.
F. Clinical features.
1. Symptoms related to intermittent (e.g., positional headaches) or prolonged increased intracranial pressure. Occasionally sudden ventricular obstruction may cause "drop attack," coma, or sudden death.
2. Treatment includes observation, ventricular shunting, stereotactic aspiration, open resection, and endoscopic surgery. Curative if completely resected or aspirated.

G. Imaging.
  1. CT.
     a. Discrete, smoothly rounded, hyperdense (2/3) midline mass at foramen of Monro. Less commonly isodense (1/3).
     b. No calcification.
     c. Usually enhancement absent, although occasional peripheral rim enhancement.
     d. May have associated obstructive hydrocephalus of lateral ventricles, usually asymmetric.
  2. MRI.
     a. Variable signal, usually hyperintense to GM on T1WI; hypointense on T2WI.
H. Differential diagnosis.
  1. Subependymal giant cell astrocytoma (moderately enhancing, heterogeneous, associated TS findings).
  2. Central neurocytoma (moderately enhancing).
  3. Intraventricular astrocytoma (rare, usually enhancing).
  4. Subependymoma (small, pedunculated may enhance).
  5. Ependymoma (commonly has extraventricular component, enhancing).
  6. CSF flow artifact at foramen of Monro (can mimic tumor, associated with ghosting artifact in phase-encoding direction).
IV. Neuroepithelial cysts.
  A. Histology.
    1. Heterogeneous group of lesions including:
       a. Choroid plexus cyst.
          (1) Variant: xanthogranuloma or xanthogranulomatous cyst: composed of xanthomatous cells that release lipid into choroid plexus (fat density/signal).
       b. Ependymal (intraventricular) cyst.
       c. Choroid fissure cyst.
       d. Parenchymal cyst (rare).
    2. Origin controversial, may arise from sequestration of neuroectodermal elements.
  B. Incidence.
    1. Uncommon, varies with location.
    2. Choroid plexus cysts most common, small choroid plexus cysts >50% autopsies; may be associated with Trisomy 18, other congenital malformations.
  C. Age and gender: any age, usually adults; no gender predilection.
  D. Location.
    1. Choroid plexus cyst: usually within choroid of trigone.
    2. Ependymal cyst: usually within trigone of lateral ventricles, separate from choroid plexus.

   3. Choroid fissure cyst: CSF space in medial temporal lobe between hippocampus and diencephalon.

   4. Parenchymal cyst: anywhere.

  E. Clinical features.

   1. Usually asymptomatic, discovered incidentally.

   2. Large intraventricular cysts can cause ventricular obstruction.

  F. Imaging.

   1. U/S.

    a. Hypoechoic choroid plexus cysts commonly seen in utero; most spontaneously resolve by birth.

   2. CT.

    a. Small, discrete, rounded CSF-density cystic mass.

    b. No calcification or enhancement.

   3. MRI.

    a. Resembles CSF-signal.

    b. No surrounding edema or gliosis, stable between serial studies.

    c. Choroidal fissure cysts are ovoid or spindle-shaped on sagittal images, anatomic relationship to choroidal fissure best demonstrated on coronal images.

  G. Differential diagnosis.

   1. Choroidal fissure region lesions.

    a. Arachnoid cyst (usually in Sylvian fissure, lateral to temporal lobe).

    b. Large perivascular (Virchow-Robin) space (located in parenchyma above choroidal fissure).

    c. Dermoid (usually resembles fat density/signal).

    d. Epidermoid (often slightly hyperintense to CSF).

   2. Parenchymal cyst.

    a. Lacunar infarct.

    b. Perivascular or Virchow-Robin space.

    c. Demyelinating lesion.

    d. Cystic tumor.

V. Endodermal (neurenteric or enterogenous) cyst.

  A. Histology.

   1. Probably results from persistence of embryologic neurenteric canal between notochord and foregut; of endodermal origin. Cyst lined by columnar ciliated or goblet-cell containing epithelium.

   2. Immunopositive for EMA, cytokeratin.

  B. Incidence: rare.

  C. Age: any age.

  D. Location.

1. More common in spine (80%); intradural extramedullary, usually ventral to cord.
2. Uncommon in cranium (10% to 15%); usually posterior fossa (CPA or midline ventral to medulla).

E. Clinical features.
1. Small lesions usually asymptomatic, larger lesions present with symptoms related to mass effect.
2. Prognosis dependent on operability. Incompletely resected lesions prone to recurrence.

F. Imaging.
1. CT.
   a. Discrete round or lobulated hypodense mass.
   b. No calcification or enhancement.
   c. Often associated with anterior dysraphism or vertebral body cleft; rarely Klippel-Feil, segmentation anomalies, diastematomyelia, posterior dysraphism.
2. MRI.
   a. Signal varies with cyst content. Usually isointense or mildly hyperintense to CSF on T1WI; moderately hyperintense on PD and T2WI.

VI. Pineal cyst.
A. Histology.
1. Cyst lined by normal pineal cells, glial cells, gliosis, and occasionally ependyma. May contain protein, hemorrhagic products.
2. Origin controversial.
   a. Small cavity probably from failure of obliteration of embryologic third ventricular diverticulum.
   b. Subsequent enlargement into larger cyst may be due to degenerative change, hemorrhagic expansion, hormonal influences (e.g., pregnancy).

B. Incidence: 40% of autopsies, 1% to 5% of MR studies.
C. Age: any age, average 30 years.
D. Gender: slight female predilection.
E. Location: pineal gland.
F. Clinical features.
1. Usually small, asymptomatic, discovered incidentally.
2. Larger cysts (usually >1 cm) may present with Parinaud syndrome, symptoms due to obstructive hydrocephalus (cerebral aqueduct compression), increased intracranial pressure (vein of Galen compression), or endocrinopathy.
3. Treatment for symptomatic cysts includes ventricular shunting, open resection, and stereotactic aspiration; usually curative.

G. Imaging.
  1. CT.
     a. Typically small, well-circumscribed, round, homogeneous, cystic mass. Usually hypodense, can be hyperdense due to hemorrhage.
     b. Peripheral calcification uncommon.
     c. May be difficult to detect on CT.
  2. MRI.
     a. Usually CSF-signal but often hyperintense to CSF on both T1WI and T2WI. Signal also varies with hemorrhage.
     b. Sagittal images demonstrate flattening of quadrigeminal plate, compression of cerebral aqueduct.
     c. Septation or multiloculation uncommon.
     d. Rim enhancement common (60%), probably due to normal displaced pineal parenchyma, which lacks blood-brain barrier.
     e. Delayed imaging may show subsequent homogeneous intracystic enhancement, mimicking solid tumor.
H. Differential diagnosis.
  1. Pineocytoma (usually solid, when cystic may be indistinguishable).
  2. Cystic masses (dermoid, epidermoid, arachnoid cyst) in quadrigeminal cistern or velum interpositum (displace pineal and tectum inferiorly).
  3. Cavum velum interpositum (triangle-shaped, contiguous with quadrigeminal plate cistern).
VII. Lipoma.
  A. Pathogenesis.
    1. Previously thought to be mesodermal neoplasm but probably result of malformation of meninx primitiva.
    2. May be associated with other brain malformations: callosal dysgenesis, frontal lobe anomalies, absent septum pellucidum, and cephaloceles.
    3. Two forms.
       a. Tubulonodular: usually associated with callosal dysgenesis.
       b. Curvilinear: corpus callosum usually normal or near-normal.
  B. Incidence: uncommon, <1% of primary intracranial tumors; 5% of corpus callosum tumors.
  C. Age: any age.
  D. Location: usually midline (80% to 95%).
    1. Dorsal pericallosal most common (50%).
       a. Tubulonodular: usually along anterior corpus callosum.

   b. Curvilinear: usually along mid- and posterior corpus callosum.

  2. Other intracranial sites: quadrigeminal/ambient, suprasellar, CPA cisterns.

  3. Spinal: usually thoracic; 30% associated with other spine anomalies such as tethered cord, spina bifida, or meningomyelocele.

 E. Clinical features.

  1. Usually asymptomatic, discovered incidentally.

  2. More likely to present from other associated brain malformations.

  3. Does not increase in size.

  4. Often intimately associated with vessels and nerves and virtually unresectable.

 F. Imaging.

  1. Plain film: occasionally may see lucent midline lesion surrounded by "comma-shaped" calcification.

  2. U/S: neonatal cranial sonography may show midline pericallosal echodense mass with or without callosal dysgenesis.

  3. CT.

   a. Fat-density nonenhancing mass.

   b. Calcification   common   (tubulonodular > curvilinear forms).

   c. Hemorrhage or degeneration uncommon.

   d. May see associated brain malformations.

  4. MRI.

   a. Fat-signal mass: hyperintense on T1WI, hypointense on T2WI (note that hyperintensity will persist on FSE T2WI unless fat suppression used). Chemical shift artifact may be seen.

   b. May see prominent vessels, encasement of ACA, or engulfed nerves.

VIII. Hypothalamic hamartoma.

 A. Histology: nonneoplastic abnormal growth and organization of mature neuronal and glial tissues. Resembles gray matter.

 B. Incidence: rare. May be associated with other cerebral anomalies including microgyria, heterotopia, and callosal dysgenesis. Extracranial congenital anomalies also reported, including polydactyly, facial anomalies, heart defects.

 C. Age: childhood.

 D. Gender: male predilection.

 E. Location: tuber cinereum, between infundibulum and mammillary bodies.

 F. Clinical features.

      1. May present with precocious puberty, gelastic (laughing) seizures, behavioral abnormalities.

      2. Benign, resection may relieve symptoms.

  G. Imaging.

      1. CT.

         a. Discrete, rounded, isodense, suprasellar mass.

         b. No enhancement or calcification.

         c. Rarely cystic areas.

      2. MRI.

         a. Typically sessile or pedunculated suprasellar mass between infundibulum and mammillary bodies, may extend to interpeduncular cistern or bulge upward into third ventricle.

         b. Isointense to GM on T1WI and PD; hyperintense on T2WI.

  H. Differential diagnosis.

      1. Chiasmatic-hypothalamic glioma (usually enhancing).

      2. Craniopharyngioma (usually calcified, heterogeneously enhancing, partly solid/cystic mass).

      3. Germinoma (homogeneously enhancing).

      4. Langerhans cell histiocytosis (usually enhancing).

      5. Sarcoidosis (may have focal hypothalamic enhancing mass or infundibular thickening/enhancement, uncommon in children).

      6. Lymphoma (rarely suprasellar enhancing mass, uncommon in children).

 IX. Dysplastic gangliocytoma of cerebellum (see Chapter 28).

SUGGESTED READINGS

Ahmadi J, Savabi F, Apuzzo MLJ, Segall HD, Hinton D: Magnetic resonance imaging and quantitative analysis of intracranial cystic lesions: surgical implications, *Neurosurg* 35:199-207, 1994.

Boyko OB, Scott JA, Muller J: Intradiploic epidermoid cyst of the skull: case report, *Neuroradiol* 36:226-227, 1994.

Brooks BS, Duvall ER, El Gammal T, et al: Neuroimaging features of neuroenteric cysts: analysis of nine cases and review of the literature, *AJNR* 14:735-746, 1993.

Burger PC, Scheithauer BW: *Atlas of tumor pathology (third series , fascicle 10): tumors of the central nervous system,* Washington, 1994, Armed Forces Institute of Pathology.

Fain JS, Tomlinson FH, Scheithauer BW, et al: Symptomatic glial cysts of the pineal gland, *J Neurosurg* 80:454-460, 1994.

Fleege MA, Miller GM, Fletcher GP, et al: Benign glial cysts of the pineal gland: unusual imaging characteristics with histologic correlation, *AJNR* 15:161-166, 1994.

Garcia Santos JM, Martinez-Lage J, Gilabert Ubeda A, Capel Aleman A, Climent Oltra V: Arachnoid cysts of the middle cranial fossa: a consideration of their origins based on imaging, *Neuroradiol* 35:355-358, 1993.

Golzarian J, Baleriaux D, Bank WO, Matos C, Flament-Durand J: Pineal cyst: normal or pathological? *Neuroradiol* 35:251-253, 1993.

Gormley WB, Tomecek FJ, Qureshi N, Malik GM: Craniocerebral epidermoid and dermoid tumours: a review of 32 cases, *Acta Neurochir* 128:115-121, 1994.

Graziani N, Dufour H, Figarella-Branger D, et al: Do the suprasellar neurenteric cyst, the Rathke cleft cyst and the colloid cyst constitute a same entity? *Acta Neurochir* 133:174-180, 1995.

Harrison MJ, Morgello S, Post KD: Epithelial cystic lesions of the sellar and parasellar region: a continuum of ectodermal derivatives? *J Neurosurg* 80:1018-1025, 1994.

Higashi S, Takinami K, Yamashita J: Occipital dermal sinus associated with dermoid cyst in the fourth ventricle, *AJNR* 16:945-948, 1995.

Inoue Y, Saiwai S, Miyamoto T, Katsuyama J: Enhanced high-resolution sagittal MRI of normal pineal glands, *J Comp Assist Tomog* 18:182-186, 1994.

Kash F, Osborn AG, Smirniotopoulos JG: Radiologic spectrum of intracranial lipoma, *International J Radiol* (in press).

Lewis AI, Crone KR, Taha J, et al: Surgical resection of third ventricle colloid cysts: preliminary results comparing transcallosal microsurgery with endoscopy, *J Neurosurg* 81:174-178, 1994.

McAndrew PT, Land N, Sellar RJ: Case report: a case of intracranial septated arachnoid cyst, *Clin Radiol* 50:502-503, 1995.

Nassar SI, Haddad FS, Abdo A: Epidermoid tumors of the fourth ventricle, *Surg Neurol* 43:246-251, 1995.

Osborn AG: Miscellaneous tumors, cysts, and metastases. In *Diagnostic radiology,* St Louis, 1994, Mosby, pp 626-670.

Russell DS, Rubinstein LJ: Tumours and tumour-like lesions of maldevelopmental origin. In *Pathology of tumours of the nervous system,* ed 5, Baltimore, 1989, Williams and Wilkins, pp 664-765.

Sakamoto Y, Takahashi M, Ushio Y, Korogi Y: Visibility of epidermoid tumors on steady-state free precession images, *AJNR* 15:1737-1744, 1994.

Tatter SB, Ogilvy CS, Golden JA, et al: Third ventricular xanthogranulomas clinically and radiologically mimicking colloid cysts: report of two cases, *J Neurosurg* 81:605-609, 1994.

Tien RD, Felsberg GJ, Lirng J-F: Variable bandwidth steady-state free-precession MR imaging: a technique for improving characterization of epidermoid tumor and arachnoid cyst, *AJR* 164:689-692, 1995.

Valdueza JM, Cristante L, Dammann O, et al: Hypothalamic hamartomas: with special reference to gelastic epilepsy and surgery, *Neurosurg* 34:949-958, 1994.

Vinchon M, Pertuzon B, Lejeune J-P, et al: Intradural epidermoid cysts of the cerebellopontine angle: diagnosis and surgery, *Neurosurg* 36:52-57, 1995.

SECTION V
Aneurysms, Vascular Malformations, and Other Vascular Lesions

35

Intracranial Aneurysms

Key Concepts

1. The three major types of intracranial aneurysms are:
   a. Saccular aneurysm (most common).
   b. Fusiform aneurysm (usually manifestation of atherosclerosis).
   c. Dissecting aneurysm (traumatic or spontaneous).
2. Saccular aneurysms are not congenital lesions but represent degenerative changes induced by hemodynamic stresses on vessel walls.
3. The vast majority of saccular aneurysms are located on the circle of Willis or at the middle cerebral artery (MCA) bifurcation.
4. Distal aneurysms are often secondary to trauma, infection, high-flow states (e.g., arteriovenous malformation or fistula).
5. The most common presentation of intracranial aneurysm is subarachnoid hemorrhage (SAH).

Intracranial aneurysms are usually silent until they rupture, and when they rupture the clinical consequences are often devastating. Subarachnoid hemorrhage from aneurysm rupture has a significant morbidity and mortality rate exceeding 50%. With improved noninvasive screening procedures such as high-resolution standard MR imaging and MR angiography, finding an unruptured aneurysm is an increasingly common event in radiologic practice.

In this chapter we discuss the pathology, etiology, clinical presentation, and imaging of intracranial aneurysms. Although there are three distinct types of intracranial aneurysms (saccular, fusiform, and dissecting), each with its own distinct pathologic features and imaging spectrum, saccular or "berry" aneurysms are by far the most common. We will therefore focus most of the discussion on these important lesions (box).

   I. Saccular aneurysm.

      A. Pathology (Fig. 35-1).

         1. Rounded, "berry"-shaped outpouching.

         2. Most often arises at vessel bifurcation (lateral wall is a less common site).

         3. True aneurysm, that is, dilatation of vascular lumen due to weakness of all vessel wall layers.

         4. Deficient, collagenized tunica muscularis protrudes through defect in internal elastic membrane (IEM).

         5. Wall of aneurysm typically consists of only intima, adventitia.

         6. Lumen may contain thrombotic debris.

      B. Etiology, pathogenesis.

         1. No evidence for congenital origin.

Intracranial Saccular Aneurysms: The Essentials

Aneurysm wall composed of intima, adventitia
90%-95% are acquired, arise from hemodynamic stresses
5%-10% caused by trauma, infection, tumor, high flow
2%-8% prevalence in general population
Incidence increased with:
  Polycystic kidney disease
  Aortic coarctation, anomalous vessels
  Vasculopathy (FMD, Marfan, connective tissue disorder)
  Family history of intracranial aneurysm (first-degree relative)
Peak age 40 to 60 years; <2% in children
90% located on anterior circulation; 10% vertebrobasilar
Rupture risk estimated 1%-2% per year, cumulative
Most common presentation is SAH
Results in death or disability in 2/3 to 3/4 of cases

2. Between 90% and 95% of all intracranial aneurysms arise from hemodynamically induced degenerative vascular injury.
3. Mechanical shear stresses are greatest at vessel bifurcation points, hence most aneurysms arise at these sites.
4. Less common causes of aneurysm formation.
   a. Trauma.
      (1) Causes between 0.2% and 1% of aneurysms.
      (2) Can result from penetrating trauma, skull fracture, or closed head injury.
      (3) Common sites: intracavernous ICA, distal ACA, cortical MCA branches.
   b. Infection.
      (1) Represent 2.5% to 4.5% of aneurysms.
      (2) Infective endocarditis, drug abuse may be contributory causes.
      (3) *Streptococcus viridans, Aspergillus* common organisms.
      (4) Affects distal cerebral vessels.

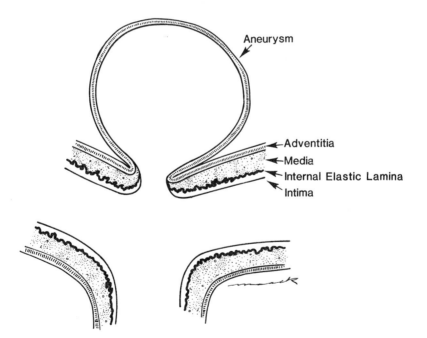

Fig. 35-1   Anatomic diagram depicts histology of intracranial saccular bifurcation aneurysm. Note termination of the media and internal elastic lamina at the aneurysm neck. The sac wall is thin and consists only of intima and adventitia (thickness of vessel wall and layers are exaggerated for purposes of illustration).

    c. Tumor.

        (1) Rare cause of intracranial aneurysm (<0.1%).

        (2) Pituitary adenoma, high-grade astrocytoma, metastases (atrial myxoma, choriocarcinoma).

        (3) Invade vessel directly or arise from tumor emboli.

    d. Drug abuse.

    e. High-flow states (AVM, AVF).

        (1) May represent up to 5% of all intracranial aneurysms.

        (2) Can be located within lesion ("intranidal aneurysm"), on feeding vessel ("pedicle aneurysm"), or elsewhere ("remote aneurysm").

        (3) Pedicle or remote aneurysm seen in 10% to 12% of cases; superselective angiography demonstrates intranidal aneurysm in 60% of cases.

        (4) Intranidal aneurysm increases hemorrhage risk.

C. Incidence.

  1. From 2% to 8% incidental finding at autopsy; 7% in patients undergoing cerebral angiography performed for indications other than SAH.

    a. At least 2% of general population harbors intracranial aneurysm.

    b. 1% will rupture; in 0.5%, cause of death will be aneurysm.

  2. Recent studies show much higher incidence in patients with family history of aneurysm (up to 20%).

    a. 10% at MR angiography.

    b. Nearly 30% when both mother and sibling have an aneurysm.

  3. Associated conditions with known increased incidence of intracranial aneurysm (box on p. 340).

    a. Polycystic kidney disease (PKD).

        (1) 10% to 12% overall.

        (2) 26% if family history of PKD with aneurysm.

    b. Aortic coarctation.

    c. Anomalous vessels (e.g., persistent trigemal artery).

    d. Vasculopathies, connective tissue disorders.

        (1) Fibromuscular dysplasia (FMD).

        (2) Ehlers-Danlos.

        (3) Marfan syndrome.

        (4) Systemic lupus erythematosus (SLE).

        (5) High-flow states such as AVM or AVF (aneurysm can be on remote vessel, pedicle, or within nidus).

        (6) Deficiency of Type III collagen, elevated lipoprotein reported in some cases.

     e. So-called "spontaneous dissections" have an increased incidence of associated aneurysm.

     f. Familial intracranial aneurysms (FIA).

  4. Multiplicity.

     a. 70% to 80% solitary; 15% to 30% multiple.

     b. Multiple aneurysms.

       (1) 75% have two.

       (2) 15% have three.

       (3) 10% have four or more.

D. Age at presentation.

  1. Rare in children (<2% of all aneurysms), but can occur at any age.

     a. Often larger.

     b. Frequent association with trauma, infection.

     c. Location in posterior fossa, distal to circle of Willis common.

     d. Often large (average = 17 mm).

  2. Peak age 40 to 60 years.

  3. FIAs have earlier rupture (aneurysms often smaller).

E. Location (Fig. 35-2).

  1. Vast majority arise on circle of Willis plus MCA bifurcation.

     a. 90% on anterior circulation (includes posterior communicating arteries).

       (1) Internal carotid-posterior communicating artery (IC-PC) junction accounts for one third of all aneurysms.

       (2) Anterior communicating artery (ACoA) accounts for 30% to 35%.

       (3) MCA bifurcation accounts for approximately 20%.

     b. 10% on posterior (vertebrobasilar) circulation.

       (1) Approximately 5% of all aneurysms arise from basilar artery (BA) bifurcation.

       (2) 1% to 5% from other sites (e.g., superior, posterior, inferior cerebellar arteries).

     c. Miscellaneous sites.

       (1) Distal ACA bifurcation.

       (2) Anterior choroidal artery origin.

       (3) Other distal, unusual sites should arouse suspicion of infection, trauma.

F. Clinical presentation.

  1. Most common initial presentation is subarachnoid hemorrhage (SAH).

     a. 80% to 90% of nontraumatic SAH is caused by aneurysm rupture.

     b. Graded according to clinical status.

     c. Hunt and Hess scale.

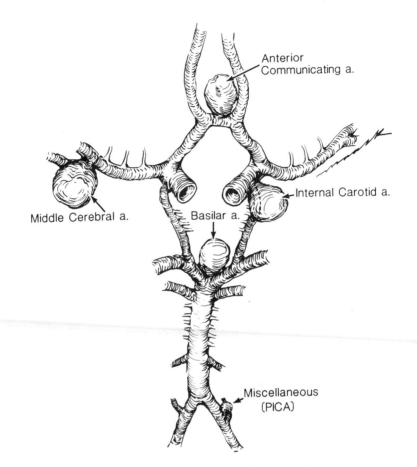

Fig. 35-2 Anatomic diagram depicts common locations of intracranial saccular aneurysms. Approximately 90% are located on the "anterior" circulation, whereas only 10% are found on the "posterior" (vertebrobasilar) circulation.

(1) Grade 0 = unruptured.
(2) Grade 1 = asymptomatic or mild headache.
(3) Grade 2 = moderate/severe headache, no neurologic deficit (except cranial nerve palsy).
(4) Grade 3 = drowsy, confused, mild focal neurologic deficit.
(5) Grade 4 = stupor, moderate/severe hemiparesis.
(6) Grade 5 = comatose, decerebrate posturing, moribund.
2. Cranial neuropathy.
  a. Pupil-involving oculomotor nerve (CN III) palsy is most common, typically caused by IC-PC aneurysm.

   b. CNs III, IV, VI, and $V_{1,2}$ may be involved by intracavernous IC aneurysm.
   3. Stroke (embolic debris, vasospasm with late or recurrent SAH).
   4. Seizure (mass effect usually associated with "giant" aneurysm, i.e., >2.5 cm).
G. Outcome.
   1. Death or significant neurologic disability in two thirds to three quarters of all cases.
      a. One third mortality (50% if unclipped aneurysm rehemorrhages).
      b. One third morbidity (vasospasm is leading cause).
H. Natural history and predicting aneurysm rupture.
   1. Rupture risk estimated 1% to 2% per year, cumulative.
      a. 2.5% if aneurysm is 7 mm or greater.
      b. 1.1% if aneurysm is less than 7 mm.
   2. Rupture risk increases with size.
   3. Some authorities suggest between 4 and 7 mm is the "critical size."
   4. But there is no known "safe" size below which aneurysm will not rupture.
   5. Irregular, lobulated configuration correlates with increased rupture risk.
   6. Drug abuse (e.g., cocaine) both increases risk of rupture from preexisting aneurysm, may increase likelihood of forming new aneurysms.
I. Flow dynamics and aneurysm growth (Fig. 35-3).
   1. Vessel bifurcation is site of maximum hemodynamic stress in vascular networks.
   2. Wall shear stresses, degeneration probably initiate aneurysm formation.
   3. Hemodynamic forces govern progression, growth of aneurysms.
   4. Intraaneurysmal flow dynamics.
      a. "Inflow zone": flow typically enters aneurysm at distal aspect of ostium.
      b. "Outflow zone": flow exits proximal ostium.
      c. "Slowflow zone": central slow-flow vortex.
   5. "Giant" aneurysms (>2.5 cm) often enlarge by recurrent intramural hemorrhage.
J. Complications of aneurysm rupture (Fig. 35-4).
   1. Vasospasm with cerebral ischemia, infarction is leading cause of death, disability.
   2. Parenchymal hematoma.

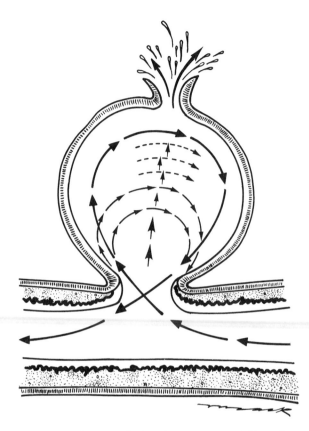

Fig. 35-3 Anatomic diagram depicts intraaneurysmal flow dynamics (heavy black lines with large arrows) and typical growth patterns (smaller, dotted arrows). Note the inflow zone is typically along the distal wall of the ostium, whereas the outflow zone is at the proximal aspect of the aneurysm. A slower-flow vortex is often found in the central part of an aneurysm. The usual rupture site is at the apex (dome) of the aneurysm and is indicated by the droplets of extravasated blood.

      3. Embolic stroke.
      4. Sudden death (12% of patients die before reaching medical attention). Typical case has:
         a. Intraventricular hemorrhage.
         b. Pulmonary edema.
         c. Ruptured posterior circulation aneurysm.
    K. Imaging.
      1. Conventional angiography.
         a. Remains imaging "gold standard" for evaluating presence of intracranial aneurysm.

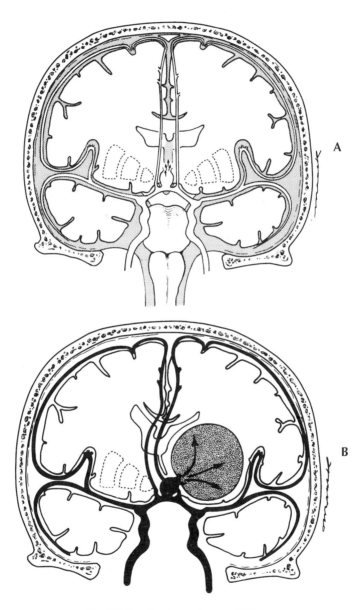

Fig. 35-4   For legend see p. 348.

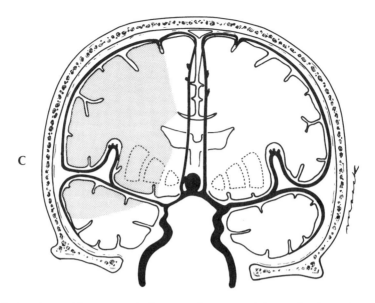

C

Fig. 35-4, cont'd   Anatomic diagrams show potential complications of aneurysm rupture. An anterior communicating artery aneurysm with superior rupture into the interhemispheric fissure and third ventricle is depicted.

A, The most common immediate complication is subarachnoid hemorrhage (dotted areas).

B, Another acute complication is paraaneurysmal intraparenchymal hematoma (shaded area). Note mass effect with ventricular displacement, subfalcine herniation.

C, Serious delayed complications include vasospasm (with narrowed vessels on right side, shown in black; compare normal vessels on left side, shown for comparison) and ischemia or infarction (dotted area depicts middle cerebral artery territory infarction).

   b. Goals in imaging patient with suspected aneurysm:
      (1) Identify aneurysm(s).
      (2) Delineate relationship to parent vessel, penetrating branches.
      (3) Define collateral circulation.
      (4) Detect complications (vasospasm, infarct, mass effect).
   c. Technical considerations.
      (1) Visualize entire intracranial circulation (including anterior, posterior communicating arteries, both posterior inferior cerebellar arteries).
      (2) Use cross-compression if necessary.
      (3) Multiple views (including obliques).
      (4) Subtraction studies (film or digital).

    d. Risks, benefits of angiography.

       (1) Need for definitive imaging to permit early surgery.

       (2) Overall risk of cerebral aneurysm rerupture related to angiography is 1.4%.

       (3) Emergency angiography performed within 6 hours of initial rupture is associated with rerupture rate of 4.8%.

       (4) Spontaneous rerupture of aneurysm in patient with acute SAH is 9.7%.

       (5) Therefore risk of delay usually outweighs risk of emergency angiography.

    e. Findings.

       (1) Contrast-filled outpouching from arterial bifurcation or lateral wall.

       (2) Thrombosed aneurysm may have negative angiogram or show avascular mass effect.

       (3) Aneurysm "mimics."

          (a) Vascular loop.

          (b) PCoA infundibulum (should be 2 mm or less in diameter, smooth funnel shape, with PCoA arising from apex).

    f. The "negative" angiogram.

       (1) Most common cause is incomplete study.

       (2) 15% negative in complete study.

          (a) "Microaneurysm" rupture.

          (b) Aneurysm may be thrombosed.

          (c) Repeat angiography positive in 10% to 20%.

       (3) SAH may be "nonaneurysmal."

          (a) Occult vascular malformation.

          (b) Neoplasm.

          (c) Nonaneurysmal perimesencephalic hemorrhage (focal SAH in prepontine, interpeduncular or ambient cisterns, probably caused by spontaneous rupture of small pontine or perimesencephalic veins).

2. Computed tomography.

    a. Subarachnoid hemorrhage.

       (1) NECT scans within 24 to 48 hours of rupture show SAH in approximately 95% of cases.

       (2) Pattern of SAH is sometimes helpful in localizing aneurysm.

          (a) Interhemispheric SAH (ACoA aneurysm).

          (b) Sylvian fissure (MCA aneurysm).

          (c) Fourth ventricle (PICA aneurysm).

          (d) Suprasellar (PCoA, basilar aneurysm).

    b. Parenchymal hemorrhage.
      (1) Occurs with 20% to 30% of ruptured aneurysms.
    c. Subdural hematoma.
      (1) Rare (<5%).
      (2) Usually associated with MCA aneurysm.
    d. Hydrocephalus.
      (1) Occurs in at least 10% of patients.
      (2) May develop rapidly.
    e. Patent aneurysm.
      (1) Isodense to slightly hyperdense on NECT.
      (2) Intense, uniform enhancement.
      (3) CT angiography (CTA) using spiral or helical scans helpful.
      (4) CECT 97% positive when aneurysm is 3 mm or larger.
    f. Partially or completely thrombosed aneurysm.
      (1) Variably hyperdense, often calcified.
      (2) Variable enhancement.
      (3) Giant "serpentine" aneurysms (>2.5 cm) can mimic neoplasm on MR, CT.
  3. MR.
    a. Appearance variable, often complex.
    b. Signal depends on presence, direction, rate, turbulence of flow.
    c. Presence of hematoma, calcification can complicate appearance.
    d. Typical patent aneurysm with rapid flow shows "flow void" (high-velocity signal loss).
      (1) Slow or turbulent flow may appear isointense.
      (2) Pulsation causes phase-encoding artifact.
    e. Partially or completely thrombosed aneurysm.
      (1) Complex, multilayered signal in wall.
      (2) "Flow void" in patent lumen.
  4. MR angiography (MRA).
    a. Time-of-flight (TOF) sequences use flow-related enhancement to identify moving spins.
    b. Phase-contrast (PC) sequences use velocity-induced phase shifts of flowing blood to separate blood from background (stationary) tissue.
    c. Sensitivity of MRA.
      (1) 87% sensitive for aneurysms 5 mm or larger using high-resolution TOF.
      (2) 75% using PC.
    d. MRA is accurate, feasible, noninvasive screening for

aneurysm in patients with increased familial risk, although conventional angiography is still necessary before operative treatment.

II. Fusiform aneurysms.
  A. Pathology.
    1. Exaggerated arterial ectasia due to severe atherosclerosis.
    2. More focal areas of fusiform or even saccular enlargement, aneurysmal dilatation.
    3. Intraluminal clots, disturbed flow patterns common.
  B. Clinical.
    1. Patients are usually older (>60 years).
    2. SAH rare.
    3. Symptoms usually due to mass effect, thrombosis of vessel, embolization of clot.
  C. Imaging.
    1. CT.
      a. Usually slightly hyperdense on NECT.
      b. Calcification common in both parent vessel, aneurysm.
      c. Patent lumen enhances strongly.
    2. MR.
      a. Heterogeneous signal due to hemorrhages (often of different ages), slow or turbulent flow.
      b. Secondary changes (ischemia, mass effect) depicted.

III. Dissecting aneurysms.
  A. Pathology, etiology.
    1. Tear of intima, internal elastic lamina.
    2. Plane of dissection usually within media.
    3. Intramural clot often compresses true lumen of artery.
    4. Dissection may extend toward adventitia and form a saclike focal outpouching, that is, a dissecting aneurysm is formed (see Fig. 22-1).
  B. Etiology.
    1. Spontaneous (no trauma, underlying vasculopathy).
    2. Trauma.
    3. Underlying vasculopathy (e.g., fibromuscular dysplasia).
  C. Location.
    1. Extracranial ICA.
      a. Midcervical segment to skull base most common site.
      b. Typically spares common carotid artery, carotid bulb.
    2. Vertebral artery (VA).
      a. C2 to skull base most common site.
      b. C6 (site where VA typically enters foramen transversarium).
      c. Mid-VA (injury with cervical fracture/subluxation).

D. Incidence.
  1. Found in approximately 0.2% of cervicocephalic angiograms.
E. Natural history.
  1. During initial (acute) phase, dissecting aneurysms may form and continue to enlarge for several weeks.
  2. In chronic phase, aneurysm may remain unchanged, grow smaller, or resolve (continued enlargement or rupture is rare).
  3. Dissecting aneurysm may become nidus for distal thromboembolism.
F. Imaging.
  1. Angiography shows elongated ovoid or saccular contrast collection that extends beyond vessel lumen.
  2. CT, MR show intravascular or perivascular hematoma.

SUGGESTED READINGS

Alberico RA, Patel M, Casey S, Jacobs B, et al: Evaluation of the circle of Willis with three-dimensional CT angiography in patients with suspected intracranial aneurysms, *AJNR* 16:1571-1578, 1995.

Bolger C, Philips J, Gilligan S, et al: Elevated levels of lipoprotein (a) in association with cerebrovascular saccular aneurysmal disease, *Neurosurg* 37:241-245, 1995.

Bosmans H, Wilms G, Marchal G, et al: Characterization of intracranial aneurysms with MR angiography, *Neuroradiol* 37:262-266, 1995.

Dippel DWJ, Habbema JDF: Natural history of unruptured aneurysms (letter), *J Neurosurg* 80:772-773, 1994.

Dorsch NWC, Young N, Kingston RJ, Compton JS: Early experience with spiral CT in the diagnosis of intracranial aneurysms, *Neurosurg* 36:230-238, 1995.

Huston J III, Nichols DA, Luetmer PH, et al: Blinded prospective evaluation of sensitivity of MR angiography to known intracranial aneurysms: importance of aneurysm size, *AJNR* 15:1607-1614, 1994.

Juvela S, Porras M, Heiskanen O: Natural history of unruptured aneurysms (reply), *J Neurosurg* 80:773-774, 1994.

Juvela S, Porras M, Heiskanen O: Natural history of unruptured intracranial aneurysms: a long-term follow-up study, *J Neurosurg* 79:174-182, 1993.

King JT, Berlin JA, Flamm ES: Morbidity and mortality from elective surgery for asymptomatic, unruptured, intracranial aneurysms: a meta-analysis, *J Neurosurg* 81:837-842, 1994.

Litt AW: MR angiography of intracranial aneurysms: proceed, but with caution (commentary), *AJNR* 15:1615-1616, 1994.

Mawad ME, Klucznik RP: Giant serpentine aneurysms: radiographic features and endovascular treatment, *AJNR* 16:1053-1060, 1995.

Nakagawa T, Hashi K: The incidence and treatment of asymptomatic, unruptured cerebral aneurysms, *J Neurosurg* 80:217-223, 1994.

Obuchowski NA, Modic MT, Magdinec M: Current implications for the efficacy of noninvasive screening for occult intracranial aneurysms in patients with a family history of aneurysms, *J Neurosurg* 83:42-49, 1995.

Osborn AG: Intracranial aneurysms: clinicopathologic correlations. In *Core curriculum in neuroradiology, part I: vascular lesions and degenerative diseases,* Chicago, 1995, American Society of Neuroradiology, pp 5-10.

Perata HJ, Tomsick TA, Tew JM Jr: Feeding artery pedicle aneurysms: association with parenchymal hemorrhage and arteriovenous malformation in the brain, *J Neurosurg* 80:631-634, 1994.

Rinne J, Hernesniemi J, Puranen M, Saari T: Multiple intracranial aneurysms in a defined population: prospective angiographic and clinical study, *Neurosurg* 35:803-808, 1994.

Ronkainen A, Hernesniemi J, Tromp G: Special features of familial intracranial aneurysms: report of 215 familial aneurysms, *Neurosurg* 37:43-47, 1995.

Ronkainen A, Puranen MI, Hernesniemi JA, et al: Intracranial aneurysms: MR angiographic screening in 400 asymptomatic individuals with increased familial risk, *Radiol* 195:35-40, 1995.

Saitoh H, Hayakawa K, Nishimura K, et al: Rerupture of cerebral aneurysms during angiography, *AJNR* 16:539-542, 1995.

Schievink WI, Piepgras DG, McCaffrey TV, Mokri B: Surgical treatment of extracranial internal carotid artery dissecting aneurysms, *Neurosurg* 35:809-816, 1994.

Schievink WI, Wijdicks EFM, Parisi JE, et al: Sudden death from aneurysmal subarachnoid hemorrhage, *Neurol* 45:871-874, 1995.

Tampieri D, Leblanc R, Oleszek J, et al: Three-dimensional computed tomographic angiography of cerebral aneurysms, *Neurosurg* 36:749-755, 1995.

Tatter SB, Crowell RM, Ogilvy CS: Aneurysmal and microaneurysmal "angiogram-negative" subarachnoid hemorrhage, *Neurosurg* 37:48-55, 1995.

Turjman F, Massoud TF, Vinuela F, et al: Aneurysms related to cerebral arteriovenous malformations: superselective angiographic assessment in 58 patients, *AJNR* 15:1601-1605, 1994.

36

Intracranial Vascular Malformations

Key Concepts

1. Four classic types of intracranial vascular malformations.
   a. Arteriovenous malformations.
   b. Venous vascular malformations ("venous angiomas").
   c. Capillary telangiectasias.
   d. Cavernous angiomas.
2. Venous "angioma" is an anatomic variant (developmental anomaly of cerebral venous system or "DVA"), not a true malformation.
3. Venous "angioma" is the most common brain vascular malformation.
4. Intracranial vascular malformations are often histopathologically heterogeneous (cavernous angioma is the most common type that occurs with other malformations).
5. The terms "cryptic" or "occult" vascular malformation should be discarded. These are nonspecific terms that refer to malformations not imaged on cerebral angiography.

Cerebrovascular malformations are developmental abnormalities that affect the brain blood vessels. Postmortem studies suggest that approximately 4% of the population harbor such lesions. These malformations are a heterogeneous group with varied histopathology, clinical significance, and imaging appearance. In this chapter we consider the four classic types of intracranial vascular malformations: arteriovenous malformations (AVM, AVF), venous "angiomas" or developmental venous anomalies (DVAs), capillary telangiectasias, and cavernous angiomas.

I. Arteriovenous malformations. Arteriovenous malformations are subdivided into brain parenchymal (pial) malformations (AVMs) and dural malformations and fistulae (AVFs). Mixed pial-dural AVMs may occur when a large parenchymal malformation recruits vascular supply from dural vessels.

   A. Parenchymal (pial) AVM (Fig. 36-1).
      1. Pathology.
         a. Congenital lesion with four main anatomic components.
            (1) Enlarged arterial feeders.
            (2) Arterial collaterals.
            (3) Nidus (core of AVM).
               (a) Thick-walled shunting arterioles.
               (b) Connect to thin venous channels.
               (c) No intervening capillary bed.
               (d) Absent or only gliotic brain in nidus.
               (e) Intranidal "aneurysms" in nearly 60%.
            (4) Venous outflow channels.
               (a) Collector veins.
               (b) Dilated draining veins.
               (c) Enlarged cortical veins.
               (d) May form varix.
               (e) Stenosis or occlusion may occur.
         b. Adjacent brain.
            (1) Hemorrhagic residua.
            (2) Dystrophic calcification.
            (3) Atrophy, ischemic changes.
      2. Location.
         a. 80% to 85% cerebral hemispheres.
         b. 10% to 15% posterior fossa.
      3. Shape.
         a. Usually cone-shaped or wedge-shaped.
         b. Broad base at cortical surface.
         c. Apex at ventricle.
      4. Incidence.

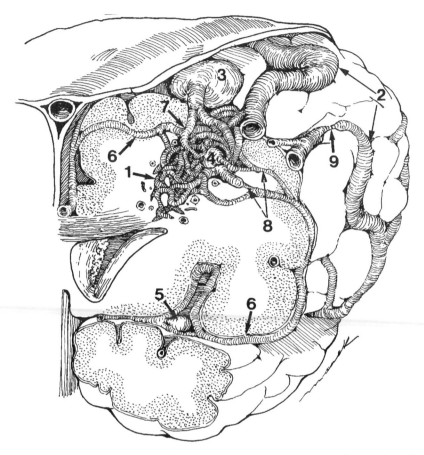

Fig. 36-1 Anatomic diagram that depicts some features of a typical parenchymal AVM. The AVM is a cone-shaped mass of arteries and veins with its base at the brain surface and its apex extending toward the lateral ventricle. 1, AVM nidus. 2, Enlarged cortical draining veins. 3, Venous varix. 4, Intranidal aneurysm. 5, Flow-related aneurysm at middle cerebral artery (MCA) bifurcation. 6, Enlarged ACA and MCA feeding arteries. 7, Arteriovenous fistula. 8, High flow vasculopathy with focal stenosis of feeding arteries. 9, Vasculopathic change in draining vein. (From Osborn AG: *Diagnostic neuroradiology,* St Louis, 1994, Mosby.)

    a. Estimated between .02% and .14% in general population (one seventh to one tenth that of saccular aneurysms).
    b. Solitary in 98%.
    c. 2% multiple.
       (1) Rendu-Osler-Weber syndrome (skin, mucosal capillary telangiectasias with pulmonary AVFs, brain AVMs).
       (2) Wyburn-Mason syndrome (ocular, brain AVMs).

5. Age at presentation.
   a. Peak between 20 and 40 years.
   b. 25% have hemorrhaged by age 15.
   c. 80% to 90% are symptomatic by age 50.
6. Clinical presentation.
   a. 50% hemorrhage.
      (1) Can be parenchymal, intraventricular, subarachnoid, or combination.
      (2) Mortality 10% to 17%.
      (3) Morbidity with significant neurologic deficit approximately 10%.
   b. 25% seizure.
      (1) Larger, more superficial lesions.
      (2) More likely to present early (<20 years of age).
   c. 25% miscellaneous.
   d. Isolated SAH rare.
7. Natural history and hemorrhage risk.
   a. Estimated 3% to 4% per year, cumulative.
   b. Spetzler classification.
      (1) Grades AVMs from 1 to 5, using points for size (1 = <3 cm, 2 = 3 to 6 cm, 3 = >6 cm), eloquence of adjacent brain (0 = noneloquent, 1 = eloquent), and pattern of venous drainage (0 = superficial only, 1 = deep).
      (2) Outcome correlates with score (1 = best).
      (3) Spetzler grade 6 is considered inoperable.
   c. Increased risk of hemorrhage.
      (1) Periventricular or intraventricular location.
      (2) Associated aneurysm (remote, pedicle, or intranidal).
      (3) Central or deep venous drainage.
      (4) Stenosis or occlusion of draining vein.
   d. Decreased risk of hemorrhage.
      (1) "Angiomatous" change (multiple dilated cortical vessels feed AVM with collateral supply from arteries—either cortical or leptomeningeal—that do not directly supply the nidus).
      (2) Peripheral or mixed venous drainage.
8. Imaging (Table 36-1).
   a. Cerebral angiography.
      (1) Tightly packed mass of vessels ("bag of worms").
      (2) Enlarged feeding arteries.
      (3) Dilated draining veins.
      (4) Little mass effect compared with lesion size (unless

Table 36-1   Imaging of Intracranial Vascular Malformations*

Malformation	Angiography	Computed Tomography	Magnetic Resonance Imaging
AVMs			
Parenchymal (pial)			
Patent	Enlarged arteries, veins AV shunting, "early" draining veins Minimal mass effect	Iso/hyperdense on NECT Strong serpentine enhancement on CECT ± hematoma, edema, mass effect Calcification 25% to 30%	Tightly packed flow voids Gliosis (hyperintense on T2WI) Hemorrhage (variable signal) MRA shows vessels, nidus
Thrombosed	May be normal + mass effect "stagnant" flow Subtle AV shunting	Calcification frequent Variable enhancement	Mixed signal lesion
Dural	Enlarged dural arteries AV shunting Stenotic/occluded dural sinus common	May be normal + enlarged dural sinus, venous varix	May be normal PC MRA can show flow direction in fistulae
Capillary telangiectasias	Often normal Racemose type may show faint blush ROW has vascular "nests" in nasopharyngeal mucosa	Normal/hyperdense on NECT Variable calcification Variable enhancement Usually no mass effect, edema	Racemose type may show curvilinear faint enhancement Cavernous type often hypointense, like cavernous angiomas
Cavernous angiomas	Usually normal	Iso/hyperdense on NECT Variable calcification Minimal/no enhancement on CECT Edema, mass effect usually absent	Mixed signal reticulated core, hemosiderin/ferritin rim "Blooms" on T2WI, GRE 50% to 80% multiple

Venous malformations			
Venous angioma (developmental venous anomaly)	Arterial phase normal ± blush in capillary phase "Medusa head" of enlarged medullary veins Enlarged transcortical or subependymal draining vein	NECT normal CECT shows tuft of vessels near ventricle, dilated draining vein	Tubular and stellate vessels, variable signal Strong enhancement 10% to 15% have gliotic, hemorrhagic changes in adjacent brain
Vein of Galen malformation	Enlarged choroidal/thalamoperformating arteries Aneurysmal enlargement of vein of Galen Accessory/falcine sinus common May have atretic straight sinus, slow flow, and thrombosis	Iso/hyperdense posterior third ventricular mass on NECT Strong enhancement on CECT Obstructive hydrocephalus, encephalomalacia common	Mixed signal from turbulent flow common along with areas of high-velocity signal loss
Venous varices	Coexisting high-flow AVM or AVF, less often venous angioma Saccular or fusiform enlargement of cortical/deep veins May have sinus pericranii	Iso/hyperdense serpentine or saccular vessels on NECT Strong uniform enhancement on CECT	Ovoid/fusiform vessels often with high-velocity signal loss

*Used with permission from Osborn AG: *Diagnostic neuroradiology*, St Louis, 1994, Mosby.

acute hemorrhage has occurred or large venous varix is present).

(5) Superselective studies delineate internal angioarchitecture (e.g., presence of intranidal aneurysm) and draining veins (stenosis, occlusion).

(6) Thrombosed AVMs may have normal angiogram or show only subtle changes (minimal arteriovenous shunting, stagnating arteries, early draining vein).

(7) Differential diagnosis: highly vascular neoplasm (anaplastic astrocytoma, glioblastoma multiforme).

b. Computed tomography.

(1) Isointense to slightly hyperintense on NECT.

(2) Calcification in 25% to 30%.

(3) Strong, uniform enhancement of serpentine feeding and draining vessels, nidus.

(4) Secondary changes.

  (a) Hematoma, mass effect.

  (b) Atrophy.

c. Magnetic resonance imaging.

(1) Signal varies depending on:

  (a) Flow rate, direction.

  (b) Pulse sequence.

  (c) Presence and age of hemorrhage.

(2) Typical uncomplicated AVM.

  (a) "Honeycomb" of "flow voids."

  (b) Little or no mass effect.

  (c) No normal brain inside AVM.

  (d) Adjacent gliosis, atrophy.

d. Magnetic resonance angiography.

(1) Gross delineation of AVM.

(2) Useful for treatment follow-up.

9. Treatment options.

a. Endovascular (embolization) therapy.

b. Surgery.

c. Stereotactic radiosurgery.

d. Combination of techniques.

B. Dural AVM/AVF (Fig. 36-2).

1. Pathology, etiology.

a. Considered acquired, not congenital, malformation.

b. Feeding arteries are dural or leptomeningeal, not pial.

c. "Nidus" is a network of microfistulae in dural sinus wall.

d. Draining structures are dural sinuses, cortical veins, or both.

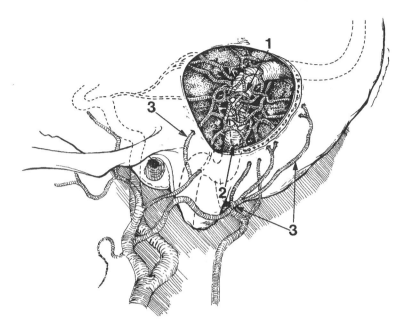

Fig. 36-2   Anatomic diagram of a transverse sinus AVM. The calvarium over the transverse and sigmoid sinuses has been removed to show the vascular malformation. 1, Tangle of dural arteries and draining veins in the transverse and sigmoid sinus wall forms the dural AVM. 2, Dotted line shows the sinus lumen is occluded. 3, Transosseous feeders arise from the occipital, posterior auricular, and vertebral arteries to supply the AVM. (Used with permission from Osborn AG: *Diagnostic neuroradiology,* St Louis, 1994, Mosby.)

   e. Often accompanied or caused by dural sinus thrombosis or occlusion, recanalization.
  2. Location.
   a. Infratentorial location is typical.
    (1) Transverse, sigmoid sinus most common sites.
   b. Other sites.
    (1) Cavernous sinus.
    (2) Anterior skull base.
    (3) Tentorium.
  3. Incidence.
   a. Account for 10% to 15% of intracranial vascular malformations.
   b. 6% of supratentorial AVMs.
   c. 35% of infratentorial AVMs.

4. Age, gender.
   a. Usually become symptomatic between 40 and 60 years.
   b. Males, females equally affected.
   c. Exception: cavernous sinus dural AVFs (strong female preponderance).
5. Clinical presentation.
   a. Varies with location.
   b. Bruit, nonspecific headache (transverse, sigmoid sinus DAVM).
   c. Proptosis, vision loss (cavernous sinus DAVM).
   d. Cranial nerve palsy.
   e. Venous congestive hypertension can cause neurologic deficit.
   f. If DAVM has cortical or deep venous drainage, can cause hemorrhage, seizure, neurologic deficit.
6. Hemorrhage risk.
   a. Rare compared with parenchymal (pial) AVM.
   b. Increased with retrograde flow into cortical veins.
7. Imaging (Table 36-1).
   a. Cerebral angiography.
      (1) One or more dural arteries drains directly into venous sinus.
      (2) Most common vessels involved:
         (a) Occipital artery.
         (b) Middle meningeal artery.
         (c) Meningohypophyseal trunk.
      (3) Dural venous sinus stenosis, occlusion is common.
      (4) May have venous varix.
      (5) Angiographic classification and clinical correlation.
         (a) Type I: DAVF drains into a sinus with normal antegrade flow (benign clinical course).
         (b) Type II: DAVF drains into sinus, but retrograde venous drainage is present. Intracranial hypertension in 20%; reflux into cortical veins induces hemorrhage in 10%.
         (c) Type III: DAVF drains directly into cortical vein without venous ectasia. Hemorrhage occurs in 40% of these cases.
         (d) Type IV: DAVF drains into cortical vein with ectasia >5 mm. Hemorrhage occurs in 65% of these cases.
         (e) Type V: Intracranial DAVF drains into spinal perimedullary veins. Progressive myelopathy in 50%.
   b. Computed tomography.
      (1) Often normal.
      (2) May show enlarged dural sinus (e.g., prominentcavernous sinus with dilated superior ophthalmic vein).

    c. Magnetic resonance imaging.
      (1) Often normal.
      (2) Dilated cortical veins without apparent nidus suggests DAVM with venous stenosis or occlusion.
      (3) MR angiography underestimates arterial feeders.
      (4) 2DPC MRA with flow quantitation can be used to evaluate hemodynamics.
  C. Mixed pial-dural AVMs.
    1. Pathology.
      a. Large parenchymal AVM recruits dural vascular supply.
      b. Dural, leptomeningeal supply occurs in approximately 10% of AVMs.
    2. Imaging.
      a. Cerebral angiography.
        (1) Pial supply (from cortical vessels).
        (2) Dural supply (usually from meningeal arteries).
II. Venous malformations.
  A. Venous "angioma" (Fig. 36-3).
    1. Pathology.
      a. Dilated cerebral or cerebellar medullary (white matter) veins form "caput medusae."
      b. Enlarged transcortical draining "collector vein."
      c. Normal brain is present between the enlarged tributary veins.
    2. Etiology.
      a. Faulty embryogenesis may cause occlusion or maldevelopment of venous drainage.
      b. Represents extreme anatomic variant or developmental venous anomaly (DVA) rather than true malformation.
      c. Common association with anomalies of neuronal migration.
    3. Incidence.
      a. Most common brain vascular malformation.
      b. Found in 3% of autopsies.
      c. Usually solitary (exception: blue rubber bleb nevus syndrome).
    4. Age, gender.
      a. Can be found at any age.
      b. Slight male preponderance (56% of cases).
    5. Location.
      a. Supratentorial 65%.
        (1) Frontal lobe is most common site (40%).
        (2) Typically near frontal horn of lateral ventricle.
      b. Infratentorial 35%.
        (1) Cerebellar hemispheres.

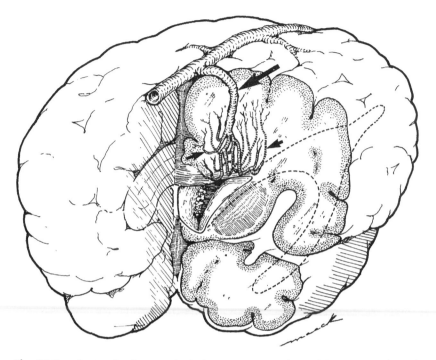

Fig. 36-3   Anatomic diagram depicting a venous angioma. Numerous enlarged medullary veins *(small arrows)* within the deep white matter converge near the ventricular angle and drain into an enlarged transcortical "collector vein" *(large arrow)*. The collector vein then empties into the superior sagittal sinus. The brain parenchyma in between the enlarged venous channels is normal. The prominent medullary veins form the familiar "Medusa head" that is seen on cerebral angiograms of venous angiomas. (Used with permission from Osborn AG: *Diagnostic neuroradiology,* St Louis, 1994, Mosby.)

        (2) Typically near fourth ventricle.
    6. Clinical presentation.
      a. Debatable.
      b. No clear correlation between venous angiomas and symptoms or signs; symptoms may be caused by associated lesion (e.g., cavernous angioma).
        (1) Asymptomatic patients (60%).
        (2) Symptomatic patients (40%).
          (a) Headache (15% to 30%).
          (b) Seizure (50%).
          (c) Hemorrhage, focal neurologic deficit (5% to 15%).
    7. Imaging (Table 36-1).
      a. Cerebral angiography.

(1) Arterial phase normal.

(2) Late capillary or early venous phase blush.

(3) Dilated medullary veins ("Medusa head").

(4) Enlarged transcortical draining vein.

    (a) Superficial venous drainage in 70%.

    (b) Deep (subependymal) in 20% to 30%.

(5) Focal stenosis of draining vein may lead to hemorrhagic or ischemic complications.

  b. Computed tomography.

    (1) NECT scans usually normal.

    (2) CECT scans:

      (a) Enhancing tuft near angle of ventricle.

      (b) Dilated collector vein (usually shown in serial sections).

  c. Magnetic resonance imaging.

    (1) T1-, T2WI may be normal or show linear area of high-velocity signal loss.

    (2) Postcontrast studies show radially arranged dilated tributaries, enlarged collector vein.

    (3) Hemorrhage suggests associated cavernous angioma or venous restrictive disease.

  d. Associated anomalies.

    (1) Cavernous angioma in 23%, other malformations (e.g., AVM) rare.

    (2) Venous varix (rare).

    (3) Sinus pericranii (extracranial vein that communicates directly with intracranial vein or dural sinus via emissary or diploic channel).

    (4) Blue rubber bleb nevus syndrome.

B. Vein of Galen (V of G) malformation ("aneurysm").

  1. Terminology.

    a. Used to encompass diverse group of vascular anomalies.

    b. Common feature is dilatation of vein of Galen.

  2. Pathology, etiology.

    a. Normally, V of G is conduit between deep parenchymal venous system and venous sinuses.

    b. Arterial tributaries.

      (1) Posterior choroidal arteries most common primary feeders.

      (2) Anterior cerebral arteries second most common source of supply.

      (3) Others:

        (a) Thalamoperforating arteries.

        (b) Perimesencephalic vessels.

        (c) Posterior cerebral artery branches.
- c. Nearly 70% of cases have venous anomalies.
  - (1) Absent, hypoplastic, or interrupted straight sinus.
  - (2) Persistent falcine sinus.
- 3. Categories.
  - a. Type I.
    - (1) Direct arteriovenous connection (fistula) between arteries and V of G.
  - b. Type II.
    - (1) Thalamic AVM with Galenic drainage.
    - (2) May present in older children.
  - c. Type III.
    - (1) Complex lesion; mixture of types I and II.
    - (2) Usual presentation is neonate with intractable high-output congestive heart failure and cranial bruit.
  - d. Type IV.
    - (1) AVM drains into veins that then empty into V of G.
- 4. Imaging.
  - a. U/S.
    - (1) Color Doppler typically shows complex blood flow within an enlarged V of G.
    - (2) Third ventricle anteriorly displaced.
    - (3) Hydrocephalus is common.
  - b. Cerebral angiography.
    - (1) Provides definitive diagnosis.
    - (2) Delineates arterial supply.
    - (3) Defines venous drainage (including anomalies, outflow stenosis).
  - c. CT.
    - (1) Round mass in quadrigeminal cistern.
    - (2) Strong, uniform enhancement (unless thrombosed).
    - (3) Hydrocephalus.
    - (4) Encephalomalacia.
  - d. MR.
    - (1) Mass posterior to third ventricle.
    - (2) Delineates presence, direction of flow.
    - (3) Thrombosis, secondary parenchymal changes defined.
    - (4) MR angiography shows gross features; cerebral angiography needed for detailed delineation of feeders and venous outflow.
- 5. Associated anomalies.
  - a. Turner syndrome.
  - b. Blue rubber bleb nevus syndrome.
- C. Venous varix (enlarged vein with focal dilatation; usually associ-

ated with AVM or AVF but occasionally occurs as isolated lesion).

III. Capillary malformations.
  A. Capillary telangiectasias.
    1. Pathology.
      a. Nests or racemose collections of dilated capillaries with abnormal walls (lack smooth muscle, elastic fibers).
      b. Contain normal brain.
      c. May contain blood storage products from previous hemorrhage.
    2. Location.
      a. Anywhere in brain, spinal cord.
      b. Pons, medulla, spinal cord are favored sites.
    3. Incidence.
      a. Second most common intracranial vascular malformation identified at autopsy (venous angiomas are the most common type).
      b. Multiple lesions are the rule.
    4. Clinical presentation.
      a. Most are clinically silent.
      b. May hemorrhage, especially if associated with cavernous angioma.
    5. Imaging.
      a. Cerebral angiography is usually normal.
      b. NECT usually normal; CECT scans may show faint areas of increased density.
      c. MR.
        (1) Multifocal areas of decreased signal on T2WI, gradient-refocused scans.
        (2) May occasionally show poorly delineated enhancement.
    6. Associated abnormalities.
      a. May coexist with cavernous angioma.
  B. Radiation-induced hemorrhagic vasculopathy.
    1. Pathology.
      a. Large, irregular capillary telangiectasias with proliferation of small blood vessels in white matter.
      b. Perivascular hemosiderin.
      c. Intracranial hemorrhage (25% of cases).
    2. Etiology.
      a. Unknown.
      b. Theories.
        (1) Vascular endothelial damage.
        (2) Possible immune-mediated hypersensitivity response.
    3. MR.
      a. Hemorrhagic foci.

(1) Usually small (<5 mm).
(2) 45% multiple.
(3) Seen as hypointense foci on T2WI, gradient-refocused sequences.

C. Hereditary hemorrhagic telangiectasia (HHT; also known as Rendu-Osler-Weber disease).
  1. Inheritance.
    a. Autosomal dominant neurocutaneous syndrome.
  2. Vascular lesions.
    a. Capillary telangiectasias (in skin and mucosa, *not* brain).
    b. Cerebral vascular malformations (found in 23% of patients with HHT).
      (1) 4% are typical AVMs.
      (2) 6% are venous malformations.
      (3) 12.5% are indeterminate lesions, namely cavernous angiomas or "micro" AVMs.
      (4) Multiple AVMs common; may be difficult to detect with MR but can be delineated with high-resolution conventional angiography.
    c. Visceral vascular malformations, fistulae.
      (1) AVM of liver (30% of cases).
      (2) Pulmonary AVFs (15% to 20%).
  3. Clinical presentation.
    a. Epistaxis in 85%.
    b. Neurologic complications.
      (1) 50% are caused by pulmonary AVF (e.g., emboli).
      (2) Others caused by intracranial vascular malformation, hepatic encephalopathy, cerebral abscess.

IV. Cavernous malformations.
  A. Cavernous angioma (parenchymal) (Fig. 36-4).
    1. Pathology.
      a. Gross, surgical examination shows multilobulated purple lesion that is well demarcated from adjacent brain.
      b. Histology.
        (1) "Honeycomb" of large endothelial-lined sinusoidal spaces that lack muscular or elastic layers.
        (2) Fibrous septae separate vascular spaces.
        (3) Slow-flowing blood, intravascular thrombi.
        (4) Hemorrhagic residua (recent, remote), calcification common.
        (5) No normal brain within lesion.
        (6) Adjacent brain surrounding lesion is often hemosiderin-stained, gliotic.

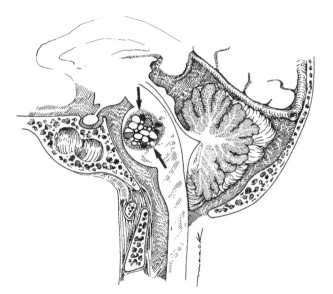

Fig. 36-4   Anatomic diagram of pontine cavernous anigoma. The lesion has a reticulated core with multiple cavities containing blood degradation products. The angioma is surrounded by a hemosiderin/ferritin rim *(arrows)*. (Used with permission from Osborn AG: *Diagnositic neuroradiology,* St Louis, 1994, Mosby.)

    2. Inheritance.
      a. Sporadic form.
        (1) Characterized by isolated lesions.
        (2) 10% to 15% multiple.
      b. Familial form.
        (1) Autosomal dominant, variable penetrance.
        (2) Characterized by multiple lesions (75%).
        (3) Dynamic disease; MR imaging discloses changes in lesion number, size, and imaging characteristics.
    3. Incidence.
      a. Represent about 15% of cerebrovascular malformations at autopsy.
      b. Affect between 0.5% and 0.7% of population.
    4. Location.
      a. 80% supratentorial.
      b. Approximately one third of all cases are multiple.
      c. Occasionally occur in dura, venous sinuses (see below).
    5. Age, gender.
      a. Peak presentation between 20 and 40 years.

   b. No gender predilection.
6. Clinical presentation.
   a. Often asymptomatic (found on 0.4% of MR scans).
   b. Seizure (usually seen in patients <40 years).
   c. Neurologic deficit (especially with posterior fossa lesion).
7. Hemorrhage risk.
   a. Familial form: 1.1% per lesion per year.
   b. Sporadic form: 0.5% to 1% per lesion per year.
   c. Female hormonal factors may play possible role.
8. Imaging.
   a. Cerebral angiography.
      (1) Usually normal because these are slow-flow lesions.
      (2) Faint blush on late capillary or early venous phase can sometimes be identified.
   b. CT.
      (1) Isodense to moderately hyperdense on NECT.
      (2) Calcification common.
      (3) Variable enhancement.
   c. MR.
      (1) Reticulated "popcorn-like" lesion with mixed-signal core, low-signal rim.
      (2) Gradient-refocused scans may detect multiple lesions.
9. Associated abnormalities.
   a. Most common vascular malformation coexisting with other vascular malformations.
      (1) 23% of venous angiomas.
      (2) Can also occur with capillary telangiectasias, AVMs.
   b. A few cases of cavernous angiomas with skin angiomas and arachnoid cysts have been reported.
   B. Extracerebral cavernous malformations.
      1. Location.
         a. Cavernous sinus most common site.
         b. Dura.
      2. Imaging.
         a. Angiography.
            (1) Enlarged dural arteries.
            (2) Dense, prolonged vascular stain.
         b. CT, MR.
            (1) Dural-based mass resembles meningioma.
V. "Cryptic" or "occult" vascular malformation.
   A. Terminology.
      1. Misnomer.
         a. Outdated term.

   b. Prior to advent of CT and MR, was used to refer to vascular malformations that were angiographically occult.
   c. Angiography in such cases was normal because of absent or very slow flow in the lesion.
   2. Term should probably be discarded because vascular malformations that are normal on conventional cerebral angiography are usually delineated on MR.
B. Vascular malformations that are so-called occult (angiographically normal) include:
   1. Thrombosed AVM (approximately 40% to 50%).
   2. Cavernous angioma (between 30% and 35%).
   3. Venous angioma (7% to 10%).
   4. Capillary telangiectasia (4%).
   5. Mixed or unclassified lesions (1% to 3%).

SUGGESTED READINGS

Aiba T, Tanaka R, Koike T, et al: Natural history of intracranial cavernous malformations, *J Neurosurg* 83:56-59, 1995.

Awad IA, Robinson JR Jr, Mohanty S, Estes ML: Mixed vascular malformations of the brain: clinical and pathogenetic considerations, *Neurosurg* 33:179-188, 1993.

Borden JA, Wu JK, Schucart WA: A proposed classification for spinal and cranial dural arteriovenous fistulous malformations and implications for treatment, *J Neurosurg* 82:166-179, 1995.

Chaloupka JC, Fulbright RK, Putman CM, et al: Cerebral vascular malformations detected by screening MRI/MRA in patients with hereditary hemorrhagic telangiectasia. Presented at the American Society of Neuroradiology Annual Scientific Meeting, Chicago, Illinois, April 23-27, 1995.

Cognard C, Gobin YP, Pierot L, et al: Cerebral dural arteriovenous fistulas: clinical and angiographic correlation with a revised classification of venous drainage, *Radiol* 194:671-680, 1995.

Crercco M, Floris R, Vidiri A, et al: Venous angiomas: plain and contrast-enhanced MRI and MR angiography, *Neuroradiol* 37:20-24, 1995.

Gaensler EHL, Dillon WP, Edwards MSB, et al: Radiation-induced telangiectasia in the brain simulates cryptic vascular malformations at MR imaging, *Radiol* 193:629-636, 1994.

Hoang T-A, Hasso AN: Intracranial vascular malformations, *Neuroimaging Clin North Am* 4:823-847, 1994.

Horowitz MB, Jungreis CA, Quisling RG, Pollack I: Vein of Galen aneurysms: a review and current perspective, *AJNR* 15:1486-1496, 1994.

Kelly KJ, Rockwell BH, Raji MR, et al: Isolated cerebral intraaxial varix, *AJNR* 16:1633-1635, 1995.

Luker GD, Siegel MJ: Sinus pericranii: sonographic findings, *AJR* 165:175-176, 1995.

Meyer B, Stangl AP, Schramm J: Association of venous and true arteriovenous malformation: a rare entity among mixed vascular malformations of the brain, *J Neurosurg* 83:141-144, 1995.

Mullan S, Mojtahedi S, Johnson DL: Radiological anatomy of arteriovenous malformations [Abstract], *J Neurosurg* 82:371A-372A, 1995.

Muller-Forell W, Valavanis A: How angioarchitecture of cerebral arteriovenous malformations should influence the therapeutic considerations, *Minim Invas Neurosurg* 38:32-40, 1995.

Osborn AG: Intracranial vascular malformations. In *Diagnostic neuroradiology*, St Louis, 1994, Mosby, pp 284-329.

Poussaint TY, Siffert J, Barnes PD, et al: Hemorrhagic vasculopathy after treatment of central nervous system neoplasia in childhood: diagnosis and follow-up, *AJNR* 16:693-699, 1995.

Strother CM: Vascular malformations of the central nervous system. In *Core curriculum in neuroradiology part I: vascular lesions and degenerative diseases,* Chicago, 1995, American Society of Neuroradiology, pp 27-29.

Tew JM Jr, Lewis AI, Reichert KW: Management strategies and surgical techniques for deep-seated supratentorial arteriovenous malformations, *Neurosurg* 36:1065-1072, 1995.

Uchino A, Hasuo K, Matsumoto S, et al: Varix occurring with cerebral venous angioma: a case report and review of the literature, *Neuroradiol* 37:29-31, 1995.

Wagner BJ, Richardson KJ, Moran AMM, Carrier DA: Intracranial vascular malformations, *Sem U/S, CT, MRI* 16:253-268, 1995.

Willinsky R, Terbrugge K, Montanera W, et al: Venous congestion: an MR finding in dural arteriovenous malformations with cortical venous drainage, *AJNR* 15:1501-1507, 1994.

Wilms G, Bleus E, Demaerel P, et al: Simultaneous occurrence of developmental venous anomalies and cavernous angiomas, *AJNR* 15:1247-1254, 1994.

Zabramski JM, Wascher TM, Spetzler RF, et al: The natural history of familial cavernous malformations: results of an ongoing study, *J Neurosurg* 80:422-432, 1994.

37

Stroke

Key Concepts

1. "Stroke" is a lay term that encompasses a heterogeneous group of cerebro-vascular disorders characterized by sudden onset of an acute neurologic event.
2. The four major types of "stroke" are:
   a. Cerebral infarction.
   b. Primary intracerebral hemorrhage.
   c. Subarachnoid hemorrhage.
   d. Veno-occlusive disorders.
3. The concept of a "therapeutic window" in acute ischemic stroke implies there is a short period (usually less than 6 hours) during which there may be still-viable cerebral tissue that can be salvaged by appropriate and timely intervention.
4. Imaging studies play a key role in the evaluation and treatment of cerebral ischemia.

Stroke has a high prevalence, illness burden, and economic cost. Although stroke is ideally suited for prevention, it remains a major cause of disability among adult Americans and is the third leading cause of death in this age group (after cardiovascular disease and cancer). With promising new therapies for treating stroke continually evolving, appropriate and timely imaging studies are playing an increasingly prominent role in the evaluation of cerebral ischemia and infarction.

"Stroke" is actually a lay term that means sudden onset of an acute neurologic event. The term is used to designate a heterogeneous group of cerebrovascular disorders with widely different clinical and imaging presentations, pathophysiology, etiology, prognosis, and treatment.

There are four major types of "stroke": (1) cerebral ischemia and infarction; (2) primary intracerebral hemorrhage (ICH); (3) subarachnoid hemorrhage (SAH); and (4) venous occlusions. Primary intracerebral hemorrhage in middle-aged and older adults is most often hypertensive in origin (see Chapter 23). Nearly 85% of nontraumatic SAH cases are secondary to ruptured aneurysm (see Chapter 23).

In this chapter we discuss the demographics, pathophysiology, anatomy, and imaging of cerebral arterial ischemia and infarction. Cerebral veno-occlusive disorders are discussed in Chapter 40; atherosclerosis and nonatheromatous stenosis are considered in Chapters 38 and 39.

I. Stroke demographics.
   A. Prevalence.
      1. Three million stroke survivors in the United States.
      2. 400,000 to 500,000 new or recurrent strokes each year.
      3. Third leading cause of death among adult Americans (after cardiovascular disease and cancer).
      4. Estimate of "preventable" strokes is as high as 80%.
   B. Cost.
      1. Estimated $30 billion dollars spent annually in United States.
      2. Targeted for cost containment by managed health care systems.
   C. Risk factors.
      1. Hypertension.
         a. Most important treatable risk factor for stroke.
         b. Relative stroke risk three to four times that in normotensive population.
      2. Cardiac disease.
         a. Independent predictors of ischemic stroke.
            (1) Coronary heart disease.
            (2) Left ventricular hypertrophy.
            (3) Congestive heart failure.
            (4) Atrial fibrillation.
      3. Systemic, metabolic disorders.

       a. Diabetes mellitus.

         (1) Independent risk factor for ischemic stroke (large artery type).

         (2) Risk factor in both men, women (especially older women).

       b. Blood lipid levels (still uncertain).

       c. Cigarette smoking.

       d. Heavy alcohol consumption.

    4. Asymptomatic carotid stenosis.

       a. Increasing vascular death, stroke, cardiac events associated with increasing severity of asymptomatic carotid stenosis.

         (1) 75% or less: annual stroke rate of 1.3%.

         (2) >75%: annual stroke rate of 3.3%.

    5. Transient ischemic attack (TIA).

       a. TIA precedes atherothrombotic brain infarction in 10% to 12% of cases.

       b. Estimated overall 5-year risk of stroke following TIA is approximately 33%.

  D. Outcome.

    1. Poor outcome.

       a. Related to age, clinical CNS status.

         (1) 10% in patients <70 years with good initial CNS score.

         (2) 90% in patients >70 years with poor initial CNS score.

       b. Large infarct, coma.

II. Acute cerebral ischemia and infarction.

  A. Pathophysiology in a nutshell.

    1. Diminished blood flow.

       a. Can be global, regional, or focal.

       b. Ischemia causes energy depletion, which in turn causes:

         (1) Loss of ion homeostasis.

         (2) Influx of Na^+, Cl^-, Ca^{++}, water into cells.

         (3) Metabolic acidosis.

         (4) Extracellular glutamate accumulation.

    2. Ischemic "cascade."

       a. Cell membrane integrity is lost.

       b. Cell death.

       c. Edema, mass effect.

    3. Selective vulnerability.

       a. Different cell types in CNS are variably susceptible to ischemic damage.

       b. Neurons most vulnerable, especially cells in:

         (1) CA_1 area of hippocampus.

         (2) Cortex, basal ganglia.

      c. Relatively less susceptible to ischemic damage.
        (1) Astrocytes.
        (2) Oligodendrocytes.
        (3) Vascular endothelial cells.
    4. Ischemic area.
      a. Densely ischemic central focus.
        (1) Cell damage is usually irreversible.
        (2) All cell types affected.
        (3) Typically progresses to frank infarction.
      b. Less densely peripheral ischemic "penumbra."
        (1) Cells may remain viable for several hours.
        (2) Salvage therapies directed at rescuing these at-risk areas.
B. Imaging.
    1. Cerebral angiography.
      a. Limited role during hyperacute stage unless intraarterial thrombolysis is considered.
      b. Findings.
        (1) Occluded vessel (45% to 50%).
        (2) Slow antegrade flow/delayed arterial emptying (15%).
        (3) Retrograde filling of vessel distal to occlusion via collateral flow (15% to 25%).
        (4) Hyperemia, seen as vascular blush or "luxury perfusion" (15% to 25%).
        (5) Arteriovenous shunting, seen as "early draining vein" (10% to 15%).
        (6) Nonperfused ("bare") areas (5% to 10%).
        (7) Variable mass effect.
    2. Transcranial Doppler ultrasonography (TCD).
      a. Useful for detecting major vessel occlusion, detecting reperfusion.
      b. Findings.
        (1) Proximal middle cerebral artery (MCA) occlusion indicated by absence of MCA flow signal.
        (2) Distal occlusion seen as asymmetric MCA flow velocity.
        (3) Distal branch occlusions only episodically detectable.
    3. CT.
      a. Usually initial imaging procedure because of accessibility, rapidity.
      b. Used to diagnose/exclude intracerebral hematoma, detect stroke "mimics."
        (1) Clinical diagnosis of ischemic stroke may be incorrect.
        (2) Nonvascular lesions cause 1% to 2% of acute stroke syndromes.

        (a) Subdural hematoma.

        (b) Hemorrhagic vascular malformation.

        (c) Neoplasm.

  c. Findings (NECT).

    (1) Hyperacute (<6 hours).

        (a) May be normal (25% to 50%) or only subtly abnormal.

        (b) Hyperattenuating artery (indicates acute thrombus) in 25% to 50%.

        (c) Mild parenchymal hypodensity, seen as subtle decreased density of subcortical gray matter (obscuration of lentiform nuclei).

    (2) Acute (12 to 24 hours).

        (a) Low-density basal ganglia.

        (b) Loss of gray-white matter interfaces (insular ribbon sign, obscuration of cortex-medullary white matter border).

        (c) Sulcal effacement (early mass effect).

    (3) Late acute (1 to 3 days).

        (a) Wedge-shaped low-density area.

        (b) Affects both gray, white matter.

        (c) Mass effect increases.

        (d) Hemorrhagic transformation may occur (basal ganglia, cortex common sites).

4. MRI.

  a. Increased sensitivity compared with CT.

  b. Findings.

    (1) Immediate.

        (a) Absence of normal "flow void" in affected vessel.

        (b) T1WI: intravascular contrast enhancement (reflects slow flow) in 75%.

        (c) MRA: occluded vessel in 80%.

        (d) Diffusion MRI: hyperintense; reduced apparent diffusion coefficient of water.

    (2) Hyperacute (1 to 6 hours).

        (a) T1WI: sulcal effacement, gyral swelling, loss of gray-white interfaces.

        (b) T2WI: may be normal.

    (3) Acute (6 to 24 hours).

        (a) T1WI: mass effect increases; meningeal enhancement adjacent to infarct may occur; visualization of enhancement improved with magnetization transfer (MT).

        (b) T2WI: increased signal intensity in affected area.

        (c) MR spectroscopy: elevation of lactate peak (highly correlated with both acute stroke severity, eventual clinical outcome), depressed N-acetylaspartate peak.

    (4) Late acute (1 to 3 days).

        (a) T1WI: mass effect increases, intravascular/meningeal enhancement diminish as early parenchymal enhancement becomes apparent; visualization improved with MT sequences.

        (b) T2WI: hyperintense; hemorrhagic transformation may be hypointense.

        (c) ADC values on day 2 increase, may be associated with vasogenic edema and cell lysis.

III. Subacute, chronic infarction.

  A. Pathophysiology.

    1. Continued evolution of infarct.

  B. Imaging.

    1. CT.

      a. Useful for detecting hemorrhagic transformation.

      b. Findings.

        (1) Early subacute (4 to 7 days).

          (a) Mass effect, edema persist.

          (b) Hemorrhagic transformation (HT) may become apparent.

          (c) Gyral enhancement after contrast administration may occur.

        (2) Late subacute (1 to 8 weeks).

          (a) Mass effect resolves.

          (b) Transient calcification may occur (children).

          (c) Gyral enhancement persists.

        (3) Chronic (months to years).

          (a) Atrophy, encephalomalacia.

          (b) Ventricles, sulci enlarge.

          (c) Calcification very rare.

          (d) No enhancement following contrast administration.

    2. MR.

      a. Useful for detecting HT.

      b. Findings.

        (1) Early subacute (4 to 7 days).

          (a) T1WI: parenchymal enhancement with contrast.

          (b) T2WI: hemorrhage in 25%; subcortical hyperintensity in 15%; acute Wallerian degeneration (high signal intensity in descending corticospinal tract).

      (2) Late subacute (1 to 8 weeks).

          (a) T1WI: parenchymal enhancement may persist; mass effect resolves; foci of subacute hemorrhage detected in slightly >50% of cases (80% are petechial).

          (b) T2WI: decrease in abnormal signal sometimes occurs ("fogging effect").

      (3) Chronic (months to years).

          (a) T1WI: volume loss, atrophy; Wallerian degeneration (ipsilateral peduncle, pons show atrophy).

          (b) T2WI: encephalomalacia, hemorrhagic residua (low signal).

IV. Strokes in specific vascular distributions (Fig. 37-1).

  A. Supratentorial infarcts.

    1. Middle cerebral artery (MCA).

      a. 75% to 80% of all strokes occur in MCA distribution.

      b. Complete MCA infarct.

        (1) Basal ganglia.

        (2) Large wedge-shaped area extending from lateral ventricle to cortex (involves both gray, white matter).

      c. MCA infarct distal to lenticulostriate arteries.

        (1) Spares basal ganglia.

        (2) Wedge-shaped area from lateral ventricle to cortex.

      d. Branch occlusion.

        (1) Focal wedge-shaped area involving cortex, underlying subcortical white matter.

    2. Posterior cerebral artery (PCA).

      a. Second most common site of stroke.

      b. Variable distribution.

        (1) Posterior one third of convexity.

        (2) Occipital lobe.

        (3) Inferomedial temporal lobe.

        (4) Thalamoperforating, posterior choroidal branches.

          (a) Thalamus.

          (b) Posterior limb of internal capsule.

          (c) Midbrain tegmentum.

    3. Anterior cerebral artery (ACA).

      a. Rare site of stroke (0.5% to 1%).

      b. Complete ACA infarct.

        (1) Anterior two thirds of convexity (to parietooccipital sulcus).

        (2) Inferomedial frontal lobe.

        (3) Recurrent artery of Heubner, medial lenticulostriate arteries.

          (a) Septum pellucidum.

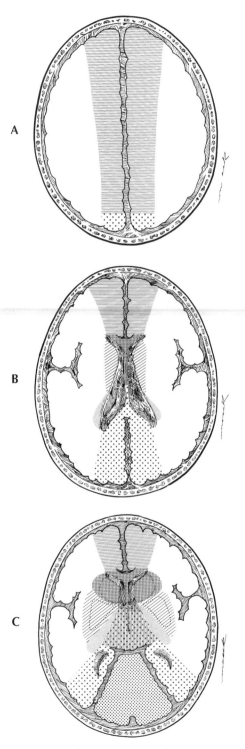

For legend see opposite page.

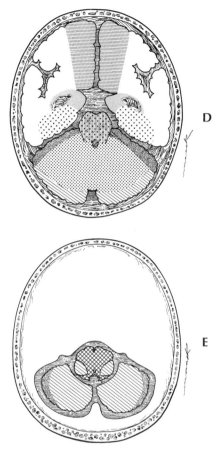

D

E

BRAIN VASCULAR TERRITORIES

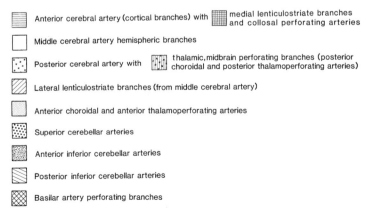

Anterior cerebral artery (cortical branches) with medial lenticulostriate branches and collosal perforating arteries

Middle cerebral artery hemispheric branches

Posterior cerebral artery with thalamic, midbrain perforating branches (posterior choroidal and posterior thalamoperforating arteries)

Lateral lenticulostriate branches (from middle cerebral artery)

Anterior choroidal and anterior thalamoperforating arteries

Superior cerebellar arteries

Anterior inferior cerebellar arteries

Posterior inferior cerebellar arteries

Basilar artery perforating branches

Fig. 37-1   Axial anatomic drawings depict the brain vascular territories and infarctions in specific arterial distributions.

        (b) Corpus callosum genu.

        (c) Head of caudate nucleus.

        (d) Anterior limb of internal capsule.

    c. Distal ACA infarct (pericallosal, callosomarginal).

      (1) Convexity.

      (2) May occur secondary to severe subfalcine herniation.

4. Miscellaneous supratentorial infarcts.

    a. Lenticulostriate arteries (LSAs).

      (1) Common site of "lacunar" infarcts (<1 cm).

      (2) Territory.

        (a) Medial LSAs (including recurrent artery of Heubner from ACA): head of caudate nucleus, anterior limb of internal capsule, region inferolateral to frontal horn of lateral ventricle.

        (b) Lateral LSAs (from MCA): putamen, genu, and superior aspect of posterior limb of internal capsule.

      (3) Differential diagnosis = dilated perivascular (Virchow-Robin) spaces.

    b. Anterior choroidal artery.

      (1) Arcuate zone between corpus striatum anterolaterally, thalamus posteromedially.

      (2) Globus pallidus, inferior aspect of posterior limb of internal capsule.

    c. Thalamotuberal, thalamoperforating arteries (TPAs).

      (1) Less common site of "lacunar" infarcts.

      (2) Territory.

        (a) Anterior TPAs (from PCoA): posterior hypothalamus, anterior pole of thalamus.

        (b) Posterior TPAs (from basilar bifurcation, PCAs): midbrain, posteromedial thalamus.

    d. "Border zone" ("watershed") infarcts.

      (1) Premature infants.

        (a) Deep (periventricular, central white matter); may cause periventricular leukomalaia.

        (b) Common even in absence of asphyxia.

      (2) Term infants, children, and adults.

        (a) Peripheral (cortex between adjacent vascular territories, e.g., MCA/PCA, ACA/PCA, ACA/MCA; may also cause generalized cortical or "pseudolaminar" necrosis).

        (b) Usually caused by focal/global hypoperfusion secondary to decreased cardiac output (basal ganglia also commonly affected).

(c) Earliest change may be loss of normal low T2-signal intensity in precentral, postcentral gyri.
  e. Complete global ischemia.
    (1) Profound neonatal asphyxia.
      (a) Affects ventrolateral thalami, posterolateral lentiform nuclei, posterior mesencephalon, hippocampi, and perirolandic cerebral cortex.
      (b) Basal ganglia, brainstem may enhance following contrast administration.
    (2) Cardiac arrest with reperfusion.
      (a) Bilateral, symmetric lesions in basal ganglia, thalami, substantia nigra.
B. Infratentorial infarcts.
  1. Basilar artery.
    a. "Top of basilar" infarct.
      (1) Both posterior thalami.
      (2) Mesencephalon.
      (3) Occipital, temporal lobe (PCA distribution).
    b. Pontine perforating branches.
      (1) Patchy pontine lesions.
      (2) May cause "locked-in" syndrome.
  2. Superior cerebellar artery (SCA).
    a. Only 2% to 3% of acute brain infarcts affect the cerebellum; approximately 50% are in the SCA territory.
    b. Vermian branch occlusion.
      (1) Ipsilateral superior vermis.
      (2) Quadrangular shape, medial location, sagittal orientation.
    c. Hemispheric branch occlusion.
      (1) Superolateral hemisphere with variable involvement of white matter, brachium pontis, dentate nuclei.
      (2) Oblique orientation paralleling folia.
  3. Posterior inferior cerebellar artery (PICA).
    a. High anatomic variation (absent or anomalous PICA).
    b. Accounts for slightly less than 50% of cerebellar infarcts.
    c. May cause Wallenberg syndrome.
      (1) Loss of pain, temperature on ipsilateral face/contralateral body.
      (2) Horner's sign.
      (3) Ataxia, nystagmus.
      (4) Dysphagia, dysphonia.
    d. Variable involvement.
      (1) Dorsolateral medulla.

(2) Posteroinferior cerebellum.
(3) Tonsil.
(4) Inferior vermis.
4. Anterior inferior cerebellar artery (AICA).
  a. Very rare site of isolated posterior fossa infarct (<1% of cerebellar infarcts).
  b. Usually occurs in diabetic, hypertensive patients.
  c. Anterolateral (petrosal) surface of cerebellar hemisphere.

SUGGESTED READINGS

Castillo M, Smith JK, Mukherji SK: MR appearance of cerebral cortex in children with and without a history of perinatal anoxia, *AJR* 164:1481-1484, 1995.

Cinnamon J, Viroslav AB, Dorey JH: CT and MRI diagnosis of cerebrovascular disease: going beyond the pixels, *Sem U/S, CT, MRI* 16:212-236, 1995.

Drayer BP: Brain infarction: localization. In *Core curriculum in neuroradiology, part I: vascular lesions and degenerative disease,* Chicago, 1995, American Society of Neuroradiology, pp 105-111.

Fiorelli M, Alperovitch A, Argentino C, et al: Prediction of long-term outcome in the early hours following acute ischemic stroke, *Arch Neurol* 52:250-255, 1995.

Gorelick PB: Stroke prevention, *Arch Neurol* 52:347-355, 1995.

Graham GD, Kalvach P, Blamire AM, et al: Clinical correlates of proton magnetic resonance spectroscopy findings after acute cerebral infarction, *Stroke* 26:225-229, 1995.

Hasso AN, Stringer WA, Brown KD: Cerebral ischemia and infarction, *Neuroimaging Clin North Am* 4:733-752, 1994.

Ida M, Mizunuma K, Hata Y, Tada S: Subcortical low intensity in early cortical ischemia, *AJNR* 15:1387-1393, 1994.

Johnson BA, Heiserman JE, Drayer BP, Keller PJ: Intracranial MR angiography: its role in the integrated approach to brain infarction, *AJNR* 15:667-673, 1994.

Johnson MH, Christman CW: Posterior circulation infarction: anatomy, pathophysiology, and clinical correlation, *Sem U/S, CT, MR* 16:237-252, 1995.

Lang EW, Daffertshofer M, Daffertshofer A, et al: Variability of vascular territory in stroke: pitfalls and failure of stroke pattern interpretation, *Stroke* 26:942-945, 1995.

Mathews VP, Barker PB, Blackband SJ, et al: Cerebral metabolites in patients with acute and subacute strokes: concentrations determined by quantitative proton MR spectroscopy, *AJR* 165:633-638, 1995.

Mehta RC, Pike GB, Haros SP, Enzmann DR: Central nervous system tumor, infection, and infarction: detection with gadolinium-enhanced magnetization transfer MR imaging, *Radiol* 195:41-46, 1995.

Nakano S, Yokogami K, Ohta H, et al: CT-defined large subcortical infarcts: correlation of location with site of cerebrovascular occlusive disease, *AJNR* 16:1581-1586, 1995.

Osborn AG: Stroke. In *Diagnostic neuroradiology,* St Louis, 1994, Mosby, pp 330-398.

Takahashi S, Suzuki M, Matsumoto K, et al: Extent and location of cerebral infarcts on multiplanar MR images: correlation with distribution of perforating arteries on cerebral angiograms and on cadaveric microangiograms, *AJR* 163:1215-1222, 1994.

terPenning B: Pathophysiology of stroke, *Neuroimaging Clin North Am* 2:389-408, 1992.

Toni D, Fiorelli M, Gentile M, et al: Progressing neurological deficit secondary to acute ischemic stroke: a study on predictability, pathogenesis, and prognosis, *Arch Neurol* 52:670-675, 1995.

Warach S, Gaa J, Siewert B, et al: Acute human stroke studied by whole brain echo planar diffusion-weighted magnetic resonance imaging, *Ann Neurol* 37:231-241, 1995.

Weingarten K: Computed tomography of cerebral infarction, *Neuroimaging Clin North Am* 2:409-419, 1992.

You R, McNeil JJ, O'Malley SRN, et al: Risk factors for lacunar infarction syndromes, *Neurol* 45:1483-1487, 1995.

Zanette EM, Roberti C, Mancini G, et al: Spontaneous middle cerebral artery reperfusion in ischemic stroke. A follow-up study with transcranial Doppler, *Stroke* 26:430-433, 1995.

38

Atherosclerosis

Key Concepts

1. Atherosclerosis is the most common cause of craniocervical vessel stenosis.
2. Atherosclerosis and its complications account for over 90% of cerebral thromboembolic events.
3. Modified "response-to-injury" pathogenesis of atherosclerosis.
   a. Endothelial injury is initiating event.
   b. Fatty streaks are earliest visible lesions.
   c. Fatty streak is converted into fibrotic cap composed of smooth-muscle cells, connective tissue, "foam" cells (transformed smooth-muscle cells, macrophages).
   d. Focal loss of endothelial cells over cap.
   e. Advanced lesion is complex (plaque ulceration, hemorrhage, with platelet aggregation).

Diseases of the heart and blood vessels cause nearly 50% of deaths in the United States. Most of these deaths can be attributed to atherosclerotic vascular disease (ASVD) and its ensuing complications such as thromboembolic stroke. In this chapter we discuss atherosclerosis and its pathogenesis and imaging manifestations. In Chapter 39 we consider the less common, nonatheromatous causes of vascular stenosis and occlusion such as vasculopathy and vasculitis.

  I. Pathophysiology of atherosclerosis.
    A. Etiology and pathogenesis.
      1. Normal arterial endothelium.
        a. Retards development of atherosclerosis.

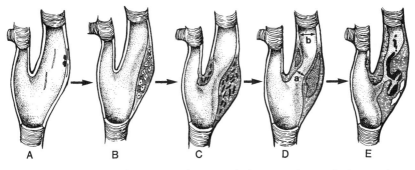

Fig. 38-1   Anatomic diagrams and gross pathology specimens depict craniocerebral atherosclerotic vascular disease (ASVD). **A** to **E,** Development of atherosclerotic plaque at the common carotid artery (CCA) bifurcation and internal carotid artery (ICA) origin is shown schematically. **A,** Intimal fatty streaks are present. Some platelet adhesion to the intima is noted but the carotid artery is otherwise normal. **B,** Monocyte-derived macrophages and smooth-muscle cells proliferate under the intima, becoming lipid-filled foam cells. **C,** Foam cell necrosis produces a thickened plaque with cellular debris and cholesterol crystals. **D,** Intraplaque subintimal hemorrhage occurs, further narrowing the vessel lumen. Stenosis calculation is performed by measuring the narrowest diameter of the diseased artery *(a)* and subtracting from the normal ICA diameter *(b)* distal to the bulb beyond the angiographically recognizable diseased segment. This gives the calculated stenosis diameter. To obtain the percentage stenosis, stenosis is divided by the normal lumen diameter and multiplied by 100. For example, if the normal ICA is 8 mm at *b* and the residual lumen is 2 mm at *a,* the stenosis diameter is 6 mm ($6 \div 8 \times 100 = 75\%$ stenosis). According to the North American Symptomatic Carotid Endarterectomy Trial (NASCET), symptomatic lesions with 70% to 99% stenosis are clinically significant. **E,** Plaque rupture produces intimal ulceration with platelet thrombi that may embolize distally. (Used with permission from Osborn AG: *Diagnostic neuroradiology,* St Louis, 1994, Mosby.)

b. Provides nonthrombogenic surface (inhibits platelet deposition).
c. Provides surface to which monocytes, lymphocytes cannot adhere.
2. Modified "response-to-injury" hypothesis of atherogenesis (Fig. 38-1).
a. Injured endothelium becomes dysfunctional.
b. Inflammatory cells, smooth-muscle cells are recruited to sites of injury.
c. Monocytes are transformed to macrophages, ingest lipoproteins.
d. Fatty streaks are earliest visible atherosclerotic lesions and are initially found at arterial branch points.
e. Fatty streak is converted into fibrotic lesion consisting of smooth-muscle cells (SMCs) that migrate from subendothelium, media to surface of lesion and ingest lipoproteins, becoming foam cells.
f. Foam cells undergo necrosis, forming pools of extracellular cholesterol, calcium.
g. Vasa vasorum vascularize wall of atherosclerotic artery.
h. Fibrotic lesion is eventually converted into advanced, complex lesion.
(1) Superficial plaque ulceration, fracture.
(a) Platelet adhesion, aggregation.
(b) Activation of coagulation cascade.
(c) Thrombus forms, may embolize.
(2) Intraplaque hemorrhage.
(a) Ruptured vasa vasorum.
(b) Release of matrix-degrading enzymes by macrophages.
(3) Luminal narrowing occurs from subintimal hemorrhage.
3. Alternate hypotheses.
a. Immune-mediated response.
b. Herpesvirus-mediated cell transformation.
c. Carcinogens, mutagens.
d. Monoclonal hypothesis (smooth-muscle cells within atherosclerotic lesion are derived from a stable transformed cell population).
B. Location.
1. Most common extracranial site: internal carotid artery (ICA) at/above common carotid bifurcation.
2. Most common intracranial sites: vertebrobasilar system, carotid siphon (paracavernous internal carotid artery).
3. "Tandem" lesions, i.e., distal stenosis, occurs in approximately

2% of patients with hemodynamically significant cervical ICA stenosis.

4. Intracranial ASVD.
   a. Compared with extracranial atherosclerosis, ASVD distal to circle of Willis is relatively uncommon.
      (1) Severe intracranial atherosclerosis present on angiograms in slightly >10% of patients undergoing angiographic assessment of carotid stenosis.
      (2) ASVD is the most common cause of an "arteritis-like" pattern on cerebral angiograms (see below).
   b. May cause thrombosis.
      (1) Occlusions occur at site of greatest luminal compromise or just distal to it.
      (2) Plaque rupture or intraplaque hemorrhage not required for cerebral artery thrombosis.
      (3) Nonocclusive mural thrombi may occur in absence of plaque rupture, eventually leading to local occlusion or distal embolization.

II. Imaging of atherosclerosis.
   A. Noninvasive methods.
      1. Standard sonography.
         a. Duplex scanning with combination of real-time, color Doppler imaging (CDI) is considered most reproducible, complete technique.
         b. Advantages of CDI with spectral analysis compared with standard duplex sonography include better definition of arterial anatomy and enhanced detection of the residual lumen in nearly occluded vessels.
         c. With CDI, the principal method for assessing lumenal narrowing is the measurement of flow velocity elevation in the stenotic portion of the artery.
            (1) Flow velocity increases with increasing stenosis.
            (2) Waveform broadens, flattens with increasing stenosis.
         d. Arterial stenosis is depicted on CDI.
            (1) Flowing blood has frequency shifts, whereas stationary objects do not.
            (2) Directional-dependent color assignment.
               (a) Flow towards probe assigned red.
               (b) Flow away from probe assigned blue.
               (c) Nonlaminar flow shows mixture of color.
               (d) Flow reversal in posterior carotid bulb is normal.
            (3) Color saturation is directly related to flow velocity; velocity is proportional to severity of obstruction, but only *average* velocities are shown. Reliance on spectral

Doppler for quantitative measurements that infer different levels of stenosis is still necessary.

   (a) Elevated flow velocity shifts color (varies with different systems; e.g., from dark red to light pink or from red to yellow to white).

  e. Stenosis determination in symptomatic patients comparable to angiography, with exception of occlusion and mild-to-moderate stenosis (<50%).

2. Transcranial Doppler sonography (TCD).

  a. Delineates anterior, middle, posterior cerebral arteries through temporal window, carotid siphon and ophthalmic artery through transorbital approach.

  b. Demonstrates blood flow velocities, direction.

3. Computed tomography.

  a. NECT scans.

    (1) Calcification.

      (a) Carotid siphon most common site.

      (b) Vertebral arteries next most common.

      (c) Rare in anterior or middle cerebral arteries, basilar artery.

    (2) Ectasia.

      (a) Carotid siphon, basilar artery most common sites.

  b. CECT scans.

    (1) Contrast-filled lumen is narrowed.

    (2) Arterial wall abnormalities.

      (a) Circumferential or eccentric lucent areas represent atherosclerotic plaque with or without subintimal hemorrhage.

      (b) Peripheral enhancement may occur with vasa vasorum proliferation.

  c. CT angiography (CTA).

    (1) Visualization of arterial anatomy using intravenous administration of contrast bolus, timed rapid image acquisition ("spiral") techniques.

    (2) Careful examination of both source images, three-dimensional display is necessary.

    (3) Visualization of extracranial vessels, circle of Willis equivalent to MR angiography.

  d. Spin-echo MR imaging.

    (1) Arterial patency, stenosis may be difficult to assess.

    (2) Intraluminal thrombus may be isointense or hyperintense.

    (3) Presence of normal "flow void" in intracranial vessels does not exclude extracranial stenosis.

(4) In-plane or slow flow can mimic intraluminal thrombi.

  e. MR angiography (MRA).

    (1) Uses differences between moving blood, stationary background tissue.

    (2) Time-of-flight (TOF) MRA.

      (a) Based on flow-related enhancement coupled with suppression of background signal.

      (b) Three-dimensional TOF techniques useful for intracranial vessel delineation, less useful for slow-flow lesions; parenchymal hemorrhage may obscure vessels.

      (c) Two-dimensional TOF techniques useful for extracranial vessel delineation, useful for slow-flow lesions.

    (3) Phase-contrast (PC) MRA.

      (a) Based on phase shifts of moving spins.

      (b) Two-dimensional PC excellent for slow-flow lesions, providing directional information, quantifying flow; will not show hemorrhage.

B. Invasive methods.

  1. Cerebral angiography.

    a. Remains most precise technique for evaluating the cerebral vasculature.

    b. Little agreement between angiography and surgical observation in detecting carotid plaque ulceration.

    c. Stenosis determination (Fig. 38-2).

      (1) North American Symptomatic Carotid Endarterectomy Trial (NASCET) method.

        (a) Two views (AP, lateral).

        (b) Luminal diameter of maximal stenosis is compared with diameter at normal part of internal carotid artery beyond bulb.

        (c) Greatest value for percent diameter stenosis from the two views is used.

        (d) NASCET showed surgical benefit in symptomatic patients with >70% stenosis.

        (e) Asymptomatic Carotic Atherosclerosis Study (ACAS) showed surgical benefit in asymptomatic patients with 60% or greater stenosis.

        (f) No surgical benefit for stenosis <30%.

        (g) Ongoing trial is evaluating data in mild-moderate cases (30% to 60% stenosis).

      (2) European Carotid Surgery Trial (ECST) method.

        (a) Smallest diameter of residual lumen is compared

PERCENT STENOSIS

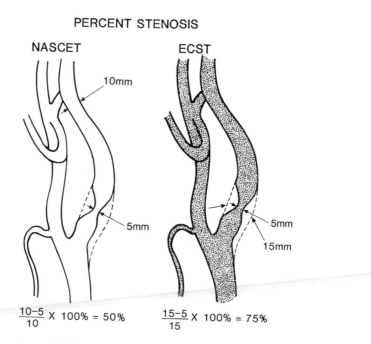

Fig. 38-2   Anatomic diagram compares NASCET (North American Symptomatic Carotid Endarterectomy Trial) and ECST (European Carotid Surgery Trial) stenosis calculations. NASCET calculations compare the point of maximum stenosis with the nonstenotic distal internal carotid artery. ECST calculations compare the stenosis with the estimated diameter of the carotid artery at the level of the stenosis. Therefore, with a 5 mm residual lumen and normal 10 mm distal ICA diameter, NASCET calculation results in 50% stenosis. The ECST calculation, given a projected normal diameter of 15 mm at the site of stenosis, yields a 75% stenosis.

with that of estimated original vessel at same site.

(b) Requires extrapolation of natural convex curvature of carotid bulb.

(c) Seems to correlate better with visual observations of stenosis at surgery.

(d) ECST calculations give higher percentage stenosis compared with NASCET.

(3) Carotid stenosis index (CSI) estimates bulb dimensions using diameter of the common carotid artery, then calculates stenosis similarly to ECST. Consensus may be emerging to use CSI method.

d. Plaque morphology.

(1) NASCET showed that presence of plaque ulceration in conjunction with stenosis significantly increases stroke risk in patients with 70% to 99% stenosis who are treated medically.

    (2) Significance of intraplaque hemorrhage as predictor of ischemic symptoms is unclear.

    (3) Little agreement exists between angiography and surgical observation in detecting carotid plaque ulceration.

III. Collateral circulation.

  A. Adequacy extremely important in event of hemodynamically significant vessel stenosis or occlusion.

  B. Major potential pathways.

    1. Extracranial to intracranial.

      a. External carotid artery (ECA).

        (1) Angular branch of facial artery to ophthalmic artery to intracranial ICA.

        (2) Internal maxillary branches to lateral mainstem branch of cavernous ICA.

        (3) Ascending pharyngeal artery to odontoid branches of vertebral artery (VA).

        (4) Occipital artery to cervical branches of VA.

        (5) Transosseous branches to leptomeningeal ICA branches.

      b. Vertebral artery.

        (1) Contralateral VA to basilar artery to occluded VA ("subclavian steal syndrome").

    2. Intracranial anastomoses.

      a. Circle of Willis.

        (1) Only 25% of cases have "complete" or "balanced" circle of Willis.

        (2) Communicating arteries often hypoplastic or absent.

        (3) Horizontal anterior cerebral artery (A1) segment often hypoplastic/absent; both ACAs fill from same carotid artery.

      b. Pial collaterals.

        (1) Across so-called vascular watershed or border zone.

        (2) Between anterior and middle, middle and posterior, and posterior and anterior cerebral arteries.

      c. Microvasculature collaterals.

        (1) Interdigitating supply between vessels in subcortical white matter, external capsule.

        (2) Cortex has short arterioles from single source.

        (3) Basal ganglia have large, long, single penetrating vessels that have few collaterals and are thus vulnerable sites for atherosclerosis and hypoxic injury.

SUGGESTED READINGS

Anzola GP, Gasparotti R, Magoni M, Prandini F: Transcranial Doppler sonography and magnetic resonance angiography in the assessment of collateral hemispheric flow in patients with carotid artery disease, *Stroke* 26:214-217, 1995.

Aoki S, Shirouzu I, Sasaki Y, et al: Enhancement of the intracranial arterial wall at MR imaging: relationship to cerebral atherosclerosis, *Radiology* 194:477-481, 1995.

Barnett HJM, Eliasziw M, Meldrum HE: The identification by imaging methods of patients who might benefit from carotid endarterectomy, *Arch Neurol* 52:827-831, 1995.

Berman SS, Devine JJ, Erdoes LS, Hunter GC: Distinguishing carotid artery pseudo-occlusion with Color-flow Doppler, *Stroke* 26:434-438, 1995.

Consigny PM: Advances in clinical medicine: pathogenesis of atherosclerosis, *AJR* 164:553-558, 1995.

de Bray JM, Galland F, Lhoste P, et al: Colour Doppler and duplex sonography and angiography of the carotid artery bifurcations, *Neuroradiol* 37:219-224, 1995.

Fox AJ: Update on NASCET. *Core Curriculum in Neuroradiology, part I: Vascular Lesions and Degenerative Disease*, Chicago, 1995, American Society of Neuroradiology, pp 121-122.

Griffiths PD, Worthy S, Gholkar A: Incidental intracranial vascular pathology in patients investigated for carotid stenosis [Abstract], *Neuroradiol* 37:167-168, 1995.

Heiserman JE: The evaluation of carotid arteriosclerosis. In *Core curriculum in neuroradiology, part I: vascular lesions and degenerative disease*, Chicago, 1995, American Society of Neuroradiology, pp 99-104.

Hu H-H, Luo C-L, Sheng W-Y, et al: Transorbital color Doppler flow imaging of the carotid siphon and major arteries at the base of the brain, *AJNR* 16:591-598, 1995.

Katz DA, Marks MP, Napel SA, et al: Circle of Willis: evaluation with spiral CT angiography, MR angiography, and conventional angiography, *Radiol* 195:445-449, 1995.

Loftus CM, Quest DO: Technical issues in carotid artery surgery 1995, *Neurosurg* 36:629-647, 1995.

Ogata J, Masuda J, Yutani C, Yamaguchi T: Mechanisms of cerebral artery thrombosis: a histopathological analysis on eight necropsy cases, *J Neurol Neurosurg Psychiatr* 57:17-21, 1994.

Savy LE, Moseley IF: The incidence of intracranial arterial calcification and ectasia [Abstract], *Neuroradiol* 37:167-168, 1995.

Srinivasan J, Mayberg MR, Weiss DG, Eskridge J: Duplex accuracy compared with angiography in the Veterans Affairs Cooperative Studies Trial for Symptomatic Carotid Stenosis, *Neurosurg* 36:648-655, 1995.

Stock KW, Radue EW, Jacob AL, et al: Intracranial arteries: prospective blinded comparative study of MR angiography and DSA in 50 patients, *Radiol* 195:451-456, 1995.

Streifler JY, Eliasziw M, Fox AJ, et al: Angiographic detection of carotid plaque ulceration, *Stroke* 25:1130-1132, 1994.

Vanninen RV, Manninen HI, Koivisto K, et al: Carotid stenosis by digital subtraction angiography: reproducibility of the European Carotid Surgery Trial and the North American Symptomatic Carotid Endarterectomy Trial measurement methods and visual interpretation, *AJNR* 15:1635-1641, 1994.

Vanninen RL, Manninen HI, Partanen PLK, et al: Carotid artery stenosis: clinical efficacy of MR phase-contrast flow quantification as an adjunct to MR angiography, *Radiol* 194:459-467, 1995.

39

Nonatheromatous Causes of Arterial Stenosis and Occlusion

Key Concepts

1. Common nonatheromatous causes of arterial narrowing.
   a. Congenital hypoplasia (e.g., horizontal or A1 anterior cerebral artery segment).
   b. Dissection (traumatic or spontaneous).
   c. Vasospasm (e.g., with subarachnoid hemorrhage).
   d. Vasculopathy (e.g., fibromuscular dysplasia).
   e. Tumor encasement (e.g., nasopharyngeal squamous cell carcinoma).
2. Uncommon nonatheromatous causes of arterial stenosis.
   a. Neurocutaneous syndrome (NF 1 most common).
   b. Idiopathic progressive arteriopathy of childhood (moyamoya).
   c. Sickle cell disease.
   d. Vasculitis.
3. Approximately 3% of cerebral infarcts occur in young individuals.
4. Common causes of stroke in children, young adults.
   a. Dissection.
   b. Moyamoya syndrome.
   c. Migraine.
   d. Cardiac pathology (congenital lesion with cerebral thromboembolism, acquired disease such as endocarditis).
   e. Drug abuse.

Atherosclerosis is by far the most common cause of craniocervical arterial narrowing and occlusion in middle-aged and older adults (see Chapter 38). In this chapter we consider both the congenital and acquired nonatheromatous causes of arterial narrowing (box). The diverse causes of arterial ischemia and infarction among adolescents and young adults are also considered here; sinovenous occlusive disease is considered in Chapter 40.

  I. Congenital causes of nonatheromatous arterial narrowing.
    A. Aplasia/hypoplasia.
      1. Common sites.
        a. Horizontal (A1) segment, anterior cerebral artery (ACA).
        b. Horizontal (P1) segment, posterior cerebral artery (PCA).
        c. Vertebral artery.
          (1) With normal origin (may terminate in posterior inferior cerebellar artery).
          (2) With aberrant origin (from aortic arch).

Nonatherosclerotic Arterial Stenoses

Dissection
  Traumatic
  Spontaneous (no underlying vasculopathy)
  Underlying vasculopathy (e.g., FMD)
Vasospasm
  Chemical (SAH)
  Mechanical
  Infection
  Migraine
Vasculopathy
  FMD
  Radiation
  Compression (osteophyte, trauma, tumor)
  Flow-related degenerative changes (AVM/AVF/venous angioma)
Vasculitis
  Infection
  Primary angiitis of the CNS
  SLE and other collagen-vascular diseases
  Giant cell arteritides (temporal, Takayasu arteritis)
  Granulomatous angiitis
  Sarcoid
  Drug-induced vasculitis (cocaine, amphetamine, phenylpropanolamine, ginseng)

2. Rare sites.
   a. Extracranial internal carotid artery (ICA).
     (1) Absent bony carotid canal.
   b. Horizontal (M1) segment, middle cerebral artery (MCA).
B. Neurocutaneous syndromes.
  1. Neurofibromatosis type 1 (NF-1).
   a. Most common neurocutaneous syndrome associated with vascular abnormalities.
   b. Causes extracranial vascular stenoses (e.g., renal artery, celiac trunk).
   c. Uncommonly affects cerebral vasculature.
   d. May cause progressive basal arterial stenoses (with moya-moya pattern of collateral blood flow).
  2. Tuberous sclerosis.
   a. Rare cause of vascular abnormality.
   b. Aneurysms, ectasias of extracranial vessels.
   c. Progressive stenosis of internal carotid artery has been reported.
C. Idiopathic progressive arteriopathy of childhood (moyamoya is the Japanese term that means puff of smoke and was originally used to describe the whiff of contrast in the basal collateral vascular channels seen during fluoroscopy for cerebral angiography).
  1. Pathology, etiology.
   a. Unknown etiology.
   b. Relentless, progressive thickening of walls of intracranial arteries.
   c. Multiple infarcts, brain atrophy.
  2. Location.
   a. Typically involves distal ICA, basilar artery, ACA, PCA, MCA.
   b. Prominent parenchymal (lenticulostriate, thalamoperforating arteries), leptomeningeal, dural collateral vessels develop.
  3. Note: Moyamoya is not a disease; the term represents the striking pattern of collateral circulation that can be seen with any slowly progressive occlusive arteriopathy (atherosclerosis, radiation arteritis, sickle-cell disease).
D. Sickle cell disease (SCD).
  1. Stroke complicates approximately 5% to 15% of patients with SCD.
  2. Most common pattern of vasculopathy is progressive occlusion of supraclinoid carotid, proximal ACA, MCA.
  3. Moyamoya type of collateral circulation may develop.

II. Acquired causes of arterial narrowing, occlusion.
   A. Dissection.
      1. Etiology.
         a. Spontaneous.
         b. Trauma.
         c. Underlying vasculopathy (e.g., fibromuscular dysplasia).
         d. Other predisposing conditions.
            (1) Migraine headache.
            (2) Hypertension.
            (3) Oral contraceptives.
            (4) Drug abuse.
      2. Clinical manifestations.
         a. Can be asymptomatic.
         b. Neck, posterior occipital pain.
         c. Headache.
         d. Postganglionic Horner syndrome.
         e. Stroke (manifestations can be delayed for days up to 2 or 3 weeks).
      3. Location.
         a. Extracranial (common).
            (1) ICA, between bulb and skull base.
            (2) Vertebral artery between C1-C2, C1 and skull base.
         b. Intracranial (rare).
            (1) Supraclinoid ICA.
            (2) Circle of Willis.
      4. Pathology.
         a. Intramural hematoma splits media; often occurs under intima or adventitia.
         b. If aneurysmal dilatation occurs, dissecting aneurysm is formed (see Chapter 22).
      5. Imaging.
         a. U/S.
            (1) Occlusion.
               (a) Absent flow in internal carotid artery.
               (b) Spares bulb, shows lack of atherosclerosis.
               (c) Biphasic (stump) flow in bulb.
               (d) High-resistance flow in ipsilateral common carotid artery.
               (e) Collateral flow across circle of Willis.
               (f) Low flow in middle cerebral artery.
            (2) Stenosis.
               (a) Tapered ICA lumen.
               (b) Membrane crossing, dividing lumen into false and true segments.

           (c) Spares bulb, shows lack of atherosclerotic changes.

    b. Cerebral angiography.

       (1) Irregular or tapered vessel lumen.

       (2) May be occluded.

       (3) Intimal tear may permit contrast to penetrate wall (false lumen).

    c. CT.

       (1) May be normal.

       (2) CT angiography shows narrowed vessel.

       (3) Complications.

          (a) Cerebral ischemia, infarction.

          (b) Cranial nerve palsies.

    d. MR.

       (1) Subacute intramural hematoma (hyperintense on T1WI).

       (2) Reduced or absent flow void.

       (3) MRA shows focal or long segment arterial stenosis.

B. Vasospasm.

  1. Etiology.

    a. Chemical.

       (1) Intrathecal (subarachnoid) hemorrhage.

       (2) Ergot derivatives.

       (3) Eicosanoids (e.g., in preeclampsia/eclampsia).

    b. Mechanical.

       (1) Penetrating or blunt trauma.

       (2) Catheter spasm during angiography.

       (3) Distal flow reduction (e.g., massively increased intracranial pressure).

    c. Migraine headache.

  2. Imaging.

    a. Transcranial doppler U/S.

       (1) Increased vascular resistance.

    b. Cerebral angiography.

       (1) Segmental vessel narrowing.

C. Vasculopathy.

  1. Fibromuscular dysplasia (FMD).

    a. Unknown etiology.

    b. Intimal or medial proliferative changes.

    c. Location.

       (1) 75% cervical ICA (between bulb, skull base).

       (2) 25% cervical VA (C2-C3 level).

    d. Imaging studies show string-of-beads or long segment narrowing.

    e. Increased prevalence of intracranial aneurysm, embolic stroke.

    2. Flow-related vasculopathy.
      a. Intimal thickening, degenerative changes in vessel wall.
      b. Most commonly seen in afferent arteries to AVM, AVFs.
      c. Occasionally causes efferent (outflow) stenosis in veins that drain AVM, venous angioma.
    3. Radiation vasculopathy.
      a. Rare, late complication of radiation therapy for intracranial, head and neck neoplasms.
      b. Pathology.
        (1) Accelerated atherosclerotic changes.
        (2) Internal elastic lamina, endothelial degenerative changes with progressive stenosis.
        (3) Intraluminal thrombi.
        (4) Mineralizing microangiopathy (cerebral white matter).
        (5) Angiomatous changes may resemble cavernous angiomas and capillary telangiectasias with multifocal petechial hemorrhages.
      c. Imaging.
        (1) Progressive arterial stenoses.
        (2) Moyamoya pattern of collateral circulation may develop.
        (3) Calcifying (mineralizing) changes in cerebral white matter.
        (4) White matter gliosis, necrosis.
        (5) Multifocal hemorrhages.
    4. Compressive vasculopathy.
      a. Trauma.
        (1) Cervical fracture-subluxation.
          (a) Foramen transversarium fracture with VA laceration or dissection.
          (b) Extrinsic compression secondary to rotational subluxation.
        (2) Skull base fracture.
          (a) Carotid canal.
        (3) Paravascular hematoma (if cavitates and communicates with vessel lumen, may form pseudoaneurysm).
      b. Degenerative spine disorders.
        (1) Osteophyte.
      c. Neoplasm.
        (1) Squamous cell carcinoma.
        (2) Pituitary adenoma.
        (3) Meningioma.

D. Vasculitis.
  1. General pathology, etiology.
    a. Inflammation, necrosis of blood vessels.
    b. Alternating areas of stenosis, dilatation.
    c. May cause thrombosis, abnormalities in adjacent brain parenchyma.
    d. Variety of causes (see box on p. 396).
  2. Infectious vasculitides.
    a. Tuberculous arteritis (TB).
      (1) Usually secondary to TB meningitis.
      (2) Typically affects vessels at base of brain.
      (3) Imaging studies show multifocal areas of narrowing.
      (4) Complications include occlusion with cerebral ischemia, infarction.
    b. Fungal vasculitis.
      (1) Angioinvasive fungus (e.g., aspergillus, mucor).
      (2) Multifocal occlusions with hemorrhagic infarcts are characteristic.
  3. Noninfectious vasculitides: immune complex diseases.
    a. Primary angiitis of the central nervous system (PACNS and its variants).
      (1) Idiopathic granulomatous arteritis.
      (2) Most commonly affects small to medium-sized arteries of brain.
      (3) Nonspecific angiographic findings (multiple segmental narrowings, less often "beaded" vessel).
    b. Polyarteritis nodosa (PAN).
      (1) Most common systemic necrotizing vasculitis with CNS manifestations.
      (2) Primarily involves small, medium-sized vessels.
      (3) Predilection for arterial bifurcations with propensity to form microaneurysms.
      (4) Less often causes segmental stenoses, thrombosis.
    c. Systemic lupus erythematosus (SLE).
      (1) Multisystem disease.
      (2) CNS involvement in 50%.
      (3) Focal cerebral infarcts can result from cardiac emboli, coagulopathy, antiphospholipid antibody syndrome.
      (4) Lupus "vasculitis" is uncommon.
        (a) Multifocal cortical, subcortical areas of increased signal on T2WI.
        (b) May enhance following contrast administration.

4. Noninfectious vasculitides: cell-mediated disorders.
   a. Temporal arteritis.
      (1) Form of giant cell arteritis.
      (2) Panarteritis characterized by mononuclear cell infil-
          trates, giant cells in vessel walls.
      (3) 95% are over age 50.
      (4) Classic presentation is headache, fever, anemia, elevated
          sedimentation rate, polymyalgia rheumatica syndrome.
      (5) Predilection for branches of the carotid artery, especially
          superficial temporal branch.
      (6) May involve ophthalmic artery, cause blindness.
      (7) Cerebral angiography shows nonspecific segmental ste-
          noses.
   b. Takayasu arteritis.
      (1) Another form of giant cell arteritis.
      (2) High prevalence in young women, Asians.
      (3) Affects aortic arch, great vessels, and major branches
          (carotid artery is most common site).
          (a) Most common manifestation is symmetric long-
              segment stenosis.
          (b) May eventually occlude vessels.
          (c) Rarely, ectasia or aneurysmal dilatations are iden-
              tified.
   c. Other vasculitides.
      (1) Granulomatous angiitis.
      (2) Sarcoidosis.
      (3) Wegener granulomatosis.
      (4) Drug-induced, chemical vasculitis.
          (a) Reported with cocaine, sympathomimetics (amphet-
              amines, phenylpropanolamine), ginseng.
      (5) Behcet disease.
          (a) Oral ulcers, genital ulcers, ocular inflammation (two
              of these three features).
          (b) CNS disease (neuro-Behcet) in 10% to 25% of cases.
          (c) Ocular involvement in 70% to 85%.
          (d) Vasculitis (arterial occlusions, thromboses, aneu-
              rysms, venous occlusions)
          (e) Predilection for brainstem, diencephalon.
      (6) Lymphomatoid granulomatosis.
III. Ischemic stroke in children, young adults <40 years of age (see box
     on p. 403).
   A. Undetermined cause 35%.
   B. Atherosclerosis (large artery disease) 10%.

Causes of Stroke in Children, Young Adults

Cardioembolism
Dissection
Trauma
Migraine headache
Drug abuse
Pregnancy and its complications
Hematologic disorder
Collagen-vascular disease (e.g., SLE, APLA syndrome)
Vasculopathy (e.g., FMD)
Atherosclerosis

    C. Cardioembolism 18%.
       1. Paradoxic embolism.
       2. Prosthetic valve.
       3. Rheumatic heart disease.
       4. Cardiomyopathy.
       5. Infective endocarditis.
    D. Miscellaneous causes of stroke in young patients 30%.
       1. Dissection.
       2. Idiopathic progressive arteriopathy of childhood.
       3. Migraine.
       4. Drug, alcohol abuse.
       5. Collagen-vascular disorder.
          a. SLE.
          b. Antiphospholipid antibody syndrome (APLA).
       6. Trauma.
       7. Vasculitis.
       8. Fibromuscular dysplasia.
       9. Pregnancy and its complications.
      10. Hematologic disorder.
          a. Clotting factor abnormalities.
          b. Hypercoagulability syndromes.

SUGGESTED READINGS

Adams HP Jr, Kappelle LJ, Biller J, et al: Ischemic stroke in young adults, *Arch Neurol* 52:491-495, 1995.

Bitzer M, Topka H: Progressive cerebral occlusive disease after radiation therapy, *Stroke* 26:131-136, 1995.

Ehsan T, Hasan S, Powers JM, Heiserman JE: Serial magnetic resonance imaging in isolated angiitis of the central nervous system, *Neurol* 45:1462-1465, 1995.

Harris KG, Yuh WTC: Intracranial vasculitis. *Neuroimaging Clinics North Am* 4:773-797, 1994.

Ito T, Sakai T, Inagawa S, et al: MR angiography of cerebral vasospasm in preeclampsia, *AJNR* 16:1344-1346, 1995.

Osborn AG: Nonatheromatous causes of arterial narrowing and occlusion. In *Diagnostic neuroradiology,* St Louis, 1994, Mosby, pp 369-384.

Ozdemir H, Atilla H, Atilla S, et al: Diagnosis of ocular involvement in Behcet's disease, *AJR* 164:1223-1227, 1995.

Perler BA: Hypercoagulability and the hypercoagulability syndromes, *AJR* 164:559-564, 1995.

Ryu S-J, Chien Y-Y: Ginseng-associated cerebral arteritis, *Neurol* 45:829-830, 1995.

Sturzenegger M, Mattle HP, Rivoir A, Baumgartner RW: Ultrasound findings in carotid artery dissection, *Neurol* 45:691-698, 1995.

Yamada I, Suzuki S, Matsushima Y: Moyamoya disease: Comparison of assessment with MR angiography and MR imaging versus conventional angiography, *Radiol* 196:211-218, 1995.

40

Venous Occlusions

Key Concepts

1. Venous sinus occlusive disease (VSOD) is a diagnostically elusive, potentially lethal lesion that often has a confusing clinical presentation.
2. Common conditions that predispose to VSOD include:
   a. Infection.
   b. Dehydration.
   c. Drugs (including oral contraceptives).
   d. Pregnancy and its complications.
   e. Coagulopathy.
   f. Tumor, trauma.
3. The superior sagittal sinus is the most commonly thrombosed dural venous sinus.
4. Differences between VSOD and arterial occlusive disease.
   a. Absence of abnormal arterial, parenchymal enhancement is typical in VSOD.
   b. Brain swelling may be persistent and is often greater than associated area of signal abnormality.
   c. Signal abnormalities in VSOD do not follow arterial distribution.
   d. Hemorrhage is more common in VSOD than in typical thromboembolic arterial infarct.
5. Deep cerebral vein thrombosis is a rare but important cause of bithalamic low-density/low-signal intensity.
6. Venous collagenosis may cause nonthrombotic stenosis and occlusion of periventricular veins and be responsible for deep white matter disease in elderly patients.

Venous disease plays an increasingly well-recognized role in many CNS disorders. The potential role of venous mechanisms in benign intracranial hypertension, hydrocephalus, dural sinus occlusion and venous infarction, hemorrhage in vascular malformations, and deep white matter disease in the elderly has been emphasized by numerous authors. In this chapter we focus on dural sinus occlusion, superficial cortical and deep vein occlusions, venous infarcts, and the possible role of periventricular venous occlusion in the development of deep white matter disease.

I. Dural sinus and cortical venous occlusive disease.
  A. Dural sinus thrombosis.
    1. Pathology.
      a. Thrombus forms in dural sinus.
      b. May progress to involve tributary superficial cortical veins.
      c. Venous infarction often ensues.
    2. Etiology and predisposing conditions.
      a. Common causes of venous sinus occlusion (box).
      (1) Pregnancy and delivery.

Dural Sinus/Cerebral Venous Occlusions: Predisposing Conditions

Common
    Pregnancy, postpartum state
    Infection
        Focal (mastoiditis, sinusitis)
        Systemic
    Dehydration
    Coagulopathy, blood dyscrasia
    Mechanical disruption
        Trauma
        Tumor
    Drugs
        Oral contraceptives
        Drug abuse
Uncommon
    Inflammatory bowel disorder
        Chron's disease
        Ulcerative colitis
    Vasculitis
        Behçet disease
    Systemic lupus erythematosus
    Primary antiphospholipid syndrome
    Malignancy
        Paraneoplastic syndrome

(2) Infection.
    (a) Paranasal sinuses.
    (b) Middle ear or mastoid.
    (c) Systemic infection.
(3) Dehydration.
(4) Drugs.
    (a) Oral contraceptives.
    (b) Drug abuse.
(5) Coagulopathy, blood dyscrasia.
(6) Neoplasm.
    (a) Meningioma.
    (b) Metastasis.
    (c) Paraneoplastic syndrome.
(7) Trauma.
b. Uncommon causes of sinovenous occlusive disease.
    (1) Inflammatory bowel disease.
        (a) Crohn's disease.
        (b) Ulcerative colitis.
    (2) Behçet disease.
    (3) Systemic lupus erythematosus (SLE).
    (4) Primary antiphospholipid syndrome.
3. Clinical presentation (correlation with outcome, imaging findings).
    a. Stage I.
        (1) Mild signs, symptoms.
            (a) Headache.
            (b) Papilledema.
            (c) Normal mentation.
        (2) Imaging.
            (a) "Delta sign" on CECT (see below).
            (b) No parenchymal change.
        (3) Outcome generally good.
    b. Stage II.
        (1) Moderate signs.
            (a) Very drowsy.
            (b) Poor mentation.
        (2) Additional imaging findings.
            (a) Moderate brain swelling with sulcal effacement and mass effect.
            (b) Dural sinus pressures mildly elevated (20 to 25 mm Hg).
            (c) Hemorrhage generally absent.
        (3) Outcome good with thrombolysis.
    c. Stage III.

(1) Obtunded or semicomatose, may have seizure.

(2) Dural sinus pressures moderately elevated (30 to 40 mm Hg), but hemorrhage generally absent.

(3) Outcome good with thrombolysis.

   d. Stage IV.

(1) Comatose, hemiparesis; may have seizure.

(2) Imaging.

     (a) Severe edema with or without parenchymal hemorrhage.

     (b) Dural sinus pressures up to 50 mm Hg.

(3) Outcome variable.

   e. Stage V.

(1) Deep coma.

(2) Massive edema, hemorrhage, or both.

(3) Nearly always fatal.

4. Location.

   a. Superior sagittal sinus (SSS) most common site.

   b. Transverse, sigmoid, cavernous sinuses.

5. Imaging.

   a. Cerebral angiography.

(1) Absent filling of sinus.

(2) Prominent collateral channels in adjacent dura, brain.

   b. Sonography.

(1) Absence of flow in affected sinus.

(2) Flow in adjacent cortical veins, collateral channels can sometimes be identified.

(3) Differentiation between very slow flow, occlusion can be difficult; some authors suggest gentle compression and release of jugular veins (e.g., in infants with veno-arterial extracorporeal membrane oxygenation therapy ECMO—and suspected dural sinus occlusion).

   c. NECT.

(1) Hyperdense venous sinus (caution: dural sinuses are normally slightly hyperdense compared to brain).

(2) Hyperdense falx ("falx sign") (caution: dura is normally slightly hyperdense compared to brain).

(3) Patchy cortical, subcortical hemorrhages (venous infarcts).

(4) Variable cerebral edema.

     (a) Sulcal effacement.

     (b) Mass effect.

     (c) Small ventricles.

(5) Differential diagnosis and mimics of dural sinus occlusion.

        (a) Normal flowing blood in dural sinus.

        (b) Unmyelinated brain in neonate makes sinuses appear unusually dense.

        (c) High-splitting tentorium.

d. CECT.

  (1) "Empty delta sign."

        (a) Nonenhancing clot is surrounded by enhancing dura.

        (b) Seen in <50% of dural sinus occlusions.

        (c) Subarachnoid, subdural blood along tentorium, falx can mimic empty delta sign (NECT scans).

  (2) Thickened, enhancing dura (especially in subacute or chronic thrombosis).

e. MR.

  (1) Normal "flow void" is replaced by intraluminal clot with signal intensity that varies with clot age.

  (2) Acute occlusion.

        (a) Clot is isointense on T1WI, hypointense on T2WI.

        (b) Parenchymal edema, hemorrhage in more severe cases.

        (c) Gradient-refocussed scans show absent or reduced flow.

        (d) Contrast-enhanced T1WI show thrombus as nonenhanced central area of intermediate intensity surrounded by enhanced rim of dura, collateral venous channels.

  (3) Subacute occlusion.

        (a) Clot is hyperintense on both T1WI, T2WI.

  (4) Chronic occlusion.

        (a) Clot is isointense on T1WI, hyperintense on T2WI.

        (b) Fibrotic clot typically enhances.

        (c) Thickened, enhancing dura may surround nonenhancing clot in very long-standing cases.

        (d) Partial recanalization may cause inhomogeneous signal.

        (e) Brain swelling can persist up to 2 years with or without abnormal signal on T2WI.

  (5) Problems in MR imaging of sinus thrombosis.

        (a) Normal high signal from entry phenomenon on T1WI can mimic subacute thrombus.

        (b) Even-echo rephasing artifacts.

        (c) Flow-compensation techniques can cause high signal in venous sinuses.

        (d) Deoxyhemoglobin of acute thrombus may mimic flow void on T2WI.

(6) Solutions in MR imaging of sinus thrombosis.
   (a) Use asymmetric first, second echo T2WI.
   (b) Turn off gradient moment nulling (gradient moment refocusing, flow compensation).
   (c) Include a blood flow sequence ("MR venography").
   (d) Use inferior saturation band to reduce effects of arterial signal.
   (e) Use orthogonal planes (e.g., with suspected SSS occlusion, use both sagittal and coronal planes).

f. MR angiography.
   (1) Procedure of choice for diagnostic evaluation, follow-up of VSOD.
   (2) Recommended techniques include oblique or coronal two-dimensional TOF MRA, sagittal 2D PC MRA.
   (3) Pitfalls and mimics (see above).
      (a) On three-dimensional TOF sequences, subacute thrombus can mimic flow (appears high signal on gradient-echo scans but generally does not acquire the very high signal intensity seen with true flow).
      (b) Signal loss in areas of flow that course parallel to imaging plane.
      (c) Incorrect placement of saturation bands.
      (d) Incorrect selection of velocity-encoding (VENC) gradient in PC MRA.

B. Cortical vein occlusion.
1. Location.
   a. Usually seen in presence of VSOD and occurs in adjacent brain.
   b. Isolated cortical vein thrombus can cause focal peripheral (cortical/subcortical) hematoma.
2. Imaging.
   a. Cerebral angiography.
      (1) Persistent collection of cordlike contrast.
      (2) Slow filling, emptying (veins appear to "hang in space").
      (3) Intraluminal thrombi sometimes seen as filling defects, menisci.
      (4) Adjacent dural sinus is typically occluded.
      (5) Collateral flow through enlarged deep medullary veins is common.
   b. NECT.
      (1) "Cord sign" (tubular high density collection).
      (2) May cause focal parenchymal hematoma.
   c. CECT.

              (1) Adjacent sinus may demonstrate "empty delta" sign.

              (2) Parenchymal enhancement is uncommon.

       d. MR/MR angiography.

              (1) Focal cortical/subcortical hematoma may suggest diagnosis.

              (2) Adjacent VSOD is usually present.

C. Deep cerebral vein thrombosis.

  1. Underdiagnosed cause of neurologic deterioration.

  2. Location.

     a. Internal cerebral veins (ICVs).

     b. May extend into vein of Galen, straight sinus.

  3. Imaging.

     a. Cerebral angiography.

        (1) ICVs are not visualized.

        (2) Vein of Galen, straight sinus may fail to opacify.

     b. NECT.

        (1) High density in ICVs ("cord sign").

        (2) Low density in thalami, basal ganglia.

        (3) May cause patchy petechial hemorrhages.

     c. CECT.

        (1) Dilated medullary, subependymal veins may enhance.

        (2) Deep venous infarcts may show patchy enhancement.

     d. MR/MRA.

        (1) Mass effect, signal alterations in thalami, basal ganglia.

           (a) Low intensity on T1WI.

           (b) Patchy hyperintensity on T2WI.

        (2) Variable signal in ICVs.

           (a) Absent "flow void."

           (b) Acute thrombus may be isointense with brain on T1WI.

        (3) MRA shows absent flow in ICVs.

II. Periventricular venous collagenosis and its potential role in the aging brain.

A. Primary nonthrombotic intraparenchymal cerebral venous stenosis.

  1. Pathology.

     a. Collagen deposition in venules thickens walls, narrows lumen.

     b. Collagen "balls" may occlude venules.

     c. Occluded or severely stenotic periventricular venules are associated with deep white matter spongiosis (sometimes called "leukoaraiosis").

     d. Increasing evidence indicates that these deep white matter lesions are not arterial vascular-ischemic in origin.

2. Imaging.
   a. CT.
      (1) Diminished attenuation in deep cerebral white matter.
   b. MR.
      (1) Multifocal patchy or confluent periventricular foci of increased signal intensity on T2WI.

SUGGESTED READINGS

Crawford SC, Digre KB, Palmer CA, Bell DA, Osborn AG: Thrombosis of the deep venous drainage of the brain in adults: analysis of seven cases with review of the literature, *Arch Neurol,* 1995 (in press).

Curé JK, Van Tassel P: Congenital and acquired abnormalities of the dural venous sinuses, *Sem U/S, CT, MRI* 15:520-539, 1994.

Dean LM, Taylor GA: The intracranial venous system in infants: normal and abnormal findings on Duplex and Color Doppler sonography, *AJR* 164:151-156, 1995.

Dormont D, Sag K, Biondi A, et al: Gadolinium-enhanced MR of chronic dural sinus thrombosis, *AJNR* 16:1347-1352, 1995.

Laine FJ: Questions and answers: pulse sequences in superior sagittal sinus thrombosis, *AJR* 164:763, 1995.

Lewin JS, Masaryk TJ, Smith AS, et al: Time-of-flight intracranial MR venography: evaluation of the sequential oblique section technique, *AJNR* 15:1657-1664, 1994.

Moody DM, Brown WR, Challa VR, Anderson RL: Periventricular venous collagenosis: association with leukoaraiosis, *Radiol* 194:469-476, 1995.

Osborn AG: Venous occlusions. In *Diagnostic Neuroradiology,* pp 385-395, St Louis, 1994, Mosby.

Perkin GD: Cerebral venous thrombosis: developments in imaging and treatment, *J Neurol Neurosurg Psychiatr* 59:1-3, 1995.

Provenzale JM, Ortel TL: Anatomic distribution of venous thrombosis in patients with antiphospholipid antibody: imaging findings, *AJR* 165:365-368, 1995.

Streifler JY, Eliasziw M, Benavente OR, et al: Lack of relationship between leukoaraiosis and carotid artery disease, *Arch Neurol* 52:21-24, 1995.

Takahashi S, Higano S, Kurihara N, et al: Contrast-enhanced MR imaging of dural sinus thrombosis: Demonstration of the thrombosis and collateral venous channels, *Clin Radiol* 49:639-644, 1994.

Tsai FY, Wang A-M, Matovich VB, et al: MR staging of acute dural sinus thrombosis: correlation with venous pressure measurements and implications for treatment and prognosis, *AJNR* 16:1021-1029, 1995.

Vogl TJ, Bergman C, Villringer A, et al: Dural sinus thrombosis: value of venous MR angiography for diagnosis and follow-up, *AJR* 162:1191-1198, 1994.

Yuh WTC, Simonson TM, Wang A-M, et al: Venous sinus occlusive disease: MR findings, *AJNR* 15:309-316, 1994.

SECTION VI
Intracranial Infections and Inflammation

41

Congenital and Neonatal Infections

Key Concepts

1. The classic TORCH infections include:
   a. Toxoplasmosis.
   b. Rubella.
   c. Cytomegalovirus (CMV).
   d. Herpes simplex virus (HSV) type 2.
2. CMV infection and toxoplasmosis are the first and second most common TORCH infections, respectively.
3. Transmission can occur through three major routes:
   a. Hematogenous/transplacental (toxoplasmosis, most viruses except HSV type 2).
   b. Ascending cervical infection (most bacteria).
   c. During delivery through birth canal (HSV type 2).
4. Although there is overlap, first-trimester and second-trimester infections usually result in brain malformations, whereas third trimester infections usually result in encephaloclastic lesions.
5. Although the pattern of dystrophic calcification is not entirely specific, CMV calcifications are usually central with predilection for periventricular location, whereas toxoplasmosis calcifications are more widespread with slight predilection for basal ganglia.
6. Herpes simplex virus (HSV) type 2 is responsible for congenital CNS infection, whereas HSV type 1 is responsible for childhood and adult encephalitis.
7. Congenital HIV infection is becoming an increasing cause of morbidity/mortality in pediatric population.
8. Unlike adult HIV infection, superimposed CNS infection or neoplasm is uncommon in congenital HIV infection.

I. General comments.
  A. Congenital and neonatal infections have different sequelae than that of childhood or adult CNS infections.
    1. The immature brain is unable to respond to injury with gliosis; rather the immune response removes damaged cells.
    2. The gestational age of the fetus is the most important factor determining degree of damage. Generally, infections during the first two trimesters result in brain malformations, whereas infections during the last trimester result in destructive lesions. However, there is overlap, and severe encephaloclastic lesions can occur at any gestational stage.
  B. The classic TORCH infections refer to the most commonly implicated organisms including toxoplasmosis, rubella, cytomegalovirus, and herpes simplex virus (HSV) type 2.
  C. Other congenital infections that can involve CNS include HIV, syphilis, varicella, listeriosis, papovavirus, and HSV type 1.
  D. Transmission can occur through three major routes.
    1. Hematogenous/transplacental: toxoplasmosis, most viruses except HSV type 2.
    2. Ascending cervical infection: most bacteria.
    3. During delivery through birth canal: HSV type 2.
II. Cytomegalovirus (CMV).
  A. Organism.
    1. Ubiquitous virus belonging to herpes virus group.
    2. Maternal infection usually due to reactivation of latent virus, although can be via primary gestational infection.
    3. In utero transmission via hematogenous/transplacental route.
  B. Incidence.
    1. Most common cause of congenital CNS infection, 1% to 2% of live births.
    2. Two to three times more frequent than toxoplasmosis (next most common infection).
    3. 50% to 85% of women of childbearing age are seropositive for CMV.
    4. 40% of neonates born to infected mothers are infected.
  C. Pathophysiology.
    1. CNS involvement most common (70%).
      a. Affinity for germinal matrix and/or associated vascular insult results in periventricular tissue necrosis and dystrophic calcification as well as cortical abnormalities.
      b. Associated migrational abnormalities range from lissencephaly to focal cortical dysplasia or heterotopia.

      c. Encephaloclastic lesions include porencephaly and hydranencephaly.

      d. Ocular abnormalities include chorioretinitis, optic atrophy, and microphthalmia.

  2. Extracranial involvement less common (30%).

      a. Cardiac anomalies.

      b. Hepatosplenomegaly.

      c. Anemia, thrombocytopenia.

      d. Inner ear abnormalities.

D. Clinical course.

  1. CMV-infected fetuses often born prematurely.

  2. Severity of CNS disease correlates with time of infection; the earlier the insult the greater the CNS impairment.

  3. 10% of infected neonates are symptomatic at birth (microcephaly, jaundice, hepatosplenomegaly, petechiae); of these, 10% do not survive beyond several months, 90% will show CNS involvement within several years.

  4. 10% to 15% of asymptomatic infected neonates will develop neurologic or developmental abnormalities within first year of life.

  5. Late manifestations include microcephaly, seizures, growth and mental retardation, neuromuscular disorder, visual impairment, sensorineural hearing loss.

  6. CMV may also remain latent with possibility of reactivation at later time, especially if become immunosuppressed.

  7. Diagnosis made by viral isolation from body fluids or positive serum titers of CMV antibodies.

  8. No prevention or treatment currently available.

E. Imaging.

  1. Plain film: microcephaly with eggshell-like periventricular calcifications.

  2. U/S.

      a. Antenatal U/S may demonstrate periventricular echogenicity and architectural distortion due to necrotizing inflammation and/or linear echogenicities in basal ganglia and thalami due to perivascular inflammatory infiltrates.

      b. Microcephaly, ventriculomegaly.

      c. Subependymal and porencephalic cysts may be seen.

      d. Periventricular or parenchymal calcifications seen at or after birth.

  3. CT.

      a. Microcephaly.

    b. Calcifications are typically periventricular, although can also occur in other locations such as basal ganglia.

    c. Variable cerebral and cerebellar atrophy with prominent sulci, ventricular enlargement, and enlarged subarachnoid spaces.

    d. Neuronal migration anomalies frequent (see below).

 4. MRI.

    a. MRI not as sensitive as CT for detection of calcifications, although may occasionally observe small foci of hypointensity on T1 and T2WI.

    b. Migrational abnormalities include lissencephaly, pachygyria, polymicrogyria, focal cortical dysplasia, and heterotopias.

    c. May see delayed myelination.

    d. Generally degree of abnormal findings are greater with early gestational infection:

      (1) First-trimester infection: lissencephaly, marked ventriculomegaly, cerebellar hypoplasia, delayed myelination, and significant periventricular calcification.

      (2) Second-trimester infection: polymicrogyria or focal cortical dysplasia, moderate ventricular dilatation, variable cerebellar hypoplasia, and moderate calcification.

      (3) Third-trimester infection: normal gyral pattern, mild ventricular or sulcal prominence, scattered periventricular calcification.

III. Toxoplasmosis.

 A. Organism.

   1. Toxoplasma gondii is ubiquitous protozoan parasite; up to 70% of general population are seropositive.

   2. Maternal infection usually due to ingestion of poorly cooked meat containing tissue cysts or by direct/indirect exposure to oocysts in cat feces.

   3. Congenital transmission is hematogenous/transplacental and occurs only if mother acquires organism during pregnancy.

   4. Frequency of transmission greater during later stages of gestation, although severity of disease greater if infected during earlier stages of gestation (prior to 26 to 30 weeks).

 B. Incidence.

   1. Second only to CMV in causing congenital CNS infections; 1 in 1000 to 1 in 3500 live births, and up to 1% of pregnancies (including stillbirths).

   2. 35% of neonates born to women infected during pregnancy are infected.

C. Pathophysiology.
  1. CNS.
      a. Severity of disease generally greater with earlier gestational age.
      b. Calcifications occur in basal ganglia, periventricular, peripheral locations. Unlike CMV, involvement is more widespread and does not have predilection for periventricular areas.
      c. Hydrocephalus results from ependymitis and periaqueductal necrosis occluding aqueduct.
      d. Unlike CMV, usually not associated with migrational anomalies.
      e. Ocular involvement such as chorioretinitis common.
  2. Extracranial.
      a. Anemia, thrombocytopenia.
      b. Hepatosplenomegaly.
      c. Pneumonitis.
      d. Maculopapular rash.
D. Clinical course.
  1. Recent/acute maternal infection usually subclinical, diagnosed by serum specific antibodies.
  2. Congenital infection diagnosed by viral isolation from placenta, cord blood or CSF; or analysis of specific antibodies in cord or neonatal sera.
  3. Majority of infected infants are asymptomatic (70% at birth) or only have chorioretinitis (10%); although later tend to manifest mental retardation, spasticity, or seizures.
  4. 20% have generalized CNS and systemic disease at birth; fulminating course may result in death within days to months.
  5. Overall mortality up to 15%.
  6. Pyrimethamine and sulfadiazine used to treat infants. If diagnosed in utero, treatment is limited as pyrimethamine is potentially teratogenic in first trimester.
E. Imaging.
  1. Plain film: microcephaly, scattered calcifications.
  2. U/S.
      a. Microcephaly, ventriculomegaly.
      b. Scattered punctate calcifications with slight predilection for basal ganglia.
      c. May see multicystic encephalomalacia, porencephaly, or hydranencephaly.
  3. CT.
      a. Microcephaly.

b. Variable hydrocephalus with obstruction at level of aqueduct.

c. Multifocal diffusely scattered calcifications common in basal ganglia and cortex, although can occur anywhere.

4. MRI.

a. No migrational anomalies, although may see porencephaly or hydranencephaly.

b. Severity of findings generally greater with earlier gestational infection.

(1) <20 weeks: encephaloclastic lesions (porencephaly, hydranencephaly), hydrocephalus, extensive calcifications.

(2) 20 to 30 weeks: moderate hydrocephalus and calcifications.

(3) >30 weeks: milder degrees of calcification, rarely associated with hydrocephalus.

IV. Herpes Simplex Virus (HSV).

A. Organism.

1. HSV has two main serotypes.

a. HSV type 1 (orofacial herpes): usually causes encephalitis in children or adults (see Chapter 44); rarely causes neonatal infection.

b. HSV type 2 (genital herpes): 75% to 90% of all neonatal infection.

2. Infection is rare during fetal development, possibly because degree of damage results in spontaneous abortion.

3. Most neonatal infections are transmitted during delivery by direct contact of the infant's skin, eyes or oral cavity with maternal herpetic lesions in the cervix or vagina.

B. Incidence.

1. Between 1 in 2000 and 1 in 5000 live births.

2. CNS involvement in 30% to 50% of infections.

C. Pathophysiology.

1. CNS involvement.

a. Acute neonatal HSV infection results in diffuse brain involvement.

b. Unlike pediatric and adult infection (HSV type 1), does not have predilection for limbic system.

c. Organism has predilection for endothelial cells, resulting in vascular thrombosis and hemorrhagic infarction. Sequelae include multicystic encephalomalacia and atrophy.

d. Ocular lesions include chorioretinitis and microphthalmia.

2. Extracranial involvement.

a. Hepatitis.

   b. Pneumonitis.
   c. Disseminated intravascular coagulopathy.
D. Clinical course.
   1. Neonatal herpetic infections are divided into three categories.
      a. Mucocutaneous lesions.
         (1) Skin, eye, and mouth lesions (vesicles) are mildest manifestation and most common (40%).
         (2) Death is uncommon in this group but if untreated, can progress to disseminated or CNS disease in 75% of infants.
      b. CNS infections.
         (1) Isolated CNS involvement is present in approximately 30% of infected infants.
         (2) Symptoms include lethargy, hypotonia, apnea, and seizures, beginning 2 to 4 weeks after birth.
         (3) Overall mortality of 50%.
      c. Disseminated disease (with visceral organ involvement).
         (1) Disseminated disease presents like severe bacterial sepsis.
         (2) CNS manifestations are present in 50% of cases.
         (3) Mortality approaches 80% in untreated and 50% in treated infants.
   2. Diagnosis made by viral isolation, usually from vesicles or CSF. Occasionally may require brain biopsy.
   3. Therapy: vidarabine or acyclovir.
E. Imaging.
   1. U/S.
      a. Parenchymal hemorrhage.
      b. Cystic encephalomalacia.
      c. Scattered parenchymal calcification.
   2. CT.
      a. Initially patchy focal white matter hypodensity, which becomes more prominent and diffuse.
      b. Subsequent accentuation of relative hyperdensity of cortex.
      c. May see hemorrhagic infarction.
      d. Loss of brain substance occurs as early as third week.
      e. Sequelae include multicystic encephalomalacia, diffuse atrophy, and punctate or gyriform parenchymal calcification.
   3. MRI.
      a. May be difficult to distinguish diffuse white matter edema in neonatal brain from unmyelinated white matter.
      b. As disease progresses often observe increased T1 signal of cortical gray matter, may persist for weeks to months.

      c. May see patchy parenchymal or meningeal enhancement in some subacute cases.

V. Rubella.
  A. Organism.
    1. Infection of fetus occurs if primary maternal infection occurs during pregnancy or up to 3 months prior to conception.
    2. Virus transmitted through hematogenous/placental route.
    3. Frequency and severity of infection greater with early gestation.
    4. Congenital rubella syndrome usually results from first-trimester and second-trimester infections.
  B. Incidence.
    1. Prior to widespread rubella immunization, congenital rubella infection occurred in up to 2% of neonates.
    2. Incidence has since markedly diminished and is rare in developed countries.
  C. Pathophysiology.
    1. Organism causes cellular damage as well as endothelial necrosis.
    2. CNS effects.
      a. Organism thought to interfere with cellular multiplication, especially progenitor cells in germinal matrix, resulting in micrencephaly and possibly delayed myelination.
      b. Meningoencephalitis involves meninges and perivascular spaces. Endothelial necrosis may result in ischemic vasculopathy and infarct.
      c. Perivascular necrosis and microcalcification most common in centrum semiovale, corpus callosum, and basal ganglia.
      d. Ocular: cataracts, glaucoma, chorioretinitis, microphthalmia.
    3. Extracranial involvement.
      a. Anemia, thrombocytopenia.
      b. Hepatosplenomegaly.
      c. Pneumonitis.
      d. Lymphadenopathy.
      e. Cardiac malformations include pulmonary artery hypoplasia and patent ductus arteriosis.
      f. Musculoskeletal abnormalities.
      g. Inner ear pathology.
      h. Dental abnormalities.
  D. Clinical course.
    1. Maternal infection suggested by recent seroconversion.
    2. Infection can result in spontaneous abortion or spectrum of fetal damage.

3. Frequency and severity of infection greatest if gestation <8 to 12 weeks, whereas third-trimester infection is relatively mild.
4. Classic rubella syndrome includes cardiac, ocular, and hearing defects.
5. Presentation at birth may include low birth weight, hypotonia, jaundice, cyanosis, petechiae/purpura, hepatosplenomegaly, pneumonitis, adenopathy, osteitis, retinopathy, or cataracts.
6. Diagnosis made by viral isolation from body fluids (infants usually shed virus for about 6 months) or analysis of specific antibodies.
7. There is no treatment; prevention is most important.

E. Imaging.
  1. U/S.
    a. Subependymal cysts in caudate nucleus and striothalamic regions may be seen but are nonspecific.
    b. Echogenic foci in basal ganglia may represent mineralizing vasculitis with calcification.
  2. CT.
    a. Microcephaly, atrophy, ventriculomegaly.
    b. Near-total brain destruction may be seen in severe infections.
    c. Parenchymal calcifications (mostly microcalcification) less prominent than other TORCH infections, often in cortex and basal ganglia.
  3. MRI.
    a. Deep and subcortical white matter lesions may be caused by vascular injury and ischemic necrosis.
    b. Delayed myelination may be seen.

VI. Congenital HIV infection.
  A. Organism.
    1. Human immunodeficiency virus—type 1 (HIV-1) is a lymphotropic retrovirus that infects T4 helper cells but is also neurotropic and affects central and peripheral nervous system.
    2. In infants and children, CNS manifestations are due to primary encephalitis and less commonly due to secondary infections (e.g., toxoplasmosis) or development of tumors (e.g., lymphoma), which are more common in adults.
  B. Incidence.
    1. In US, 2% of AIDS patients are children; worldwide incidence is 5% to 25%.
    2. 80% of all childhood infections are maternally transmitted; 30% of neonates born to HIV-positive mothers are infected.
    3. Transfusion-acquired HIV is decreasing.

4. AIDS is now ninth highest ranking cause of death in children between 1 and 4 years.
C. Pathophysiology: see Chapter 45.
D. Clinical course.
  1. General symptoms include failure to thrive, weight loss, chronic fever.
  2. Other signs include lymphadenopathy, oral thrush, chronic diarrhea, dermatitis, and repeated infections.
  3. 80% of infants with AIDS do not survive beyond first year of life.
  4. 30% to 50% develop progressive encephalopathy with developmental delay, cognitive and psychomotor impairment (spastic quadriparesis, ataxia).
  5. Superimposed CNS infection or neoplasm are uncommon: PML is most often reported, lymphoma occurs in 5%, toxoplasmosis and other infections rare.
E. Imaging.
  1. CT.
    a. Diffuse cerebral atrophy most common finding (90%).
    b. Unlike adult infection, basal ganglia calcifications are frequent (30%) but usually not seen until after 1 year of age.
    c. Hemorrhage may be seen with underlying thrombocytopenia.
    d. Unlike adult infection, opportunistic infections uncommon (15%).
  2. MRI.
    a. May see foci of increased signal on T2WI in peripheral and deep white matter.
    b. May have delayed myelination or white matter hypoplasia.
    c. Occasionally see cerebral infarcts.

SUGGESTED READINGS

Barkovich AJ: Infections of the nervous system. In *Pediatric neuroimaging,* New York, 1995, Raven Press, pp 541-568.
Barkovich AJ, Lindan CE: Congenital cytomegalovirus infection of the brain: imaging analysis and embryologic considerations, *AJNR* 15:703-715, 1994.
Becker LE: Infections of the developing brain, *AJNR* 13:537-549, 1992.
Fitz CR: Inflammatory diseases of the brain in childhood, *AJNR* 13:551-567, 1992.
Osborn AG: Infection, white matter abnormalities, and degenerative diseases. In *Diagnostic radiology,* St Louis, 1994, Mosby, pp 671-715.

42

Infectious Meningitis, Subdural Empyema and Epidural Abscess

Key Concepts

1. Meningitis is the most common form of CNS infection.
2. Infectious meningitis can be divided into three general categories.
   a. Acute pyogenic meningitis (mostly bacterial).
   b. Lymphocytic meningitis (usually viral).
   c. Chronic meningitis (e.g., tuberculosis, coccidiomycosis).
3. Complications of meningitis include:
   a. Hydrocephalus.
   b. Infarct.
   c. Subdural/epidural empyema.
   d. Parenchymal infection.
   e. Ventriculitis/ependymitis.
4. Sterile subdural effusions are common in infantile meningitis.
5. Epidural/subdural empyema are more commonly due to postcraniotomy infection or sinusitis rather than meningitis.
6. Diagnosis of menigitis is generally made clinically; imaging is reserved for evaluating complications of meningitis.

I. General comments.
   A. Meningitis is the most common form of CNS infection.
   B. Infectious meningitis can be divided into three general categories.
      1. Acute pyogenic meningitis (mostly bacterial).
      2. Lymphocytic meningitis (usually viral).
      3. Chronic meningitis (e.g., tuberculosis and coccidiomycosis).
   C. Incidence of causative organism is affected by various factors, including age, immune status, other underlying illness.
II. Acute bacterial (pyogenic) meningitis.
   A. Organisms, incidence and age.
      1. 80% of cases caused by three organisms.
         a. Neisseria meningitidis.
         b. Hemophilus influenzae.
         c. Streptococcus (Diplococcus) pneumoniae.
      2. Nonepidemic meningitis is most common in neonates, infants, and children; fifth most common cause of death in children between 1 and 4 years of age.
      3. Organisms distributed by age.
         a. Neonates: group B streptococcus and E. coli account for 70%, Listeria less common >> Staphylococcus, Proteus, Pseudomonas.
         b. Infants: N. meningitidis.
         c. Young children (1 to 7 years): H. influenzae.
         d. Older children: N. meningitidis.
         e. Adults: S. pneumoniae.
      4. Organisms also distributed by underlying illness or patient population.
         a. Pneumococcus meningitis: alcoholism, sinusitis, otomastoiditis, pneumococcal pneumonia, sickle cell anemia, and asplenism.
         b. Gram-negative meningitis (esp. E. coli, Klebsiella, Enterobacter): CNS surgery/trauma, GU manipulation, nosocomial infection, elderly, and immune-compromised.
         c. Staphylococcal meningitis: CNS surgery/trauma, endocarditis.
         d. Listeria meningitis: neonates, elderly, and chronic renal failure.
   B. Pathophysiology.
      1. Bacteria reach meninges from various routes.
         a. Hematogenous spread most common.
         b. Extension from adjacent infected structures less common (e.g., otitis media, mastoiditis, sinusitis).

      c. Communication of CSF with exterior uncommon (e.g., myelomeningocele, dermal sinus tract, CSF leak).

      d. Direct implantation infrequent (e.g., penetrating head injury or comminuted skull fracture).

      e. Rupture of superficial cortical abscesses are rare.

  2. Purulent exudate covers brain or located within basilar cisterns and brain becomes congested, edematous.

  3. Complications.

      a. Venous stasis (increased risk with dehydration) and thrombophlebitis may result in venous thrombosis.

      b. Perivascular inflammation may cause vasospasm and secondary arterial or venous infarction.

      c. Exudate in basilar cisterns may damage cranial nerves or cause extraventricular (communicating) obstructive hydrocephalus.

      d. Hydrocephalus (more common in neonates than in children or adults) may develop secondary to obstruction at cisterns or due to ventriculitis/ependymitis.

      e. Subdural (sterile) effusions are common in infantile meningitis (20% to 50%); 2% become secondarily infected, resulting in subdural empyema. Most resolve spontaneously.

      f. Subdural empyema and epidural empyema/abscess may be complications of meningitis (15%) although are more commonly related to postcraniotomy infection or sinusitis. May result in secondary cortical vein thrombosis and venous infarction.

      g. Infection may spread to cerebral parenchyma and result in cerebritis or abscess.

      h. Ventriculitis more likely in neonatal meningitis (especially with gram-negative enteric bacilli).

      i. Late sequelae include encephalomalacia and atrophy.

C. Clinical.

  1. Often preceded by prodromal respiratory illness or pharyngitis.

  2. Onset of meningitis may occur within 24 hours in adults, possibly sooner in children.

  3. Acute adult meningitis typically presents with fever, headache, stiff neck, nausea and vomiting, followed by progressive decrease in level of consciousness.

  4. Acute infantile meningitis may present with fever, irritability, vomiting, seizures, and bulging fontanelle.

  5. Meningococcal meningitis often accompanied by petechial/purpural rash.

6. Diagnosis made by CSF studies.
7. Treatment: antibiotics.
8. Cerebral infarction, edema, and ventriculitis are predictive of poor outcome.
9. Overall 10% mortality; 20% to 40% mortality for adult bacterial meningitis; 15% to 60% mortality for neonatal meningitis (Group B streptococcus meningitis has better prognosis than gram-negative enteric meningitis).
10. Hearing impairment due to labyrinthitis is frequent complication of childhood meningitis.

D. Imaging.
   1. Neonatal U/S.
      a. May see increased echogenicity and widening of sulci and fissures.
      b. Mild to moderate hypoechoic extraaxial fluid may be seen over convexity or in widened interhemispheric fissure.
      c. May see focal hyperechoic areas, which may represent vasculitis, infarct, or cerebritis.
   2. CT.
      a. Commonly normal.
      b. Basal cisterns and sulci may be poorly visualized or effaced on NECT due to isodense exudate.
      c. Less than 50% of children with documented meningitis will have abnormally enhancing meninges on CECT.
      d. Ventricles may be enlarged due to hydrocephalus or small due to diffuse cerebral edema.
      e. Crescentic low-density extraaxial collections representing subdural effusions are common in infantile meningitis.
      f. Less commonly see extraaxial fluid collections in adults, imaging studies unable to distinguish between sterile or infected fluid, although associated rim enhancement usually implies latter.
      g. Sinus thrombosis may be recognized by "delta" sign on CECT due to central triangular nonenhancing thrombus marginated by contrast-enhanced flowing blood or vasa vasorum.
      h. May see hemorrhagic venous infarction or development of cerebritis and/or abscess.
   3. MRI.
      a. Obliterated cisterns may be difficult to detect on routine non-contrast MRI.
      b. Meninges may enhance diffusely after contrast administration.

   c. MRI more sensitive than CT in detecting early complications of meningitis.
   d. Neonatal meningitis particularly prone to hydrocephalus, ventriculitis, infarction, subdural effusions, and abscess.
   e. MR venography can be used to detect dural venous sinus thrombosis.
   f. Venous infarcts are usually subcortical, hypointense on T1 and hyperintense on T2, often hemorrhagic (25%), and occur in characteristic locations.
      (1) Parasagittal: due to sagittal sinus thrombosis.
      (2) Thalamic: due to straight sinus or vein of Galen thrombosis.
      (3) Temporal lobe: due to vein of Labbe or transverse/sigmoid sinus thrombosis.
III. Acute lymphocytic (aseptic) meningitis.
   A. Organisms.
      1. Virus isolated in 70% of cases.
      2. Enteroviruses (echoviruses, coxsackieviruses) responsible for 50% to 80% of viral meningitides.
      3. Other viruses include mumps, varicella zoster, herpes virus types 1 and 2, Epstein-Barr, arbovirus, HIV.
   B. Incidence.
      1. Annual reported incidence 10 to 30 cases per 100,000; over 7000 cases reported annually in United States (actual number probably higher due to underreporting).
      2. Most cases of viral meningitis occur in children and adults; uncommon in neonates.
   C. Pathophysiology.
      1. Viruses can cause meningitis or encephalitis (see Chapter 44).
      2. Viral meningitis is result of hematogenous infection.
   D. Clinical.
      1. Symptoms (fever, headache, and meningismus) are usually less severe than bacterial meningitis.
      2. Diagnosis suggested by sterile CSF with mild pleocytosis and normal CSF glucose; occasionally may isolate virus or viral antigen directly from CSF.
      3. Usually benign and self-limited, requiring only supportive treatment.
      4. Development of associated encephalitis may result in alteration in consciousness, seizures, paresis.
      5. Permanent CNS impairment more likely in infants.
   E. Imaging (CT/MRI): rarely see enhancing meninges.
IV. Chronic meningitis.

A. Etiology and incidence.
1. Infectious.
   a. TB most common (see Chapter 46); TB meningitis in children usually accompanies generalized miliary TB.
   b. Other frequent organisms include Coccidiomycosis and Cryptococcus (see Chapter 47).
   c. Less common organisms include Candida, Actinomyces, and Aspergillus (see Chapter 47).
2. Noninfectious granulomatous disease (see Chapter 46): especially sarcoid; less commonly Wegener's granulomatosis, Langerhans cell histiocytosis, rheumatoid pachymeningitis.
B. Pathophysiology.
1. Chronic meningitis has predilection for basal cisterns, although other locations may also be involved.
2. Thick fibrinous exudate obliterates cisterns.
3. Complications include hydrocephalus, infarction, atrophy, and dystrophic calcifications.
C. Clinical.
1. Symptoms less severe and evolve more slowly than acute pyogenic meningitis. Fever may be minimal.
2. Diagnosis suggested by CSF lymphocytic pleocytosis and low glucose, and occasionally made by CSF culture (e.g., TB) or antigen detection (e.g., cryptococcal).
3. Definitive diagnosis may ultimately require meningeal or cortical biopsy (best yield in enhancing lesions).
4. Overall mortality in TB meningitis is 25% to 30%; long-term morbidity ranges from 65% to 90% of survivors.
D. Imaging.
1. CT.
   a. NECT scans may demonstrate "en-plaque" dural thickening, which enhances after contrast administration.
   b. May see "popcorn"-like dystrophic calcifications, especially around basal cisterns.
   c. May see sequelae of meningitis including hydrocephalus, infarction, and atrophy.
2. MRI.
   a. Inflammatory exudate generally isointense to brain and often difficult to detect without contrast administration.
   b. Contrast-enhanced studies typically show basal meningeal enhancement but can also show convexity meningeal enhancement.
V. Subdural empyema and epidural abscess.
A. Etiology and incidence.

1. Comprise 20% to 40% of intracranial infections.
2. Postoperative infection may now be most common cause in developed countries.
    a. Although incidence of infection after craniotomy still relatively low (1%), the frequency of craniotomies have greatly increased.
    b. Risk factors in patients include repeated procedures, older age, lack of fever, evidence of wound infection.
    c. Organisms: usually gram-negative bacteria, Streptococcus, or Staphylococcus.
3. Sinusitis, especially frontal and ethmoid, was previously most common cause. Frequency and severity of sinusitis-related complications are decreasing in developed countries due to earlier and improved treatment.
4. Meningitis (15%) is less common cause.
5. Uncommon causes include orbital infections, skull osteomyelitis, chronic otitis media, mastoiditis, skull fractures, primary brain parenchymal infection.

B. Pathophysiology.
1. Often extraaxial purulent collections are both intradural and extradural. However, sometimes collections will be confined to one space.
2. Epidural empyema or abscess.
    a. Collections of suppurative fluid between skull and dura.
    b. Like other epidural collections (e.g., hematoma), is usually restricted by dural attachments at sutures.
    c. Can cross falx, often bilateral.
3. Subdural empyema.
    a. Collection of infected fluid in potential space between dura and arachnoid.
    b. Like subdural hematoma, is not restricted by dural attachments at sutures.
    c. Unable to cross falx, usually unilateral.
    d. May occur over convexities or within interhemispheric fissures (parafalcine).

C. Clinical.
1. Symptoms nonspecific but may correlate with location.
    a. Epidural abscess often presents with headache, fever, and manifestations of primary infection (e.g., sinusitis).
    b. Subdural empyema more likely to develop encephalopathy, focal neurologic signs, or seizures.
2. Poor prognostic factors include older age, encephalopathy, delayed treatment.

3. Estimated 10% of patients with epidural abscess will develop subdural empyema; and 20% to 25% of patients with subdural empyema will develop brain abscess.
4. Complications include cortical or dural venous thrombosis and infarction.
5. Overall mortality 20%.
6. Treatment: antibiotic therapy with possible surgical debridement/drainage.

D. Imaging.
  1. CT.
    a. Hypodense extraaxial fluid collections, often unable to distinguish intradural or extradural location. However, generally:
      (1) Subdural: typically unilateral, crescentic collection over convexity or within interhemispheric fissure.
      (2) Epidural: typically bilateral, lentiform collection over convexities.
    b. CECT may show enhancing rim after 1 to 3 weeks.
  2. MRI.
    a. Signal is similar to or slightly hyperintense to CSF on T1 and T2WI.
    b. May see T2-hyperintense cerebral edema.
    c. May see complications including venous infarction, cerebritis, abscess (see Chapter 43).

SUGGESTED READINGS

Anderson M: Management of cerebral infection, *J Neurol Neurosurg Psych* 56:1243-1258, 1993.

Ashwal S, Tomasi L, Schneider S, Perkin R, Thompson J: Bacterial meningitis in children: pathophysiology and treatment, *Neurol* 42:739-748, 1992.

Baltas I, Tsoulfa S, Sakellariou P, et al: Posttraumatic meningitis: bacteriology, hydrocephalus, and outcome, *Neurosurg* 35:422-427, 1994.

Brennan M: Subdural empyema, *Amer Fam Phys* 51:157-162, 1995.

Cheng TM, O'Neill BP, Scheithauer BW, Piepgras DG: Chronic meningitis: the role of meningeal or cortical biopsy, *Neurosurg* 34:590-596, 1994.

Eustace S, Buff B: Magnetic resonance imaging in drug-induced meningitis, *Can Assoc Radiol J* 45:463-465, 1994.

Hlavin ML, Kaminski HJ, Fenstermaker RA, White RJ: Intracranial suppuration: a modern decade of postoperative subdural empyema and epidural abscess, *Neurosurg* 34:974-981, 1994.

Lambert HP: Meningitis, *J Neurol Neurosurg Psych* 57:405-415, 1994.

Mamelak AN, Kelly WM, Davis RL, Rosenblum ML: Idiopathic hypertrophic cranial pachymeningitis, *J Neurosurg* 79:270-276, 1993.

Masson C, Henin D, Hauw JJ, et al: Cranial pachymeningitis of unknown origin: a study of seven cases, *Neurol* 43:1329-1334, 1993.

Osborn AG: Infection, white matter abnormalities, and degenerative diseases. In *Diagnostic radiology,* St Louis, 1994, Mosby, pp 671-715.

Pfister H-W, Feiden W, Einhaupl K-M: Spectrum of complications during bacterial meningitis in adults: results of a prospective clinical study, *Arch Neurol* 50:575-581, 1993.

River Y, Averbuch-Heller L, Weinberger M, et al: Antibiotic induced meningitis, *J Neurol Neurosurg Psych* 57:705-708, 1994.

43

Cerebritis, Abscess, and Ventriculitis/Ependymitis

Key Concepts

1. Pyogenic or bacterial parenchymal infections are relatively uncommon in developed countries.
2. Pyogenic brain abscess evolves from focal cerebritis in predictable stages.
   a. Early cerebritis (up to 3 to 5 days): typically ill-defined nonenhancing focus.
   b. Late cerebritis (from 4 to 14 days): patchy enhancement and developing edema.
   c. Early capsule (begins at about 2 weeks): thin enhancing rim may or may not be sharply marginated.
   d. Late capsule (may last for weeks/months): discrete enhancing rim becomes thicker.
   e. Resolution of imaging findings lags behind clinical improvement.
3. Complications of pyogenic abscess include:
   a. Formation of satellite or "daughter" abscesses.
   b. Ventriculitis, ependymitis, choroid plexitis.
   c. Purulent leptomeningitis.
4. Nonpyogenic abscesses are more likely to occur in immunocompromised populations and include the following organisms: toxoplasma, mycobacterium, fungi, nocardia, actinomyces.
5. Ventriculitis/ependymitis is more likely to occur from surgical procedures than from ruptured brain abscess or meningitis.

I. Cerebritis.
  A. Etiology.
    1. Cerebritis is the earliest stage of purulent brain infection.
    2. Various causes.
      a. Most common cause is hematogenous spread from extra-cranial primary infection (e.g., cardiac, pulmonary, IV drug abuse).
      b. Direct spread from adjacent otomastoid or sinus infections may result in meningitis, empyema, and parenchymal infection.
      c. Trauma (e.g., direct penetrating injury, comminuted skull fracture, or postsurgical) is not uncommon.
      d. Congenital or acquired dural defect or dermal sinus tracts are uncommon.
    3. Organisms are variable (see below).
  B. Incidence: uncommon in developed countries.
  C. Pathophysiology.
    1. Cerebritis and abscess generally do not occur in normal brain, often underlying injury such as infarction results in necrotic tissue, which is susceptible to superimposed infection.
    2. Location: usually cortical/subcortical (gray/white matter) junction.
    3. Stages in cerebritis.
      a. Early cerebritis.
        (1) Up to 3 to 5 days.
        (2) Infection is focal but not yet localized.
        (3) Pathology shows unencapsulated mass of edema, hyperemia, perivascular polymorphonuclear cell infiltrates, petechial hemorrhage, and minimal necrosis.
      b. Late cerebritis.
        (1) From 4 to 14 days.
        (2) Infection becomes more localized.
        (3) Pathology shows coalescing central necrotic zones surrounded by ill-defined ring of inflammatory cells, macrophages, granulation tissue, and fibroblasts.
  D. Clinical.
    1. Treatment: antibiotics.
    2. Surgery is generally contraindicated for cerebritis.
    3. If treatment is unsuccessful, cerebritis progresses to abscess (see below).
  E. Imaging.
    1. Neonatal U/S: may see focal areas of increased echogenicity (indistinguishable from vasculitis, infarct).

2. CT.
   a. Ill-defined subcortical low-density lesion.
   b. Early cerebritis may not enhance (may resemble low-grade astrocytoma).
   c. Late cerebritis may show patchy, gyriform, or ill-defined peripheral enhancement. Delayed scans may show subsequent enhancement of central region.
3. MRI.
   a. Focal but ill-defined heterogeneous lesion with mild hypointensity to GM on T1WI and mild hyperintensity on T2WI.
   b. Usually shows some patchy enhancement.
   c. Moderate to marked edema and mass effect in later stage.
II. Pyogenic abscess.
   A. Etiology.
      1. Evolves from focus of cerebritis (see above).
      2. Organisms are variable.
         a. Most abscesses are produced by single pyogenic organism, although in one third of cases, more than one organism is responsible.
            (1) Most frequently isolated organisms are steptococci (aerobic and anaerobic) and staphylococci.
            (2) Gram-negative organisms are increasing in frequency.
         b. Organisms also dependent on underlying illness or patient population.
            (1) Sinus infection: Bacteroides, Streptococcus.
            (2) Otomastoid infection: Enterobacter, Streptococcus, Bacillus.
            (3) Dental infection: Streptococcus, Bacteroides, Fusobacterium.
            (4) Penetrating head trauma/surgery: Staphylococcus, Streptococcus, Clostridium, and gram-negative organisms.
            (5) Pneumonia: Streptococcus, gram-negative organisms.
            (6) Immunosuppression: TB (see Chapter 46), Nocardia, Actinomyces, fungi (see Chapter 47).
            (7) Neonates: Citrobacter, Proteus, Pseudomonas, Serratia, and Staphylococcus.
   B. Incidence.
      1. Intracranial abscesses are uncommon in developed countries.
      2. Risk factors include septicemia, endocarditis, sinusitis, otomastoiditis, immunosuppression, diabetes, congenital heart disease, trauma, and surgery.

      3. Most abscesses in neonates and infants occur as complications of meningitis.

C. Pathophysiology.

      1. Routes of spread are same as for cerebritis (see above).

      2. Location.

         a. Abscesses generally occur at subcortical location (gray/white junction).

         b. Location is also dependent on underlying primary infection:

            (1) Abscess due to frontal sinusitis usually located in frontal lobe.

            (2) Abscess due to otomastoid infection usually located in temporal lobe or cerebellum.

            (3) Abscess due to direct penetrating injury, fracture, or craniotomy located adjacent to affected site.

      3. Stages of abscess formation (evolve from cerebritis).

         a. Early capsule.

            (1) Begins at about 2 weeks.

            (2) Collagen and reticulin form a capsule around core of liquefied necrotic and inflammatory debris.

            (3) Early capsule is thin-walled and surrounded by edema.

         b. Late capsule.

            (1) May last for weeks or months.

            (2) As more collagen is laid down, capsule becomes thicker.

            (3) Capsule wall tends to be thinner on medial side, presumably due to relatively less blood supply to white matter compared with gray matter.

            (4) Surrounding edema and mass effect subsides.

            (5) Gliosis develops around abscess periphery.

         c. Abscess in immunosuppressed individuals tends to have less edema and thinner capsule.

D. Clinical course.

      1. With improved diagnostic imaging, antibiotic therapies and neurosurgical care, mortality of intracranial abscess has decreased from 40% to 50% to under 5%.

      2. Treatment.

         a. Antibiotics preferred for small, multiple, or critically situated (e.g., dominant hemisphere) abscesses.

         b. Surgery performed for confirmation of diagnosis, poor response to antibiotic therapy, and relief of mass effect of large lesion(s). Complete excision usually not necessary, aspiration can be performed with stereotactic guidance.

      3. Complications of abscess include:

         a. Formation of satellite or "daughter" abscesses.

b. Ventriculitis, ependymitis, or choroid plexitis.
c. Purulent leptomeningitis.
4. Intraventricular rupture associated with poor outcome.
E. Imaging.
1. Nuclear imaging: SPECT studies or radiolabeled IgG antibody may be helpful in distinguishing between brain abscess, neoplasm, or postoperative changes.
2. CT.
a. Ring-enhancing subcortical lesion.
b. Early capsule has relatively thin enhancing rim that may or may not be sharply marginated, surrounded by marked edema.
c. Late capsule has discrete thicker wall; edema and mass effect begin to subside.
d. Medial/inner margin of capsule often thinner than outer margin (50%).
e. Rim enhancement may lag behind clinical improvement, persisting for months after clinical resolution.
3. MRI.
a. Central area of necrosis is typically hypointense or isointense to GM on T1WI and hyperintense on PD and T2WI.
b. Surrounding capsule appears isointense to mildly hyperintense to GM on T1WI and hypointense or isointense on T2WI.
c. Marked enhancement of capsule is seen after contrast administration.
d. Abscess in immunocompromised patients tends to have less edema, thinner wall, and minimal or absent enhancement.
e. May see evidence of complications.
(1) Satellite or daughter abscesses.
(2) Ventriculitis/ependymitis: enhancing ventricular margins.
(3) Choroid plexitis: bulky enhancement of choroid plexus.
(4) Leptomeningitis: diffuse meningeal enhancement.
F. Differential diagnosis (see box on p. 439).
III. Nonpyogenic brain abscesses.
A. Etiology: organisms other than common bacteria can cause brain abscess including:
1. Toxoplasma (see Chapter 45).
2. Mycobacterium (see Chapter 46).
3. Fungi (see Chapter 47).
4. Actinomycetaceae (Nocardia, Actinomyces) (see Chapter 47).
B. Incidence: less common than pyogenic brain abscess.

   C. Pathophysiology: usually require some impairment in host immunity.
   D. Clinical: see corresponding chapters.
   E. Imaging (CT/MRI).
       1. Often do not follow typical sequence of bacterial abscess.
       2. More likely to be multiple, thicker walled, multiloculated.
IV. Ventriculitis/ependymitis.
   A. Etiology and incidence.
       1. Usually follows shunting procedures, intraventricular surgery, placement of in-dwelling prosthetic devices, intrathecal chemotherapy.
       2. Risk factors for shunt infection include young age (especially <2 weeks of age), lengthy procedure, and open neural tube defect.
       3. Less commonly due to ruptured paraventricular brain abscess or meningitis (latter more common in neonatal meningitis).
   B. Organisms.
       1. Most common organisms are related to shunt infections and include S. epidermidis, S. aureus, and gram-negative bacilli.
       2. Neonates: E. coli, S. hemoliticus, and gram-negative bacilli common.
       3. Cytomegalovirus frequently causes ependymitis in AIDS population.

Differential Diagnosis of Ring-enhancing Lesions

Common:

Primary brain tumor (e.g., high-grade astrocytoma)
Metastatic brain tumor
Abscess
Granuloma
Resolving hematoma
Subacute infarct

Less Common:

Thrombosed vascular malformation
Active demyelinating lesion (e.g., multiple sclerosis)

Uncommon:

Thrombosed aneurysm
Other primary brain tumors (e.g., primary lymphoma in AIDS)
Radiation necrosis

C. Clinical.
   1. Symptoms nonspecific, especially in neonates and infants (e.g., lethargy, irritability).
   2. Definitive diagnosis of shunt infection made by shunt tap.
   3. Treatment: antibiotics; shunt revision if related to ventricular shunt.
D. Imaging.
   1. Neonatal U/S.
      a. Hydrocephalus.
      b. May see hyperechoic, shaggy ependymal lining.
      c. Echogenic debris, septations, and loculations frequently seen.
   2. CT/MRI.
      a. Ependymal enhancement in the appropriate clinical setting is diagnostic of ventriculitis/ependymitis.
      b. May see hydrocephalus with obstruction at foramen of Monro or aqueduct.
      c. Frequently see adhesions or septations resulting in loculated areas; intraventricular contrast can be administered through shunt to evaluate noncommunicating loculations.
      d. Demonstration of increasing ventriculomegaly on serial studies is consistent with shunt failure.
E. Differential Diagnosis (see box below).

Differential Diagnosis of Ependymal Enhancement

Common:

Ventriculitis/ependymitis (bacterial, fungal, parasitic)
Primary brain tumor
    Anaplastic astrocytoma, GBM
    Lymphoma/leukemia
    Pineal tumors (germinoma, pineoblastoma)
    PNET/medulloblastoma
    Ependymoma

Uncommon:

Neurosarcoidosis
Collateral venous drainage pathway (Sturge-Weber, dural sinus occlusion, vascular malformation)
Primary brain tumor (choroid plexus tumor)
Metastatic tumor (especially lung, breast, melanoma)

SUGGESTED READINGS

Anderson M: Management of cerebral infection, *J Neurol Neurosurg Psych* 56:1243-1258, 1993.

Hatta S, Mochizuki H, Kuru Y, et al: Serial neuroradiological studies in focal cerebritis, *Neuroradiol* 36:285-288, 1994.

Lo WD, Wolny A, Boesel C: Blood-brain barrier permeability in staphylococcal cerebritis and early brain abscess, *J Neurosurg* 80:987-905, 1994.

Mamelak AN, Mampalam TJ, Obana WG, Rosenblum ML: Improved management of multiple brain abscesses: a combined surgical and medical approach, *Neurosurg* 36:76-86, 1995.

Osborn AG: Infection, white matter abnormalities, and degenerative diseases. In *Diagnostic radiology*, St Louis, 1994, Mosby, pp 671-715.

Sharma BS, Khosla VK, Vak VK, et al: Multiple pyogenic brain abscesses, *Acta Neurochir* 133:36-43, 1995.

Yen P-T, Chan S-T, Haung T-S: Brain abscess: with special reference to otolaryngologic sources of infection, *Otolaryngol Head Neck Surg* 113:15-22, 1995.

Yuh WTC, Nguyen HD, Gao F, et al: Brain parenchymal infection in bone marrow transplantation patients: CT and MR findings, *AJR* 162:425-430, 1994.

Zeidman SM, Geisler FH, Olivi A: Intraventricular rupture of a purulent brain abscess: case report, *Neurosurg* 36:189-193, 1995.

44

Encephalitis and Post-Infectious Syndromes

Key Concepts

1. Encephalitis refers to an acute nonfocal inflammatory disease of the brain due to direct invasion (usually viral) or to immune-mediated hypersensitivity initiated by virus or other foreign protein.
2. Viruses can cause various CNS manifestations (often overlap).
    a. Meningitis (see Chapter 42): e.g., echovirus, coxsackievirus, mumps, HIV.
    b. Encephalitis: e.g., HSV, HIV, arbovirus, measles, rhabdovirus.
    c. Leukoencephalitis (predominantly involving white matter): e.g., Subacute sclerosing panencephalitis (SSPE), Progressive multi-focal leukoencephalitis (PML), and equine encephalitis.
    d. Vasculitis and infarct: e.g., rubella, varicella zoster virus, coxsackievirus, echovirus, and arbovirus.
    e. Myelitis: e.g., poliovirus, HSV, varicella zoster virus.
3. Herpes simplex virus-type 1 encephalitis is the most common fatal non-epidemic encephalitis in the nonneonatal population.
4. Postinfectious encephalitides include: acute disseminated encephalomyelitis (ADEM), and Lyme disease.

I. General comments.
  A. Encephalitis is a diffuse, nonfocal brain parenchymal inflammatory disease that can be caused by a variety of agents, although usually viral.
  B. Viruses can spread hematogenously or via peripheral nerves (e.g., Herpes simplex type 1).
  C. Viruses can cause various CNS manifestations (often overlap).
    1. Meningitis (see Chapter 42): e.g., echovirus, coxsackievirus, mumps, HIV.
    2. Encephalitis: e.g., HSV, HIV, arbovirus, measles, rhabdovirus.
    3. Leukoencephalitis (predominantly involving white matter): e.g., Subacute sclerosing panencephalitis, Progressive multifocal leukoencephalitis, and equine encephalitis.
    4. Vasculitis and infarct: e.g., rubella, varicella zoster virus, coxsackievirus, echovirus, and arbovirus.
    5. Myelitis: e.g., poliovirus, HSV, varicella zoster virus.
  D. Most viral encephalitides result in a nonspecific increase in water content of affected parenchyma, which can be observed on imaging. A few viral infections have more specific clinical or radiologic features.
  E. Primary acute viral encephalitides include:
    1. Sporadic.
      a. Most commonly caused by herpes simplex type 1.
      b. Others include HIV, herpes simplex type 2, varicella zoster, mumps, measles, rhabdovirus.
    2. Epidemic: usually caused by arboviruses (e.g., equine), coxsackievirus, and poliovirus.
  F. Nonviral infectious encephalitides may be caused by tick-borne pathogens such as Lyme disease or Rocky Mountain spotted fever encephalitis.
  G. Postinfectious or secondary encephalitides include:
    1. Acute disseminated encephalomyelitis.
    2. Lyme disease.
  H. Other encephalitides of uncertain etiology.
    1. Creutzfeldt-Jakob disease.
    2. Rasmussen encephalitis.
    3. Reyes syndrome.
II. Herpes simplex encephalitis (nonneonatal).
  A. Organism.
    1. Herpes simplex encephalitis caused by two major types.

        a. Type 1 (orofacial herpes): usually responsible for childhood or adult encephalitis.

        b. Type 2 (genital herpes): usually responsible for neonatal encephalitis (see Chapter 41).

B. Incidence.

    1. Estimated annual incidence of 1 in 750,000 to 1 in million.

    2. Most common cause of fatal nonepidemic viral encephalitis.

    3. Common in both children and adults.

    4. Approximately one third of patients are <20 years old.

C. Pathophysiology.

    1. During oral herpes infection, virus is transported along sensory nerve fibers to gasserian ganglion.

    2. Encephalitis results from retrograde spread to brain.

    3. Active virus may occur with primary infection, reinfection, or reactivation of latent virus.

    4. HSV causes fulminant hemorrhagic, necrotizing meningoencephalitis, and vasculitis.

    5. Location.

        a. HSV type 1 encephalitis has predilection for limbic system: temporal lobes, insular cortex, subfrontal area, cingulate gyri.

        b. Often appears unilateral initially but subsequently becomes bilateral.

        c. Less common areas of involvement include cranial nerves (particularly trigeminal nerve), midbrain, and pons (mesenrhombencephalitis) presumably from retrograde spread along trigeminal nerve.

D. Clinical.

    1. Typically present with altered mental status or seizures. Symptoms may localize to temporal or frontal lobe pathology. Often afebrile.

    2. Direct isolation of virus from CSF is rare. Diagnosis can be made by demonstrating specific antibodies in serum or CSF, although may remain normal until second week and therefore not useful for early detection.

    3. Definitive diagnosis made by identification of virus or viral antigen on brain biopsy.

    4. Treatment: intravenous acyclovir now preferred over vidarabine.

    5. Mortality rate between 50% and 70%.

    6. Significant long-term morbidity often occurs in surviving patients.

E. Imaging.

1. Nuclear imaging.
   a. SPECT studies may demonstrate increased activity in temporal lobes.
2. CT.
   a. May be normal early in disease (usually not abnormal until 3 to 5 days).
   b. Initially ill-defined low-density lesion with mild mass effect seen in temporal lobe(s).
   c. CECT may show ill-defined patchy or gyriform enhancement, especially later in course.
   d. Later in disease may see hemorrhagic foci, although still relatively uncommon (12%).
   e. Note that lesion can mimic tumor or even pyogenic brain abscess. Because early treatment is essential, maintain high index of suspicion for lesions of the frontal and temporal lobes.
   f. Late sequelae include encephalomalacia, atrophy, and dystrophic calcifications.
3. MRI.
   a. MRI is more sensitive than CT in detecting early findings.
   b. Initially observe gyral edema on T1WI and ill-defined T2 hyperintensity in temporal lobe or cingulate gyrus.
   c. Signal abnormalities often extend to insular cortex but characteristically spare putamen (resulting in exaggerated sharp lateral margin of putamen).
   d. Patchy or gyral enhancement and petechial hemorrhage often seen later in course.
III. Lyme disease.
   A. Etiology.
      1. Organism is a tick-borne spirochete, Borrelia burgdorferi.
      2. Lyme disease occurs worldwide; in United States the most common geographic regions are New England, the Pacific states, Minnesota, and Wisconsin.
   B. Incidence.
      1. Highest incidence of infection in children <15 years and young adults between 25 and 45 years of age.
      2. CNS involvement in 15% to 20% of infections.
   C. Pathophysiology.
      1. Multisystem disease involving skin, joints, heart, eyes, and nervous system.
      2. Pathogenesis uncertain, possibly due to immune complex mechanisms (as in ADEM), vasculitis, or both.
      3. Organism is neurotropic and can produce acute symptom-

atic neurologic disease or remain dormant in CNS for long periods.

4. Pathology reveals perivascular inflammatory infiltrates with multiple areas of demyelination (resembling ADEM).
5. CNS involvement can have various forms.
   a. Lymphocytic meningitis: response to direct invasion of bacteria into subarachnoid space.
   b. Meningoencephalitis: may result in vasculitis and ischemia/infarct.
   c. Cranial neuritis: especially CN VII.
   d. Radiculitis.
   e. Peripheral neuritis.

D. Clinical.
1. Lyme disease has three clinical stages (may overlap):
   a. Stage 1 (acute, localized): flulike illness, arthralgia, and erythema chronicum migrans.
   b. Stage 2 (acute, disseminated): cardiac, ocular, and neurologic manifestations.
   c. Stage 3 (chronic, disseminated): arthritis and chronic neurologic symptoms.
2. Common CNS findings include headache, papilledema, behavioral changes, facial palsy, radiculopathy, and peripheral neuropathy.
3. Organism is notoriously difficult to isolate or culture.
4. Demonstration of specific antibodies in CSF thought to be fairly specific for CNS infection, although not necessarily sensitive.
5. Treatment: various antibiotics.

E. Imaging.
1. CT.
   a. Often normal.
   b. Occasionally may show focal areas of hypodensity.
2. MRI.
   a. 25% will show focal areas of T2 hyperintensity in periventricular and deep white matter, occasionally in thalami and pons, some of which may represent infarcts due to vasculitis.
   b. Some lesions may show enhancement.
   c. Occasionally may see diffuse leptomeningeal enhancement of brain or spinal cord.

F. Differential diagnosis.
1. Multiple sclerosis.
2. ADEM (may be indistinguishable).

        3. SSPE.

        4. PML.

IV. Poliovirus.

  A. Etiology.

      1. Poliovirus is an enterovirus transmitted by direct/indirect contact with infected feces or oropharyngeal secretions.

      2. Most poliovirus infections are asymptomatic or nonspecific febrile illness (abortive poliomyelitis).

  B. Incidence.

      1. Most common in children, especially with poor hygiene.

      2. Rare in developed countries and is primarily due to vaccine-associated infection. Three risk groups:

        a. Recipients of live attenuated oral vaccine.

        b. Persons in contact with recipients of oral vaccine.

        c. Immunosuppressed children.

      3. In United States, approximately 10 cases per year.

      4. CNS complications occur in <1% of infected patients.

  C. Pathophysiology.

      1. Aseptic meningitis or nonparalytic poliomyelitis.

      2. Spinal poliomyelitis (most common): neuronal loss, gliosis, and inflammation involving lower motor neurons; affects gray matter of spinal cord, particularly ventral horns.

      3. Bulbar polio (10% to 15%): affects reticular formation and cranial nerves (CNs IX, X, XI > CNs V, VII, XII).

      4. Encephalitis: may involve motor cortex, globus pallidus, thalamus, cerebellum.

  D. Clinical.

      1. Incubation of 1 to 3 weeks; nonspecific symptoms of sore throat, fever, abdominal pain.

      2. Spinal poliomyelitis presents with flaccid paralysis.

      3. Bulbar polio may present with lower cranial neuropathy (e.g., hoarseness, dysphagia, airway obstruction).

      4. Encephalitis may present with altered level of consciousness or seizures.

  E. Imaging (CT/MRI).

      1. Spinal poliomyelitis: T2 hyperintensity and enlargement of ventral horns of spinal cord, with enhancement of ventral roots.

      2. Bulbar polio: may see foci of T2 hyperintensity in brainstem; or enhancement of cranial nerves (see above).

      3. Encephalitis: may see nonspecific T2 hyperintensity in motor cortex of cerebral hemispheres, globus pallidus, thalamus, or cerebellum.

V. Subacute sclerosing panencephalitis (SSPE).
   A. Etiology.
      1. Progressive encephalitis thought to be caused by reactivation of measles virus.
      2. In most cases, patients have had clinical measles before the age of 3.
   B. Incidence.
      1. Rare, approximately 1 per million.
      2. With advent of measles vaccination, significant reduction in incidence in developed countries.
      3. Occurs more commonly in children (5 to 15 years of age) but can also occur in young adults.
   C. Pathophysiology.
      1. Thought to result from reactivation of latent virus.
      2. Gross atrophy of brain typical.
      3. Gray matter shows neuronal loss, gliosis, perivascular lymphocytic infiltrates.
      4. White matter shows patchy demyelination and gliosis.
      5. Pathologic changes also seen in basal ganglia, thalamus, pons, and cerebellum.
   D. Clinical.
      1. Initially presents with slowly progressive intellectual and behavioral deterioration; followed by development of myoclonus or ataxia, and eventually severe dementia, quadraparesis, and autonomic instability.
      2. Diagnosis suggested by specific antibodies in CSF and serum.
      3. Average survival 2 to 6 years.
      4. Occasionally disease is more rapidly progressive, fulminant.
      5. No known treatment, although interferon and interferon-isoprinosine therapy reported to be successful in some cases.
   E. Imaging.
      1. CT.
         a. May be normal early in disease.
         b. May show multiple hypodense foci in subcortical and periventricular white matter as well as basal ganglia.
         c. Later in course generalized atrophy is common.
      2. MRI.
         a. May see multifocal lesions that are hypointense or isointense to GM on T1WI and hyperintense on T2WI in cerebral or cerebellar white matter and basal ganglia.
         b. Lesions do not enhance.
   F. Differential diagnosis.
      1. Multiple sclerosis.

2. ADEM.
3. PML.
VI. Progressive multifocal leukoencephalitis/leukoencephalopathy (PML).
  A. Organism.
    1. Caused by ubiquitous JC polyomavirus of the papovirus group (named after first reported patient and not to be confused with Jakob-Creutzfeld disease).
    2. By puberty, 70% of general population are seropositive.
    3. Disease occurs in patients with abnormal cell-mediated immunity.
  B. Incidence.
    1. Uncommon.
    2. Patient population includes: AIDS (see Chapter 45), leukemia/lymphoma, congenital immunodeficiency syndromes, organ transplant, systemic lupus erythematosis, tuberculosis, sarcoidosis, Whipple's disease, nontropical sprue.
  C. Pathophysiology.
    1. Probably initial childhood inoculation but actual disease does not occur until immunity becomes impaired.
    2. Organism infects and destroys oligodendroglia, resulting in multifocal areas of demyelination.
    3. Location.
      a. Most commonly frontal and parieto-occipital subcortical white matter then spreads to deep white matter.
      b. Lesions tend to be more peripheral rather than periventricular (unlike multiple sclerosis).
      c. Any myelinated areas can be involved, including corpus callosum, thalami, basal ganglia.
      d. Brainstem or cerebellar involvement uncommon.
      e. Cortical gray matter usually spared.
  D. Clinical.
    1. Typically presents with slowly progressive mental deterioration, sensory deficits, visual loss, paralysis, and ataxia.
    2. Diagnosis in non-AIDS population may require biopsy.
    3. No proven effective therapy.
    4. Average survival less than 6 months.
  E. Imaging.
    1. CT.
      a. Single or multiple areas of low density in white matter (particularly frontal and parieto-occipital).
      b. No mass effect or enhancement.
    2. MRI.
      a. MRI more sensitive in detecting lesions than CT.

      b. Lesions typically hypointense or isointense to GM on T1WI and hyperintense on T2WI.

      c. Later in course, lesions may become confluent or show cavitation.

      d. Rarely, lesions may enhance peripherally.

  F. Differential diagnosis.

    1. Multiple sclerosis.

    2. ADEM.

    3. SSPE.

VII. Acute disseminated encephalomyelitis (ADEM) (see Chapter 53).

  A. Etiology.

    1. Probable immune-mediated response to preceding viral infection or vaccination.

    2. Occurs in several settings.

      a. Shortly after specific (usually viral) illness, especially measles or chickenpox, but also reported after rubella, mumps, smallpox, infectious mononucleosis, herpes zoster, influenza, herpes simplex encephalitis, coxsackie, legionella, leptospirosis, lyme disease.

      b. Following upper respiratory infection (presumably viral).

      c. Following vaccination against diptheria, pertussis, measles, rubella, tetanus, influenza, rabies, smallpox, typhoid, or polio.

      d. Spontaneously (possibly due to preceding subclinical viral infection).

  B. Incidence.

    1. True incidence unknown (as high as 1 in 300 after rabies vaccination and as low as 45 in 5 million after smallpox vaccination).

    2. Usually occurs in children between 5 to 10 years of age, although can occur at any age.

  C. Pathophysiology.

    1. Probably autoimmune reaction to myelin triggered by a virus or viral particle and mediated by antigen-antibody complexes.

    2. Multifocal perivascular (especially around venules) inflammation resulting in zones of demyelination.

    3. Perivascular astrocytosis occurs as disease resolves.

    4. Location.

      a. Most commonly subcortical white matter.

      b. Deep white matter, brainstem, and cerebellum often affected.

      c. Lesions are bilateral and widely distributed.

      d. Although typically a disease of white matter, involvement

of the basal ganglia and thalami have been reported (deep gray nuclei also contain oligodendrocytes and myelin).
  e. May involve cranial nerves (especially optic nerves).
  f. May also involve spinal cord.
D. Clinical.
  1. Typically presents 4 days to 3 weeks after initial infection with abrupt onset and monophasic course.
  2. Initial symptoms may be mild (fever, headache, drowsiness) but rapidly progress to seizures, focal neurologic deficits, and coma. Spinal cord involvement may present with symptoms of transverse myelitis.
  3. CSF studies may be normal or show only mild abnormality. No viral particles are isolated from CSF.
  4. Typical course lasts from several days to several weeks and results in complete recovery. Less common outcomes are permanent neurologic deficit (10% to 20%) or death (15% to 20%).
  5. Treatment: steroids.
E. Imaging.
  1. CT.
    a. May appear normal in early stages.
    b. May see bilateral ill-defined moderate to large low-density lesions without significant mass effect in subcortical white matter.
  2. MRI.
    a. MRI is superior to CT in detecting lesions.
    b. Typically observe multiple bilateral discrete T2-hyperintense areas in subcortical white matter, deep white matter, basal ganglia, thalami, brainstem, or cerebellum.
    c. Some lesions may show patchy, nodular, gyriform, or ring enhancement.
    d. May see optic nerve enhancement consistent with optic neuritis.
F. Differential diagnosis.
  1. Multiple sclerosis (lesions generally smaller, characteristic periventricular location).
  2. PML.
  3. SSPE.
VIII. Rasmussen encephalitis.
  A. Etiology.
    1. Chronic progressive localized encephalitis.
    2. Etiology not known, thought to be viral in origin.
  B. Incidence.

1. Rare.
2. Usually occurs in children (85% have onset <10 years of age), occasionally reported in adults.
C. Pathophysiology.
   1. Viral DNA from the herpesvirus family (e.g., cytomegalovirus, HSV type 1, EBV) have been demonstrated in affected brains, suggesting viral etiology, although to date no viral inclusions have been documented nor any virus successfully cultured from affected tissues.
   2. Pathology shows nonspecific diffuse inflammatory changes consistent with viral encephalitis, typically confined to one hemisphere.
D. Clinical.
   1. Typically progressive hemiplegia, psychomotor deterioration, and severe intractable seizures.
   2. Seizures may be of continuous nature (epilepsia partialis continua or generalized status epilepticus).
   3. May require biopsy for definitive diagnosis.
   4. In severe cases hemispherectomy may be only option for seizure control.
E. Imaging.
   1. CT.
      a. Initially may appear normal.
      b. May see progressive atrophy confined to one hemisphere.
   2. MRI.
      a. MRI is more sensitive than CT in detecting pathology.
      b. May see focal area(s) of T2-hyperintensity in affected brain, usually confined to one hemisphere.
F. Differential diagnosis: Dyke-Davidoff-Mason syndrome (may require biopsy for definitive diagnosis).
IX. Reyes Syndrome.
   A. Etiology.
      1. Disease of unknown cause.
      2. Associated with toxic agents including salicylates, aflatoxin, insectides.
   B. Incidence: usually affects children between 6 months and 16 years of age.
   C. Pathophysiology.
      1. Current theories postulate interaction of viral infection (e.g., varicella) and toxin.
      2. Pathology demonstrates severe diffuse brain edema.
      3. Liver failure in all cases.
   D. Clinical.

   1. Symptoms usually develop while patient is recovering from presumed viral illness.
   2. Initial symptoms include lethargy and vomiting but progress to seizures and coma.
   3. Death may occur as rapidly as within several days due to increased intracranial pressure.
   4. Mortality is approximately 20%.
   E. Imaging (CT/MRI): diffuse cerebral edema most common finding.
X. Creutzfeldt-Jakob disease (CJD) (see Chapter 54).
   A. Etiology.
      1. Thought to be transmitted by prions (proteinaceous infectious particles containing no nucleic acids).
      2. However, recent studies have also shown familial pattern, with up to 15% of cases occurring in autosomal dominant pattern.
   B. Incidence.
      1. Rare, approximately 1 per million.
      2. Onset is symmetrically distributed around a peak of 60 years (rarely occurs below age 40 or beyond age 80).
   C. Pathophysiology.
      1. Actual route of infection unknown. Only known cases of documented horizontal transmission have been with direct contact with infected organs, tissues, or instruments.
      2. Genetic studies have reported mutations on a gene (PRNP) that encodes for an essential protein component (PrP) often found in amyloid plaques of affected brains.
      3. Pathology shows spongiform encephalopathy with neuronal vacuolization, degeneration and gliosis; often with aggregates of PrP in the form of amyloid plaques.
      4. Predilection for cerebral cortex and basal ganglia, but all parts of CNS may be involved.
   D. Clinical.
      1. In early stages behaves like Alzheimer's disease.
      2. May have prodromal symptoms of visuo-spatial disorders or memory loss.
      3. Gradual onset of dementia with development of weakness as well as myoclonus, tremors, rigidity, and ataxia.
      4. Spectrum of disease.
         a. Typical generalized encephalopathy.
         b. Variant forms with predominant involvement localized to particular area: occipital lobe, striatum, thalamus, cerebellum, mesencephalon, or long white matter tracts.

    c. Gertsmann-Straussler-Scheinker syndrome (now felt to be a variant of CJD): cerebellar ataxia, dementia.

    d. Atypical forms: absence of spongiform change, long duration or spastic paralysis without significant cerebellar component.

  5. Disease is usually rapidly progressive, average survival less than 1 year (80%).

  6. Occasionally atypical forms may have more chronic course with survival exceeding several years (20%).

  7. Note: routine sterilizing procedures do not inactivate agent, requires steam autoclaving or immersion in sodium hydroxide or sodium hypochlorite.

  8. Diagnosis made by brain biopsy.

  9. No known treatment.

E. Imaging (CT/MRI).

  1. Imaging often normal.

  2. MRI may show foci of T2 hyperintensity in basal ganglia.

  3. May see diffuse cerebral and cerebellar atrophy later in disease.

SUGGESTED READINGS

Baganz MD, Dross PE, Reinhardt JA: Rocky mountain spotted fever encephalitis: MR findings, *AJNR* 16:919-922, 1995.

Baram TZ, Gonzalez-Gomez I, Xie Z-D, et al: Subacute sclerosing panencephalitis in an infant: diagnostic role of viral genome analysis, *Ann Neurol* 36:103-108, 1994.

Baum PA, Barkovich AJ, Koch TK, Berg BO: Deep gray matter involvement in children with acute disseminated encephalomyelitis, *AJNR* 15:1275-1283, 1994.

Belman AL, Iyer M, Coyle PK, Dattwyler R: Neurologic manifestations in children with North American Lyme disease, *Neurol* 43:2609-2614, 1993.

Defer G, Levy R, Brugieres P, Postic D, Degos JD: Lyme disease presenting as a stroke in the vertebrobasilar territory: MRI, *Neuroradiol* 35:529-531, 1993.

Demaerel P, Wilms G, Van Lierde S, Delanote J, Baert A: Lyme disease in childhood presenting as primary leptomeningeal enhancement without parenchymal findings on MR, *AJNR* 15:302-304, 1994.

Jay V, Becker LE, Otsubo H, et al: Chronic encephalitis and epilepsy (Rasmussen's encephalitis): detection of cytomegalovirus and herpes simplex virus 1 by the polymerase chain reaction and in situ hybridization, *Neurol* 45:108-117, 1995.

Leber SM, Brunberg JA, Pavkovic IM: Infarction of basal ganglia associated with California encephalitis virus, *Ped Neurol* 12:346-349, 1995.

McLachlan RS, Girvin JP, Blume WT, Reichman H: Rasmussen's chronic encephalitis in adults, *Arch Neurol* 50:269-274, 1993.

Osborn AG: Infection, white matter abnormalities, and degenerative diseases. In *Diagnostic radiology,* St Louis, 1994, Mosby, pp 671-715.

Reik L Jr: Stroke due to Lyme disease, *Neurol* 43:2705-2707, 1993.

Richardson EP, Masters CL: The nosology of Creutzfeldt-Jakob disease and conditions related to the accumulation of PrP^{CJD} in the nervous system, *Brain Pathol* 5:33-41, 1995.

Soo MS, Tien RD, Gray L, Andrews PI, Friedman H: Mesenrhomben-cephalitis: MR findings in nine patients, *AJR* 160:1089-1093, 1993.

Tien RD, Ashdown BC, Lewis DV Jr, Atkins MR, Burger PC: Rasmussen's encephalitis: neuroimaging findings in four patients, *AJR* 158:1329-1332, 1992.

Tien RD, Felsberg G, Osumi AK: Herpesvirus infections of the CNS: MR findings, *AJR* 161:167-176, 1993.

van der Meyden CH, de Villiers JFK, Middlecote BD, Terblanche J: Gadolinium ring enhancement and mass effect in acute disseminated encephalomyelitis, *Neuroradiol* 36:221-223, 1994.

Vinters HV, Wang R, Wiley CA:Herpesviruses in chronic encephalitis associated with intractable childhood epilepsy, *Hum Pathol* 24:871-879, 1993.

45

CNS Manifestations of HIV Infection

Key Concepts

1. CNS diseases in AIDS are primarily infectious or neoplastic.
2. Common organisms responsible for infectious CNS diseases include:
   a. HIV.
   b. Toxoplasma.
   c. Cryptococcus.
   d. Papovavirus (progressive multifocal encephalopathy).
   e. Cytomegalovirus.
3. Common neoplastic diseases involving CNS include:
   a. Primary CNS lymphoma.
   b. Secondary CNS lymphoma.
4. Other CNS manifestations include:
   a. Stroke.
   b. Hypoxic encephalopathy.
   c. Metabolic encephalopathy.
   d. Drug neurotoxicity.
5. AIDS dementia complex (ADC) describes a triad of cognitive, motor, and behavioral deterioration predominantly due to HIV encephalopathy although initially thought to be due to CMV.

I. General comments.
  A. CNS manifestations are frequently a secondary AIDS-defining illness and are presenting diseases in 5% to 10% of AIDS patients.
  B. Overall neurologic disease associated with HIV infection probably exceeds 50%.
  C. Only 5% of AIDS patients will have a normal brain at autopsy.
  D. AIDS dementia complex (ADC).
    1. Describes a clinical constellation of symptoms and signs rather than an established disease entity of specific etiology (although most studies now support predominant role of HIV).
    2. Key features.
      a. No alteration in level of alertness.
      b. Triad of cognitive, motor, and behavioral dysfunction.
    3. Classification or staging is based on ability to function. Two main schemes.
      a. AIDS dementia complex (ADC) stages: from 0 to 4, representing spectrum between normal function to nearly vegetative state.
      b. American Academy of Neurology AIDS Task Force: divided mainly into mild impairment (HIV-1 associated minor cognitive/motor disorder) and major impairment (HIV-1 associated cognitive/motor complex).
  E. Infection is most common pathologic process involving CNS:
    1. Infections can be caused by the following organisms:
      a. Common.
        (1) HIV.
        (2) Toxoplasma.
        (3) Cryptococcus.
        (4) Papovavirus (progressive multifocal encephalopathy).
        (5) Cytomegalovirus.
      b. Uncommon.
        (1) Coccidiodes.
        (2) Aspergillus.
        (3) Histoplasma.
        (4) Mycobacterium.
        (5) Treponema (syphilis).
        (6) Herpes simplex virus (types 1 or 2).
        (7) Varicella zoster.
        (8) Candida.
        (9) Nocardia.
    2. Infections manifest as specific processes.

    a. Meningitis (see box below).

      (1) Most commonly HIV or cryptococcal meningitis.

      (2) Less commonly tuberculous meningitis, syphilitic-meningitis, histoplasmosis, coccidiodomycosis.

      (3) Note: lymphoma can also cause meningitis.

    b. Parenchymal brain disease.

      (1) Diffuse involvement (see box on p. 459).

        (a) HIV.

        (b) PML.

        (c) CMV.

      (2) Focal involvement (mass lesion) (see box on p. 460).

        (a) Toxoplasma.

        (b) Tuberculous abscess.

        (c) Cryptococcoma.

        (d) Syphilitic gumma.

        (e) Candida abscess.

        (f) Nocardia abscess.

    c. Myelopathies.

      (1) Commonly caused by varicella zoster virus, cytomegalovirus, and toxoplasma.

      (2) Note: spinal lymphoma can also cause myelopathy.

  F. Neoplastic diseases involving CNS include:

    1. Primary neoplasms.

      a. Primary CNS lymphoma.

      b. Glioblastoma multiforme.

    2. Secondary neoplasms.

      a. Lymphoma.

      b. Immunoblastic sarcoma.

      c. Plasmacytoma.

      d. Karposi's sarcoma.

Differential Diagnosis of Leptomeningeal Enhancement in AIDS

Common

HIV aseptic meningitis
Cryptococcal meningitis
Tuberculous meningitis

Uncommon

Lymphoma (usually secondary)
Neurosyphilitic meningitis
Other fungal meningitis: candida, aspergillus, coccidiodomycosis

G. Other CNS manifestations include:
1. Stroke.
2. Hypoxic encephalopathy.
3. Metabolic encephalopathy.
4. Drug neurotoxicity.
II. HIV infection of the CNS.
A. Organism.
1. Human immunodeficiency virus (HIV) type 1 is a lymphotropic retrovirus that infects T4 helper cells, causing acquired immunodeficiency syndrome (AIDS), but is also neurotropic and can directly involve the peripheral and central nervous systems.
2. HIV is the most common CNS pathogen in AIDS patients, followed by Toxoplasma and Cryptococcus.
B. Incidence.
1. Early in the course of HIV infection, CNS infection may be asymptomatic.
2. HIV encephalopathy is noted at initial AIDS diagnosis in 10% and eventually develops in up to 65% of patients.
C. Pathophysiology.
1. AIDS encephalopathy was previously thought to be due to superimposed opportunistic infection (especially CMV) but now known to be primarily due to HIV organism.
2. Pathology reveals two major types of brain disease (although frequently overlap).
a. HIV encephalitis: multiple foci composed of microglial nodules, macrophages, multinucleated giant cells, and inflammatory infiltrates.
b. HIV leukoencephalopathy: diffuse white matter injury with myelin loss, reactive astrogliosis, macrophages, and multinucleated giant cells but little or no inflammatory infiltrates.

Differential Diagnosis of White Matter Lesions in AIDS

Common

HIV encephalitis
Progressive multifocal leukoencephalopathy

Uncommon

Vasculitis due to neurosyphilis, varicella zoster virus, aspergillosis or candidiasis

3. Location.
   a. Brain involvement.
      (1) Commonly involves periventricular white matter or centrum semiovale (especially frontal lobes).
      (2) Lesions usually bilateral.
      (3) Less commonly involves cerebellum or brainstem.
      (4) Gray matter usually spared.
   b. Meninges.
   c. Spinal cord.
   d. Peripheral nerves.
D. Clinical.
   1. HIV encephalopathy (previously known as subacute encephalitis, HIV dementia, and AIDS dementia) responsible for most cases of AIDS dementia complex.
   2. Other neurologic manifestations include:
      a. Meningitis (acute or chronic).
      b. Myelopathy.
      c. Peripheral neuropathy.
   3. Zidovudine (AZT) is the only studied therapy for CNS disease caused directly by HIV.
E. Imaging.
   1. CT.
      a. Asymptomatic HIV infection usually associated with normal imaging.
      b. Most common finding is diffuse cerebral and cerebellar atrophy.

Differential Diagnosis of Intracranial Mass Lesion in AIDS

Common

Toxoplasmosis
Lymphoma

Uncommon

Cryptococcoma
Tuberculoma or tuberculous abscess
Fungal abscess
Nocardia abscess
Neurosyphilitic gumma
Kaposi's sarcoma
Glioblastoma multiforme

       c. Multifocal bilateral hypodense areas in deep white matter also common.

  2. MRI.

      a. MR spectroscopy may be a more sensitive indicator of CNS involvement in early disease; findings include:

         (1) Reductions in N-acetyl aspartate (located solely in neurons and axons), consistent with neuronal loss.

         (2) Increased levels of choline (found in glial cells) in white matter, which may reflect astrocytosis or microglial proliferation.

      b. On conventional MRI typically observe ill-defined focal or confluent patches of T2-hyperintensity in deep white matter, especially in frontal lobes. Presence of focal lesions do not necessarily correlate with ADC (can be seen in asymptomatic patients), although severe white matter involvement is more likely to be symptomatic.

      c. Lesions do not enhance with contrast administration.

      d. Focal lesions may be seen in brainstem or cerebellum, although usually later in disease.

III. Toxoplasmosis.

  A. Organism.

    1. Toxoplasma gondii is a protozoan parasite that can cause infection in immunosuppressed populations or congenital infection (see Chapter 41).

    2. Chronic positive serology as high as 70% in general population.

    3. Organism is acquired by ingestion of poorly cooked meat containing tissue cysts or by direct/indirect exposure to oocysts in cat feces.

  B. Incidence.

    1. Toxoplasmosis is the most common superimposed opportunistic infection in AIDS patients.

    2. Encephalitis develops in up to 30% of AIDS patients who have toxoplasma antibodies.

    3. At autopsy 10% to 30% of AIDS patients have cerebral toxoplasmosis.

  C. Pathophysiology.

    1. Following acute inoculation, the organism assumes a latent form that later reactivates and becomes invasive (tachyzoites) when host experiences a decline in cell-mediated immunity.

    2. Toxoplasma lesions are characterized by three distinct zones and no capsule.

      a. Central zone of coagulative necrosis and few organisms.

      b. Intermediate zone of hypervascularity, inflammatory cells, and organisms (free tachyzoites > encysted forms).

      c. Peripheral zone mostly composed of encysted organisms.

      d. Usually surrounded by vasogenic edema.

  3. Location.

      a. Usually involves corticomedullary junction of frontal lobe or basal ganglia.

      b. Other sites (in descending order of frequency) include parietal lobe, occipital lobe, temporal lobe, cerebellum, centrum semiovale, thalamus.

  4. More commonly have multiple rather than solitary lesions (whereas lymphoma is more likely to have solitary lesion), although by itself is not a useful distinguishing feature.

D. Clinical.

  1. Toxoplasmic encephalitis in AIDS almost always represents reactivation of chronic (latent) infection; therefore the presence of IgG Toxoplasma antibodies in an AIDS patient must be regarded as a marker for potential development of disease.

  2. May have initial prodrome of fever and malaise, days to weeks before onset of neurologic illness.

  3. Subsequent focal neurologic symptoms (mild hemiparesis), seizures or confusion develop over 1 to 2 weeks (more rapid course than AIDS dementia complex or PML).

  4. Appearance of chorea in AIDS patients is highly suggestive of toxoplasmosis.

  5. Diagnosis suggested by clinical/radiologic improvement with antitoxoplasmosis therapy.

  6. Use of steroids should be avoided during therapeutic trials to differentiate between toxoplasmosis and lymphoma (both will demonstrate improvement).

  7. Definitive diagnosis often requires biopsy.

  8. Average survival 1 year after diagnosis.

E. Imaging.

  1. Nuclear imaging: SPECT studies may distinguish between toxoplasmosis and lymphoma (latter demonstrates intense activity on early and delayed images).

  2. CT.

      a. Usually show solitary or multiple hypodense or isodense ring-enhancing masses with peripheral edema. Often have "target" appearance. Enhancing portion probably corresponds to intermediate zone with hyperemia.

      b. Lesions generally range from 1 to 3 cm in diameter.

    c. Hemorrhage is uncommon (more likely in lymphoma), although may be seen in treated lesions.

    d. Upon institution of antitoxoplasmosis therapy, usually see decrease in size, number and edema of lesions over 2 to 4 weeks; time to complete resolution varies from 3 weeks to 6 months.

    e. Persistent enhancing areas after treatment may be at greater risk for recurrence.

    f. Follow-up scans may show calcification of treated lesions, focal atrophy, or encephalomalacia.

  3. MRI.

    a. Lesions typically slightly hypointense or isointense to GM on T1WI and hyperintense on T2WI; with surrounding edema.

    b. Focal nodular or ring-enhancement patterns can be seen.

 F. Differential diagnosis: Lymphoma (Table 45-1).

IV. Cryptococcosis (see also Chapter 47).

 A. Organism: Cryptococcus neoformans is ubiquitous fungus that enters body via respiratory tract.

 B. Incidence.

  1. Cryptococcus is the third most frequent CNS pathogen in AIDS patients, exceeded only by HIV and toxoplasma.

  2. 5% to 25% of AIDS patients develop cryptococcosis.

 C. Pathophysiology.

  1. Spreads hematogenously after entry.

  2. Spectrum of involvement.

Table 45-1 Differentiating Imaging Features of Toxoplasmosis and Lymphoma in AIDS

	Toxoplasmosis	Lymphoma
No. of lesions	Usually multiple	Usually one or two lesions
Size of lesions	Usually 1 to 3 cm	Usually larger than 3 cm
CT density	Hypodense or isodense	Often hyperdense
Hemorrhage	Rare	Occasional
White matter location	Usually corticomedullary junction or basal ganglia	Usually periventricular or corpus callosum
Response to antitoxoplasmosis therapeutic trial	Decrease in size, number and edema over 2 to 4 weeks	Rapid progression of disease

    a. Meningeal infiltration most common.

    b. Organisms may then infiltrate and dilate perivascular spaces with gelatinous mucoid material.

    c. Further spread along perivascular spaces into brain parenchyma can result in larger focal lesions consisting of organisms, inflammatory cells, and gelatinous mucoid material (cryptococcomas or cryptococcal pseudocysts).

D. Clinical.

  1. In AIDS patients, organism usually results in disseminated infection, unlike immunocompetent individuals where infection is usually limited to meningitis.

  2. Symptoms of meningitis are mild and insidious with low-grade fever, altered mentation, or behavior changes. Symptoms of meningeal irritation are minimal.

  3. Focal brain lesions may present with focal neurologic deficits.

  4. Diagnosis of cryptococcal meningitis can be made by identification of organism (India ink preparation) or cryptococcal antigen in serum or CSF; or by culture from body fluid or tissue.

  5. Treatment: various antifungal agents.

E. Imaging.

  1. CT.

    a. CT findings may be minimal; usually unable to detect meningeal pathology.

    b. May see small foci of hypodensity in basal ganglia or midbrain that represent dilated perivascular spaces or cryptococcal pseudocysts (cryptococcomas).

  2. MRI.

    a. Most common findings are small multifocal lesions in basal ganglia and midbrain; signal usually hypointense on T1WI and hyperintense on T2WI.

    b. Enhancement variable.

    c. Meningitis not usually detectable with imaging.

V. Progressive multifocal leukoencephalopathy (see also Chapter 44).

A. Etiology.

  1. Organism is ubiquitous JC polyomavirus of the papovavirus group (named after first reported patient, not to be confused with Jakob-Creutzfeldt disease).

  2. By puberty 70% of general population are seropositive.

B. Incidence.

  1. Generally occurs in immunocompromised population (see Chapter 44).

   2. Occurs in up to 5% of AIDS patients.
C. Pathophysiology.
   1. Organism preferentially infects and destroys oligoden-
      droglia.
   2. Pathology reveals areas of demyelination with areas of frank
      necrosis.
   3. Viral antigen or particles are demonstrated within intranuclear
      inclusions.
   4. Location.
      a. Most commonly frontal and parieto-occipital subcortical
         white matter, then spreads to deep white matter including
         internal and external capsules.
      b. Lesions tend to be more peripheral rather than periven-
         tricular.
      c. Any myelinated areas can be involved, including corpus
         callosum, thalami, basal ganglia.
      d. Brainstem or cerebellar involvement uncommon.
      e. Cortical gray matter usually spared.
D. Clinical.
   1. Slowly progressive mental deterioration, sensory deficits, vi-
      sual loss, paralysis, and ataxia.
   2. Usually no associated dementia.
   3. Prognosis worse with brainstem or cerebellar involvement.
   4. Diagnosis in AIDS setting can usually be made by clinical and
      radiologic findings.
   5. No proven effective therapy.
   6. Average survival less than 6 months, although rare cases of
      survival for several years.
E. Imaging.
   1. CT.
      a. Single or multiple areas of ill-defined low density in white
         matter.
      b. Usually no mass effect, edema, or enhancement.
   2. MRI.
      a. MRI more sensitive in detecting lesions than CT.
      b. Lesions typically hypointense or isointense to GM on
         T1WI and hyperintense on T2WI.
      c. Later in course, lesions may become confluent or show
         cavitation.
      d. Subcortical lesions usually involve U-fibers, resulting in a
         scalloped appearance.
      e. Although bilateral, lesions are asymmetric with one hem-

isphere often showing greater involvement (unlike metabolic or inherited white matter diseases).

    f. Rarely, lesions may show faint peripheral enhancement.

VI. Cytomegalovirus.

  A. Organism: cytomegalovirus is a member of the herpesvirus family.

  B. Incidence.

    1. Was recognized as one of the major opportunistic infections associated with HIV shortly after initial description of AIDS.

    2. Initially thought to be primarily responsible for AIDS dementia, but recent studies have shown a direct role of HIV itself.

    3. Is still thought to cause a subacute encephalitis that may be difficult to distinguish from HIV encephalopathy; therefore actual incidence unknown.

  C. Pathophysiology.

    1. Pathology reveals scattered microglial nodules predominantly in cortical gray matter, with occasional characteristic intranuclear inclusion bodies or evidence of CMV antigens, nucleic acid, or both.

    2. Location of involvement.

      a. Brain.

        (1) Encephalitis.

        (2) Necrotizing ependymitis.

        (3) Vasculitis.

      b. Cranial nerves.

      c. Spinal cord.

      d. Spinal nerves.

      e. Peripheral nerves.

  D. Clinical.

    1. Neurologic manifestations.

      a. CMV encephalitis and ependymitis often occur simultaneously (CMV ventriculoencephalitis): symptoms resemble that of HIV encephalopathy and may be difficult to distinguish.

      b. Some reports suggest that CMV encephalopathy is associated with later onset, more acute presentation, and shorter overall survival than HIV encephalopathy.

      c. Vasculitis: may present with focal neurologic defects due to ischemia/infarct.

      d. Polyradiculomyelitis: ascending weakness and hyporeflexia resembling Guillain-Barre syndrome.

      e. Radiculitis: involving cranial or spinal nerves.

      f. Peripheral neuropathy.

g. Chorioretinitis.
2. Presence of coexistent CMV infection of the eye or other organs may suggest diagnosis.
3. Diagnosis made by positive CSF cultures or biopsy.
E. Imaging.
1. CT.
a. May see generalized atrophy (as in HIV encephalopathy).
b. May see periventricular low-density changes.
c. Subependymal enhancement may be observed.
2. MRI.
a. Typically see confluent periventricular rim enhancement, resembling lymphoma (although latter tends to be thicker, irregular, and nodular) (see box below).
VII. Neurosyphilis.
A. Organism: Treponema pallidum is a spirochete that is responsible for one of the most common worldwide sexually transmitted diseases.
B. Incidence.
1. Positive serology in 1% to 3% of HIV-infected patients.
2. Syphilis is known to be associated with increased risk for HIV infection (presumably due to similar at-risk sexual practices); although it is unknown if HIV infection increases the risk of acquiring syphilis.
3. Syphilis in HIV patients tends to present younger than in immunocompetent populations.
C. Pathophysiology.
1. Organism is believed to be more aggressive in immunosuppressed HIV-infected patients than in immunocompetent individuals.
2. Two main pathologic processes.
a. Meningovasculitis: resulting in meningeal and perivascu-

Differential Diagnosis of Ependymal Enhancement in Aids

Common

Lymphoma
Cytomegalovirus ependymitis

Uncommon

Ependymitis due to intraventricular rupture of abscess or retrograde spread of basilar meningitis.
Glioblastoma multiforme

lar inflammatory infiltration and small-to-medium vessel arteritis.

   b. Focal lesions (gummas): circumscribed masses with granulation tissue that occur near cerebral convexities usually arising from pia or dura.

D. Clinical.

   1. CNS disease may occur at any stage of syphilis, although usually within 3 to 18 months in AIDS population. Acute syphilitic meningitis is most common manifestation in HIV-infected patients. Chronic encephalitis and tabes dorsalis generally not seen in AIDS population.

   2. Spectrum of manifestations.

      a. Acute syphilitic meningitis (usually within 2 years of infection): headache, meningismus, and cranial nerve abnormalities.

      b. Meningovascular neurosyphilis (5- to 7-year latent period): focal neurologic defects related to vascular insult.

      c. Chronic encephalitis or general paretic form due to involvement of cerebral cortex (10- to 20-year latent period): insidious progressive dementia, tremors, and weakness.

      d. Tabes dorsalis due to involvement of posterior columns and dorsal root ganglia of spinal cord (15- to 20-year latent period): lightning pains, dysuria, ataxia, Argyll-Robertson pupils, areflexia, loss of proprioception.

      e. Syphilitic meningomyelitis: e.g., spastic paraparesis.

      f. Syphilitic polyradiculopathy: e.g., progressive leg pain and weakness.

      g. Ocular manifestations: uveitis, chorioretinitis, retrobulbar neuritis.

      h. Otologic manifestation: sensorineural hearing loss.

   3. Diagnosis made by CSF treponemal tests.

   4. Treatment: penicillin.

E. Imaging (intracranial).

   1. CT.

      a. May see infarcts in basal ganglia or middle cerebral artery territory.

      b. May see isolated, peripherally located circumscribed contrast-enhancing masses (gummas) with moderate to marked edema. May be associated with adjacent dural thickening and enhancement (mimicking meningioma).

   2. MRI.

      a. MRI more sensitive than CT, better able to detect small infarcts (especially in brainstem).

       b. May detect leptomeningeal enhancement.

       c. May detect cranial nerve involvement with enhancement particularly of optic and vestibulocochlear nerves.

VIII. Mycobacterium (see also Chapter 46).

  A. Organisms.

    1. Mycobacterium tuberculosis.

    2. Mycobacterium avium intracellulare (MAI).

    3. Atypical mycobacteria.

  B. Incidence.

    1. HIV infection now thought to be most important risk factor for subsequent M. tuberculosis infection.

    2. 30% of all TB patients are HIV-positive; 5% to 10% of AIDS patients have TB.

    3. CNS tuberculosis occurs in up to 20% of AIDS patients, specific incidence varies with subpopulations.

    4. 90% of TB cases in AIDS occur in IV drug abusers; two thirds of these cases initially present with TB.

    5. Disseminated MAI infection reported in 5% of AIDS patients; CNS involvement probably rarer.

  C. Pathophysiology.

    1. Most tuberculosis in AIDS probably due to reactivation of latent infection rather than progression of primary infection.

    2. Mycobacterium tuberculosis can produce spectrum of craniospinal disease.

      a. Tuberculous meningitis is most common (see Chapter 42).

      b. Tuberculoma, tuberculous abscess (see Chapter 46).

      c. Subacute encephalitis.

      d. Spondylitis (Pott's disease).

    3. MAI and other atypical mycobacteria more commonly result in intracerebral mass lesions (granuloma or abscess).

  D. Clinical.

    1. Tuberculous meningitis often occurs concurrently with brain granulomas or abscesses, and therefore symptoms may reflect both focal and diffuse disease.

    2. Parenchymal lesions may require biopsy for definitive diagnosis.

    3. Treatment for TB consists of combination antituberculous therapy.

    4. Newer strains of M. tuberculosis and atypical mycobacterial infections are notoriously resistant to standard therapy.

  E. Imaging.

    1. Communicating hydrocephalus due to obstruction of basal

cisterns by dense inflammatory exudate is most common finding (50%).

2. Basilar meningeal enhancement frequent (40%).
3. Parenchymal involvement is less common.
    a. Tuberculoma (25%).
        (1) Often multiple (35%), less than 1 cm.
        (2) MRI.
            (a) Early tuberculomas are isointense on T1WI and hypointense on T2WI; more solidly enhancing.
            (b) Mature tuberculomas hypointense centrally with isointense capsule on T2WI; occasionally hyperintense centrally with hypointense rim.
    b. Tuberculous abscess (20%).
        (1) Usually appears as ring-enhancing lesion with moderate edema, which may be indistinguishable from toxoplasma lesion, lymphoma, or pyogenic abscess.
4. Infarcts (particularly of basal ganglia) occur in 25%.

IX. Primary CNS lymphoma.
    A. Etiology: usually B cell NHL.
    B. Incidence: occurs in 6% of AIDS patients.
    C. Pathophysiology.
        1. Tendency to necrosis, unlike disease in immunocompetent individuals (see Chapter 32).
        2. Usually located in periventricular white matter or basal ganglia.
    D. Clinical.
        1. Usually present with progressive focal or multifocal neurologic deficits.
        2. Course is slightly slower than toxoplasmosis.
        3. Corticosteroids should be avoided if considering therapeutic trial to differentiate between toxoplasmosis and lymphoma.
        4. Definitive diagnosis made by biopsy.
        5. Treatment: radiation therapy.
        6. Poor prognosis, average survival 3 months (even shorter than in immunocompetent population).
    E. Imaging (CT/MRI).
        1. Although microscopically multicentric, imaging studies often only show one or two lesions with predilection for periventricular white matter or corpus callosum.
        2. Unlike lesions in immunocompetent individuals, more likely to have ring-enhancing pattern rather than homogeneous enhancement.
        3. May occasionally see hemorrhage (more common than in toxoplasmosis).

    4. May see ependymal enhancement, which is usually irregular, thick, and more nodular than CMV ependymitis.

   F. Differential diagnosis: Toxoplasmosis (Table 45-1).

X. Secondary CNS lymphoma.

   A. Etiology: usually systemic high-grade B-cell NHL (immunoblastic lymphoma, Burkitt's lymphoma).

   B. Incidence: occurs in 2% to 3% of AIDS patients.

   C. Pathophysiology: meningeal involvement is more frequent in AIDS-related systemic lymphomas (10% to 25% at initial presentation) than disease in immunocompetent populations.

   D. Clinical: prognosis is poor, average survival of 5 weeks.

   E. Imaging (CT/MRI): may see diffuse meningeal enhancement.

XI. Glioma.

   A. Etiology: astrocytoma, glioblastoma multiforme, and astroblastoma.

   B. Incidence: rare.

   C. Pathophysiology: studies suggest that RNA retroviruses may have a role in activation of dominant oncogenes and inactivation of tumor suppressor genes, resulting in genesis of gliomas.

   D. Clinical: present with focal neurologic signs.

   E. Imaging (CT/MRI): identical to tumors in immunocompetent patients (see Chapter 25).

SUGGESTED READINGS

Bacellar H, Munoz A, Miller EN, et al: Temporal trends in the incidence of HIV-1-related neurologic diseases: multicenter AIDS cohort study, 1985-1992, *Neurol* 44:1892-1900, 1994.

Barker PB, Lee RR, McArthur JC: AIDS dementia complex: evaluation with proton MR spectroscopic imaging, *Radiol* 195:58-64, 1995.

Bertoli F, Espino M, Arosemena JR, Fishback JL, Frenkel JK: A spectrum in the pathology of toxoplasmosis in patients with acquired immunodeficiency syndrome, *Arch Pathol Lab Med* 119:214-224, 1995.

Brightbill TC, Ihmeidan IH, Post MJD, Berger JR, Katz DA: Neurosyphilis in HIV-positive and HIV-negative patients: neuroimaging findings, *AJNR* 16:703-711, 1995.

Broderick DF, Wippold FJ II, Clifford DB, Kido D, Wilson BS: White matter lesions and cerebral atrophy on MR images in patients with and without AIDS dementia complex, *AJR* 161:177-181, 1993.

Chang L, Cornford ME, Chiang FL, et al: Radiologic-pathologic correlation: cerebral toxoplasmosis and lymphoma in AIDS, *AJNR* 16:1653-1664, 1995.

Chong WK, Paley M, Wilkinson ID, et al: Localized cerebral proton MR spectroscopy in HIV infection and AIDS, *AJNR* 15:21-25, 1994.

Cortey A, Jarvik JG, Lenkinski RE, et al: Proton MR spectroscopy of brain abnormalities in neonates born to HIV-positive mothers, *AJNR* 15:1853-1859, 1994.

Enting RH, Esselink RAJ, Portegies P: Lymphomatous meningitis in AIDS-related systemic non-Hodgkin's lymphoma: a report of eight cases, *J Neurol Neurosurg Psych* 57:150-153, 1994.

Falangola MF, Reichler BS, Petito CK: Histopathology of cerebral toxoplasmosis in human immunodeficiency virus infection: a comparison between patients with early-onset and late-onset acquired immunodeficiency syndrome, *Hum Pathol* 25:1091-1097, 1994.

Hawkins CP, McLaughlin JE, Kendall BE, McDonald WI: Pathological findings correlated with MRI in HIV infection, *Neuroradiol* 35:264-268, 1993.

Holland NR, Power C, Mathews VP, et al: Cytomegalovirus encephalitis in acquired immunodeficiency syndrome (AIDS), *Neurol* 44:507-514, 1994.

Laissy JP, Soyer P, Parlier C, et al: Persistent enhancement after treatment for cerebral toxoplasmosis in patients with AIDS: predictive value for subsequent recurrence, *AJNR* 15:1773-1778, 1994.

Manji H, McAllister R, Valentine AR, et al: Serial MRI of the brain in asymptomatic patients infected with HIV: results from the UCMSM/Medical Research Council neurology cohort, *J Neurol Neurosurg Psych* 57:144-149, 1994.

Olson EM, Healy JF, Wong WHM, Youmans DC, Hesselink JR: MR detection of white matter disease of the brain in patients with HIV infection: fast spin-echo vs conventional spin-echo pulse sequences, *AJR* 162:1199-1204, 1994.

Osborn AG: Infection, white matter abnormalities, and degenerative diseases. In *Diagnostic radiology,* St Louis, 1994, Mosby, pp 671-715.

Post MJD, Berger JR, Duncan R, et al: Asymptomatic and neurologically symptomatic HIV-seropositive subjects: results of long-term MR imaging and clinical follow-up, *Radiol* 188:727-733, 1993.

Ruiz A, Ganz WI, Post JD, et al: Use of thallium-201 brain SPECT to differentiate cerebral lymphoma from toxoplasma encephalitis in AIDS patients, *AJNR* 15:1885-1894, 1994.

Sweeney BJ, Manji H, Miller RF, et al: Cortical and subcortical JC virus infection: two unusual cases of AIDS associated progressive multifocal leukoencephalopathy, *J Neurol Neurosurg Psych* 57:994-997, 1994.

von Giesen H-J, Arendt G, Neuen-Jacob E, et al: A pathologically distinct new form of HIV associated encephalopathy, *J Neurology Sci* 121:215-221, 1994.

Wheeler AL, Truwit CL, Kleinschmidt-DeMasters BK, Byrne WR, Hannon RN: Progressive multifocal leukoencephalopathy: contrast enhancement on CT scans and MR images, *AJR* 161:1049-1051, 1993.

Whiteman M, Espinoza L, Post MJD, Bell MD, Falcone S: Central nervous system tuberculosis in HIV-infected patients: clinical and radiographic findings, *AJNR* 16:1319-1327, 1995.

Whiteman MLH, Post MJD, Berger JR, et al: Progressive multifocal leukoencephalopathy in 47 HIV-seropositive patients: neuroimaging with clinical and pathologic correlation, *Radiol* 187:233-240, 1993.

Winstanley P: Drug treatment of toxoplasmic encephalitis in acquired immunodeficiency syndrome, *Postgrad Med J* 71:404-408, 1995.

46

Granulomatous Diseases

Key Concepts

1. There is an increasing prevalence of tuberculosis in developed countries due to HIV, IV drug abuse, immunocompromised states, homelessness, crowded conditions in confined populations (e.g., prisons and nursing homes), and immigration from endemic areas.
2. Newer strains of mycobacterium are more resistant to conventional therapy.
3. CNS tuberculosis can cause:
   a. Chronic meningitis.
   b. Encephalitis.
   c. Tuberculoma or abscess.
4. Chronic meningitis is the most common manifestation of CNS tuberculosis.
5. Miliary pattern is uncommon except in children with tuberculosis meningitis.
6. Noninfectious granulomatous diseases of the CNS include:
   a. Neurosarcoidosis.
   b. Wegener's granulomatosis.
   c. Langerhans cell histiocytosis.

I. Tuberculosis.
  A. Organism.
    1. Mycobacterium tuberculosis is responsible for most mycobacterium infections, including that of the CNS.
    2. Mycobacterium avium-intracellulare (MAI) complex rarely involves the CNS.
  B. Incidence.
    1. Increasing prevalence of tuberculosis in the United States and other developed countries probably due to HIV (see Chapter 45), IV drug abuse, immunocompromised states, homelessness, crowded conditions in confined populations (e.g., prisons and nursing homes), and immigration from endemic areas. Newer strains also more resistant to conventional therapy.
    2. Childhood tuberculosis accounts for 5% of cases in the United States; most patients are less than 5 years of age and are from minority groups (especially blacks and Hispanics).
    3. Highest incidence of adult tuberculosis occurs in the elderly population.
    4. 25% to 50% of cases in the United States are related to immigrant populations.
    5. Outbreaks frequently occur in crowded populations.
    6. Tuberculosis remains important public health problem worldwide.
  C. Pathophysiology.
    1. Most pediatric infections are primary.
    2. Most adult infections (including those in HIV-infected populations) are due to reactivation, although with changing epidemiology, 10% to 30% of adult tuberculosis now due to primary infection.
    3. CNS infection results from hematogenous spread from a primary focus, usually pulmonary tuberculosis.
    4. Craniospinal infection has various manifestations.
      a. Chronic meningitis (see Chapter 42): most common.
      b. Encephalitis.
      c. Tuberculoma, tuberculous abscess: account for up to 30% of intracranial mass lesions in developing countries, rare in developed countries.
        (1) Tuberculoma.
          (a) Solid granuloma with minimal central caseating necrosis surrounded by epitheloid cells, multinucleated giant cells, and mononuclear inflammatory cells. Few bacilli are seen.
          (b) Location.

(i) Cerebrum (periventricular or corticomedullary junctions), cerebellum, subarachnoid space, subdural space, or epidural space.
(ii) Brainstem and ventricles are uncommon sites.
(iii) Lesions in adults are usually supratentorial; lesions in children are frequently infratentorial (60%).
(c) Usually solitary although 10% to 35% multiple.
(d) Usually unilocular and less than 1 cm.
(e) Miliary pattern is uncommon except in children with tuberculous meningitis.
(2) Tuberculous abscess.
(a) Central caseating necrosis and semiliquid pus with numerous bacilli. Wall lacks giant cell epitheliod reaction.
(b) Typically solitary, multiloculated, and usually larger than 1 cm.
d. Spondylitis (Pott's disease): common.
D. Clinical.
1. Symptoms dependent on involved location.
a. Meningitis usually presents with headache and low-grade fever.
b. Tuberculomas and tuberculous abscesses often do not result in symptoms, although large lesions may be associated with focal neurologic deficit.
2. Antituberculous drug therapy remains predominant treatment.
3. Adjunctive steroid therapy may lower incidence of neurologic sequelae.
4. Surgical intervention includes shunting procedures for obstructive hydrocephalus and biopsy of mass lesions.
5. Overall mortality in TB meningitis is 25% to 30%; long-term morbidity ranges from 65% to 90% of survivors.
E. Imaging.
1. Angiography.
a. May see vessel irregularities, stenoses, or occlusion, particularly at distal supraclinoid internal carotid artery.
b. Signs of infarct involving lenticulostriates or MCA territory.
2. CT.
a. Meningitis usually results in obliteration of basal cisterns on NECT; enhancement of thickened meninges on CECT.
b. May see "popcorn"-like dystrophic calcifications around basal cisterns.
c. Sequelae of meningitis include hydrocephalus, infarc-

tion (especially in basal ganglia and MCA territory), and atrophy.

   d. Tuberculomas and tuberculous abscesses may be indistinguishable on imaging studies, however:

     (1) Tuberculomas are generally small (<1 cm) lesions with nodular or ring enhancement, and often multiple.

     (2) Tuberculous abscesses are generally larger (>1 cm) with more typical ring enhancement pattern, and usually solitary.

   e. May see multiple small (miliary) nodules at corticomedullary junction and in distribution of perforating vessels (thalami, basal ganglia, brainstem), especially in pediatric patients.

   f. Healed tuberculomas often calcify.

  3. MRI.

   a. Exudate in basal cisterns may be difficult to see on non-contrast studies.

   b. Early tuberculomas are usually isointense on T1WI and hypointense on T2WI (latter probably due to greater amount of fibrosis, gliosis, and inflammatory cellular infiltrate).

   c. Mature tuberculomas are hypointense centrally with isointense capsule on T2WI; occasionally hyperintense centrally with hypointense rim.

   d. Tuberculous abscesses are usually ring-enhancing lesions with less edema than pyogenic abscesses.

   e. Miliary nodules appear as multiple small foci of T2 hyperintensity with nodular enhancement.

   f. Radiologic improvement may lag behind clinical improvement; may even occasionally see paradoxic enlargement of tuberculomas during therapy, which may not correlate with clinical improvement (phenomenon may represent effects of host immune response).

II. Neurosarcoid.

  A. Etiology: unknown.

  B. Incidence.

   1. Sarcoidosis is most prevalent in young (20 to 40 years), female black population.

   2. CNS involvement usually occurs with systemic disease: 5% by clinical presentation, up to 15% by autopsy.

   3. 3% neurosarcoidosis occurs without systemic disease.

   4. CNS manifestations generally occur in more aggressive disease.

  C. Pathophysiology.

1. CNS manifestations: noncaseating granulomatous involvement of:
   a. Meninges.
   b. Brain: parenchymal and perivascular (may result in vasculitis and infarct).
   c. Ependyma.
   d. Cranial nerves: especially CNs VII, II, and VIII.
   e. Spinal cord: intramedullary or extramedullary (latter resembling meningioma).
2. Head and neck.
   a. Orbital involvement: ocular globe, conjunctiva, extraocular muscles, retrobulbar fat, lacrimal gland.
   b. Adenopathy.
3. Peripheral nerves.
D. Clinical.
1. 50% of CNS involvement is subclinical.
2. CNS symptoms are location-dependent, may include headache, cranial neuropathy (e.g., optic neuritis), hypothalamic/pituitary dysfunction (e.g., diabetes insipidus), hearing loss (due to CPA disease) focal neurologic deficits or cauda equina syndrome.
3. Seizures are rare (should suggest other pathology).
4. Diagnosis suggested by elevated serum angiotensin-converting enzyme (ACE) or systemic disease (e.g., pulmonary). CSF ACE levels may be elevated, although actual sensitivity unknown. May require biopsy.
5. Treatment: steroids.
E. Imaging.
1. Angiography: nonspecific vessel irregularities, stenoses, and mild dilatations.
2. CT.
   a. May see diffuse or focal meningeal thickening that enhances strongly. Basal cisterns commonly involved.
   b. Sequelae include hydrocephalus and infarcts.
3. MRI.
   a. Often more sensitive than CT.
   b. Diffuse or focal leptomeningeal enhancement common.
   c. Periventricular high signal lesions on T2WI also common, may resemble multiple sclerosis. Occasionally periaqueductal high signal observed.
   d. Less commonly observe focal parenchymal mass (granuloma) with patchy or nodular enhancement.
   e. May see thickened infundibulum, chiasm, or both.
   f. May see cranial nerve enhancement (especially CNs II, VII).

      g. Optic nerve(s) may demonstrate enhancement (may mimic optic nerve sheath meningioma) or atrophy.

      h. Small infarcts, especially brainstem lesions, are better seen on MRI.

      i. May see ependymal enhancement.

      j. Ventricular enlargement may be due to hydrocephalus (communicating, or obstruction at aqueduct), or atrophy.

      k. Rarely observe dural-based mass(es) that may mimic meningioma. Often isointense on T1WI and hypointense on T2WI (may be due to hypercellularity and fibrous stroma).

III. Wegener's granulomatosis.

  A. Etiology.

    1. Etiology unknown: theories include autoimmune diseases or delayed hypersensitivity reaction to unknown antigen or organism.

    2. Disease classification and staging (current concept).

      a. Purely granulomatous Wegener's granulomatosis (PGWG): primarily involving ears, nose, throat, eyes, or lungs.

      b. Limited Wegener's granulomatosis (not to be confused with lethal midline granuloma): confined to one organ (frequently kidney). Note: previous use of this designation was for nonrenal disease.

      c. Classic Wegener's granulomatosis: chronic multisystem disorder usually involving the respiratory tract, kidneys, eyes, and skin.

  B. Incidence.

    1. Wegener's granulomatosis is uncommon disease, usually occurring in young or middle-age Caucasians.

    2. Head and neck involvement common.

    3. CNS involvement occurs in 15% to 30% of cases.

  C. Pathophysiology.

    1. Pathology reveals necrotizing granulomatous vasculitis due to neutrophilic infiltration and fibrinoid necrosis.

    2. CNS manifestations.

      a. Direct granulomatous invasion from contiguous lesions in nose and paranasal sinuses.

      b. Primary intracranial lesions: meningeal, focal parenchymal granulomas.

      c. Vasculitis: small-vessel arteritis.

    3. May have peripheral nerve involvement.

  D. Clinical.

    1. Systemic symptoms nonspecific (e.g., fever, malaise). Nasal/paranasal sinus involvement may present with symptoms of

sinusitis, epistaxis, and destructive nasal deformity (saddle nose). CNS symptoms include headache, cranial neuropathy, hearing loss.

   2. Diagnosis suggested by serum anti-neutrophil cytoplasmic antibody (ANCA). Definitive diagnosis made by biopsy (e.g., nasal, lung, renal).

   3. Treatment: steroids, cyclophosphamide. Plasmapheresis may be used in rapidly progressive disease.

E. Imaging.

   1. Angiography: nonspecific arterial wall irregularities and occlusions.

   2. CT/MRI.

     a. May see diffuse nodular, thickened enhancing meninges.

     b. May see focal infarcts.

     c. Rarely see enhancing parenchymal granulomas.

IV. Langerhans cell histiocytosis.

A. Etiology.

   1. Multisystem disease characterized by nonmalignant proliferation of histiocytic granulomas in tissues.

   2. Exact etiology unknown; theories include immune reaction to unknown antigen and autoimmune disease.

B. Incidence.

   1. Primarily a disease of childhood; rare in adults.

   2. CNS manifestations occur predominantly in chronic, recurring disseminated form also known as Hand-Schuller-Christian disease (90%).

   3. Calvarial lesions occur predominantly in acute form also known as eosinophilic granuloma.

C. Pathophysiology.

   1. Histology reveals Langerhans cells, which are unique histiocytes that stain for S-100 protein and contain Birbeck granules on electron microscopy.

   2. More common cranial involvement is of calvarium.

   3. CNS manifestations involve:

     a. Infundibulum/hypothalamus.

     b. Meninges: leptomeninges >> dura.

     c. Cranial nerves.

     d. Brain parenchyma: cerebral hemispheres, basal ganglia, brainstem, cerebellum: rare.

     e. Spinal cord: rare.

D. Clinical.

   1. Symptoms include hypothalamic/pituitary dysfunction (e.g., diabetes insipidus), visual disturbances, ataxia.

    2. Treatment: low-dose radiation therapy.
E. Imaging.
  1. CT.
    a. May see infundibular thickening.
    b. Focal masses are of variable density on NECT and enhance strongly and uniformly on CECT.
  2. MRI.
    a. MRI more sensitive than CT.
    b. May see infundibular thickening or focal hypothalamic mass.
    c. Focal parenchymal masses usually isointense to GM on T1WI and T2WI and enhance homogeneously (multiple lesions may mimic metastases).
    d. May observe absence of posterior pituitary "bright spot."
    e. May see diffuse thick, nodular leptomeningeal enhancement; occasionally focal dural-based mass (may mimic meningioma).
    f. May see cranial nerve enlargement and enhancement.

SUGGESTED READINGS

Afghani B, Lieberman JM: Paradoxical enlargement or development of intracranial tuberculomas during therapy: case report and review, *Clin Infect Dis* 19:1092-1099, 1994.

Burlacoff SG, Wong FSH: Wegener's granulomatosis—the great masquerade: a clinical presentation and literature review, *J Otolaryng* 22:94-105, 1993.

Carmody RF, Mafee MF, Goodwin JA, Small K, Haery C: Orbital and optic pathway sarcoidosis: MR findings, *AJNR* 15:773-783, 1994.

Goldberg-Stern H, Weitz R, Zaizov R, Gornish M, Gadoth N: Progressive spinocerebellar degeneration "plus" associated with Langerhans cell histiocytosis: a new paraneoplastic syndrome? *J Neurol Neurosurg Psych* 58:180-183, 1995.

Gropper MR, Schulder M, Duran HL, Wolansky L: Cerebral tuberculosis with expansion into brainstem tuberculoma: report of two cases, *J Neurosurg* 81:927-931, 1994.

Kioumehr F, Dadsetan MR, Rooholami A, Au A: Central nervous system tuberculosis: MRI, *Neuroradiol* 36:93-96, 1994.

Lexa FJ, Grossman RI: MR of sarcoidosis in the head and spine: spectrum of manifestations and radiographic response to steroids, *AJNR* 15:973-982, 1994.

Nishino H, Rubino FA, Parisi JE: The spectrum of neurologic involvement in Wegener's granulomatosis, *Neurol* 43:1334-1337, 1993.

Osborn AG: Infection, white matter abnormalities, and degenerative diseases. In *Diagnostic radiology,* St Louis, 1994, Mosby, pp 671-715.

Poe LB, Dubowy RL, Hochhauser L, et al: Demyelinating and gliotic cerebellar lesions in Langerhans cell histiocytosis, *AJNR* 15:1921-1928, 1994.

Tishler S, Williamson T, Mirra SS, et al: Wegener granulomatosis with meningeal involvement, *AJNR* 14:1248-1252, 1993.

Weinberger LM, Cohen ML, Remler BF, Naheedy MH, Leigh RJ: Intracranial Wegener's granulomatosis, *Neurol* 43:1831-1834, 1993.

Wilson JD, Castillo M, Van Tassel P: MRI features of intracranial sarcoidosis mimicking meningiomas, *Clin Imag* 18:184-188, 1994.

47

Fungal and Parasitic Infections

Key Concepts

1. Fungal and parasitic infections of the CNS are generally uncommon and often require impairment of host immune system.
2. Frequent fungal CNS infections in the immunocompromised ("opportunistic" infections) include:
   a. Aspergillosis.
   b. Candidiasis.
   c. Cryptococcosis.
   d. Mucormycosis.
3. CNS manifestation of fungal infection are generally of three forms (although pattern varies with different fungi).
   a. Meningitis.
   b. Granuloma or abscess.
   c. Encephalitis.
4. Aspergillus and mucorales are angio-invasive and are prone to arterial, venous, or cavernous sinus thrombosis and infarct.
5. Parasitic CNS infections in North America include toxoplasmosis, cysticercosis, and echinococcus.
6. Neurocysticercosis typically occurs in four stages.
   a. Vesicular stage: live larvum.
   b. Colloidal vesicular stage: larvum dies, inciting inflammatory reaction.
   c. Granular nodular stage: cyst degenerates, edema diminishes, and scolex begins to calcify.
   d. Nodular calcified stage: lesion completely calcifies.

I. Fungal infections.
  A. General comments.
    1. Fungi are ubiquitous single-celled organisms that are distinctly different from bacteria.
    2. Most fungal infections require some decrease in normal host resistance (i.e., "opportunistic" infections).
      a. Aspergillosis.
      b. Candidiasis.
      c. Cryptococcosis.
      d. Mucormycosis.
    3. Some fungal infections can occur in immunocompetent individuals.
      a. Histoplasmosis.
      b. Coccidiomycosis.
      c. Blastomycosis.
      d. Aspergillosis.
    4. Fungal infection of the CNS is uncommon, although a recent rise has occurred due to more aggressive chemotherapy, immunosuppressive therapy, and AIDS.
    5. CNS manifestation usually of three forms (although pattern varies with different fungi).
      a. Meningitis.
      b. Granuloma or abscess.
      c. Encephalitis.
  B. Aspergillosis.
    1. Organism: Aspergillus fumigatus is acquired by inhaling spores.
    2. Incidence.
      a. Immunosuppressed (including diabetics) populations >> immunocompetent populations.
      b. Cerebral aspergillosis occurs in 10% to 15% of infections.
    3. Pathophysiology.
      a. Spread.
        (1) Usually spreads hematogeneously from primary pulmonary focus of infection.
        (2) May spread contiguously from paranasal sinus mycetoma.
      b. Patterns of involvement.
        (1) Direct contiguous spread may result in focal adjacent dural infiltration. (Diffuse meningitis is rare).
        (2) Tends to be angio-invasive, affecting medium and large vessels, resulting in:
          (a) Mycotic aneurysm.
          (b) Thrombosis and infarct.

(i) Often of MCA or lenticulostriate arteries.

(ii) Commonly hemorrhagic.

(c) Thrombosis of cavernous sinus.

(3) Subsequent parenchymal infection (aspergilloma or abscess) can develop at site of infarct, thereby converting sterile infarct to septic infarct. Predilection for cortical-subcortical junction, basal ganglia, and cerebellum.

4. Clinical.

   a. Symptoms commonly include seizures or stroke. Cavernous sinus syndrome may present with exophthalmos, headache, and papilledema.

   b. CSF findings nonspecific, organism rarely cultured from CSF.

   c. Diagnosis suggested by pulmonary infection. Definitive diagnosis may require biopsy.

   d. Mortality of cerebral aspergillosis >90% in immunosuppressed populations.

   e. Treatment: aggressive antifungal therapy; occasionally surgical aspiration of abscess performed.

5. Imaging.

   a. Angiography: may see mycotic aneurysm, thrombosis, secondary signs of infarct.

   b. CT.

      (1) Typically see multiple low-density subcortical lesions with minimal mass effect representing areas of ischemia/infarction.

      (2) Hemorrhage may occur in mycetomas or infarcts.

      (3) Granulomas are typically ring or nodular enhancing lesions (usually implies intact host defense system and therefore more commonly seen in immunocompetent population). Thickness of ring-enhancing wall often thicker, more irregular than pyogenic abscess.

      (4) May see focal dural enhancement adjacent to areas of contiguous spread, frequently inferior frontal or temporal areas.

      (5) Healed parenchymal lesions may calcify.

   c. MRI.

      (1) Parenchymal lesions often hypointense on T1WI and isointense on PD and T2WI, surrounded by edema.

      (2) May also see hypointense rim on T2WI, which has been attributed to dense population of hyphal elements, presence of iron, magnesium or manganese, or presence of hemorrhagic products.

C. Mucormycosis.
  1. Organism: ubiquitous saprophyte belonging to order Muco-
     rales.
  2. Incidence.
     a. Overall incidence low.
     b. 90% of mucormycosis occurs in immunosuppressed popu-
        lation, including HIV-infected, diabetics, patients on steroids
        or who abuse IV drugs.
  3. Pathophysiology.
     a. Spread.
        (1) Usually spreads contiguously (e.g., perineural or peri-
            vascular) from nasal/paranasal sinus infection—rhino-
            cerebral mucormycosis.
            (a) Through cribriform plate into inferior frontal lobes.
            (b) Through orbital apex into cavernous sinus.
        (2) Less common is hematogenous spread (e.g., IV drug
            abuse).
     b. Patterns of involvement.
        (1) Tends to be angio-invasive: causing both arterial and ve-
            nous thrombosis/infarct or cavernous sinus thrombosis.
        (2) May form parenchymal fungal abscesses.
  4. Clinical.
     a. Symptoms nonspecific, similar to aspergillosis.
     b. Infection is rapidly progressive.
     c. Diagnosis suggested by nasal/paranasal disease. Definitive
        diagnosis may require biopsy.
     d. Treatment: aggressive antifungal therapy.
  5. Imaging (CT/MRI).
     a. May see infarcts particularly in inferior frontal or temporal
        lobes.
     b. May see nodular or ring-enhancing fungal abscess(es).
D. Cryptococcosis or Torulosis.
  1. Organism: Cryptococcus neoformans (also known as Torula
     histolytica) is ubiquitous fungus that enters body via respiratory
     tract.
  2. Incidence: increased incidence in HIV-infected population (see
     Chapter 45).
  3. Pathophysiology.
     a. Spreads hematogenously after entry.
     b. Spectrum of CNS involvement.
        (1) Meningeal infiltration: most common.
        (2) Perivascular infiltration and dilatation with gelatinous
            mucoid material.

(3) Formation of gelatinous parenchymal lesions (crypto-coccomas or gelatinous pseudocysts) with predilection for basal ganglia. True granulomas are rare.

4. Clinical.
   a. Symptoms of meningitis are mild and insidious with low-grade fever, minimal meningeal irritation, altered mentation or behavioral changes.
   b. Focal brain lesions may present with focal neurologic deficits.
   c. Diagnosis made by isolation of organism (India ink preparation) or cryptococcal antigen in CSF, positive CSF cultures, or biopsy.
   d. Treatment: various antifungal agents.

5. Imaging.
   a. CT.
      (1) CT findings may be minimal.
      (2) May see small foci of hypodensity in basal ganglia or midbrain, which represent dilated perivascular spaces or cryptococcal pseudocysts (cryptococcomas).
   b. MR.
      (1) Most common findings are small multifocal lesions in basal ganglia and midbrain; signal usually hypointense on T1WI and hyperintense on T2WI.
      (2) Enhancement variable.
      (3) Meningitis not usually detectable with imaging.

E. Candidiasis.
   1. Etiology: Candida albicans is a ubiquitous fungus.
   2. Incidence.
      a. Superficial candidiasis is universal.
      b. Invasive or systemic disease occurs in chronically ill or immunosuppressed population.
   3. Pathophysiology.
      a. Spread: hematogenously from superficial sources; patients with in-dwelling catheters are particularly at risk.
      b. CNS manifestations.
         (1) Meningitis.
         (2) Fungal abscess or "fungus balls."
         (3) Diffuse cerebritis with microabscesses.
         (4) Vasculitis with subsequent ischemia, infarct or hemorrhage.
   4. Clinical.
      a. CNS symptoms nonspecific, may present with symptoms of meningitis.
      b. Diagnosis made by blood or CSF cultures.

      c. Treatment: antifungal therapy.

   5. Imaging (CT/MRI).

      a. Meningitis resembles other granulomatous meningitides with thickened, enhancing basilar meninges.

      b. Candidal abscesses tend to have thicker, less sharply defined walls than bacterial abscesses.

      c. Diffuse cerebritis may result in focal or diffuse edema.

      d. May see areas of infarct or hemorrhage.

F. Coccidiodomycosis.

   1. Organism: Coccidiodes imatans acquired by inhalation of spores from soil.

   2. Incidence.

      a. Endemic in southwestern United States (especially San Joaquin valley of California, and parts of Arizona).

      b. CNS involvement rare, occurs only with disseminated disease.

   3. Pathophysiology.

      a. Spread: hematogenous from primary pulmonary source.

      b. CNS manifestations.

         (1) Basilar meningeal inflammation common (see Chapter 42).

         (2) Granulomas, abscess less common.

         (3) Vasculitis can occasionally cause infarction.

   4. Clinical.

      a. Symptoms include headache, meningismus, cranial neuropathy, or stroke.

      b. Diagnosis suggested by primary pulmonary infection. Definitive diagnosis made by isolation of organism from CSF or biopsy.

      c. Treatment: antifungal therapy.

   5. Imaging.

      a. CT.

         (1) May see thickened, enhancing basilar meninges and hydrocephalus.

         (2) Rarely may see focal granuloma or abscess, typically in basal cisterns.

         (3) Infarcts uncommon.

      b. MRI.

         (1) Inflammatory exudate in basal cisterns may not be detectable on noncontrast MRI.

         (2) May occasionally see infarcts secondary to vasculitis.

II. Actinomycetaceae (features resembling mycobacterium as well as fungi).

   1. Nocardiosis.

a. Organism.
   (1) Nocardia asteroides (most common).
   (2) Transmission not well understood but probably inhaled with subsequent hematogenous spread.
b. Incidence.
   (1) Many patients (>30%) are chronically ill (e.g., alveolar proteinosis) or immunosuppressed (e.g., AIDS), although disease can occur in healthy individuals.
   (2) Incidence is rising due to more aggressive immunosuppressive therapies and AIDS, although actual incidence in AIDS probably underestimated because treatment for toxoplasmosis is also effective for nocardiosis.
   (3) CNS involvement in 15% to 45% of systemic infections.
   (4) Nocardial abscesses account for 2% of all brain abscesses.
c. Pathophysiology.
   (1) Most cases of disseminated nocardiosis begin as pulmonary infections that subsequently spread hematogenously to brain, kidneys, skin.
   (2) Can result in meningitis or brain abscess.
d. Clinical.
   (1) Symptoms nonspecific.
   (2) Diagnosis made by isolation of organism in tissue or culture.
   (3) Mortality due to nocardial brain abscess is greater in immunosuppressed population compared with immunocompetent individuals.
   (4) Treatment: sulfonamides.
   (5) More aggressive (e.g., surgical) therapies instituted in immunosuppressed population.
e. Imaging (CT/MRI).
   (1) Nocardial brain abscesses are frequently multiple (40%), often multiloculated, and have thicker wall than pyogenic abscess.
   (2) Rarely see enhancing meninges.
2. Actinomycosis.
   a. Organism: Actinomyces israelii (most common).
   b. Incidence.
      (1) Unlike nocardia, actinomycetes are not opportunists and primarily infect healthy individuals.
      (2) CNS actinomycosis is rare.
   c. Pathophysiology.
      (1) Chronic suppurative infection usually localized to neck, lung, or abdomen.

(2) Pathology is characteristic for sulfur granules.
(3) Routes of spread to CNS include:
    (a) Hematogenous spread from cervicofacial, pulmonary, or genitourinary focus.
    (b) Direct extension from otomastoid or sinus infection.
(4) CNS manifestations include:
    (a) Actinomycoma or brain abscess (75%).
    (b) Meningitis or meningoencephalitis (15%).
    (c) Subdural empyema, epidural abscess (10%).
d. Clinical.
  (1) Symptoms nonspecific.
  (2) Treatment: penicillin.
e. Imaging (CT/MRI).
  (1) Similar to nocardial abscess.
  (2) Typically thick-walled, multiloculated, rim-enhancing abscess.
  (3) However, may also have solid appearance with homogeneous enhancement (mimicking meningioma).

III. Parasitic infections.
  A. General comments.
    1. More frequent (North American) CNS infections include:
      a. Toxoplasmosis (see Chapters 41, 45).
      b. Cysticercosis
    2. Other parasites with possible CNS involvement (although less common in North America) include: echinococcus, schistosomiasis, amebiasis, paragonomiasis, sparganosis, toxocariasis.
  B. Neurocysticercosis.
    1. Organism.
      a. Pork tapeworm, Taenia solium.
      b. Humans can be definitive host by ingestion of larval forms in undercooked pork (intermediate hosts), which only results in asymptomatic gastrointestinal adult tapeworm infection (taeniasis).
      c. However, ingestion of ova in contaminated food/water (by feces of intermediate hosts: pig or man) or autoinfection results in embryos invading intestinal mucosa and spreading hematogenously to other organs where larval forms encyst (cysticercosis).
    2. Incidence.
      a. Neurocysticercosis is most common CNS parasitic infection worldwide.
      b. Endemic in Mexico, Central and South America, Eastern Europe, Africa, and parts of Asia.

    c. Most cases in developed countries occur in immigrants from endemic areas.

    d. CNS involvement occurs in 60% to 90% of infected patients.

3. Pathology.

    a. CNS manifestations typically occur in four stages.

        (1) Vesicular stage: live larvum (cysticercus) consists of central scolex enclosed in a fluid-containing bladder and surrounded by thin capsule without inflammatory reaction.

        (2) Colloidal vesicular stage: immediately after larvum dies, capsule thickens and cyst degenerates, releasing metabolic products that incite inflammatory response and edema.

        (3) Granular nodular stage: cyst retracts, capsule thickens further and scolex begins to calcify; surrounding edema begins to diminish.

        (4) Nodular calcified stage: granulomatous lesion completely calcifies (may take 1 to 10 years), active inflammation and edema resolve.

    b. Four principal patterns of location (may be mixed).

        (1) Parenchymal.

            (a) Commonly in cortical gray matter (cerebrum > cerebellum).

            (b) Single or multiple (from one to thousands of lesions, although usually under 10 lesions).

            (c) Range from 3 to 15 mm in size.

        (2) Intraventricular.

            (a) May adhere to ependymal surface or may be free within ventricular space.

            (b) Most commonly in fourth ventricle, although can occur anywhere in ventricular system.

            (c) Can acutely obstruct ventricular system.

        (3) Leptomeningeal.

            (a) Cysts may occur free in subarachnoid cisterns or burrow under pia into cortex.

            (b) May have inflammatory exudate involving basilar cisterns.

            (c) Common complications include hydrocephalus and vasculitis.

        (4) Racemose.

            (a) Grapelike clusters of cysts that lack scoleces may occur in basal cisterns.

            (b) Can cause obstructive hydrocephalus.

4. Clinical.

a. Seizures are most common symptom (50% to 70%).
b. Morbidity usually results from dying larvae that incite intense host inflammatory response.
c. Occasionally intraventricular lesions may cause acute ventricular obstruction with sudden death.
d. Cysticercotic encephalitis is a particularly severe form in which hundreds of cysticerci cause intense inflammation.
e. Diagnosis made by combination of typical imaging findings and/or analysis of serum or CSF antibody titers by enzyme-linked studies.
f. Treatment: praziquantel or (more recently) albendazole. Steroids may be adjunctive for decreasing inflammatory response.
g. Surgery may be performed for removal of intraventricular cysts, ventricular shunting, or both.

5. Imaging (CT/MRI).
a. Stages of cysticercus.
   (1) Vesicular stage.
       (a) Typically see round CSF-like cyst(s) with small mural nodule (scolex) which is slightly hyperdense or hyperintense to adjacent fluid on T1WI.
       (b) No associated edema or mass effect.
   (2) Colloidal vesicular stage.
       (a) Cyst fluid becomes turbid and is hyperdense or hyperintense to CSF.
       (b) Commonly see ring enhancement.
       (c) Marked edema and mass effect.
   (3) Granular nodular stage.
       (a) On CT cyst may be isodense to brain, with hyperdense calcifying scolex.
       (b) On MRI cyst is usually isointense on T1WI and isointense or hypointense on T2WI.
       (c) Nodular or ring enhancement may be seen.
       (d) May have "target" or "bulls-eye" appearance due to central dense scolex with surrounding ring enhancement.
       (e) Edema persists.
   (4) Nodular calcified stage.
       (a) On CT a small calcified nodule without mass effect or enhancement is typical.
       (b) May be difficult to distinguish on routine MRI. Gradient echo imaging may be helpful due to magnetic susceptibility of calcification.
b. Patterns of involvement.

        (1) Parenchymal: calcifications more often seen in adults, usually occur in cortical gray matter.

        (2) Leptomeningeal: more often in children, observe basilar meningeal enhancement.

        (3) Intraventricular: MRI is superior to CT in detecting cysts with small soft-tissue nodule of scolex, although CT can be performed after instillation of intraventricular water-soluble contrast to detect filling defects.

        (4) Racemose: multilocular cysts without scoleces in basilar, suprasellar, cerebellopontine, or Sylvian cisterns.

    c. Associated findings: hydrocephalus, infarcts (lacunar or large-vessel distribution).

C. Echinococcus.
  1. Organism.
    a. Echinococcal infection (hydatid disease), is caused by a tapeworm of sheep or cattle: Echinococcus granulosis (Australia, New Zealand, Central/South America, and parts of Europe, Africa, or United Kingdom) or Echinococcus multilocularis (Northern Canada and Alaska). The latter tends to be more invasive.
    b. Human infection is caused by ingestion of ova from dog feces that hatch in gastrointestinal tract; resulting embryos spread through portal or systemic circulation to other organs where they develop into cystic larvae or hydatid cysts.
  2. Incidence.
    a. Cerebral hydatid cysts occur in 2% of infections.
    b. Hydatid cysts account for 1% to 5% of intracranial mass lesions in endemic areas.
  3. Pathophysiology.
    a. CNS involvement may be primary or secondary to ruptured extracranial cyst (usually cardiac). Rupture of intracranial cysts rare.
    b. Primary cyst usually solitary.
    c. Secondary cyst(s) usually multiple.
    d. Involved locations include parenchyma (supratentorial > infratentorial), intraventricular, and meningeal.
  4. Clinical.
    a. CNS involvement may present with seizures or focal deficits if lesions are large.
    b. Treatment primarily surgical resection of intact cyst (rupture can result in allergic reaction or recurrence) as drug therapy is not effective for CNS infection.
  5. Imaging (CT/MRI).

    a. Typically single thin-walled spheric CSF-density cyst (supratentorial > infratentorial) with absent or minimal enhancement.

    b. Multilocular or multiple lesions rare.

    c. Occasionally wall calcifies.

SUGGESTED READINGS

Ashdown BC, Tien RD, Felsberg GJ: Aspergillosis of the brain and paranasal sinuses in immunocompromised patients: CT and MR findings, *AJR* 162:155-159, 1994.

Breadmore R, Desmond P, Opeskin K: Intracranial aspergillosis producing cavernous sinus syndrome and rupture of internal carotid artery, *Australas Radiol* 38:72-75, 1994.

Coleman JM, Hogg GG, Rosenfeld JV, Waters KD: Invasive central nervous system aspergillosis: cure with liposomal amphotericin B, itraconazole, and radical surgery—case report and review of the literature, *Neurosurg* 36:858-863, 1995.

Del Brutto OH: Single parenchymal brain cysticercus in the acute encephalitic phase: definition of a distinct form of neurocysticercosis with a benign prognosis, *J Neurol Neurosurg Psych* 58:257-249, 1995.

Funaki B, Rosenblum JD: MR of central nervous system actinomycosis, *AJNR* 16:1179-1180, 1995.

Gollard R, Rabb C, Larsen R, Chandrasoma P: Isolated cerebral mucormycosis: case report and therapeutic considerations, *Neurosurg* 34:174-177, 1994.

Kim DG, Hong SC, Kim HJ, et al: Cerebral aspergillosis in immunologically competent patients, *Surg Neurol* 40:326-331, 1993.

Levy AS, Lillehei KO, Rubinstein D, Stears JC: Subarachnoid neurocysticercosis with occlusion of the major intracranial arteries: case report, *Neurosurg* 36:183-188, 1995.

Mamelak AN, Obana WG, Flaherty JF, Rosenblum ML: Nocardial brain abscess: treatment strategies and factors influencing outcome, *Neurosurg* 35:622-631, 1994.

Mendel E, Milefchik EN, Amadi J, Gruen P: Coccidioidomycosis brain abscess: case report, *J Neurosurg* 81:614-616, 1994.

Miaux Y, Ribaud P, Williams M, et al: MR of cerebral aspergillosis in patients who have had bone marrow transplantation, *AJNR* 16:555-562, 1995.

Osborn AG: Infection, white matter abnormalities, and degenerative diseases. In *Diagnostic radiology,* St Louis, 1994, Mosby, pp 671-715.

Siddiqi SU, Freedman JD: Isolated central nervous system mucormycosis, *South Med J,* 87:997-1000, 1994.

Ward BA, Parent AD, Raila F: Indications for the surgical management of central nervous system blastomycosis, *Surg Neurol* 43:379-388, 1995.

SECTION VII
Metabolic, White Matter, and Degenerative Diseases

48

Normal Myelination

Key Concepts

1. Normal brain myelination begins during the fifth fetal month and continues throughout life.
2. Myelination occurs in predictable, predetermined patterns and generally progresses.
   a. From caudad to cephalad.
   b. From dorsal to ventral.
   c. From central to peripheral.
3. Sensory tracts generally myelinate earlier than motor tracts.
4. Myelination of the human brain occurs mainly after birth, but high-signal intensity in the dorsal midbrain on T1WI can be seen as early as 23 gestational weeks.
5. The brain myelinates rapidly during the first 18 months, essentially achieving an adult pattern by age 2.
6. Association fiber tracts around ventricular trigones often do not myelinate completely until age 30.

To understand the inherited metabolic and degenerative disorders that can affect the human brain, it is necessary first to review briefly normal myelination patterns and their typical appearance on imaging studies.

Normal brain myelination is a dynamic but orderly, highly predictable process. Microscopic myelination is detectable at 20 weeks; on imaging studies myelination is detectable as early as the fifth fetal month and is largely completed by age 2. In general, MR imaging reflects the progress of histogenesis and myelination quite accurately and can readily depict departures from expected patterns of normal development (see Chapters 49-51).

In this chapter we briefly discuss the imaging appearance of normal brain myelination and maturation from the fifth fetal month to adulthood. Signal intensity of unmyelinated and myelinated white matter with respect to gray matter depends on magnetic field strength and the pulse sequence used. For the first few months of life, the signal intensities of gray and white matter are the reverse of those seen in the mature brain. White matter is largely unmyelinated and therefore has a lower signal intensity than gray matter on T1WI and a higher signal intensity on T2-weighted sequences.

Brain maturation as depicted on MR scans lags a few weeks behind histologic myelination timetables. It also appears substantially different depending on the pulse sequence selected. Changes in signal intensity on T2-weighted scans generally lag somewhat behind those seen on T1WI. We therefore delineate the appearance of the normal developing brain on standard T1-weighted and T2-weighted spin echo sequences separately. Where appropriate, special techniques such as short-inversion-time inversion-recovery (STIR) sequences and MR spectroscopy (MRS) are also included.

For imaging the developing brain, our typical short TR/short TE or "T1-weighted scan" requires a TR of 500 to 600 msec and a TE of 20 msec. We use very long TRs (between 3000 and 4000 msec) and TEs (between 80 and 120 msec) for our typical T2-weighted scans in newborns and infants.

   I. Fetal brain maturation.
      A. 21 to 28 gestational weeks.
         1. Sulci, ventricles.
            a. Brain appears nearly agyric.
            b. Sylvian fissures wide, vertically oriented.
            c. Parieto-occipital fissure, olfactory and cingulate sulci present.
            d. Rolandic sulcus appears between 18 and 22 weeks, followed by prerolandic and other sulci.
            e. Ventricles are large.
         2. Parenchyma.
            a. T1WI.

        (1) Multilayered pattern at 23 weeks.
          (a) High-signal cortical ribbon.
          (b) Intermediate layer (migrating glia).
          (c) Low-signal white matter.
        (2) High-signal intensity within dorsal brainstem appears at approximately 23 weeks (Fig. 48-1).
          (a) Represents earliest myelination.
          (b) Sensory tracts of pons, medulla.
        (3) High signal in basal ganglia.
          (a) Reflects increased cellularity.

B. 28 to 35 gestational weeks.
    1. Sulci, ventricles.
      a. Gyri, sulci develop.
      b. Cavum septi pellucidi, cavum Vergae prominent.
      c. Ventricles small.
    2. Parenchyma.
      a. T1WI.
        (1) Multilayered pattern disappears.
        (2) High signal in posterior limb of internal capsule at 31 weeks.
        (3) High signal within central white matter at 35 weeks.
      b. T2WI.
        (1) Allows differentiation of cortex, white matter.
        (2) Cortical ribbon seen as low-signal intensity between high-signal subarachnoid spaces, unmyelinated white matter.
        (3) Ventrolateral thalamus appears hypointense.

II. Birth.
  A. Term infant.
    1. Sulci, ventricles.
      a. By 38 to 40 weeks, brain sulci resemble adult pattern.
      b. Cavum septi pellucidi, Vergae remain prominent.
    2. Parenchyma.
      a. T1WI (see box on p. 501; Figs. 48-1, 48-2).
        (1) High signal.
          (a) Dorsal medulla, brainstem.
          (b) Posterior limb, internal capsule.
          (c) Inferior, superior cerebellar peduncles.
          (d) Ventrolateral thalami.
        (2) Low signal.
          (a) Cerebral white matter.
      b. T2WI.
        (1) High signal.

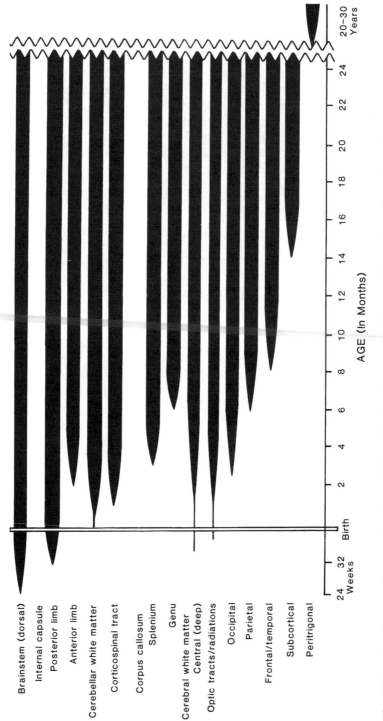

Fig. 48-1 Myelination of key marker sites as depicted by development of high-signal intensity on T1-weighted MR scans.

Normal Myelination: General Timetable[1]

Fetus

Dorsal medulla, pons
Posterior limb, internal capsule

Term infant

Dorsal medulla/midbrain
Cerebellar peduncles (inferior/superior)
Posterior limb, internal capsule
Ventrolateral thalamus

One postnatal month

Middle cerebellar peduncles
Corticospinal tracts, cerebral peduncles
Optic nerves, tracts
Precentral/postcentral gyri

Three postnatal months

Cerebellar hemispheric white matter
Ventral brainstem
Anterior limb, internal capsule
Splenium, corpus callosum
Optic radiations
Subcortical white matter (occipital lobe)

Six postnatal months

Genu, corpus callosum
Centrum semiovale (posterior to anterior, central to peripheral)

Eight postnatal months

Subcortical U fibers (except for frontotemporal)

One year to 18 months

Resembles adult

---

[1]Key myelination markers in italics

       (a) Most of cerebral white matter.
     (2) Low signal.
       (a) Dorsal medulla, brainstem.
       (b) Inferior, superior cerebellar peduncles.
       (c) Posterior limb, internal capsule.
       (d) Ventrolateral thalamus.
       (e) Perirolandic gyri.
   c. Proton MR spectroscopy (MRS).

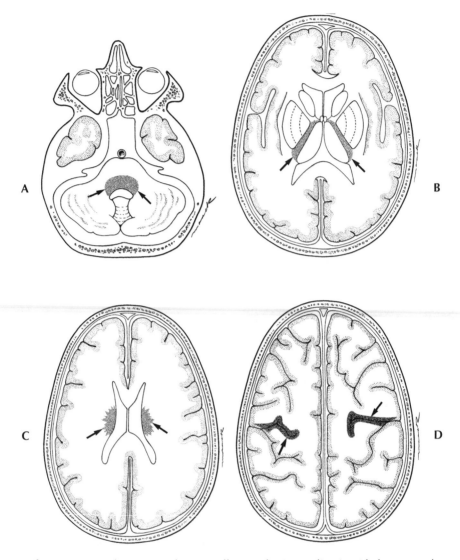

Fig. 48-2 Axial-anatomic diagrams illustrate brain myelination (dark patterned areas: arrows) present at birth. **A,** Posterior fossa myelinated areas include the dorsal midbrain (arrows), as well as the medulla and inferior and superior cerebellar peduncles. **B,** The posterior limb of the internal capsule is myelinated; some myelination also extends superiorly into the deep centrum semiovale (**C,** arrows). **D,** No myelination is present in the subcortical U (arcuate) fibers but the precentral and postcentral gyri (arrows) often appear low signal on T2-weighted MR scans by the first postnatal month. (From Osborn AG: *Diagnostic neuroradiology*, St Louis, 1994, Mosby).

        (1) NAA peak: low.

        (2) Cho peak: high.

    3. Miscellaneous.

      a. Pituitary gland.

        (1) Upwardly convex.

        (2) Uniformly hyperintense on T1WI.

III. 1 to 3 postnatal months.

  A. 1 month.

    1. Sulci, ventricles.

      a. Frontal extraaxial space may appear prominent.

    2. Parenchyma.

      a. T1WI (see box on p. 501; Fig. 48-1).

        (1) High signal now seen in:

          (a) Middle cerebellar peduncles.

          (b) Optic nerves, tracts, radiations.

          (c) Corticospinal tracts, cerebral peduncles.

          (d) White matter of precentral, postcentral gyri.

      b. T2WI.

        (1) Low signal (now seen).

          (a) Little change from birth; some hypointense areas in deep centrum semiovale may develop.

  B. 3 months.

    1. Sulci, ventricles.

      a. Frontal subarachnoid spaces may remain prominent.

    2. Parenchyma.

      a. T1WI (Figs. 48-1, 48-3).

        (1) High signal now seen in:

          (a) Subcortical cerebellar white matter.

          (b) Ventral brainstem.

          (c) Anterior limb, internal capsule.

          (d) Subcortical occipital white matter.

      b. T2WI.

        (1) Low signal now seen in:

          (a) Middle cerebellar peduncle.

          (b) Anterior limb, internal capsule.

          (c) Optic radiations.

          (d) Some parts of centrum semiovale.

      c. MRS.

        (1) Changes in NAA, Cho peaks occur earlier than changes in signal intensity on T1WI.

          (a) NAA: high.

          (b) Cho: low.

        (2) NAA/Cho and NAA/Cre ratios increase rapidly.

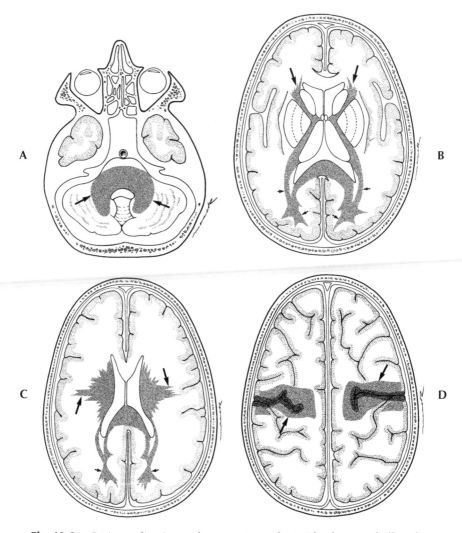

Fig. 48-3 Brain myelination at about 3 to 4 months. **A,** The deep cerebellar white matter and corticospinal tracts are myelinated. **B,** The anterior limb of the internal capsule (large arrows) and corpus callosum splenium are now at least partially myelinated. Occipital radiations and subcortical arcuate fibers are beginning to myelinate (B and C, small arrows). **C,** Myelination also extends further into the centrum semiovale (large arrows). **D,** Some arcuate fiber and centrum semiovale myelination around the precentral and postcentral gyri is present (arrows). (From Osborn AG: *Diagnostic neuroradiology*, St Louis, 1994, Mosby.)

(3) Cho/Cre ratio decreases.
d. Diffusion MR scans.
   (1) Signal depends on:
      (a) Orientation of nerve fibers.
      (b) Direction of gradients.
   (2) Diffusion-weighted imaging provides earlier detection of brain myelination compared with conventional T1WI, T2WI.
   (3) Changes of diffusional anisotropy in white matter are completed within 6 months after birth.
3. Miscellaneous.
  a. Pituitary gland.
   (1) By age 2 to 3 months, superior margin is flat.
   (2) Anterior lobe is isointense with gray matter on T1WI.
   (3) Posterior lobe (neurohypophysis) is hyperintense on T1WI.
IV. 4 to 6 postnatal months.
  A. 4 months.
    1. Sulci, ventricles.
      a. Frontal CSF spaces may still be prominent.
    2. Parenchyma.
      a. T1WI.
       (1) High signal.
         (a) Splenium, corpus callosum.
         (b) Centrum semiovale (myelination progresses from posterior to anterior and from central to peripheral).
      b. T2WI.
       (1) Low signal.
         (a) Generally little change from 3 months.
         (b) Calcarine fissure shows some low-signal intensity.
  B. 6 months.
    1. Sulci, ventricles: no change.
    2. Parenchyma.
      a. T1WI (Figs. 48-1, 48-4).
       (1) High signal.
         (a) Genu, corpus callosum.
         (b) More centrum semiovale.
      b. T2WI.
       (1) Low signal.
         (a) Splenium, corpus callosum.
         (b) More centrum semiovale.
      c. MRS.
       (1) Increases in NAA/Cho, NAA/Cre ratios and decrease in

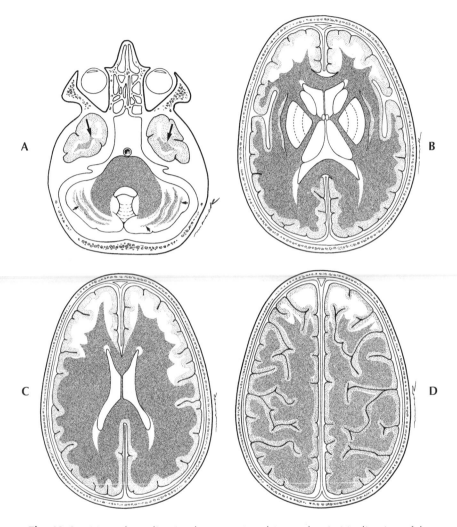

Fig. 48-4 Normal myelination between 6 and 8 months. **A,** Myelination of the cerebellar white matter is nearly completed and extends peripherally to the folia (small arrows). Temporal lobe myelination (large arrows) is present. **B,** The corpus callosum genu is also myelinated. **C** and **D,** Myelination extends through the centrum semiovale into the subcortical U fibers and is virtually complete except for some frontotemporal areas. The peritrigonal white matter may not myelinate completely until age 20 to 30 years. (From Osborn AG: *Diagnostic neuroradiology,* St Louis, 1994, Mosby.)

Cho/Cre ratio rise steeply for first 6 postnatal months, then increase more gradually in later months.

V. 8 to 12 postnatal months.
- A. 8 months.
  1. Sulci, ventricles: prominent frontal subarachnoid space may persist.
  2. Parenchyma.
     a. T1WI (see box on p. 501; Figs. 48-1, 48-4).
        (1) High signal.
            (a) Frontotemporal white matter (except for most anterior subcortical fibers).
     b. T2WI.
        (1) Low signal.
            (a) Cerebellar white matter reaches adult pattern.
            (b) Genu, corpus callosum.
            (c) Basal ganglia.
- B. 12 months.
  1. Between 12 and 18 months, brain approaches adult configuration.
  2. Sulci, ventricles are normally small.
  3. Parenchyma.
     a. T1WI.
        (1) High signal.
            (a) Little change from 8 months.
     b. T2WI.
        (1) Low signal.
            (a) Subcortical white matter.
            (b) Begins at 9 to 12 months in occipital lobe, 11 to 14 months frontally.
            (c) Temporal lobe white matter matures last.
            (d) Completed by end of second year of life.
VI. Normal areas of late/delayed myelination (Table 48-1).
- A. White matter tracts that normally show delayed myelination.
  1. Peritrigonal white matter.

Table 48-1   Normal Areas of Delayed /Diminished Myelination That Should Not be Mistaken for Disease

Location	Structure	Differential Diagnosis
Peritrigonal w.m.	Association tracts	Periventricular leukomalacia
Frontal horns	Loose myelin	Multiple sclerosis
Posterior limb, internal capsule	Corticospinal tract	Amyotrophic lateral sclerosis

a. May not myelinate completely until age 20 to 30 years.
b. Areas of poorly delineated high-signal intensity adjacent to atria of lateral ventricles can normally be seen on T2WI.
c. Differential diagnosis.
    (1) Periventricular leukomalacia (see Chapter 53).
        (a) PVL is usually sharply defined.
        (b) PVL is located more inferiorly.
        (c) PVL is associated with loss of brain tissue (diminished white matter, thinned posterior corpus callosum, irregular margins of lateral ventricles).
        (d) PVL extends to ventricular margin, whereas normal peritrigonal high-signal intensities typically do not.
    (2) Prominent perivascular spaces.
        (a) Sharply delineated.
        (b) Round or tubular.
2. Ventricular "caps."
    a. Triangle-shaped caps of high-signal intensity on T2WI are normally seen adjacent to frontal horns.
    b. Represent more loosely compacted myelinated axons with relative increase in periependymal fluid.
3. Corticospinal tracts (CST).
    a. Focal rounded or oval bilaterally symmetric areas in posterior limb of internal capsule that appear hyperintense on T2WI.
    b. Seen in 50% of normal adults.
    c. Represent large fibers with thick myelin sheaths, relatively lower axonal and myelin density compared with rest of internal capsule.
    d. Amyotrophic lateral sclerosis (ALS) often affects CSTs diffusely.

SUGGESTED READINGS

Ballesteros MC, Hansen PE, Soila K: MR imaging of the developing human brain. Part 2. Postnatal development, *Radiographics* 13:611-622, 1993.

Barkovich AJ: Normal development of the neonatal and infant brain, skull, and spine. In *Pediatric Neuroimaging,* ed 2, New York, 1995, Raven Press, pp 9-39.

Byrd SE, Darling CF, Wilczynski MA; White matter of the brain: maturation and myelination on magnetic resonance in infants and children, *Neuroimaging Clin North Am* 3:247-266, 1993.

Friedman L, Patel VH: Normal variation in MRI of the brain, *Sem US, CT, MRI* 16:175-185, 1995.

Girard N, Raybaud C, Poncet M: In vivo MR study of brain maturation in normal fetuses, *AJNR* 16:407-413, 1995.

Hansen PE, Ballesteros MC, Soila K, et al: MR imaging of the developing human brain. Part 1. Prenatal development, *Radiographics* 13:21-36, 1993.

Hittmair K, Wimberger D, Rand T, et al: MR assessment of brain maturation: comparison of sequences, *AJNR* 15:425-433, 1994.

Kimura H, Fujii Y, Itoh S, et al: Metabolic alterations in the neonate and infant brain during development: evaluation with proton MR spectroscopy, *Radiol* 194:483-489, 1995.

Nomura Y, Sakuma H, Takeda K, et al: Diffusional anisotropy of the human brain assessed with diffusion-weighted MR: relation with normal brain development and aging, *AJNR* 15:231-238, 1994.

Staudt M, Schropp C, Staudt F, et al: Myelination of the brain in MRI: a staging system, *Pediatr Radiol* 23:169-176, 1993.

Yagashita A, Nakano I, Oda M, Hirano A: Location of the corticospinal tract in the internal capsule at MR imaging, *Radiol* 191:455-460, 1994.

49

Inherited Metabolic and Degenerative Brain Disorders: Introduction, Overview, and Classification

Key Concepts

1. So-called inborn errors of metabolism are a diverse group of disorders that affect different parts of the brain in different ways and at different ages.
2. Metabolic and degenerative brain disorders have been categorized and classified in various ways, including:
   a. Inherited versus acquired disorders.
   b. *Dys*-myelinating versus *de*-myelinating disorders.
   c. Abnormal morphology or function of a particular cellular organelle (e.g., lysosomal, peroxisomal, and mitochondrial disorders).
   d. Pattern of involvement (white matter, gray matter, or both).

Metabolic, toxic, and neurodegenerative diseases are increasingly well-recognized causes of brain dysfunction. These diseases have a diverse spectrum of clinical, pathologic, and biochemical features that are both complex and confusing. A detailed discussion of the numerous inherited and acquired metabolic and degenerative disorders that affect the brain is well beyond the scope of this text. However, a brief overview of their classification and basic imaging features is worthwhile.

In this chapter we discuss various ways of categorizing metabolic and neurodegenerative brain disorders. Following the pattern established in *Diagnostic Neuroradiology,* we will primarily use the geographic or location-based approach to these diseases. In Chapter 50 we discuss inherited disorders that primarily affect white matter (the so-called leukoencephalopathies). In Chapter 51 we discuss the "inborn errors of metabolism" that affect gray matter (either primarily or exclusively).

I. Inherited versus acquired neurodegenerative diseases.
   A. Inherited metabolic and neurodegenerative disorders are sometimes referred to as "inborn errors of metabolism."
      1. One or more metabolic pathways is altered.
      2. Dysfunction may result from:
         a. Failure to produce a necessary substance or cellular component.
         b. Failure to maintain a necessary substance or cellular component that has been produced normally.
         c. Failure to metabolize a biochemical that has been produced and maintained normally.
      3. Common examples include:
         a. White matter disorders ("leukodystrophies") such as:
            (1) Adrenoleukodystrophy (ALD).
            (2) Metachromatic leukodystrophy (MLD).
            (3) Globoid cell leukodystrophy (GLD, also known as Krabbé disease).
         b. Gray matter disorders ("poliodystrophies") such as:
            (1) Mucolipidoses.
            (2) Glycogen storage diseases.
            (3) Basal ganglia diseases.
               (a) Hallervorden-Spatz disease.
               (b) Juvenile Huntington disease.
               (c) Mitochondrial disorders (see below).
   B. Acquired metabolic and neurodegenerative disorders (see Chapters 53 and 54).
      1. White matter diseases such as:
         a. Multiple sclerosis (MS).

b. Postviral autoimmune-mediated demyelination such as acute disseminated encephalomyelitis (ADEM).

c. Toxic or metabolic demyelination such as disseminated necrotizing leukoencephalopathy (DNL) and central pontine myelinolysis (CPM).

d. Age-related changes and vascular disease.

2. Gray matter diseases such as:
   a. Alzheimer dementia.
   b. Vascular dementia.
   c. Pick disease.
   d. Creutzfeld-Jacob disease.
   e. Parkinson disease.

II. *Dys*-myelinating versus *de*-myelinating disease.

A. Normal components of mature white matter include:

1. Myelinated axons (from neuronal cell bodies in gray matter).
2. Astrocytes.
3. Oligodendrocytes (responsible for production, maintenance of axonal myelin sheaths).
4. Penetrating arteries, medullary veins.

B. *Dys*-myelinating diseases.

1. Inherited disorders characterized by oligodendrocyte disfunction with abnormal myelin formation or maintenance. Examples include:
   a. ALD.
   b. MLD.
   c. GLD.

C. *De*-myelinating diseases.

1. Acquired myelinoclastic disorders characterized by destruction of normally formed myelin such as:
   a. MS.
   b. ADEM.

D. Problems with using dysmyelinating versus demyelinating disease.

1. In some inherited white matter diseases with late onset, myelin may be both initially well formed and normally maintained for a variable time period.
2. Demyelination may occur concurrently in some essentially dysmyelinating disorders.

III. Cellular organelle (abnormal morphology and/or function) (box).

A. Lysosomal disorders.

1. Etiology.
   a. Cellular enzyme deficiency (hydrolase) leads to abnormal accumulation of undigested materials of various types.
   (1) Phospholipids.

Classification of Inherited Neurodegenerative Diseases by Organelle: Common Examples

Lysosomal disorders

Metachromatic leukodystrophy
Globoid cell leukodystrophy (Krabbé disease)
Mucopolysaccharidoses (e.g., Hunter, Hurler)

Peroxisomal disorders

Adrenoleukodystrophy

Mitochondrial disorders

Leigh disease (subacute necrotizing leukoencephalopathy)
MELAS (*M*itochondrial *E*ncephalopathy with *L*actic *A*cidosis and *S*trokelike episodes)

---

        (2) Glycolipids.
        (3) Mucopolysaccharides.
        (4) Glycoproteins.
    b. Autosomal recessive inheritance.
  2. Can affect predominantly white matter, gray matter, or both.
    a. White matter.
        (1) MLD.
        (2) GLD.
    b. Gray matter or both gray, white matter.
        (1) Mucopolysaccharidoses.
           (a) Hurler.
           (b) Hunter.
           (c) San Filippo.
        (2) Mucolipidoses, lipidoses.
           (a) I-cell disease.
           (b) Niemann-Pick disease.
B. Peroxisomal disorders.
  1. Etiology.
    a. Organelles are responsible for peroxidation, metabolism of very long-chain fatty acids.
    b. Peroxisomes can be:
        (1) Absent.
        (2) Present, with decreased size or deficient numbers.
        (3) Present, single-enzyme deficiency.
        (4) Present, multiple-enzyme deficiencies.
  2. Primarily affective white matter.

       a. ALD.

       b. Zellweger syndrome.

  C. Mitochondrial disorders.

    1. Etiology.

       a. Organelles involved in oxidative respiratory cycle.

       b. Abnormal accumulation of lactate and pyruvate in blood, serum, CSF, brain, and muscle.

    2. May affect deep gray matter, cortex, white matter.

       a. Leigh disease (basal ganglia, periaqueductal gray matter, brainstem).

       b. MELAS (*M*itochondrial *E*ncephalopathy with *L*actic *A*cidosis and *S*trokelike episodes).

  D. Problems with organelle-based classification of inherited metabolic disorders.

    1. Many disorders have no known organelle basis (e.g., aminoacidurias).

    2. Some disorders (e.g., certain aminoacidemias) are involved with formation of mitochondrial proteins and also result in basal ganglia abnormalities that resemble the primary mitochondrial defects.

IV. Classification by pattern of involvement (box).

  A. Disorders that exclusively or primarily affect white matter.

    1. Characterized by complete or near-complete lack of myelination.

       a. Pelizaeus-Merzbacher disease.

       b. Macrocrania + large NAA peak on MRS = Canavan disease.

    2. Characterized by deep white matter involvement (subcortical U fibers generally spared).

       a. Occipital white matter = ALD.

       b. Periventricular (deep white matter) plus thalami also involved = Krabbé disease.

       c. Deep white matter + corticospinal tract = Suspect peroxisomal disorder.

       d. Nonspecific = MLD, aminoaciduria.

    3. Deep plus superficial white matter involvement.

       a. Frontal + macrocrania = Alexander disease.

  B. Disorders that affect gray matter.

    1. Superficial (cortical) gray matter.

       a. Ceroid lipofuscinoses (e.g., Batten disease).

       b. Glycogen storage diseases.

       c. Early-onset Alzheimer disease.

    2. Deep gray nuclei.

       a. Corpus striatum (caudate, putamen).

Classification of Inherited Neurodegenerative Diseases by Location and Pattern: Common Examples

White matter

Deep white matter
    Metachromatic leukodystrophy
    Adrenoleukodystrophy (occipital)
    Globoid cell leukodystrophy (Krabbé disease)
    Aminoaciduria
Both deep, superficial (subcortical) white matter
    Alexander disease
    Canavan disease

Gray matter

Superficial (cortical) gray matter
    Early-onset Alzheimer disease
    Batten disease
    Glycogen storage diseases
Deep gray matter nuclei
    Metabolic encephalopathy (Wilson disease)
    Hallervorden-Spatz disease
Both deep, superficial gray matter
    Huntington disease

Both white, gray matter

Superficial (cortical) gray matter
    Zellweger
Deep gray matter
    Krabbé disease
    Canavan disease
Both deep, superficial gray matter
    Mitochondrial encephalopathy (Leigh, MELAS)

---

    (1) Mitochondrial disorder (e.g., Leigh, MELAS).
    (2) Metabolic disorder (Wilson disease).
    (3) Huntington disease (also cortical, subcortical atrophy).
    (4) Acquired disorder (asphyxia, hypoglycemia).
  b. Globus pallidus.
    (1) Hallervorden-Spatz disease (hypointense on T2WI).
    (2) Methylmalonic acidemia (hyperintense on T2WI).
    (3) Acquired disorder (e.g., carbon monoxide poisoning).
C. Disorders that affect both gray, white matter.
  1. Superficial (cortical) gray matter.

   a. Peroxisomal disorder.
      (1) Zellweger (neuronal migration disorders, decreased white matter volume).
   b. Lipid storage disorders.
2. Deep gray nuclei.
   a. Thalami.
      (1) GLD (Krabbé disease).
      (2) GM$_2$ gangliosidoses.
      (3) Acquired disorders such as profound neonatal asphyxia (putamen also usually involved).
   b. Putamen, caudate.
      (1) Leigh disease.
      (2) Wilson disease.
      (3) Acquired disorders such as asphyxia or hypoglycemia.
3. Both superficial, deep gray matter.
   a. Peroxisomal disorder.
      (1) MELAS.
      (2) MERRF (*M*yoclonic *E*pilepsy with *R*agged *R*ed *F*ibers).
   b. Mucopolysaccharidoses.

SUGGESTED READINGS

Barkovich AJ: Toxic and metabolic brain disorders. In *Pediatric neuroimaging,* ed 2, New York, 1995, Raven Press, pp 55-105.

Lee BCP: Magnetic resonance imaging of metabolic and primary white matter disorders in children, *Neuroimaging Clin North Am* 3:267-289, 1993.

Medina E: Demyelinating and dysmyelinating diseases, *Riv di Neuroradiol* 6(suppl 2):33-38, 1993.

Nave K-A: Myelin genetics: new insight into old diseases, *Brain Pathol* 5:231-232, 1995.

Osborn AG: Inherited metabolic, white matter, and degenerative diseases of the brain. In *Diagnostic Neuroradiology,* St Louis, 1994, Mosby, pp 716-747.

50

Inherited Metabolic and Degenerative Brain Disorders That Primarily Affect White Matter

---

Key Concepts

1. The diagnosis of a specific inherited white matter disorder is rarely established solely on the basis of imaging abnormalities.
2. Biochemical analysis of blood or urine and sometimes histologic examination of brain, skin, or muscle is usually required for exact pathologic diagnosis of an inherited brain neurodegenerative disorder.

An exhaustive description of all the inherited white matter disorders (also sometimes called "leukodystrophies" or "dysmyelinating" diseases) is beyond the scope of this handbook. In this chapter we limit our discussion to some of the more common and important inherited metabolic disorders that exclusively or primarily involve the cerebral white matter. These "inborn errors of metabolism" are characterized by abnormal formation, maintenance, destruction, or turnover of myelin.

To simplify further our discussion of the leukodystrophies, we subdivide these disorders into two major groups. The larger of these two groups includes disorders that initially affect the deep cerebral white matter and tend to spare the subcortical regions. Examples include metachromatic leukodystrophy, adrenoleukodystrophy, globoid cell leukodystrophy (Krabbé disease), and most of the aminoacidurias.

The second group of leukodystrophies is characterized by early involvement of the peripheral (subcortical) white matter. Examples discussed here include Pelizaeus-Merzbacher, Canavan, and Alexander disease.

The definitive diagnosis of an inherited metabolic neurodegenerative disorder is rarely established solely on the basis of imaging findings. Although some patterns are suggestive of specific disorders (box), most imaging findings are nonspecific. In many cases, the precise diagnosis requires biochemical analysis of body fluids (e.g., blood or urine) or histopathologic examination of tissues such as skin fibroblasts, muscle, or even brain biopsy. Genetic linkage studies and DNA analysis are also assuming increasingly important roles in the investigation of inherited neurodegenerative disorders.

   I. Leukodystrophies that primarily affect deep white matter.
      A. Metachromatic leukodystrophy (MLD).
         1. Etiology, inheritance.
            a. Autosomal recessive.
            b. Lysosomal disorder.
               (1) Deficiency in enzyme arylsulfatase-A (MLD is diagnosed biochemically by lack of this enzyme in white blood cells and urine).
               (2) Results in abnormal breakdown, reutilization of myelin.
               (3) Lysosomes in central, peripheral nervous systems accumulate ceramide sulfatide.
         2. Pathology.
            a. Gross appearance.
               (1) Symmetric, confluent demyelination of deep (periventricular) white matter.
               (2) Subcortical U fibers initially spared.
               (3) Cerebellum often involved.
               (4) Generalized atrophy.

Diagnostic Features That May Suggest a Specific Inherited White Matter Disorder

Early, diffuse involvement of peripheral (subcortical) white matter

Pelizaeus-Merzbacher disease
Canavan disease
   Macrocephaly common
   MRS shows large NAA peak
Alexander disease
   Predilection for frontal white matter
   Enhancement with contrast

Predilection for specific location

Adrenoleukodystrophy (occipital white matter)
Alexander disease (frontal white matter)

Macrocephaly

Alexander disease
Canavan disease
Mucopolysaccharidosis Types I, II

Basal ganglia high density (CT) or hypointense (T2WI)

Globoid cell leukodystrophy (Krabbé disease)
   Deep white matter involved (subcortical spared early)

     b. Microscopic appearance.
       (1) Abnormal deposits stain "metachromatically" with acid aniline dyes.
  3. Clinical.
     a. Most common hereditary leukodystrophy.
       (1) Prevalence of 1 in 100,000 newborns.
     b. MLD is subdivided by age at onset.
       (1) Late infantile variant.
          (a) Most common form of MLD.
          (b) Initial symptoms during second year of life.
          (c) Relentless progression, death typically by age 4 to 6 years.
       (2) Juvenile form.
          (a) Symptom onset between 5 and 7 years.
          (b) Slow progression.
       (3) Adult variant.
          (a) Rarest form of MLD.
          (b) May present initially as organic brain syndrome.

4. Imaging.
   a. Findings are nonspecific.
   b. CT.
      (1) Generalized atrophy.
      (2) Confluent, symmetric decreased density of periventricular white matter.
      (3) Lesions do not enhance with contrast.
   c. MR.
      (1) Bilateral, relatively symmetric high signal in periventricular white matter on T2WI (initially patchy, then confluent).
      (2) Cerebellar involvement may be striking.
      (3) Subcortical white matter spared early.
      (4) Secondary low signal in thalami may occur late in disease course.
B. Globoid cell leukodystrophy (GLD) (Krabbé disease).
   1. Etiology and inheritance.
      a. Autosomal recessive.
      b. Lysosomal disorder.
         (1) Deficiency of galactocerebroside β-galactosidase (GLD is diagnosed by β-galactosidase assay of white blood cells or skin fibroblasts).
         (2) Cerebrosides from catabolized myelin cannot be degraded to galactose and ceramide.
         (3) Early loss of oligodendrocytes with demyelination.
         (4) Infiltration with distended macrophages ("globoid cells").
   2. Pathology.
      a. Gross pathology.
         (1) Small, atrophic brain.
         (2) Marked white matter loss.
         (3) Cortex relatively normal.
      b. Microscopic pathology.
         (1) Symmetric demyelination of centrum semiovale and corona radiata (peripheral nerves are also affected).
         (2) Subcortical arcuate fibers spared.
         (3) Myelin loss with astrogliosis.
         (4) Clusters of globoid and epithelioid cells throughout areas of demyelination.
         (5) Stippled calcifications in basal ganglia are common.
   3. Clinical.
      a. Prevalence as high as 1:50,000 in some countries (Sweden) but typically 1:100,000 to 200,000 live births in others.

b. Infantile, late infantile, adult-onset variants.
   (1) Infantile-onset most common.
      (a) Symptom onset between 3 and 6 months.
      (b) Irritability, intermittent fever.
      (c) Seizures in later stages.
      (d) Rapidly progressive, fatal.
4. Imaging.
  a. CT.
   (1) Initial studies may be normal.
   (2) Nonspecific low-density changes in periventricular, cerebellar white matter.
   (3) Hypodense white matter plus high attenuation or stippled calcifications in thalami, basal ganglia strongly suggests GLD.
   (4) Secondary generalized atrophy may become striking in later stages of the disease.
  b. MR.
   (1) Parietal region, optic pathways often affected first.
   (2) Nonspecific confluent, symmetric hyperintensity in deep cerebral, cerebellar white matter on T2WI.
   (3) Subcortical U fibers spared early but may be involved late in disease course.
   (4) Thalami, basal ganglia may be hypointense.
C. Adrenoleukodystrophy (ALD).
  1. Etiology, inheritance.
   a. Two distinct hereditary forms.
    (1) X-linked recessive ALD.
      (a) Mapped to Xq28 (terminal segment of long arm of X chromosome).
      (b) Seen exclusively in males.
    (2) Autosomal recessive ALD.
      (a) Can also affect female heterozygotes.
   b. Peroxisomal disorder.
    (1) Peroxisomes morphologically normal.
    (2) Single enzyme defect (deficiency of lignoceroyl CoA ligase).
    (3) Very long-chain saturated fatty acids (VLCFA) accumulate in brain, adrenal gland, red blood cells, plasma.
  2. Pathology.
   a. Gross pathology.
    (1) Symmetric demyelination around atria, occipital horns of lateral ventricles, and corpus callosum splenium.
    (2) Cortex spared.

b. Microscopic pathology.
(1) Inner zone of necrosis, astrogliosis, and sometimes dystrophic calcification.
(2) Intermediate zone of active demyelination and inflammation.
(3) Peripheral zone with advancing margin of active demyelination without inflammatory response.
3. Clinical.
a. Wide variation in phenotypic expression and clinical course.
b. Several forms of X-linked type recognized.
(1) Childhood cerebral phenotype.
(a) "Classic" form of ALD.
(b) Represents 50% of cases.
(c) Characterized by clinical onset between 5 and 10 years.
(d) Rapidly progressive decline and death.
(2) Adolescent cerebral phenotype.
(a) 5% of cases.
(3) Adult cerebral phenotype.
(a) 3% of cases.
(b) Severe, rapidly progressive ALD in patients 21 years or older without preceding AMN.
(4) Adrenomyeloneuropathy (AMN).
(a) 25% of cases.
(b) Involves mainly thoracic spinal cord, peripheral nerves.
(c) 20% of female heterozygotes develop neurologic disability that resembles mild form of AMN.
(5) Addison disease only.
(a) 10% of cases.
(6) Asymptomatic and presymptomatic.
(a) 8% of cases.
4. Imaging.
a. CT.
(1) Symmetric low-density lesions in peritrigonal white matter, corpus callosum splenium.
(2) May show punctate calcifications.
(3) Advancing rim enhances with contrast.
b. MR.
(1) Predominate posterior white matter involvement in 80%.
(a) Parietooccipital white matter with central to peripheral, posterior to anterior progression typical pattern.

        (b) Corpus callosum splenium (typical).

        (c) Visual, auditory pathways (frequent).

        (d) Corticospinal tracts (occasional).

    (2) Anterior white matter pattern in 15%.

        (a) Frontal white matter.

        (b) Corpus callosum genu.

        (c) Frontopontine tract.

    (3) Miscellaneous.

        (a) Cerebellum.

        (b) Projection fiber abnormalities.

    (4) AMN.

        (a) Corticospinal tract high signal on T2WI.

        (b) Parietooccipital, corpus callosum splenium hyperintensity.

        (c) Spinal cord atrophy (mainly thoracic).

  c. Proton MR spectroscopy (MRS).

    (1) Reduced N-acetyl aspartate.

    (2) Elevated choline-containing compounds.

    (3) May depict change earlier than standard spin-echo MR.

D. Organic acid disorders.

  1. Phenylketonuria (PKU).

    a. Etiology, pathology, clinical.

      (1) Most common treatable disorder of amino acid metabolism.

        (a) Classic PKU found in 1 in 7000 to 15,000 live births.

      (2) Caused by deficiency of phenylalanine 4-monooxygenase.

      (3) Autosomal recessive disorder mapped to chromosome 12q.

      (4) Early diagnosis with appropriate dietary modifications can improve long-term outcome.

    b. CT/MR findings are nonspecific.

      (1) Periventricular hypodensity.

      (2) Symmetric hyperintensity of deep white matter on T2WI.

    c. MRS can demonstrate elevated phenylalanine (Phe) levels in brain, correlation with neuropsychologic dysfunction.

  2. Maple syrup urine disease (MSUD).

    a. Etiology, pathology, clinical.

      (1) Abnormal oxidative decarboxylation of branched-chain amino acids (leucine, isoleucine, valine).

      (2) Accumulation of leucine, 2-oxoisocaproic acid.

       (3) Autosomal recessive.

       (4) Early diagnosis with appropriate dietary regimen can improve outcome.

       (5) Onset of first metabolic crisis typically occurs within 4 to 7 days after birth.

       (6) Infection can cause recurrent decompensation.

    b. Imaging.

       (1) Normal in first few days of life.

       (2) With symptom onset, severe localized edema ("MSUD edema") in cerebellar white matter, dorsal brain stem, cerebral peduncles, posterior limb of internal capsule (myelinated areas in newborns) initially appears.

       (3) Occasionally basal ganglia (globi pallidi) are involved.

       (4) Generalized hemispheric edema may appear and remain for several weeks in untreated infants.

       (5) After acute phase, periventricular white matter hypodensity/hyperintensity changes may persist.

II. Inherited leukoencephalopathies characterized by early involvement of peripheral (subcortical) white matter.

  A. Pelizaeus-Merzbacher disease (PMD).

    1. Etiology, pathology, clinical.

      a. Rare X-linked recessive leukodystrophy.

      b. Deficiency of proteolipid protein, an important component of myelin.

      c. Marked hypomyelination of both deep, superficial white matter.

      d. Clinical.

       (1) Abnormal eye movements, visual evoked potentials.

       (2) Progressive deterioration with death in late adolescence or young adulthood is typical; a more severe connatal form also occurs.

    2. Imaging.

      a. CT shows nonspecific white matter hypodensity, atrophy.

      b. MR variable.

       (1) Severe cases show near-total lack of myelination in both deep, superficial white matter (scans resemble newborn) diffuse brain atrophy.

       (2) Less severe cases of PMD may demonstrate patchy, heterogeneous white matter hyperintensities ("tigroid" pattern) on T2WI.

       (3) Secondary basal ganglia hypointensity can sometimes be identified on T2WI.

B. Canavan disease (CD) (also known as spongiform leukodystrophy).
  1. Etiology, pathology, clinical.
     a. Autosomal recessive inheritance.
     b. Deficiency of aspartoacylase with accumulation of N-acetyl-
        aspartic acid (NAA) in urine, plasma, brain.
     c. Characterized pathologically by megalencephaly with wide-
        spread demyelination, spongiform vacuolation of first pe-
        ripheral, then deep white matter.
     d. Clinical presentation is hypotonia, loss of motor activity, and
        macrocephaly.
  2. Imaging.
     a. CT shows diffuse, bilaterally symmetric hypodensity of
        cerebral, cerebellar white matter.
     b. MR.
        (1) T2WI shows diffuse hyperintensity that preferentially
            involves arcuate fibers.
        (2) Severe cases may show near-total lack of myelination
            except for internal capsule.
        (3) Basal ganglia, thalami may appear hypointense on
            T2WI.
     c. MR spectroscopy shows marked elevation of NAA peak
        (may be specific for Canavan disease).
     d. U/S shows markedly enhanced acoustic attenuation of white
        matter (reversed pattern of echogenicity of cortical gray and
        subcortical white matter).
C. Alexander disease (AD) (also known as fibrinoid leukodystrophy).
  1. Etiology, inheritance, pathology.
     a. Unknown cause, inheritance.
     b. Pathologic hallmark is accumulation of hyaline eosinophilic
        rods ("Rosenthal fibers") within swollen astrocytes accom-
        panied by variable degrees of demyelination.
        (1) *Note:* Rosenthal fibers not diagnostic of AD as they may
            be present in low-grade astrocytomas and many chronic
            nonneoplastic inflammatory or vascular diseases.
     c. Three clinical subgroups.
        (1) Infantile form presents in early life with macrocephaly,
            psychomotor retardation, spastic quadriparesis, seizures.
        (2) Juvenile-onset form presents from age 7 to 14 years with
            bulbar signs, spastic quadriparesis, ataxia but with intact
            mental status.
        (3) Adult-onset form mimics multiple sclerosis.

2. Imaging.
   a. CT.
      (1) Bilaterally symmetric low density in frontal white matter, basal ganglia, anterior limbs of internal capsules.
      (2) Basal ganglia, periventricular regions may enhance following contrast.
   b. MR.
      (1) Deep, subcortical frontal lobe white matter hyperintensity on T2WI.
      (2) Caudate, putamen, globi pallidi may be hyperintense, show enhancement following contrast administration.

SUGGESTED READINGS

Apkarian P, Kestsveld-Baart JC, Barth PG: Visual evoked potential characteristics and early diagnosis of Pelizaeus-Merzbacher disease, *Arch Neurol* 50:981-985, 1993.

Barkovich AJ: Toxic and metabolic brain disorders. In *Pediatric Neuroimaging,* ed 2, New York, 1995, Raven Press, pp 55-105.

Becker LE: Lysosomes, peroxisomes and mitochondria: Function and disorder, *AJNR* 13:609-620, 1992.

Bernardi B, Fonda C, Franzoni E, et al: MRI and CT in Krabbé's disease: Case report, *Neuroradiol* 36:477-479, 1994.

Breysem L, Smet M-H, Johannik K, et al: Brain MR imaging in dietarily treated phenylketonuria, *Eur Radiol* 4:329-331, 1994.

Brismar J, Brismar G, Gascon G, Ozand P: Canavan disease: CT and MR imaging of the brain, *AJNR* 11:805-810, 1990.

Buhrer C, Bassir C, von Moers A, et al: Cranial ultrasound findings in aspartoacylase deficiency (Canavan disease), *Pediatr Radiol* 23:395-397, 1993.

Castellote A, Vera J, Vazquez E, et al: MR in adrenoleukodystrophy: atypical presentation as bilateral frontal demyelination, *AJNR* 16:814-815, 1995.

Choi S, Enzmann DR: Infantile Krabbé disease: Complementary CT and MR findings, *AJNR* 14:1164-1166, 1993.

Cleary MA, Walter JH, Wraith JE, et al: Magnetic resonance imaging in phenylketonuria: reversal of cerebral white matter change, *J Pediatr* 127:251-255, 1995.

Felber SR, Sperl W, Chemelli A, et al: Maple syrup urine disease: Metabolic decompensation monitored by proton magnetic resonance imaging and spectroscopy, *Ann Neurol* 33:396-401, 1993.

Francis GS, Bonni A, Shen N, et al: Metachromatic leukodystrophy: Multiple nonfunctional and pseudodeficiency alleles in a pedigree, *Ann Neurol* 34:212-218, 1993.

Hittmair K, Wimberger D, Wiesbauer P, et al: Early infantile form of Krabbé disease with optic hypertrophy: Serial MR examinations and autopsy correlation, *AJNR* 15:1454-1458, 1994.

Kendall BE: Disorders of lysosomes, peroxisomes, and mitochondria, *AJNR* 13:621-653. 1992.

Kumar AJ, Kohler W, Kruse B, et al: MR findings in adult-onset adrenoleuko-dystrophy, *AJNR* 16:1227-1237, 1995.

Lee BCP: Magnetic resonance imaging of metabolic and primary white matter disorders in children, *Neuroimaging Clin North Am* 3:267-289, 1993.

Loes DJ, Hite S, Moser H, et al: Adrenoleukodystrophy: A scoring method for brain MR observations, *AJNR* 15:1761-1766, 1994.

Moser HW, Powers JM, Smith KD: Adrenoleukodystrophy: molecular genetics, pathology, and Lorenzo's oil, *Brain Pathol* 5:259-266, 1995.

Novotny EJ Jr, Avison MJ, Herschkowitz N, et al: In vivo measurement of phenylalanine in human brain by proton nuclear magnetic resonance spectros-copy, *Ped Res* 37:244-248, 1995.

Pridmore CL, Baraitser M, Harding B, et al: Alexander's disease: Clues to diagnosis, *J Child Neurol* 8:134-144, 1993.

Seitelberger F: Neuropathology and genetics of Pelizaeus-Merzbacher disease, *Brain Pathol* 5:267-273, 1995.

van der Knaap MS, Valk J: The reflection of histology in MR imaging of Pelizaeus-Merzbacher disease, *AJNR* 10:99-103, 1988.

Wang P-J, Young C, Liu H-M, et al: Neurophysiologic studies and MRI in Pelizaeus-Merzbacher disease: comparison of classic and connatal forms, *Pediatr Neurol* 12:47-53, 1995.

51

Inherited Metabolic and Neurodegenerative Disorders That Affect the Gray Matter

Key Concepts

1. Gray matter diseases that affect the cortex.
   a. Neuronal ceroid-lipofuscinosis (e.g., Batten disease).
   b. Miscellaneous (mucolipidoses, glycogen storage diseases, G_{M1} gangliosidoses).
2. Disorders of cortex plus white matter.
   a. Mucopolysaccharidoses.
   b. Generalized peroxisomal disorders.
3. Disorders that affect deep gray nuclei.
   a. Leigh disease.
   b. Huntington disease.
   c. Hallervorden-Spatz disease.
   d. Wilson disease.
4. Disorders that affect both deep gray, white matter.
   a. Globoid cell leukodystrophy (Krabbé disease).
   b. Mitochondrial disorders (MELAS, MERRF).
   c. Organic acidemias and aminoacidurias.
   d. G_{M2} gangliosidoses.
   e. Almost any late or end-stage leukodystrophy.

A broad spectrum of inherited metabolic and neurodegenerative disorders can involve the gray matter primarily or exclusively, although as a group these diseases are much less common than the leukodystrophies. Gray matter metabolic disorders can be subdivided conveniently into those that affect the cortex and those that involve the deep gray nuclei. Furthermore, each of these disorders can exist alone or in conjunction with white matter disease.

Disorders that primarily or solely involve the cortical gray matter include neuronal ceroid-lipofuscinosis (e.g., Batten disease), mucolipidoses, glycogen storage diseases, and the G_{M1} gangliosidoses. The inherited (early-onset) variety of Alzheimer disease may also belong in this category (see Chapter 54). The mucopolysaccharidoses and generalized peroxisomal disorders are examples of conditions that involve both the cortex and white matter.

Examples of inherited disorders that predominately involve the deep gray nuclei include Leigh disease, juvenile Huntington disease, Wilson disease, and Hallervorden-Spatz syndrome.

Finally, a number of leukoencephalopathies commonly involve both white matter and the basal ganglia. These include some of the mitochondrial encephalopathies such as MELAS and MERRF, globoid cell leukodystrophy (Krabbé disease), Canavan disease, and some of the organic acid disorders (e.g., methymalonic acidemia and glutaric acidemia type 1).

In this chapter we discuss briefly some of the most important "inborn errors of metabolism" that affect the cerebral gray matter, with or without concomitant white matter involvement.

I. Inherited metabolic disorders that predominately or solely affect the cortical gray matter.
  A. Neuronal ceroid-lipofuscinosis (NCL).
    1. Etiology, pathology.
      a. Group of hereditary encephalopathies characterized by progressive neural, extraneural accumulation of ceroid and lipofuscin-like storage cytosomes.
      b. Extensive loss of cortical, subcortical neurons with gross atrophy.
      c. Pathogenesis unknown.
    2. Classification into four types.
      a. Infantile NCL.
        (1) Chromosome 1.
      b. Late infantile NCL.
      c. Juvenile (Batten disease).
        (1) Chromosome 16.
      d. Adult NCL (Kufs disease).

    3. Imaging.
        a. Infantile NCL.
           (1) Variable atrophy (enlarged sulci, ventricles).
           (2) Thalami hyperdense/hypointense compared with basal ganglia.
           (3) Reversed signal intensity of peripheral white and cortical gray matter.
        b. Batten disease.
           (1) Mild to moderate atrophy.
           (2) Thin cortex.
           (3) White matter signal usually normal.
  B. Miscellaneous disorders.
    1. Mucolipidoses.
        a. Both mucopolysaccharides, lipids accumulate.
        b. Examples.
           (1) I-cell disease.
           (2) Fucosidosis, mannosidosis.
        c. Imaging manifestations.
           (1) Generalized atrophy.
           (2) Thin cortex.
           (3) Nonspecific white matter changes.
    2. Glycogen storage diseases.
        a. Abnormality of glycogen storage, synthesis, or degradation.
        b. Examples.
           (1) Pompe disease.
         c. Imaging studies show nonspecific cortical atrophy.
II. Inherited metabolic disorders that affect both cortex and white matter.
  A. Mucopolysaccharidoses (MPS).
    1. Definition.
        a. Inborn error of metabolism.
        b. Deficiency of a specific exoglycosidase prevents normal lysosomal degradation of mucopolysaccharides (glycosaminoglycans).
    2. Classification into five major types (13 syndromes or variants exist).
        a. MPS I H (Hurler).
        b. MPS I S (Scheie).
        c. MPS II (Hunter).
        d. MPS III A-D (Sanfilipo).
        e. MPS IV A and B (Morquio).
    3. Inheritance.
        a. Autosomal recessive.
        b. Exception: Hunter syndrome (X-linked recessive).

4. Pathology.
    a. Gross pathology.
        (1) Macrocephaly.
        (2) "Cribriform" deposition of glycosaminoglycans in peri-
            vascular (subendothelial) locations in CNS, other organs.
        (3) Dura may be grossly thickened.
    b. Microscopic pathology.
        (1) Cortical, cerebellar neurons develop large processes
            ("meganeurites") that contain the loaded lysosomes or
            storage bodies.
5. Clinical features variable.
    a. Large head (macrocephaly).
    b. "Gargoyle-like" facies.
    c. Dwarfism.
    d. Bone deformities.
    e. Hepatosplenomegaly.
    f. Mild to severe psychomotor retardation.
6. Imaging features.
    a. CT (nonspecific).
        (1) Enlarged ventricles.
        (2) White matter hypodensity.
        (3) Skull, odontoid dysplasia common.
        (4) Thick dura.
    b. MR.
        (1) Cortical atrophy with reduced contrast between gray,
            white matter.
        (2) Multiple cavitary lesions (perivascular "pits").
            (a) Multiple foci of prolonged T1, T2.
            (b) Radially oriented.
            (c) Found in subcortical, deep white matter.
            (d) Predominately posterior in location.
        (3) Thick dura, with or without spinal cord compression.
B. Generalized peroxisomal disorder (Zellweger syndrome).
    1. Etiology, inheritance.
        a. Also known as cerebrohepatorenal syndrome.
        b. Autosomal recessive.
        c. Deficiency of multiple peroxisomal enzymes.
    2. Imaging findings.
        a. Cortical abnormalities.
            (1) Neuronal migrational anomalies.
                (a) Pachymicrogyria, polymicrogyria.
                (b) Heterotopic gray matter.
            (2) Cortical thinning.

     b. White matter abnormalities.
       (1) Generalized hypoplasia.
       (2) Hypomyelination.

III. Inherited metabolic and neurodegenerative disorders that primarily involve the basal ganglia.
  A. Leigh disease (subacute necrotizing encephalomyelopathy).
    1. Etiology, pathology, inheritance.
      a. Mitochondrial encephalopathy.
        (1) Deficiency of multiple enzymes.
          (a) Pyruvate dehydrogenase complex.
          (b) Pyruvate carboxylase.
          (c) Defects in electron transport chain.
      b. Autosomal recessive.
      c. Pathology.
        (1) Spongiosis, demyelination, gliosis.
        (2) Symmetric necrotizing lesions.
          (a) Basal ganglia (putamina, pallidum, caudate nucleus head), thalami.
          (b) Brainstem tegmentum (periaqueductal gray matter).
          (c) Cerebellum, medulla, spinal cord.
    2. Clinical manifestations are variable.
      a. Infantile form occurs with hypotonia, vomiting, seizures.
      b. Ataxia, ophthalmoplegia.
      c. Death usually occurs from respiratory failure.
    3. Imaging.
      a. CT.
        (1) Symmetric low density of caudate, putamina.
      b. MR.
        (1) Symmetric hyperintense gray matter on T2WI.
          (a) Globi pallidi, putamena, caudate nuclei.
          (b) Periaqueductal gray, cerebral peduncles.
          (c) Cortical gray matter sometimes involved.
        (2) White matter less severely affected.
      c. MR spectroscopy shows abnormally high lactate peak, decreased NAA in basal ganglia.
  B. Huntington disease (HD).
    1. Inheritance, pathology, epidemiology.
      a. Autosomal dominant.
        (1) Mutation on short arm of chromosome 4.
        (2) Causes an expanded repeat of the trinucleotide sequence cytosine-adenine-guanine (CAG).
        (3) Individuals with fewer than 32 copies do not develop

clinical HD, whereas those with 40 or more copies do.
  b. Causes progressive caudate, cortical atrophy.
  c. Worldwide prevalence estimated at 5 to 10 cases per 100,000.
2. Clinical.
  a. Movement (choreiform) disorder, mentation abnormalities, behavioral disturbances.
  b. Statistical association between earlier age at onset and increased CAG copies.
  c. Typical age at onset is fourth or fifth decade.
  d. 5% of HD cases become symptomatic at <14 years of age with cerebellar symptoms, mental deterioration, seizures.
  e. Disease duration averages between 15 and 30 years.
3. Imaging.
  a. CT.
    (1) May be normal early in disease course.
    (2) Frontal horns of lateral ventricles appear laterally convex due to caudate atrophy.
  b. MR.
    (1) Striatum may be hyperintense or hypointense on T2WI.
    (2) Atrophy of caudate, putamen.
    (3) Cortical atrophy (especially frontal regions).
C. Wilson disease (hepatolenticular degeneration).
  1. Etiology, pathology, inheritance.
    a. Abnormal copper metabolism.
      (1) Deficiency of ceruloplasmin (serum transport protein for copper).
      (2) Deficient biliary excretion of copper.
      (3) Excessive copper deposition (liver, brain).
    b. Autosomal recessive localized to chromosome 13.
    c. Pathology.
      (1) Cirrhosis of liver.
      (2) Degenerative changes in basal ganglia.
        (a) Spongy degeneration, cavitation.
        (b) Neuronal loss with astrocytic proliferation.
  2. Clinical.
    a. Symptom onset usually between 8 and 16 years.
    b. Extrapyramidal and cerebellar signs.
    c. Dementia and psychosis.
    d. Kayser-Fleischer rings (brownish coloration on outer margin of cornea).
    e. Progressive liver disease.

3. Imaging.
  a. CT.
    (1) Bilateral putaminal low-density lesions.
    (2) Mild nonspecific atrophy.
  b. MR.
    (1) Lateral putamina, thalami hyperintense on T2WI.
      (a) Lesions usually bilateral, symmetric.
      (b) Unilateral, asymmetric involvement may occur.
    (2) Caudate, red nuclei, substantia nigra may also be affected.
    (3) Liver failure may cause high signal in pallidi, dorsal midbrain on T1WI.
    (4) Subcortical and periventricular white matter involvement may occur but is uncommon.
D. Hallervorden-Spatz disease (HSD).
  1. Etiology, pathology, inheritance.
    a. Unknown etiology.
    b. Autosomal recessive.
    c. Vacuolization, iron deposits in globi pallidi, substantia nigra.
  2. Clinical.
    a. Pyramidal, extrapyramidal signs.
      (1) Rigidity.
      (2) Choreothetoid movements.
      (3) Dysarthria.
    b. Progressive mental deterioration.
  3. Imaging.
    a. CT.
      (1) Globi pallidi may appear high or low density.
    b. MR.
      (1) Pallidonigral low signal on T2WI.
      (2) Bilateral anteromedial hyperintense foci within low-signal globus pallidus may give "eye-of-the-tiger" sign.
IV. Disorders that affect both the deep gray and white matter.
  A. Globoid cell leukodystrophy (Krabbé disease) (see Chapter 50).
  B. Mitochondrial disorders.
    1. Types.
      a. Myoclonic epilepsy with ragged red fibers (MERRF).
      b. Mitochondrial encephalomyopathy, lactic acidosis, and strokelike episodes (MELAS).
      c. Kearns-Sayre syndrome (KSS).
      d. Chronic progressive external ophthalmoplegia (CPEO).
      e. Considerable overlap.
        (1) Between MELAS and MERRF.

        (2) Between KSS and CPEO.

  2. Etiology, pathology, inheritance.

    a. CPEO, KSS caused by large-scale deletions of mitochondrial DNA (mtDNA).

    b. Point mutations of mtDNA in MELAS, MERRF.

    c. ATP production is impaired.

    d. Brain, striated muscle most commonly affected organs ("encephalomyopathy").

        (1) Spongiform encephalopathy (KSS, CPEO), external ophthalmoplegia.

        (2) Multiple infarcts (MELAS, MERRF).

        (3) Neuronal loss in dentate, olivary nuclei with widespread gliosis and degeneration of myelinated tracts (MERRF).

        (4) Ragged red fibers in striated muscle (MERRF, MELAS).

  3. Clinical.

    a. Variable presentation depending on type.

    b. Later onset than other mitochondrial disorders (Canavan, Leigh, Zellweger syndromes).

  4. Imaging.

    a. MELAS, MERRF.

        (1) Multiple small, large infarcts.

           (a) Cortex.

           (b) Subcortical white matter.

           (c) Basal ganglia.

    b. KSS, CPEO.

        (1) Cerebral, cerebellar atrophy.

        (2) Variable hyperintensities in basal ganglia, white matter on T2WI.

C. Organic acidemias and aminoacidurias.

  1. Diverse group of disorders.

  2. Variable involvement of both gray, white matter.

  3. Some examples (also see Chapter 50).

    a. Phenylketonuria (PKU).

    b. Maple syrup urine disease (MSUD).

    c. Disorders of propionate and methylmalonate metabolism.

        (1) Widened CSF spaces.

        (2) Delayed myelination.

        (3) Symmetric basal ganglia involvement.

    d. Glutaric acidemia type I.

        (1) Widely open ("batwing") operculae.

        (2) Bilateral basal ganglia lesions.

        (3) Macrocephaly.

        (4) Prominent CSF spaces.

SUGGESTED READINGS

Barkovich AJ: Toxic and metabolic brain disorders. In *Pediatric neuroimaging,* ed 2, New York, 1995, Raven Press, pp 55-105.

Barkovich AJ, Good WV, Koch TK, Berg BO: Mitochondrial disorders: analysis of their clinical and imaging characteristics, *AJNR* 14:1119-1137, 1993.

Brismar J, Ozand PT: CT and MR of the brain in disorders of the propionate and methylmalonate metabolism, *AJNR* 15:1459-1473, 1994.

Brismar J, Ozand PT: CT and MR of the brain in glutaric acidemia type I: a review of 59 published cases and a report of 5 new cases, *AJNR* 16:675-683, 1995.

Ho VB, Chuang S, Rovira MJ, Koo B: Juvenile Huntington disease: CT and MR features, *AJNR* 16:1405-1412, 1995.

Huang C-C, Wai Y-Y, Chu N-S, et al: Mitochondrial encephalomyopathies: CT and MRI findings and correlations with clinical features, *Eur Neurol* 35:199-205, 1995.

Lee C, Dineen TE, Brack M, et al: The mucopolysaccharidoses: characterization by cranial MR imaging, *AJNR* 14:1285-1292, 1993.

Magalhaes ACA, Caramelli P, Menezes JR, et al: Wilson's disease: MRI with clinical correlation, *Neuroradiol* 36:97-100, 1994.

Roh JK, Lee TG, Wie BA, et al: Initial and follow-up brain MRI findings and correlation with the clinical course in Wilson's disease, *Neurol* 44:1064-1068, 1994.

Savoiardo M, Halliday WC, Nardocci N, et al: Hallervorden-Spatz disease: MR and pathologic findings, *AJNR* 14:155-162, 1993.

Taccone A, Donati PT, Marzoli A, et al: Mucopolysaccharidosis: thickening of dura mater at the craniocervical junction and other CT/MRI findings, *Ped Radiol* 23:349-352, 1993.

Vanhanen S-L, Raininko R, Santavuori P: Early differential diagnosis of infantile neuronal ceroid lipofuscinosis, Rett syndrome, and Krabbé disease by CT and MR, *AJNR* 15:1443-1453, 1994.

Walsh LE, Moran CC: The mucopolysaccharidoses: clinical and neuroradiographic features, *Neuroimaging Clin North Am* 3:291-303, 1993.

Wray SH, Provenzale JM, Johns DR, Thulborn KR: MR of the brain in mitochondrial myopathy, *AJNR* 16:1167-1173, 1995.

52

The Normal Aging Brain

Key Concepts

1. Imaging findings in the normal aging brain include:
   a. Moderate enlargement of sulci, ventricles.
   b. Scattered white matter hyperintensities on T2WI.
   c. Periventricular high-signal rims and caps.
   d. Iron deposition in the globus pallidus, putamen.
2. The scattered foci of white matter hyperintensity in older individuals represent diverse histologic phenomena ranging from dilated perivascular spaces to microscopic foci of venous ischemia or arterial infarction.

To understand the acquired neurodegenerative disorders, it is important to understand the normal age-related changes that occur in the brain. In this chapter we delineate the age-related changes that take place in the cerebral cortex, white matter, cerebrospinal fluid (CSF) spaces, and the deep gray matter nuclei (box). In Chapter 53 we discuss acquired white matter diseases. In the concluding chapter in this section on metabolic, toxic, and neurodegenerative disorders, we discuss those disease processes that primarily affect the gray matter.

I. Normal age-related changes in the sulci, cisterns, and ventricles.
   A. Sulci and cisterns (Fig. 52-1).
      1. Generalized loss of brain volume, weight begins in late fifth decade.

Normal Age-related Changes in the Brain

Sulci, ventricles

Between age 50 and 60 years, sulci and ventricles become mildly enlarged

White matter

Overall volume remains relatively stable after age 20 years
Virchow-Robin (perivascular spaces) increase in size, number
White matter hyperintensities on T2WI are common after age >50 years, represent varied histology
    Prominent perivascular spaces
    Axonal loss
    Focal areas of myelin pallor, demyelination (may represent ischemic changes in distribution of long perforating end-arteries)
    Spongy microcystic degeneration
    Arteriosclerosis and frank lacunar infarction
    Periventricular venous collagenosis

Gray matter

Linear decline in overall volume after age 20 years
Cortical thinning with increasing sulcal prominence

Brain iron

No iron in brain at birth
Normal iron accumulation (hypointense foci on T2WI) occurs in
    Globus pallidus
    Substantia nigra
    Red nucleus
    Dentate nucleus
    Putamen (after age 80 years)

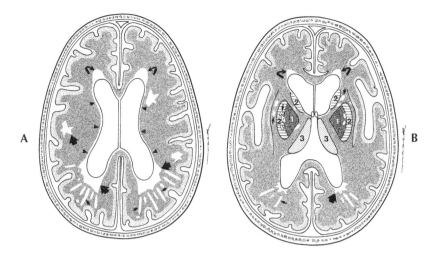

Fig. 52-1 A and **B,** Axial anatomic drawings depict basal ganglia iron deposition and white matter hyperintensities (WMHs) seen in the typical aging brain. Iron deposition is most noticeable in the globus pallidus (B, 1, black areas), less prominent in the putamen and caudate nucleus, and even less prominent in the thalamus (B, 2, 3, dotted and cross-hatched areas). Note triangular-shaped "caps" around the frontal horns (curved arrows), thin periventricular hyperintense halo (A, arrowheads), and dilated perivascular spaces, seen as punctate or linear hyperintensities (small arrows) in the subcortical white matter, centrum semiovale, and basal ganglia. Patchy periventricular and subcortical WMHs (large arrows) represent areas of myelin pallor and small vessel arteriosclerosis. (From Osborn AG: *Diagnostic neuroradiology,* St Louis, 1994, Mosby.)

   2. Significant overlap of normal brain volumetric indexes with those in demented individuals occurs.
   3. Age-related changes in subarachnoid spaces.
      a. Vermian subarachnoid spaces begin to enlarge around age 50.
         (1) Folia have prominent sulci.
         (2) Great horizontal fissures of cerebellum enlarge slightly.
      b. By late sixth decade, mild generalized enlargement of surface sulci on imaging studies is normal.
         (1) Cortical sulcal CSF volume increases curvilinearly throughout adulthood, with most striking increase occurring in the sixth to eighth decades.
         (2) Average increase in cortical CSF after age 20 is 0.6 ml per year.
   B. Age-related changes in ventricles (Fig. 52-1).

1. Overall ventricular CSF volume increases curvilinearly throughout adulthood.
   a. Average increase in ventricular CSF after age 20 is 0.3 ml per year.
   b. By early sixth decade, third ventricle appears mildly enlarged on imaging studies.
   c. Lateral ventricles in normal patients over 70 years of age are also mildly to moderately enlarged.
2. Overall ventricular size does not predict presence or progression of dementia in individual cases (see Chapter 54).

II. Normal age-related changes in white matter.
   A. White matter volume.
      1. Steadily increases from birth to 20 years.
      2. Levels off after age 20.
      3. Stable thereafter without significant fluctuation.
   B. White matter morphology.
      1. Compact white matter tracts.
         a. Age-related signal changes.
            (1) Short T1 (hyperintense on T1WI).
            (2) Short T2 (hypointense on T2WI).
         b. Caused by:
            (1) Dense, heavily myelinated fibers.
            (2) Decreasing water content.
         c. Typical locations.
            (1) Anterior commissure.
            (2) Corpus callosum.
            (3) Optic radiations.
            (4) Inferior and superior fronto-occipital fasciculi.
            (5) Uncinate and longitudinal superior fasciculi.
            (6) Internal capsules.
            (7) Mamillothalamic tracts.
            (8) Brachium pontis.
      2. Subcortical white matter (centrum semiovale).
         a. Hyperintensities (WMHs) on T2WI.
         b. Found in at least 30% to 40% of healthy elderly patients.
         c. Variable etiology (Fig. 52-1).
         d. Dilated Virchow-Robin spaces (VRSs).
            (1) Histology.
               (a) Normal pial-lined perivascular extensions of subarachnoid space.
               (b) VRSs surround penetrating arteries but are incomplete or absent around veins.

       (c) Found in basal ganglia and capsular region, cerebral cortex and subcortical white matter, and midbrain.

       (d) May extend deep into white matter (centrum semiovale).

    (2) Imaging.

       (a) Well-delineated.

       (b) Smoothly marginated.

       (c) Round, ovoid, or curvilinear.

       (d) Isointense with CSF.

       (e) Increase in size, number with age.

       (f) May be prominent (up to 2 cm in diameter), asymmetric, unilateral.

  e. Nonspecific leukoencephalopathy (NSLE).

    (1) Heterogeneous histopathology.

       (a) Reduced axonal, oligodendroglial density.

       (b) Demyelination.

       (c) Myelin pallor.

       (d) Astrocytosis and gliosis.

       (e) Spongy vacuolization or microcystic changes.

       (f) Arteriosclerosis and microvascular infarction.

    (2) Clinical correlation.

       (a) Age-related.

       (b) Extent, frequency increased with hypertension, diabetes, hyperlipidemia, cardiac disease (but overlap with normal).

    (3) Imaging.

       (a) Patchy or confluent nonenhancing low-density foci on CT.

       (b) Patchy or confluent subcortical foci of increased signal on T2-weighted MR scans.

3. Periventricular white matter lesions (Fig. 52-1).

  a. Triangle-shaped "caps" around frontal horns.

    (1) Normal finding on T2-weighted MR scans in patients of all ages.

    (2) Histopathology.

       (a) Loosely compacted myelin with relative increase in periependymal fluid.

  b. Periventricular "rims."

    (1) Normal on PD-weighted, T2-weighted MR scans in healthy elderly patients.

       (a) Smooth, thin, continuous.

       (b) Bilateral.

       (c) Symmetric.

    (2) Histopathology.

       (a) Focal loss of ependymal epithelium with mild underlying gliosis ("ependymitis granularis").

       (b) Increased periependymal CSF.

  c. Patchy, irregular focal or confluent periventricular lesions.

    (1) Found in 30% of patients >60 years old.

    (2) More common on T2WI in patients with hypertension, atherosclerosis but overlap with normal age-matched controls.

    (3) Variable histology.

       (a) Axonal loss.

       (b) Demyelination, myelin pallor.

       (c) Astrocytosis.

       (d) Spongy microcystic changes.

       (e) Periventricular venous collagenosis (see Chapter 53).

    (4) Imaging.

       (a) CT: patchy or confluent nonenhancing low-attenuation foci.

       (b) MR: isointense on T1WI; hyperintense on PD-, T2WI.

       (c) Have lower magnetization transfer ratios (MTRs) than normal white matter.

III. Normal age-related changes in gray matter.

  A. Gray matter volume.

    1. Cortical gray matter volume increases with peak at about age 4.

    2. Normal elimination during childhood of about 40% of cortical synapses ("pruning") causes subsequent decrease in cortical gray matter volume.

    3. After age 20, steady linear decline in cortical gray matter volume occurs.

  B. Gray matter morphology.

    1. Progressive age-related neuronal loss.

    2. Overlap between normal, cognitively-impaired individuals.

    3. Imaging studies.

      a. CT.

      (1) Cortical gray matter density decreases.

      (2) Surface sulci and cisterns enlarge.

       (a) Diabetes, hypertension, chronic cerebrovascular disorders, increasing number of medications as well as increasing age correlate with brain atrophy.

        (b) Overlap between normal, cognitively impaired individuals.
    b. MR.
        (1) Cortex is thinned.
        (2) Sulci become prominent.
        (3) Loss of contrast between gray, subcortical white matter (statistically significant by sixth or seventh decade).
IV. Age-related changes in brain iron.
  A. Normal age distribution of brain iron.
    1. No iron in brain at birth.
    2. Iron deposition begins shortly after birth.
      a. Non-heme iron.
        (1) Ferretin.
        (2) Hemosiderin.
      b. Location of normal iron deposition.
        (1) Globus pallidus (begins approximately 6 months after birth).
        (2) Zona reticulata of substantia nigra (beginning between 9 and 12 months).
        (3) Red nucleus (after 2 years of age).
    3. Stable iron concentration between 20 and 60 years.
      a. Detected as foci of decreased signal intensity on heavily T2-weighted MR scans (Fig. 52-1).
      b. Greatest concentration in extrapyramidal system.
        (1) Globus pallidus.
        (2) Red nucleus.
        (3) Substantia nigra.
      c. Other areas that may show shortened T2 relaxation.
        (1) Dentate nucleus.
        (2) Caudate nucleus.
    4. At age 80 years.
      a. Putamen may be as hypointense on T2WI as globus pallidus.

SUGGESTED READINGS

Autti T, Raininko R, Vanhanen SL, et al: MRI of the normal brain from early childhood to middle age. I. Appearance on T2- and proton density-weighted images and occurrence of incidental high-signal foci, *Neuroradiol* 36:644-648, 1994.

Autti T, Raininko R, Vanhanen SL, et al: MRI of the normal brain from early childhood to middle age. II. Age dependence of signal intensity changes on T2-weighted images, *Neuroradiol* 36:649-651, 1994.

Drayer BP: Degenerative disorders of the central nervous system: An integrated approach to the differential diagnosis, *Neuroimaging Clin North Am* 5:135-153, 1995.

Golomb J, Kluger A, Gianutsos J, et al: Nonspecific leukoencephalopathy associated with aging, *Neuroimaging Clin North Am* 5:33-44, 1995.

Horikoshi T, Yagi S, Fukamachi A: Incidental high-intensity foci in white matter on T2-weighted magnetic resonance imaging: frequency and clinical significance in symptom-free adults, *Neuroradiol* 35:151-155, 1993.

Magnaldi S, Ukmar M, Vasciaveo A, et al: Contrast between white and grey matter: MRI appearance with aging, *Eur Radiol* 3:513-519, 1993.

Meguro K, Yamaguchi T, Hishinuma T, et al: Periventricular hyperintensity on magnetic resonance imaging correlated with brain ageing and atrophy, *Neuroradiol* 35:125-129, 1993.

Meyer JS, Takashima S, Terayama Y, et al: CT changes associated with normal aging of the human brain, *J Neurol Sci* 123:200-208, 1994.

Mineura K, Sasajima H, Kikuchi K, et al: White matter hyperintensity in neurologically asymptomatic subjects, *Acta Neurol Scand* 92:151-156, 1995.

Ogawa T, Okudera T, Fukasawa H, et al: Unusual widening of Virchow-Robin spaces: MR appearance, *AJNR* 16:1238-1242, 1995.

Osborn AG: Acquired metabolic, white matter, and degenerative diseases of the brain. In *Diagnostic neuroradiology,* St Louis, 1994, Mosby, pp 748-779.

Pfefferbaum A, Mathalon DH, Sullivan EV, et al: A quantitative magnetic resonance imaging study of changes in brain morphology from infancy to late adulthood, *Arch Neurol* 51:874-887, 1994.

Schenker C, Meier D, Wichmann W, et al: Age distribution and iron dependency of the T2 relaxation time in the globus pallidus and putamen, *Neuroradiol* 35:119-124, 1993.

Weller RO: Anatomy and pathology of the subpial space, *Riv di Neuroradiol* 7(Suppl 4):15-21, 1994.

Wong KT, Grossman RI, Boorstein JM, et al: Magnetization transfer imaging of periventricular hyperintense white matter in the elderly, *AJNR* 16:253-258, 1995.

Ylikoski A, Erkinjuntti T, Raininko R, et al: White matter hyperintensities on MRI in the neurologically nondiseased elderly, *Stroke* 26:1171-1177, 1995.

53

Acquired Degenerative, Toxic, and Metabolic White Matter Diseases

---

Key Concepts

1. Vascular disease is the most common acquired white matter disorder but has many different possible origins.
   a. Normal age-related changes.
   b. Arteriosclerosis.
   c. Progressive occlusion of small venules (periventricular venous collagenosis).
   d. "Lacunar" and embolic infarcts.
   e. Miscellaneous vascular lesions.
      (1) Hypoxic-ischemic encephalopathy.
      (2) Hypertensive encephalopathy.
      (3) Amyloid angiopathy.
      (4) Migraine headaches.
      (5) Vasculitis and vasculopathy.
2. Multiple sclerosis is the second most common acquired demyelinating disease.
3. Viral, postviral, and postimmunization demyelination are uncommon but important causes of white matter disease.
4. Important causes of toxic demyelination include:
   a. Chronic alcoholism.
   b. Ion balance disorders (e.g., osmotic demyelination).
   c. Miscellaneous agents (e.g., organic solvents, "interval" form of carbon monoxide poisoning, inhalation of poisoned heroin).
5. Iatrogenic white matter disease can be caused by radiation, chemotherapy, or a combination of agents.
6. Secondary white matter degeneration may occur after motor neuron destruction.
   a. Amyotrophic lateral sclerosis.
   b. Wallerian degeneration.
   c. Cerebellorubral degeneration.

Many acquired neurodegenerative diseases primarily or exclusively affect the cerebral white matter. These disorders are also sometimes called myelinoclastic or *de*-myelinating disorders (to distinguish them from the inherited or so-called *dys*-myelinating disorders).

In this chapter we discuss the most common and important of the acquired white matter disorders. We begin with vascular white matter disease and its overlap with normal aging. We then turn our attention to multiple sclerosis, which is perhaps the most common and best-characterized of the nonvascular white matter disorders. We conclude our discussion by considering some less common but important immune-mediated demyelinating disorders, the toxic encephalopathies, and secondary white matter tract degeneration syndromes.

   I. Vascular causes of white matter degenerative diseases.
      A. "Normal" age-related white matter changes (also see Chapter 52) have variable histology, extensive differential diagnosis (box).
         1. Enlarged Virchow-Robin spaces (VRSs).
            a. Occur in specific locations.

Multifocal White Matter Lesions: Differential Diagnosis

Most common

Perivascular spaces
Normal aging changes
Arteriosclerosis
Periventricular venous collagenosis
Multiple sclerosis
Inflammatory lesions (e.g., cysticercosis)

Common

Emboli
Metastases
Trauma (with moderate to severe closed head injury)

Uncommon

Postviral, postimmunization demyelination
Vasculitis
Multifocal primary neoplasm (multicentric glioma, lymphoma)
Abscesses
Inherited leukoencephalopathy
Acquired leukoencephalopathy
Neurocutaneous syndromes (NF-1, tuberous sclerosis)

          (1) Basal ganglia and internal/external capsules.
          (2) Cerebral white matter.
          (3) Midbrain.
     b. Size, number increase with age but can be seen in normal patients of all ages.
     c. May become very prominent.
          (1) Sometimes called "état criblé."
          (2) Signal like CSF (hypointense on T1WI, hyperintense on T2WI).
     d. Vacuolated myelin around perivascular spaces is common in neurologically normal patients >65 years old.
2. Atherosclerosis with ischemic changes around long penetrating end arteries that have little or no collateralization.
     a. Isointense on T1WI, hyperintense on PDWI, T2WI.
     b. Typical locations.
          (1) Pons.
          (2) Thalami.
          (3) Basal ganglia, capsular region.
          (4) Deep cerebral white matter.
     c. Increase with age, history of stroke but not with severity of extracranial carotid stenosis, presence of hypertension, or history of myocardial infarction.
3. Periventricular venous collagenosis.
     a. Noninflammatory stenosis or occlusion of periventricular, subependymal veins.
     b. Strong association with advanced white matter disease ("leukoariosis").
4. "Lacunar" and embolic infarctions.
     a. Ischemic lacunar infarcts.
          (1) Histopathology shows areas of necrosis, demyelination, cystic degeneration, and axonal loss.
     b. Hemorrhagic lacunes.
          (1) Seen in hypertensive vascular disease.
          (2) Indicate higher risk of intracerebral hemorrhage.
     c. Embolic infarcts (see Chapter 37).
          (1) Often multiple.
          (2) Typical locations in basal ganglia and at junction of cortex, subcortical white matter.
5. Miscellaneous vascular causes of white matter disease.
     a. Hypoxic-ischemic encephalopathy.
          (1) Periventricular leukomalacia (PVL) in premature infants.
          (2) Watershed infarction in term infants, children, adults.

b. Hypertensive encephalopathy.
   (1) Acute.
      (a) Reversible deep white matter edema.
   (2) Eclampsia.
      (a) Symmetric cortical, subcortical, basal ganglia hyperintensities (may enhance).
      (b) Posterior circulation most severely affected.
      (c) Lesions are usually reversible.
c. Amyloid angiopathy.
   (1) Usually causes superficial lobar hemorrhages.
   (2) May cause scattered subcortical white matter lesions.
d. Migraine.
   (1) Debatable whether patients with migraine headaches have greater prevalence of single or multiple white matter lesions.
e. Vasculitis (see Chapter 39).

II. Multiple sclerosis and autoimmune-mediated demyelinating diseases.
   A. Multiple sclerosis (MS).
      1. Precise etiology unknown; suggested causes of the demyelination include:
         a. Autoimmune.
         b. Infectious.
         c. Vascular.
         d. Toxic.
      2. Pathology.
         a. MS classification.
            (1) Chronic MS.
            (2) Variants of MS.
               (a) Acute MS (Marburg type).
               (b) Neuromyelitis optica (Devic's disease).
               (c) Concentric sclerosis (Balo's disease).
         b. Gross pathology.
            (1) Acute MS plaques have pink color, soft consistency.
            (2) Older MS plaques are firmer, gelatinous, and somewhat translucent.
            (3) Atrophy, cystic changes common with chronic MS.
         c. Microscopic pathology.
            (1) Progressive destruction of both myelin and myelin-producing oligodendrocytes.
            (2) Underlying axons remain intact.
            (3) Moderate macrophage infiltration and perivascular inflammation are present in active foci.
      3. Epidemiology.

      a. Most prevalent among Northern Europeans or Americans of Northern European extraction.

      b. Individuals living in the United States have approximately a 1 in 1000 chance of developing MS.

      c. Less common in Asians.

      d. Rare in black Africans.

4. Age.

      a. Symptom onset is typically between 20 and 40 years of age.

         (1) Average age of onset is 30 years.

         (2) 85% to 95% of cases occur between ages of 18 and 50 years.

         (3) 5% to 10% of cases occur in patients >50 years.

         (4) In very rare cases, onset can be delayed until sixth or even seventh decade.

      b. <3% of all MS cases occur in children.

         (1) Rare before puberty.

         (2) Average age of onset is 13 years.

         (3) Youngest reported case is 10 months.

5. Gender.

      a. Adults: slight female predominance (60%).

      b. Children: at least twice as common in girls compared with boys.

6. Location.

      a. >85% have ovoid periventricular lesions.

         (1) Along calloseptal interface.

         (2) Oriented perpendicularly to lateral ventricles.

         (3) Located around subependymal, deep white matter medullary veins.

      b. 50% to 90% of patients with clinically definite MS have lesions in corpus callosum itself.

      c. 10% of adults have posterior fossa lesions.

      d. Gray matter (cortex, basal ganglia) lesions do occur.

      e. Spinal cord lesions.

         (1) Found at autopsy in almost all MS cases.

         (2) Cervical cord most common site.

         (3) Cord MS usually occurs with brain lesions.

         (4) Occasionally cord is sole initial site (reported in up to 10% of cases).

         (5) Cord + optic nerve without brain involvement = Devic's disease.

7. Clinical spectrum, natural history.

      a. Variable presentation; classic symptoms include:

         (1) Optic neuritis.

(2) Numbness, dysesthesia, burning sensations in arm, leg, face.

(3) Lhermitte's sign (electric, shooting, or burning sensations down back, arms, or legs when neck is flexed).

b. Course.

(1) 70% relapsing-remitting.

(2) 20% chronic progressive.

(3) Fulminant form is rare.

(4) Occasionally asymptomatic.

8. Imaging.

a. CT.

(1) Often normal early.

(2) Isodense or hypodense plaques on NECT.

(3) Active lesions may show solid or ringlike enhancement.

(4) Long-standing cases may demonstrate generalized atrophy.

b. MR.

(1) Lesions identified in 85% to 90% of clinically definite cases.

(a) T1WI: isointense to hypointense.

(b) PDWI: hyperintense.

(c) T2WI: hyperintense.

(2) Sagittal scans show lesions at callosal-septal interface.

(a) 93% sensitivity.

(b) 97% specificity.

(3) Use of contrast enhancement increases specificity of MR imaging in early diagnosis of MS.

(a) Demonstrates blood-brain barrier breakdown in inflammatory or "active" lesions.

(b) Ring-enhancing pattern is typical.

(4) Basal ganglia may appear very hypotense on T2WI (long-standing, severe MS).

(5) Magnetization transfer ratio (MTR).

(a) Decreases with diminished myelin content in brain.

(6) Atypical lesions.

(a) "Tumoral" MS (large solitary plaque can mimic neoplasm).

(b) Inhomogeneously enhancing lesion.

(c) "Target-like" lesions (central enhancement, peripheral low signal).

(d) Multisegmental MS plaque can mimic intramedullary spinal cord neoplasm.

9. MS "mimics."

a. Clinical.

   (1) Clinical overdiagnosis of MS may occur in up to 10% of patients.
   (2) CSF studies show 3% of patients with "clinically definite" MS have some diagnosis other than MS.
   (3) Some disorders that mimic MS clinically:
       (a) Single-gene disorders.
       (b) Lyme disease.
       (c) Postviral syndromes.
       (d) Vasculitis.
       (e) Sarcoid.
   b. Imaging.
   (1) Some lesions that can mimic MS on MR.
       (a) Cerebrovascular disease.
       (b) Leukodystrophy.
       (c) Vasculitis.
       (d) Encephalitis.
       (e) Sarcoidosis.
       (f) Postviral demyelination.
       (g) Multiple metastases.
   (2) Helpful features of MS on MR imaging.
       (a) Multiple lesions.
       (b) >3 mm in diameter with at least one >6 mm.
       (c) Involvement of callososeptal interface.
       (d) Presence of brainstem, cerebellar, or spinal cord lesion.
B. Viral, postviral, autoimmune demyelination (see Chapter 44).
   1. Encephalitis.
   2. Acute disseminated encephalomyelitis (ADEM).
      a. Monophasic acute or subacute illness that follows viral infection or immunization.
      b. Multifocal areas of demyelination.
      (1) Scattered hyperintense foci on T2WI.
          (a) Centrum semiovale.
          (b) Posterior fossa.
          (c) Spinal cord.
      (2) Lesions may enhance, with variable patterns.
          (a) Patchy.
          (b) Gyriform.
          (c) Ring.
      (3) Beware: Large demyelinating lesions of any etiology may cause mass effect, mimic neoplasm.
      c. ADEM may also involve deep gray nuclei (basal ganglia, thalami).
      d. Features that are helpful in distinguishing ADEM and MS.

           (1) ADEM is often subcortical or in centrum semiovale, whereas most common site for MS is callososeptal interface.

           (2) Deep gray nuclei are most often involved with ADEM.

    3. Lyme disease (CNS involvement is autoimmune-mediated).

    4. Subacute sclerosing panencephalitis (SSPE).

    5. HIV infection and its complications (see Chapter 45).

III. Toxic encephalopathies.

  A. Alcohol.

    1. Alcoholism causes a variety of neurologic disorders.

      a. Marchiafava-Bignami disease.

        (1) Due to neurotoxic effect of ethanol.

        (2) Corpus callosum demyelination but may also affect cerebral white matter.

        (3) Acute stage of demyelination may enhance.

        (4) Cystic changes, atrophy in chronic cases.

      b. Wernicke encephalopathy (WE).

        (1) Caused by nutritional thiamine deficiency.

        (2) Potentially reversible if diagnosed early, appropriate therapy instituted (parenteral thiamine).

        (3) Mainly seen in alcoholics but can occur in nonalcoholics and children.

          (a) Eating disorders, severe malnourishment.

          (b) Prolonged tube feeding.

          (c) Gastric or intestinal surgery.

          (d) Hyperemesis, diarrhea, extended fever or dehydration.

          (e) Chemotherapy, immunosuppression.

        (4) Classic symptoms.

          (a) Ataxia.

          (b) Oculomotor abnormalities.

          (c) Global confusion.

          (d) Patients who survive acute WE may develop Korsakoff's psychosis (chronic amnestic disorder).

        (5) Involves both gray, white matter.

        (6) Characteristic periventricular distribution.

          (a) Medial thalamic nuclei adjacent to third ventricle.

          (b) Mammillary bodies.

          (c) Periaqueductal region.

         (7) Lesions are hyperintense on T2WI.

        (8) Acute lesions may enhance.

      c. Other neurotoxic effects of alcohol.

(1) Atrophy.
(a) Superior vermis.
(b) Generalized (with alcoholic dementia).
(2) Central pontine myelinolysis (see below).
(3) Peripheral polyneuropathy.
(4) Acute alcoholic myopathy.
B. Altered ion balance.
1. Central pontine myelinolysis (CPM).
a. Toxic demyelination disease.
(1) Myelin loss.
(2) Relative neuron sparing.
(3) Pons is most common site.
(a) Transverse pontine fibers most severely affected.
(b) Descending corticospinal tracts relatively spared.
(4) Extrapontine involvement occurs in approximately 50% of cases (see below).
b. >75% of cases associated with two conditions.
(1) Chronic alcoholism.
(2) Rapid correction of hyponatremia.
c. Other reported clinical settings include:
(1) Chronic renal failure.
(2) Liver failure.
(3) Dehydration.
(4) Diabetes.
(5) Electrolyte imbalance.
(a) Hyponatremia.
(b) Hypernatremia.
(6) Inappropriate antidiuretic hormone secretion.
(7) Paraneoplastic syndrome.
d. Clinical manifestations.
(1) Spastic quadriparesis.
(2) Pseudobulbar palsy.
(3) May cause "locked-in" syndrome.
e. Imaging.
(1) CT.
(a) Often normal.
(b) Central pons may appear hypodense.
(2) MR.
(a) Pons appears hypointense on T1WI.
(b) Hyperintense on T2WI.
(c) Variable enhancement.
(d) May involve other sites (see below).

(e) Lesions may partially or completely resolve.
2. Extrapontine myelinolysis (EPM).
   a. EPM occurs in approximately 50% of osmotic demyelination cases.
   b. Reported sites.
      (1) Putamina.
      (2) Caudate nuclei.
      (3) Thalami.
      (4) Midbrain.
      (5) White matter (subcortical, centrum semiovale).
   c. Imaging.
      (1) Hypodense on CT.
      (2) Hyperintense on T2-weighted MR.
      (3) Combination of pontine, basal ganglionic lesions strongly suggests osmotic demyelination syndrome.
C. Miscellaneous causes of toxic demyelination.
   1. Exposure to organic toxins.
      a. Myelin has high lipid content, slow metabolic turnover.
      b. Vulnerable to lipid peroxidation, accumulation of lipophilic toxins.
      c. Examples.
         (1) Solvents.
         (2) Toluene.
   2. "Interval" form of carbon monoxide (CO) poisoning.
      a. Typical acute form of CO poisoning affects globi pallidi (see Chapter 54).
      b. Clinical characteristics of "interval" CO poisoning.
         (1) Disturbed consciousness in acute phase.
         (2) Interval recovery.
         (3) Delayed encephalopathy with recrudescence of neurologic or psychiatric symptoms after a few days to weeks.
      c. Main pathologic feature is progressive demyelination.
         (1) Occurs in approximately 1% to 3% of patients with CO poisoning.
      d. Imaging.
         (1) Bilaterally symmetric, confluent high signal on T2WI.
            (a) Periventricular white matter.
            (b) Corpus callosum.
            (c) Internal capsule.
            (d) Centrum semiovale (may involve subcortical U fibers).
            (e) Globi pallidi.

      (2) Bilateral diffuse low-signal intensity on T2WI (possibly due to iron deposition).
        (a) Thalami.
        (b) Putamina.
      (3) MR spectroscopy.
        (a) Choline elevated.
        (b) Lactate elevation with decrease in N-acetylaspartate marks irreversible neuron injury.
  3. Drug abuse.
    a. Poisoned heroin inhalation.
    b. Causes spongiform white matter degeneration.
    c. T2WI shows symmetric high-signal intensity in cerebral, cerebellar white matter with corticospinal tracts, tractus solitarius, and medial lemnisci also commonly involved.
IV. Iatrogenic causes of white matter disease.
  A. Chemotherapy.
    1. Diffuse necrotizing leukoencephalopathy (DNL).
      a. Diffuse white matter injury following chemotherapy, with or without concomitant radiation therapy.
      b. Characterized pathologically by:
        (1) Multifocal demyelination.
        (2) Coagulation necrosis.
        (3) Gliosis in periventricular, centrum semiovale white matter.
      c. Reported with many agents including:
        (1) Cyclosporin A.
        (2) Methotrexate.
        (3) Cytarabine.
        (4) 5-fluorouracil.
        (5) Levamisole.
      d. Imaging.
        (1) NECT.
          (a) Generalized atrophy is common.
          (b) Patchy or confluent hypodense white matter lesions.
          (c) Calcification in basal ganglia, subcortical white matter ("mineralizing microangiopathy") with combined chemotherapy, radiation therapy.
        (2) CECT may show single or multiple foci of rim enhancement, mimic recurrent neoplasm.
        (3) MR.
          (a) Hypodense single, multiple, or confluent lesions on T1WI; during acute phase lesions may enhance following contrast.

> (b) Demyelinated areas show increased signal intensity on T2WI.
> (c) Calcified areas show variable signal.

B. Radiation therapy.
  1. Radiation injury is arbitrarily classified according to time of symptom appearance.
     a. Early delayed radiation injury.
        (1) Occurs a few weeks to 3 months in most cases.
        (2) Often transient.
        (3) Characterized by plaques of demyelination that may resemble multiple sclerosis.
        (4) Usually reversible.
     b. Late radiation injury.
        (1) Occurs within 1 to 10 years after therapy.
        (2) Doses usually exceed 50 Gy.
        (3) Irreversible, progressive, often fatal.
        (4) Major patterns.
           (a) Focal radiation necrosis (may resemble recurrent or persistent neoplasm).
           (b) Diffuse white matter injury.
           (c) Vascular telangiectasia.
           (d) Radiation-induced neoplasm (e.g., meningioma, meningeal sarcoma).

V. Secondary white matter tract degeneration.
  A. Amyotrophic lateral sclerosis (ALS).
     1. Pathology, clinical.
        a. Progressive degeneration of motor neurons.
        b. Three clinical forms.
           (1) Classic ALS.
              (a) Upper motor neurons in cerebral cortex.
              (b) Lower motor neurons in spinal cord, brainstem.
           (2) Primary lateral sclerosis.
              (a) Only central motor neurons affected.
           (3) Primary muscular atrophy.
              (a) Peripheral motor neurons.
        c. Demographics.
           (1) Occurs as a sporadic disease.
           (2) Prevalence approximately 5 per 100,000.
           (3) Male predominance.
           (4) Peak onset between age 50 and 70 years.
     2. Imaging.
        a. Bilaterally symmetric hyperintense regions on PD, T2WI.
           (1) White matter of precentral gyrus.

(2) Posterior limb of internal capsule.
(3) Cerebral peduncles.
  b. Decreased signal in motor cortex on T2WI (not specific for ALS; can also be age-related).
B. Wallerian degeneration.
  1. Pathology.
    a. Disintegration of distal axon, myelin sheath following damage to its cell body and/or proximal axon.
      (1) Common causes include stroke, trauma.
    b. Temporal stages.
      (1) Acute demyelination.
      (2) Edema, cellular proliferation.
      (3) Fibrosis, volume loss.
  2. Imaging.
    a. Magnetization transfer (MT) MR scans more sensitive for acute stage than conventional spin-echo studies.
    b. Pyramidal tract appears hyperintense on PD, T2WI approximately 2 weeks after injury.
    c. Chronic degeneration shows atrophy of ipsilateral brainstem.
C. Cerebellorubral degeneration.
  1. Pathology.
    a. Secondary degeneration after damage to complex neural connections among dentate nuclei, contralateral red nuclei, and inferior olivary nuclei.
    b. Delayed response to surgery, trauma.
  2. Imaging.
    a. Hyperintensity in affected regions typically occurs 1 to 18 months after injury.
    b. Atrophic changes ensue.

SUGGESTED READINGS

Baum PA, Barkovich AJ, Koch TK, Berg BO: Deep gray matter involvement in children with acute disseminated encephalomyelitis, *AJNR* 15:1275-1283, 1994.

Cajade-Law AG, Cohen JA, Heier LA: Vascular causes of white matter disease, *Neuroimaging Clin North Am* 3:361-377, 1993.

Caldemeyer KS, Smith RR, Harris TM, Edwards MK: MRI in acute disseminated encephalomyelitis, *Neuroradiol* 36:216-220, 1994.

Caparros-Lefebvre D, Pruvo JP, Josien E, et al: Marchiafava-Bignami disease: use of contrast media in CT and MRI, *Neuroradiol* 36:509-511, 1994.

Chang KH, Han ML, Kim HS, et al: Delayed encephalopathy after acute carbon monoxide intoxication: MR imaging features and distribution of cerebral white matter lesions, *Radiol* 184:117-122, 1992.

Diamond I, Messing RO: Neurologic effects of alcoholism, *West J Med* 161:279-287, 1994.

Doraiswamy PM, Massey EW, Enright K, et al: Wernicke-Korsakoff syndrome caused by psychogenic food refusal: MR findings, *AJNR* 15:594-596, 1994.

Drayer BP: Degenerative disorders of the central nervous system, *Neuroimaging Clin North Am* 5:135-153, 1995.

Farlow MR, Bonnin JM: Clinical and neuropathologic features of multiple sclerosis, *Neuroimaging Clin North Am* 3:213-228, 1993.

Glasier CM, Robbins MB, Davis PC, et al: Clinical, neurodiagnostic, and MR findings in children with spinal and brain stem multiple sclerosis, *AJNR* 16:87-95, 1995.

Guttman CRG, Ahn SS, Hsu L, et al: The evolution of multiple sclerosis lesions on serial MR, *AJNR* 16:1481-1491, 1995.

Hiehle JF Jr, Grossman RI, Ramer KN, et al: Magnetization transfer effects in MR-detected multiple sclerosis lesions: comparison with gadolinium-enhanced spin-echo images and nonenhanced T1-weighted images, *AJNR* 16:69-77, 1995.

Jackson A, Fitzgerald JB, Gillespie: The callosal-septal interface lesion in multiple sclerosis: effect of sequence and imaging plane, *Neuroradiol* 35:573-577, 1993.

Laws ERJr, Stieg PE, Goumnerova L, et al: Acute presentation of an intracranial mass, *J Neurosurg* 37:109-113, 1995.

Lexa JF, Grossman RI, Rosenquist AC: MR of Wallerian degeneration in the feline visual system: characterization by magnetization transfer rate with histopathologic correlation, *AJNR* 15:201-212, 1994.

Meurice A, Fladroy P, Dondelinger RE, Reznik M: A single focus of probably multiple sclerosis in the cervical spinal cord mimicking a tumor, *Neuroradiol* 36:234-235, 1994.

Moody DM, Brown WR, Challa VR, Anderson RL: Periventricular venous collagenosis: association with leukoariosis, *Radiol* 194:469-476, 1995.

Murata T, Itoh S, Koshino Y, et al: Serial proton magnetic resonance spectroscopy in a patient with the interval form of carbon monoxide poisoning, *J Neurol Neurosurg Psychiatr* 58:100-103, 1995.

Osborn AG: Acquired metabolic, white matter, and degenerative diseases of the brain. In *Diagnostic neuroradiology,* St Louis, 1994, Mosby, pp 748-771.

Paakko E, Talvensaari K, Phytinen J, Lanning M: Late cranial MRI after cranial irradiation in survivors of childhood cancer, *Neuroradiol* 36:652-655, 1994.

Rowley HA, Dillon WP: Iatrogenic white matter diseases, *Neuroimaging Clin North Am* 3:379-404, 1993.

Scarpelli M, Salvolini U, Diamanti L, et al: MRI and pathological examination of post-mortem brains: the problem of white matter high signal areas, *Neuroradiol* 36:393-398, 1994.

Shanley DJ: Mineralizing microangiopathy: CT and MRI, *Neuroradiol* 37:331-333, 1995.

Shogry MEC, Curnes JT: Mamillary body enhancement on MR as the only sign of acute Wernicke Encephalopathy, *AJNR* 15:172-174, 1994.

Simon JH: Neuroimaging of multiple sclerosis, *Neuroimaging Clin North Am* 3:229-246, 1993.

Tan TP, Algra PR, Valk J, Wolters EC: Toxic leukoencephalopathy after inhalation of poisoned heroin: MR findings, *AJNR* 15:175-178, 1994.

Tas MW, Barkhol F, van Walderveen MAA, et al: The effect of gadolinium on the sensitivity and specificity of MR in the initial diagnosis of multiple sclerosis, *AJNR* 16:259-264, 1995.

Valk J, van der Knaap MS: Toxic encephalopathy, *AJNR* 13:747-760, 1992.

van der Meyden CH, de Villiers JFK, Middlecote BD, Terblanche J: Gadolinium ring enhancement and mass effect in acute disseminated encephalomyelitis, *Neuroradiol* 36:221-223, 1994.

Yamanouchi N, Okada S, Kodama K, et al: White matter changes caused by chronic solvent abuse, *AJNR* 16:1650-1652, 1995.

Yetkin Z, Haughton VM: Atypical demyelinating lesions in patients with multiple sclerosis, *Neuroradiol* 37:284-286, 1995.

Yuh WTC, Simonson TM, D'Alessandro MP, et al: Temporal changes of MR findings in central pontine myelinolysis, *AJNR* 16:975-977, 1995.

54

Gray Matter Neurodegenerative Disorders

Key Concepts

1. Alzheimer disease (AD) can be inherited or acquired spontaneously and is the most common brain degenerative disease.
2. There is significant overlap in many neuroimaging findings between age-related changes and AD.
3. Earliest detectable volume alterations in AD are in the hippocampus and amygdala of the medial temporal lobe; the CA1 region of Ammon's horn and the entorhinal cortex show the largest volume reductions in late AD.
4. Functional imaging studies such as positron emission tomography (PET) and MR spectroscopy (MRS) show dysfunction of multiple physiologic parameters in AD.
5. The major imaging differential diagnosis of AD is cerebral atrophy and normal pressure hydrocephalus.

By the year 2030 nearly 20% of the population in the United States will be over 65. The exact prevalence of dementia is unknown, but some estimate at least 5% of people over 65 years and 10% to 20% of those over age 80 are moderately to severely demented. Other data suggest that an even larger percentage of elderly individuals suffer some degree of mild to moderate cognitive impairment.

The social, political, and economic impact of coping with an ever-aging population cannot be overestimated. Neuroimaging may well play an increasingly important role in evaluating the cognitively impaired elderly patient, with early detection of treatable causes a major goal.

In this, the concluding chapter of the section on inherited and acquired metabolic and degenerative brain disorders, we consider gray matter neurodegenerative disorders. We begin with AD and other cortical dementias. Here we also include a discussion of the major differential diagnosis of AD, namely age-related atrophy and normal pressure hydrocephalus. Other less common causes of dementia such as Pick disease, vascular dementia, and Creutzfeld-Jacob disease are briefly delineated.

Chapter 54 also contains a discussion of extrapyramidal disorders and the subcortical dementias, then concludes with acquired disorders of the deep gray nuclei.

I. Alzheimer disease and its mimics.
  A. Alzheimer disease (AD).
    1. Pathology (definite diagnosis of AD currently requires pathologic confirmation).
      a. Gross pathology.
        (1) Diffuse atrophy.
          (a) Involves both gray, white matter.
          (b) Cortex thinned.
          (c) Temporal lobe (especially CA1 segment of Ammon's horn, entorhinal cortex, amygdala) disproportionately affected.
          (d) Ventricles enlarged (especially third ventricle, temporal horns).
          (e) Sulci widened.
      b. Microscopic pathology.
        (1) Amyloid β-protein deposition in neuropil, vascular walls is primary event in the pathologic cascade of AD.
        (2) "Senile plaques" consist of a core of extracellular amyloid surrounded by rim of dystrophic neurites, reactive microglia, and astrocytes.
        (3) Progressive neuronal degeneration and atrophy, neurofibrillary tangle formation are secondary phenomena.

(4) Lewy-body disease.
  (a) AD variant.
  (b) Prominent Parkinsonian-like features.
  (c) Accentuated frontal atrophy.
  (d) Eosinophilic cytoplasmic inclusions.
2. Prevalence, inheritance, risk factors.
  a. Most common acquired form of dementia in western industrialized nations.
  b. Causes between 60% and 70% of dementias.
  c. Affects 1% to 7% of patients over 65 years.
  d. Affects 10% to 20% of patients over age 80.
  e. Approximately 10% of AD is inherited.
  f. Except for age and positive family history, no definite risk factors.
3. Location.
  a. Early sites.
    (1) Hippocampus.
    (2) Entorhinal cortex.
    (3) Amygdala.
  b. Late.
    (1) AD plaques are ubiquitous in entire cortical ribbon.
    (2) Basal ganglia may also be involved.
4. Imaging.
  a. CT.
    (1) Best use is to screen for potentially treatable causes of dementia, including:
      (a) Subdural hematoma.
      (b) Normal pressure hydrocephalus (see below).
      (c) Neoplasm.
    (2) Findings.
      (a) Overlap with normal age-related volume loss.
      (b) Generalized cortical atrophy.
      (c) Disproportionate enlargement of sylvian fissures and anterior temporal horns.
      (d) Interuncal distance is not reliable indicator of AD.
  b. MR.
    (1) T1WI.
      (a) Generalized atrophy.
      (b) Decreased volume of amygdala, hippocampus in early AD.
      (c) Enlargement of third ventricle, temporal horns of lateral ventricles corelates with neuropsychologic impairment.

(2) T2WI.

    (a) No significant difference in white matter hyperintensities between AD, normal aging.

c. MR spectroscopy (MRS).

    (1) In vitro MRS shows elevated levels of phosphomonoesters, phosphodiesters, glutamate.

    (2) In vivo MRS shows:

        (a) Reduced N-acetyl-L-aspartate (NAA) (occurs in virtually all dementias, regardless of cause).

        (b) Increased levels of myo-inositol (MI).

        (c) MI/NAA ratio can distinguish AD from normal with comparatively high sensitivity, specificity.

        (d) MI/NAA ratio has lower specificity for distinction between AD, treatable or untreatable causes of dementia.

d. PET.

    (1) Reduced regional metabolic rates of glucose utilization correlates with dementia severity, neuropsychologic dysfunction.

e. High-resolution single-photon emission computed tomography (SPECT).

    (1) Shows reduced regional cerebral blood flow in hippocampal region in AD.

B. Normal pressure hydrocephalus (NPH).

  1. One of the few potentially treatable causes of dementia.

  2. Clinical presentation.

    a. Elderly patient.

    b. Classic triad of symptoms.

      (1) Gait disturbance (often severe apraxic gait).

      (2) Urinary incontinence.

      (3) Dementia (usually mild cognitive impairment).

  3. Imaging diagnosis (N.B.: No pathognomonic findings, nor can NPH be discriminated from AD with certainty).

    a. CT.

      (1) Severe ventricular enlargement.

        (a) Out of proportion compared with sulcal enlargement, degree of cortical atrophy.

        (b) No disproportionate enlargement of temporal horns.

        (c) Ventricular margins often show rounded margins, laterally convex bowing.

      (2) Corpus callosum often appears thinned, stretched, bowed, may show impingement by falx.

      (3) Gray-white matter discrimination normal.

  b. MR.
  (1) Ventricles disproportionately enlarged compared with sulci.
  (2) Hippocampi normal or only mildly atrophic.
  (3) Accentuated CSF "flow void" through aqueduct, third ventricle, or both may indicate NPH (some authors suggest CSF velocity, volume, and flow pattern quantification may be helpful).
  (4) Gray matter-white matter interface, signal intensity differences are well maintained.
  c. Isotope cisternography.
  (1) Findings some authors suggest indicate NPH:
    (a) Ventricular reflux.
    (b) Ventricular stasis.
  (2) Not consistently predictive of which patients will benefit from surgical shunt.
  d. PET, SPECT.
  (1) Cortical oxygen utilization, mean cortical blood flow reduced compared with age-matched controls.
  (2) AD patients have lower absolute metabolic rates in temporal, parietal lobes compared with patients with NPH.
C. Cortical atrophy.
  1. Cortical gray matter.
    a. Thinning with volume loss normally occurs with aging (see Chapter 52).
    b. No loss of gray-white matter discrimination (sometimes occurs with AD).
  2. Sulci, cisterns, ventricles.
    a. Mild to moderate enlargement.
    b. No disproportionate enlargement of third ventricle, temporal horns (seen in AD).
    c. Even with moderately severe generalized atrophy, temporal horns do not appear rounded.
    d. Combination of large ventricles, small sulci in elderly patient should raise suspicion of NPH or obstructive hydrocephalus.
    e. Ventricular walls remain parallel, do not show laterally convex bowing (as is typical with obstructive hydrocephalus and NPH).
II. Miscellaneous cortical dementias.
  A. Ischemic vascular dementia (IVD; also called multiinfarct dementia).
    1. Pathology.

    a. Multiple cortical, subcortical infarcts.
    b. Ventricles, sulci only mildly enlarged.
  2. Clinical.
    a. Second only to AD as most common cause of cognitive impairment in elderly patients.
      (1) Accounts for 10% to 30% of all dementias.
    b. Stepwise cognitive declines correlate with recurrent "silent" infarcts (versus relentless performance decline with AD).
  3. Imaging.
    a. Some overlap with age-matched controls.
    b. Compared with normal controls, patients with IVD show:
      (1) Cortical infarcts.
        (a) Large, often multifocal.
        (b) Arterial or watershed distribution.
      (2) Deep gray, white matter lacunes.
        (a) Caudate nuclei.
        (b) Thalami.
        (c) Internal capsule.
        (d) Brainstem.
      (3) Cortical, subcortical white matter lucencies or hyperintensities.
    c. PET, SPECT scans show focal asymmetric, variable regions of hypometabolism.
B. Pick disease (PD).
  1. Pathology.
    a. Gross pathology.
      (1) Striking lobar atrophy.
      (2) Frontal, anterior temporal lobe predilection.
      (3) Spares parietal, occipital lobes, posterior two thirds of superior temporal gyrus.
    b. Microscopic pathology.
      (1) "Pick bodies" (distinctive round cytoplasmic inclusions within neurons in affected areas).
  2. Clinical.
    a. Rare cause of dementia.
    b. Presenile onset (before age 65).
    c. Cognitive deficits in PD, AD similar.
  3. Imaging.
    a. MR, CT findings mirror neuropathology.
      (1) Frontal, temporal atrophy.
      (2) Caudate nuclei may appear atrophic.
      (3) Anterior interhemispheric fissure, frontal horns of lateral

ventricles appear disproportionately enlarged.
- b. PET, SPECT show diminished blood flow, hypometabolism in affected regions.
C. Creutzfeld-Jakob disease (CJD).
  1. Etiology.
    - a. One of the so-called prion diseases.
      (1) Term used to distinguish an essential, pathogenic protein (PrP) from viruses, viroids.
      (2) Term "prion" was first introduced to emphasize its "proteinaceous and infectious" nature.
      (3) Prions cause several human illnesses.
        (a) Kuru.
        (b) Creutzfeldt-Jakob disease.
        (c) Gerstmann-Straussler-Schenker syndrome (cerebellar ataxia, dementia, abundant PrP amyloid plaques).
        (d) Fatal familial insomnia.
    - b. CJD can be:
      (1) Iatrogenic (infectious and transmissible).
      (2) Sporadic (unknown cause).
      (3) Familial (caused by mutations in the PrP gene).
        (a) 15% of CJD cases.
  2. Pathology.
    - a. Neuronal loss.
    - b. Gliosis.
    - c. Spongiform change.
  3. Clinical.
    - a. Men, women equally affected.
    - b. Mean age at onset is 60 ± 9 years (contrast with AD, which increases exponentially after age 60).
      (1) Rare before age 40.
      (2) Rare after age 80.
    - c. Mean illness duration is 8 ± 11 months.
      (1) 80% die within 12 months of onset.
      (2) 20% have chronic course.
    - d. Variable signs, symptoms.
      (1) Visuo-spatial disorders.
      (2) Memory loss evolves rapidly.
      (3) Myoclonic movements.
  4. Imaging.
    - a. MR.
      (1) May be normal initially.
      (2) Hyperintensity in caudate, putamen, sometimes cerebral cortex on PDWI, T2WI.
D. Parkinson disease (PD) (see below).
  1. With increasing longevity, dementia has become an increas-

ingly common component of PD.

    a. Develops in up to 40% of patients with idiopathic PD.

  2. PD can be difficult to distinguish from AD clinically, pathologically, and epidemiologically as well as on imaging studies.

  3. Possible genetic susceptibility for dementia in the setting of PD remains controversial.

III. Subcortical dementias.

  A. Parkinson disease (PD).

    1. Pathology, etiology.

      a. Gross pathology.

        (1) Generalized atrophy.

      b. Microscopic pathology.

        (1) Loss of neuromelanin-contining neurons in substantia nigra, locus ceruleus, dorsal vagal nucleus.

          (a) Pars compacta thinned.

        (2) Iron distribution in basal ganglia generally normal or mildly elevated.

      c. May be caused by dysfunction of the mitochondrial electron transport chain.

        (1) Defect in complex I.

    2. Clinical.

      a. Bradykinesia plus one of the following:

        (1) Classic rest tremor.

        (2) Unilateral onset.

        (3) Progressive persistent asymmetry.

        (4) Excellent response to levodopa (>70%).

        (5) Levodopa-induced dyskinesias.

        (6) Continued response to levodopa for at least 5 years.

      b. With increasingly long-term survival, dementia is becoming a prominent feature of PD in many individuals.

    3. Imaging.

      a. Most common finding is nonspecific, generalized atrophy.

      b. Thinning of pars compacta.

        (1) In early stages of PD, pars compacta may appear hyperintense on long TR/short TE MR scans.

        (2) Chronic PD can be seen indirectly as smudging or blurring of the borders between the adjacent red nuclei, pars reticulata of substantia nigra (they almost seem to "touch" on T2WI).

      c. MR spectroscopy shows increased lactate.

  B. Multiple system atrophies (MSA) or "Parkinson Plus" disorders.

    1. Approximately 25% of patients with parkinsonian symptoms have more severe clinical manifestations and are drug-unresponsive.

    2. Related movement disorders.

a. Striatonigral degeneration (SND).

(1) Generalized atrophy.

(2) Putamina appear atrophic, have abnormally low signal on T2WI (equal to globus pallidus).

b. Shy-Drager syndrome.

(1) Cerebellar atrophy.

c. Olivopontocerebellar atrophy (OPCA).

(1) Cerebellar, brainstem atrophy.

(a) Small, flattened pons.

(b) Atrophic cerebellar hemispheres, vermis.

(c) Small inferior olives, medulla.

(2) Putamen hypointense on T2WI.

IV. Acquired degenerative disorders of the basal ganglia (summary).

A. Vascular causes.

1. Arterial infarction.

a. "Top of basilar" syndrome.

b. Bilateral but asymmetric thalamic lesions.

2. Hypoxic/ischemic encephalopathy.

a. Can be either ischemic or hemorrhagic.

b. Causes.

(1) Respiratory arrest.

(2) Global hypoperfusion.

3. Hypertension, renal failure.

a. Acute hypertensive encephalopathy.

(1) Fibrinoid necrosis, arteriolar thrombosis, microinfarcts.

(2) Basal ganglia, deep cerebral white matter, brainstem affected.

(3) Lesions can be ischemic or hemorrhagic.

b. Eclampsia.

c. Hemolytic-uremic syndrome.

(1) Multisystem disorder.

(2) Microthrombosis of basal ganglia.

d. Nephrotic syndrome.

4. Venous infarction.

a. Caused by internal cerebral vein thrombosis.

b. Usually bilateral.

c. Thalami most common site.

5. Vasculitis.

B. Toxic and metabolic causes.

1. Carbon monoxide poisoning.

a. Globi pallidi preferentially affected.

b. May involve remainder of basal ganglia.

c. "Interval" form involves cerebral white matter (see Chapter 53).

   2. Osmotic myelinolysis.
      a. Typical site is pons.
      b. Extrapontine sites include basal ganglia, thalami, cerebral white matter.
   3. Hypoglycemia.
      a. Manifestations resemble hypoxia.
   4. Chemotherapy, radiation therapy.
      a. May cause basal ganglia calcifications.
   5. Liver disorders.
      a. Cirrhosis.
      b. Manganese toxicity.
      c. Hemachromatosis.
   6. Miscellaneous toxins.
      a. Methanol.
         (1) Putamina, cerebellar cortex commonly affected.
      b. Cyanide.
      c. Hydrogen sulfide.
C. Infection, inflammation.
   1. Acute disseminated encephalomyelitis.
      a. Usually involves white matter.
      b. May involve basal ganglia, thalami.
   2. Bilateral striatal necrosis.
      a. Inherited causes.
         (1) Leigh disease (see Chapter 51).
         (2) Familial degeneration of striatum.
      b. Acquired causes (typically following acute systemic illness).
         (1) Often in infants, young children.
         (2) May occur as complication of viral infection.
   3. Sydenham's chorea (group A streptococcal infection).
   4. Encephalitis.
   5. Toxoplasmosis, cryptococcosis.
D. Neoplasm.
   1. Bithalamic astrocytoma.
   2. Metastases.
E. Miscellaneous.
   1. Prion disease.
      a. Creutzfeld-Jakob disease.

SUGGESTED READINGS

Albanese A, Colosimo C, Bentivoglio AR, et al: Multiple system atrophy presenting as parkinsonism: clinical features and diagnostic criteria, *J Neurol Neurosurg Psychiatr* 59:144-151, 1995.

Barboriak DP, Provenzale JM, Boyko OB: MR diagnosis of Creutzfeldt-Jakob disease: significance of high signal intensity of the basal ganglia, *AJR* 162:137-140, 1994.

Baum PA, Barkovich AJ, Koch TK, Berg BO: Deep gray matter involvement in children with acute disseminated encephalomyelitis, *AJNR* 15:12751283, 1994.

Bowen BC, Block RE, Sanchez-Ramos J, et al: Proton MR spectroscopy of the brain in 14 patients with Parkinson disease, *AJNR* 16:61-68, 1995.

Davis PC, Mirra SS, Alazraki N: The brain in older persons with and without dementia: findings on MR, PET, and SPECT images, *AJR* 162:1267-1278, 1994.

deLeon MJ, Convit A, DeSanti S, et al: The hippocampus in aging and Alzheimer's disease, *Neuroimaging Clin North Am* 5:1-17, 1995.

Drayer BP: Degenerative disorders of the central nervous system, *Neuroimaging Clin North Am* 5:135-153, 1995.

George AE, Holodny A, Golomb J, deLeon MJ: The differential diagnosis of Alzheimer's disease: cerebral atrophy versus normal pressure hydrocephalus, *Neuroimaging Clin North Am* 5:19-31, 1995.

Ho BV, Fitz CR, Chuang SH, Geyer CA: Bilateral basal ganglia lesions: pediatric differential considerations, *RadioGraphics* 13:269-292, 1993.

Lehericy S, Baulac M, Chiras J, et al: Amygdalohippocampal MR volume measurements in the early stages of Alzheimer disease, *AJNR* 15:927-937, 1994.

Marsden CD: Parkinson's disease, *J Neurol, Neurosurg, Psychiatr* 57:672-681, 1994.

Mendez MF, Selwood A, Mastri AR, Frey WH: Pick's disease versus Alzheimer's disease, *Neurol* 43:289-292, 1993.

Meyer JS, Muramatsu K, Mortel KF, et al: Prospective CT confirms differences between vascular and Alzheimer's dementia, *Stroke* 26:735-742, 1995.

Olichney JM, Hansen LA, Hofstetter R, et al: Cerebral infarction in Alzheimer's disease is associated with severe amyloid angiopathy and hypertension, *Arch Neurol* 52:702-708, 1995.

Prusiner SB: Neurodegeneration in humans caused by prions, *West J Med* 161: 264-272, 1994.

Richardson EP Jr, Masters CL: The nosology of Creutzfeldt-Jakob disease and conditions related to the accumulation of PrP[CJD] in the nervous system, *Brain Pathol* 5:33-41, 1995.

Scheltens PH, Barkhof F, Leys D, et al: Histopathologic correlates of white matter changes on MRI in Alzheimer's disease and normal aging, *Neurol* 45:883-888, 1995.

Shonk TK, Moats RA, Gifford P, et al: Probable Alzheimer disease: diagnosis with proton MR spectroscopy, *Radiol* 195:65-72, 1995.

Slansky I, Herholz K, Pietrzyk U, et al: Cognitive impairment in Alzheimer's disease correlates with ventricular width and atrophy-corrected cortical glucose metabolism, *Neuroradiol* 37:270-277, 1995.

Traill Z, Pike M, Byrne J: Sydenham's chorea: a case showing reversible striatal abnormalities on CT and MRI, *Dev Med Child Neurol* 37:270-273, 1995.

Weingarten K, Barbut D, Filippi C, Zimmerman RD: Acute hypertensive encephalopathy: findings on spin-echo and gradient-echo MR imaging, *AJR* 162:665-670, 1994.

Wisniewski HM, Wegiel J: The neuropathology of Alzheimer's disease, *Neuroimaging Clin North Am* 5:45-57, 1995.

SECTION VIII

Disease Processes by Location

55

Scalp and Calvarium

Key Concepts

1. Fluid tends to accumulate in the loose areolar layer of the scalp, such as edema (caput succedaneum in neonates) or subgaleal hematoma in adults. In the neonate, blood can also accumulate in the subperiosteal space (cephalohematoma).
2. Abnormalities in calvarial size or shape are often associated with characteristic pathology.
3. The approximate distribution of sutural involvement in craniosynostosis is:
   a. 55% sagittal.
   b. 10% unilateral coronal.
   c. 10% bilateral coronal.
   d. 7% metopic.
   e. 1% lambdoid.
   f. *Note:* unilateral coronal synostosis is a cause of "harlequin eye."
4. Delayed sutural closure or widened sutures are most commonly caused by increased intracranial pressure of various etiology.
5. Common causes of diffuse calvarial thickening are:
   a. Normal variant.
   b. Microcephaly.
   c. Chronic shunted hydrocephalus.
   d. Chronic dilantin therapy.
6. Craniolacunia or luckenshadel or lacunar skull is a bony dysplasia associated with Chiari II that usually disappears by 6 months of age. It is not caused by hydrocephalus or increased intracranial pressure.
7. Prominent convolutional markings can be normal or associated with hydrocephalus or increased intracranial pressure.

I. Scalp (see Fig. 56-1).
  A. Trauma.
    1. Outer three layers of the scalp constitute the scalp proper and usually remain together with peeling.
    2. Neonatal.
      a. Caput succedaneum.
        (1) Edematous swelling localized to the loose connective tissue layer of the scalp that may occur during birth.
        (2) Usually occurs in the region of the lambda.
        (3) Fluid is not confined by sutures.
      b. Cephalohematoma.
        (1) Due to rupture of minute periosteal arteries during birth.
        (2) Usually over a parietal bone.
        (3) Blood accumulates in subperiosteal space and is confined by sutures.
    3. Nonneonatal.
      a. Subgaleal hematoma: blood in the scalp in the nonneonatal patient tends to accumulate in the loose areolar layer.
      b. Scalp swelling: edema also tends to accumulate in loose areolar layer.
  B. Infection (e.g., cellulitis, fasciitis): associated edema tends to accumulate in loose areolar layer.
  C. Masses.
    1. Pediatric.
      a. Dermoid tumors: most common nontraumatic pediatric scalp mass.
      b. Langerhans cell histiocytosis: soft-tissue masses are more common in Hand-Schuller-Christian or Letterer-Siwe disease.
      c. Hamartoma.
      d. Hemangioma.
      e. Lymphangioma.
      f. Plexiform neurofibroma.
    2. Adult.
      a. Lipoma.
      b. Basal cell carcinoma.
      c. Lymphoma.
      d. Kaposi's sarcoma.
      e. Neurofibroma.
      f. Angioma.
  D. Other: edema may also be associated with thermal/electrical injury, hypoproteinemia, etc.

II. Calvarium (see Fig. 56-1).
  A. Cranial size.
    1. Microcephaly: common causes.
       a. Cerebral atrophy.
       b. Craniosynostosis (total).
       c. Intrauterine (TORCH) infection.
       d. Intrauterine exposure: alcohol, radiation.
       e. Trisomies: 13, 18, 21.
       f. Abnormal embryologic development: lissencephaly, holoprosencephaly.
       g. Syndromes: e.g., Menkes, Cornelia de Lange.
       h. Dysmyelinating disease: e.g., Pelizaeus-Merzbacher.
       i. Idiopathic micrencephaly.
    2. Macrocephaly: common causes.
       a. Hydrocephalus: Chiari malformations, Dandy-Walker, aqueductal stenosis, brain neoplasm, meningitis.
       b. Craniosynostosis (not total).
       c. Subdural hematoma.
       d. Dysplasias: achondrogenesis, achondroplasia, thanatophoric dysplasia, craniometaphyseal dysplasia, neurofibromatosis.
       e. Metabolic: pituitary gigantism, acromegaly, hyperphosphatasia.
       f. Mucopolysaccharidoses.
       g. Syndromes: Soto (Cerebral gigantism), Zellweger (Cerebrohepatorenal) syndromes.
       h. Dysmyelinating: Canavan's disease, Alexander's disease.
       i. Idiopathic megalencephaly.
    3. Asymmetric calvarium.
       a. Postural flattening: head positioning in infancy, cerebral palsy, scoliosis.
       b. Craniosynostosis (asymmetric).
       c. Cerebral hemiatrophy: Sturge-Weber, Dyke-Davidoff-Masson, Silver-Russell.
       d. Unilateral cerebral enlargement: hemimegalencephaly.
       e. Trauma: cephalohematoma, depressed fracture, asymmetric subdural hematoma.
       f. Postoperative.
       g. Postradiation.
       h. Other: fibrous dysplasia, neurofibromatosis, Paget disease.
  B. Sutural abnormalities.
    1. Craniosynostosis or craniostenosis: premature closure.
       a. Etiology.
          (1) Primary (idiopathic).

    (2) Secondary.

        (a) Metabolic: rickets, hypercalcemia, hyperthyroidism, hypophosphatasia, hypervitaminosis D.

        (b) Bone dysplasia: achondroplasia, thanatophoric dysplasia, chondrodysplasia punctata.

        (c) Anemia or polycythemia.

        (d) Mucopolysaccharidoses.

        (e) Craniofacial dysostosis: Carpenter, Apert, Crouzon.

        (f) Trisomies: 21, 18.

        (g) Micrencephaly.

  b. Incidence.

    (1) Sagittal: 55%.

    (2) Coronal, unilateral: 10%.

    (3) Coronal, bilateral: 10%.

    (4) Metopic: 7%.

    (5) Lambdoid: 1%.

  c. Nomenclature.

    (1) Scaphocephaly or Dolichocephaly (long, narrow head): sagittal suture closure.

    (2) Brachycephaly (short head): bilateral coronal suture closure (note: unilateral closure causes "harlequin eye").

    (3) Plagiocephaly (oblique asymmetric head): unilateral coronal or lambdoid suture closure.

    (4) Trigonocephaly (triangular anteriorly pointed head): metopic suture closure.

    (5) Oxycephaly or Turricephaly (superiorly pointed head): bilateral coronal and lambdoid suture closure.

    (6) Triphyllocephaly or Kleebattschadel or Cloverleaf skull (trilobular head): sagittal, bilateral coronal, and bilateral lambdoid suture closure.

2. Delayed closure and widened sutures: common causes.

  a. Hydrocephalus: Chiari malformations, Dandy-Walker, aqueductal stenosis, brain neoplasm, meningitis, hypervitaminosis A.

  b. Increased intracranial pressure: cerebritis, brain abscess, brain neoplasm, lead poisoning, pseudotumor cerebri.

  c. Sutural infiltration: neuroblastoma, leukemia, lymphoma.

  d. Metabolic: hypothyroidism, rickets, osteogenesis imperfecta, hyperparathyroidism, hypoparathyroidism, hypophosphatasia, hypervitaminosis A.

  e. Syndromes: Down, cleidocranial dysplasia, pyknodysostosis, pachydermoperiostosis.

f. Rebound growth: treated hypothyroidism, deprivation, or dwarfism.

3. Wormian bones: intersutural bones.
   a. Normal: up to 6 months of age.
   b. Abnormal: common causes.
      (1) Congenital: osteogenesis imperfecta, osteopetrosis, Down syndrome.
      (2) Metabolic: hypothyroidism, hypophosphatasia, Menkes (copper deficiency) syndrome.
      (3) Dysplasias: cleidocranial dysplasia, chondrodysplasia, pyknodysostosis, pachydermoperiostosis.
      (4) Other: progeria.

C. Abnormalities of calvarial thickness.
   1. Diffuse calvarial thickening (see box below).
      a. Congenital or developmental.
         (1) Normal variant.
         (2) Microcephaly.

Common Causes of a Thick Skull

Diffuse

Common
Normal variant
Chronic phenytoin (Dilantin) therapy
Microcephalic brain
Shunted hydrocephalus
Uncommon
Acromegaly
Hematologic disorders
Chronic calcified subdural hematoma

Regional/focal

Common
Hyperostosis frontalis interna
Paget disease
Fibrous dysplasia
Meningioma
Uncommon
Osteoma
Calcified cephalohematoma
Metastases (e.g., neuroblastoma, prostate)

Data from F. Guinto and R. Kumar. (From Osborn AG: *Diagnostic neuroradiology*, St Louis, 1994, Mosby.)

      (3) Osteopetrosis: osteosclerosis can cause obliteration of cranial foramina resulting in cranial nerve compression.

      (4) Infantile cortical hyperostosis (Caffey disease).

  b. Hematologic: anemias.

      (1) Any marrow-bearing portion of calvarium (usually parietal) can be affected. Occipital bones lack marrow and are therefore usually spared.

      (2) Thalassemia and sickle cell anemia: appearance varies from mottled diploic thickening to "hair on end."

      (3) Iron deficiency anemia and hereditary spherocytosis: modestly thickened calvarium most common; "hair on end" appearance is rare.

  c. Metabolic.

      (1) Treated hyperparathyroidism: usually associated with renal osteodystrophy.

      (2) Fluorosis.

      (3) Hypervitaminosis D.

      (4) Hypoparathyroidism.

  d. Iatrogenic.

      (1) Chronic shunted hydrocephalus.

      (2) Chronic dilantin therapy.

  e. Neoplastic.

      (1) Osteoblastic metastasis (especially prostate and breast): although usually not truly diffuse.

      (2) Neuroblastoma: can have "hair on end" appearance.

      (3) Leukemia, lymphoma.

  f. Other.

      (1) Acromegaly.

         (a) Location: hyperostosis of inner table, enlargement of occipital protruberance.

         (b) Additional cranial findings: enlargement of sella, enlargement of sinuses, prognathism.

      (2) Paget disease (see p. 580).

      (3) Fibrous dysplasia (see p. 579).

2. Focal or regional calvarial thickening or sclerosis (see box on p. 577).

  a. Congenital hemiatrophy.

      (1) Dyke-Davidoff-Mason.

      (2) Sturge Weber.

      (3) Silver-Russell.

  b. Benign hyperostosis: hyperostosis frontalis interna.

      (1) Location: usually frontal bones, occasionally involves entire skull.

(2) Age and sex: usually middle-aged female.
(3) Patterns.
   (a) Nodular or diffuse.
   (b) Usually bilateral and symmetric, but can be localized and unilateral.
c. Trauma.
  (1) Chronic calcified subdural hematoma can mimic calvarial thickening.
  (2) Calcified or ossified cephalohematoma.
d. Neoplasm.
  (1) Benign.
   (a) Osteoma.
    i. Juxtacortical tumor composed of membranous bone, more commonly involving outer table than inner table; can also be found in paranasal sinuses (especially frontal).
    ii. Extremely dense lesion; has appearance of periosteal thickening in profile.
   (b) Bone island.
    i. Intramedullary cortical hamartoma.
    ii. Can be associated with tuberous sclerosis.
   (c) Meningioma.
    i. Blistering hyperostosis adjacent to meningeal lesion most common.
    ii. Intraosseus meningioma is rare.
  (2) Malignant.
   (a) Osteosarcoma.
   (b) Solitary osteoblastic metastasis (e.g., prostate).
e. Infectious.
  (1) Chronic osteomyelitis (bacterial, fungal).
  (2) Tuberculosis.
  (3) Syphilis: can have extensive periosteal and endosteal proliferation.
f. Other.
  (1) Fibrous dysplasia.
   (a) Pathology: normal bone marrow replaced by fibrovascular tissue, with variable subsequent ossification.
   (b) Location: diffuse or monostotic; craniofacial involvement about 20%.
   (c) CT findings.
    i. Poorly marginated intramedullary lesion with mixed-density, inhomogeneous sclerosis (varies from "ground glass" to dense sclerosis).

ii. Thickened calvarium, expanded diploe; usually spares inner table.
(d) MRI findings.
  i. Diffuse low-signal changes (although not as hypointense as cortical bone) on T1WI and T2WI, with scattered areas of hyperintensity.
  ii. Variable enhancement.
(e) Complications.
  i. Sphenoid and frontal sinus obliteration.
  ii. Orbital deformity and proptosis.
  iii. Narrowing of skull foramina resulting in cranial nerve compression.
  iv. Malignant degeneration rare: 0.5%.
(2) Paget disease.
(a) Location: both inner and outer tables and diploe affected; less commonly involves facial bones. Can be monostotic or polyostotic, focal, or diffuse.
(b) Patterns.
  i. Osteoporosis circumscripta: lytic phase.
  ii. "Cotton wool" appearance: mixed lytic and sclerotic phase.
  iii. Sclerotic phase.
(c) Complications.
  i. Basilar invagination.
  ii. Obliteration of cranial foramina can cause cranial nerve palsies.
  iii. Giant cell tumor: skull and facial bones.
  iv. Malignant degeneration into osteosarcoma or fibrosarcoma: <5%.
3. Diffuse calvarial thinning (see box on p. 581).
  a. Congenital or developmental.
  (1) Craniolacunia or lacunar skull or lukenshadel: thinned, scalloped bone (not to be confused with prominent convolutional markings, which can be normal or associated with increased intracranial pressure).
  (a) Dysplasia of membranous skull.
  (b) Associated with but not caused by Chiari II malformation.
  (c) Not caused by hydrocephalus or increased intracranial pressure.
  (d) Spontaneously resolves after 6 months of age.
  (2) Osteogenesis imperfecta.
  (3) Down syndrome.

Common Causes of a Thin Skull

Generalized

Common
Normal (prominent convolutional markings)
Long-standing hydrocephalus
Lacunar skull (with Chiari II malformation)
Uncommon
Osteogenesis imperfecta
Rickets
Cushing's disease

Regional/focal

Common
Parietal thinning
Temporal, occipital squamae
Pacchionian (arachnoid) granulations
Uncommon
Intracranial mass (arachnoid cyst, slow-growing neoplasm)
Leptomeningeal cyst
Osteoporosis circumscripta

Data from F. Guinto and R. Kumar. (From Osborn AG: *Diagnostic neuroradiology*, St Louis, 1994, Mosby.)

      b. Chronic increased intracranial pressure.
         (1) Chronic obstructive hydrocephalus.
         (2) Intracranial neoplasm.
      c. Metabolic.
         (1) Rickets.
         (2) Hypophosphatasia.
         (3) Hyperparathyroidism.
         (4) Cushing disease.
   4. Focal calvarial thinning or lytic lesions (see box above and on p. 582).
      a. Normal.
         (1) Fissures, foramina, canals, and fontanelles.
         (2) Vascular markings: venous lakes, diploic channels.
         (3) Arachnoid or pacchionian granulations.
         (4) Temporal squamae: normally thinner calvarial bone.
      b. Variants.
         (1) Senile parietal thinning.
            (a) Outer calvarial table thinned, inner table intact.
            (b) Often in older patients.
         (2) Parietal "foramina": transmit emissary veins.

"Holes in the Skull"

Solitary

Common
Normal
　　Fissure, foramen, canal
　　Emissary venous channel
　　Pacchionian (arachnoid) granulation
　　Parietal thinning
Surgical/trauma (burr hole, shunt, surgical defect, fracture)
Dermoid
Eosinophilic granuloma
Metastasis (often multiple)
Uncommon
Osteoporosis circumscripta
Epidermoid
Hemangioma
Cephalocele
Intradiploic arachnoid cyst/meningioma
Leptomeningeal cyst (growing fracture)

Multiple

Common
Normal
　　Fissures, foramina
　　Diploic channels, venous lakes
　　Pacchionian (arachnoid) granulations
Multiple burr holes/surgical defects
Metastases
Age-related osteoporosis
Uncommon
Hyperparathyroidism
Myeloma
Osteomyelitis

(From Osborn AG: *Diagnostic neuroradiology,* St Louis, 1994, Mosby.)

　　　　　(a) Typically bilateral and symmetric.
　　　　　(b) Usually several millimeters in diameter but may reach several centimeters.
　　　(3) Sinus pericranii.
　　　　　(a) Anomalous diploic or emissary venous channels between intracranial and extracranial venous circulations.

    (b) Location: frontal bone most common, temporal bone least common.

    (c) Clinical findings: soft-tissue mass under scalp that changes in size with position, Valsalva, coughing, or sneezing.

  c. Congenital and developmental.

    (1) Cephalocele.

    (2) Dermoid: can arise in scalp or calvarium.

    (3) Cleidocranial dysostosis: large fontanelles, wormian bones.

    (4) Neurofibromatosis.

      (a) Absent greater sphenoid wing.

      (b) Lambdoidal suture defect.

    (5) Arachnoid cyst: intracranial arachnoid cyst may be associated with pressure erosion/thinning of adjacent calvarium.

  d. Trauma or surgery.

    (1) Sutural diastasis.

    (2) Skull fracture.

    (3) Leptomeningeal cyst or "growing fracture": post-traumatic herniation of meninges and CSF into fracture.

    (4) Burr hole, craniotomy, bone flap, shunt placement, other postoperative defect.

  e. Infection: osteomyelitis.

    (1) Organism: usually pyogenic, but can be secondary to fungus, tuberculosis, syphilis.

    (2) Spread: often secondary to sinusitis/mastoiditis or penetrating injury or surgery.

    (3) Appearance: usually permeative destructive lesion.

    (4) Sequestrum can occur with tuberculosis or syphilis.

    (5) Reactive sclerosis can occur with fungal infection.

 f. Necrosis.

    (1) Electric or thermal burn.

    (2) Radiation necrosis.

    (3) Failed postoperative flap.

  g. Benign neoplasm.

    (1) Epidermoid.

      (a) Can be congenital (i.e., inclusion cyst) or acquired (e.g., traumatic).

      (b) Typically well-defined, intradiploic lytic lesion with sclerotic rim, involving both inner and outer tables.

    (2) Hemangioma: well-circumscribed intradiploic lesion with "spoke-wheel" or reticulated pattern.

    (3) Langerhans cell histiocytosis: well-circumscribed lytic lesion with "beveled" edge due to asymmetric involvement of inner/outer tables (outer > inner).

h. Malignant neoplasm.

    (1) Metastasis: usually breast, lung, prostate, kidney, neuroblastoma.

    (2) Myeloma or plasmacytoma.

    (3) Leukemia/lymphoma.

    (4) Sarcoma: Ewing's, osteosarcoma, chondrosarcoma, fibrosarcoma.

i. Metabolic.

    (1) Hyperparathyroidism.

        (a) "Salt and pepper" appearance.

        (b) Brown tumor.

    (2) Osteoporosis.

j. Miscellaneous.

    (1) Paget's (see p. 580).

        (a) Osteoporosis circumscripts ·well-circumscribed, sharply marginated lytic defect.

        (b) More commonly see "cotton-wool" appearance of mixed lytic and sclerotic lesions.

    (2) Fibrous dysplasia (see p. 579).

k. Erosion or destruction by adjacent noncalvarial lesions.

    (1) Slow-growing intracranial tumor with pressure erosion/thinning of adjacent calvarium: e.g., ganglioglioma, oligodendroglioma.

    (2) Aggressive intracranial tumor with invasion: e.g., hemangiopericytoma, aggressive meningioma, or meningeal sarcoma.

l. Erosion associated with scalp masses (see p. 574).

SUGGESTED READINGS

Bourekas EC, Lanzieri CF: The calvarium, *Semin US CT MR* 15:424-453, 1994.

Harnsberger HR: *Handbook of head and neck imaging,* ed 2, Chicago, 1995, Mosby.

Osborn AG: Brain tumors and tumorlike processes. In *Diagnostic neuroradiology,* St Louis, 1994, Mosby, pp 399-528.

56

Extraaxial Pathology

Key Concepts

1. The most common extraaxial fluid collection is enlarged subarachnoid spaces due to atrophy.
2. The general differential diagnosis of extraaxial masses includes:
   a. Neoplasm: e.g., meningioma.
   b. Inflammatory process: e.g., neurosarcoidosis.
   c. Vascular lesions: e.g., vascular malformation.
   d. Traumatic lesions: e.g., calcified chronic subdural hematoma.
   e. Miscellaneous: e.g., extramedullary hematopoiesis.
3. Mimics of meningeal enhancement.
   a. Gyral enhancement should not be confused with leptomeningeal enhancement.
   b. If CT scans are obtained too quickly after contrast, strong intravascular enhancement can mimic leptomeningeal disease.
   c. Small vessels with slow flow can mimic leptomeningeal enhancement on MR if T1WI is performed with flow compensation.
4. Abnormal enhancement patterns.
   a. Dural: thickened, nodular, focal masses.
   b. Leptomeningeal: thickened, focal nodularity, continuous, base of brain, isodense or hyperdense to cavernous sinus.
5. Any process that causes meningeal irritation can cause meningeal enhancement.
6. The general differential diagnosis of abnormal meningeal enhancement includes:
   a. Infection: e.g., meningitis.
   b. Inflammation: e.g., neurosarcoidosis.
   c. Neoplasm: e.g., metastases.
   d. Trauma/surgery: e.g., postsurgical changes.
   e. Vascular: e.g., subacute infarction.
   f. Metabolic disorders: e.g., mucopolysaccharidoses.
   g. Chemicals/toxins: e.g., intrathecal medication.
   h. Benign intracranial hypotension.
   i. Idiopathic.

7. Absence of meningeal enhancement does not necessarily imply non-involvement; e.g., viral or bacterial meningitis, lymphoproliferative diseases.
8. Presence of abnormal meningeal enhancement does not necessarily imply involvement: e.g., "dural tail" of meningioma, benign leptomeningeal fibrosis after surgery.
9. Primary CNS neoplasms that can have CSF dissemination include medulloblastoma, ependymoma, germinoma, pineoblastoma, cerebral neuroblastoma, choroid plexus tumors, high-grade astrocytoma, and primary CNS lymphoma.
10. Carcinomas that may have CSF spread include breast, lung, melanoma, and gastric carcinoma.

I. Extraaxial collections (Fig. 56-1).
   A. Congenital and developmental.
      1. Normal variants.
         a. Mega-cisterna magna (see Chapter 15).
            (1) Large cisterna magna. Normal fourth ventricle, cerebellum (including vermis), and torcular Herophili. No mass effect or hydrocephalus.
            (2) Occasionally can cause scalloping of adjacent calvarium.
            (3) Possibly mildest form of Dandy-Walker variant.
         b. Benign subarachnoid collections of infancy.
            (1) Normal head circumference.
            (2) No ventricular dilatation.
            (3) Possibly due to delayed maturation of arachnoid villi.
      2. Arachnoid cyst (see Chapter 34).
         a. Most occur in pediatric patients.
         b. Location in descending order of frequency:
            (1) Middle fossa and sylvian fissure (50%).
            (2) Vermian cistern (25%).
            (3) Suprasellar cistern (10%).
            (4) CPA cistern (5% to 10%).
            (5) Quadrigeminal plate cistern (5% to 10%).
            (6) Cerebral convexity (5%).
      3. External hydrocephalus (EH).
         a. Enlarged subarachnoid spaces accompanied by abnormally increasing head circumference with minimal or no ventricular enlargement.

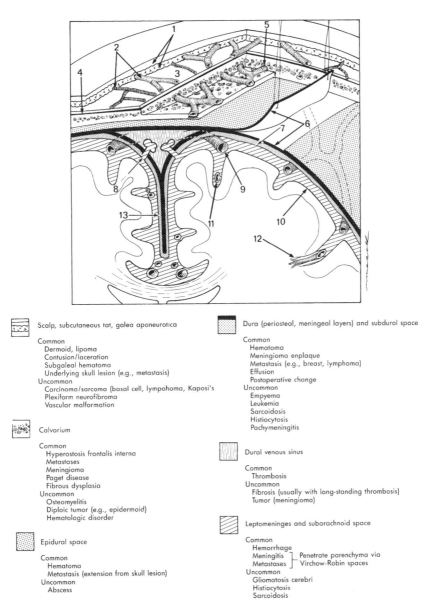

Scalp, subcutaneous fat, galea aponeurotica

Common
  Dermoid, lipoma
  Contusion/laceration
  Subgaleal hematoma
  Underlying skull lesion (e.g., metastasis)
Uncommon
  Carcinoma/sarcoma (basal cell, lymphoma, Kaposi's)
  Plexiform neurofibroma
  Vascular malformation

Calvarium

Common
  Hyperostosis frontalis interna
  Metastases
  Meningioma
  Paget disease
  Fibrous dysplasia
Uncommon
  Osteomyelitis
  Diploic tumor (e.g., epidermoid)
  Hematologic disorder

Epidural space

Common
  Hematoma
  Metastasis (extension from skull lesion)
Uncommon
  Abscess

Dura (periosteal, meningeal layers) and subdural space

Common
  Hematoma
  Meningioma enplaque
  Metastasis (e.g., breast, lymphoma)
  Effusion
  Postoperative change
Uncommon
  Empyema
  Leukemia
  Sarcoidosis
  Histiocytosis
  Pachymeningitis

Dural venous sinus

Common
  Thrombosis
Uncommon
  Fibrosis (usually with long-standing thrombosis)
  Tumor (meningioma)

Leptomeninges and subarachnoid space

Common
  Hemorrhage
  Meningitis ⎤ Penetrate parenchyma via
  Metastases ⎦ Virchow-Robin spaces
Uncommon
  Gliomatosis cerebri
  Histiocytosis
  Sarcoidosis

Fig. 56-1 Anatomic diagram depicts the scalp, skull, and meninges. The potential epidural and subdural spaces are slightly exaggerated for illustrative purposes. These spaces, and lesions that occur within them, are coded on the diagram. Important anatomic structures are listed below: 1, Scalp with subcutaneous fat. 2, Scalp arteries and veins. 3, Galea aponeurotica. 4, Periosteum (the potential subgaleal space and periosteum are shown together here as a thin black line). 5, Diploic veins in calvarium. 6, Dura (outer and inner layers are shown). 7, Arachnoid. 8, Pacchionian granulations. Note projections from subarachnoid space into superior sagittal sinus (SSS). 9, Cortical veins. These veins are shown as they course across the potential subdural space to enter the SSS. 10, Pia mater. This, the innermost layer of the leptomeninges, is closely applied to the cerebral cortex. 11, Pial arteries. 12, Virchow-Robin spaces. These are pial-lined infoldings of CSF around penetrating cortical vessels. These spaces are exaggerated for illustrative purposes. 13, Falx cerebri. Note potential subdural space adjacent to the falx. (From Osborn AG: *Diagnostic neuroradiology,* St Louis, 1994, Mosby.)

   b. Idiopathic EH usually resolves spontaneously by 3 years of age.
 B. Atrophic conditions: resulting in enlarged subarachnoid spaces.
  1. Congenital (TORCH) infections.
  2. Brain malformations: e.g., lissencephaly.
  3. Neurodegenerative disease (e.g., HIV encephalopathy, Alzheimer's disease, Pick's disease, Huntington's disease, multi-infarct dementia).
  4. Global ischemia/hypoxia.
  5. Posttraumatic.
  6. Postinflammatory.
  7. Alcohol and drug abuse.
  8. Iatrogenic (dilantin, steroids, radiation therapy, chemotherapy).
  9. Dehydration.
  10. Deprivational states.
 C. Trauma (see Chapter 20).
  1. Epidural hematoma: typically lentiform or biconvex, crosses falx but not sutures.
  2. Subdural hematoma: typically crescentic or curvilinear, crosses sutures but not falx.
  3. Subarachnoid hemorrhage.
  4. Extraaxial pneumocephalus.
 D. Infection (see Chapters 42, 47).
  1. Epidural abscess/empyema.
  2. Subdural empyema.
  3. Subdural effusion.
  4. Parasitic cysts: e.g., neurocysticercosis.
II. Focal extraaxial masses (Fig. 56-1).
 A. Neoplasm.
  1. Meningioma.
  2. Hemangiopericytoma.
  3. Sarcoma.
  4. Plasmacytoma, multiple myeloma.
  5. Lymphoma/leukemia.
  6. Metastases (osseus or dural): prostate, lung, breast, renal, neuroblastoma.
 B. Inflammatory.
  1. Neurosarcoidosis.
  2. Wegener's granulomatosis.
  3. Langerhans cell histiocytosis.
  4. Rheumatoid nodule(s).
 C. Vascular.
  1. Enlarged dural sinuses from high-flow AVMs: may resemble extraaxial mass and even cause obstructive hydrocephalus.

Abnormal Meningeal Enhancement Differential Diagnosis

Diffuse

Common
Postoperative
Infectious meningitis
Carcinomatous meningitis
Subarachnoid hemorrhage
Uncommon
Sarcoidosis
Histiocytosis
Idiopathic hypertrophic cranial pachymeningitis
Dural sinus thrombosis
Intracranial hypotension (e.g., with CSF leak)

Focal

Common
Meningioma
Postoperative (around craniotomy site)
Metastasis
Uncommon
Sarcoidosis
Histiocytosis
Rheumatoid nodules
Underlying cerebral infarction
Dural cavernous hemangioma, vascular malformation
Lymphoma/leukemia
Extramedullary hematopoiesis

(From Osborn AG: *Diagnostic neuroradiology,* St Louis, 1994, Mosby.)

   2. Giant aneurysm: can appear as extraaxial mass.
   3. Venous varix: can appear as extraaxial mass.
  D. Traumatic.
   1. Calcified chronic subdural hematoma: high attenuation on CT, typically crescentic and conforming to inner table of calvarium.
  E. Extramedullary hematopoeisis.
   1. Dural hematopoietic tissue can proliferate in anemia, myelofibrosis, or other diffuse marrow infiltrative process.
   2. Typically see multiple, isodense or hyperdense, homogeneously enhancing extraaxial masses on CT.
III. Meningeal pathology (see box above).
  A. Meningeal enhancement.
   1. Gyral enhancement should not be confused with leptomeningeal enhancement.

2. If CT scans are obtained too quickly after contrast administration, strong intravascular enhancement can mimic leptomeningeal disease. Careful examination of basal cisterns (including interpeduncular fossa) should demonstrate normal CSF around vessels.
3. Small vessels with slow flow can mimic leptomeningeal enhancement on MR if T1WI is performed with flow compensation.
4. Abnormal enhancement patterns.
   a. Dura normally enhances (see Chapter 2).
   b. Abnormal leptomeningeal enhancement usually has distinct characteristics.
      (1) Thickened.
      (2) Focal nodularity.
      (3) Long segment or continuous.
      (4) Base of brain.
      (5) Isodense or hyperdense to cavernous sinus.
B. Infection (see Chapter 42).
   1. Viral meningitis: more commonly does not demonstrate abnormal leptomeningeal enhancement.
   2. Bacterial meningitis: many uncomplicated cases of bacterial meningitis do not demonstrate findings on neuroimaging studies. Less than half of all children with clinically documented meningitis have abnormal meningeal enhancement on CECT.
   3. Tuberculous meningitis: commonly involves basilar meninges.
   4. Fungal meningitis (especially cryptococcus, coccidiodomycosis): also commonly involves basilar meninges, resembles tuberculous meningitis.
   5. Syphilitic meningitis.
C. Inflammation.
   1. Neurosarcoidosis (see Chapter 46).
      a. Of the multiple CNS manifestations, hydrocephalus is the most common abnormality, most likely secondary to arachnoiditis.
      b. Meningeal involvement (leptomeninges > dura) is more common than parenchymal involvement.
      c. Leptomeningeal involvement can be focal or diffuse; with predilection for pituitary infundibulum, optic chiasm, and cranial nerves.
      d. Dural involvement sometimes occurs, resulting in diffuse or nodular dural enhancement (latter may mimic meningioma).
      e. Enhancing parenchymal masses and gyral enhancement occurs rarely.

2. Rheumatoid pachymeningitis.
   a. CNS involvement is rare. Meningeal involvement (especially dura) occurs more often than parenchymal disease.
   b. Focal granulomatous masses in dura, subdural spaces and rarely in leptomeninges can mimic meningioma.
   c. Occasional leptomeningeal enhancement has been attributed to increased vascularity due to inflammation.
3. Langerhans cell histiocytosis: can cause diffuse or nodular leptomeningeal enhancement.
4. Wegener's granulomatosis: can have focal meningeal enhancement adjacent to extracranial disease with intracranial extension.
5. Benign leptomeningeal fibrosis.
   a. Commonly follows invasive procedures such as craniotomy, shunt placement, intrathecal chemotherapy.
   b. Probably represents inflammatory chemical arachnoiditis (e.g., bleeding into subarachnoid space).
D. Neoplastic disease.
   1. Primary meningeal neoplasm (see Chapter 31).
      a. Meningioma.
      b. Hemangiopericytoma.
      c. Hemangioblastoma.
      d. Sarcomas.
      e. Meningeal melanoma.
   2. Primary CNS tumors.
      a. Medulloblastoma, ependymoma, germinoma, pineoblastoma, choroid plexus tumors, high-grade astrocytoma, and primary CNS lymphoma can have CSF dissemination.
      b. Leptomeningeal metastases may be very subtle or inapparent even on contrast-enhanced MR studies.
   3. Metastasis.
      a. Melanoma and many carcinomas can have CSF spread, particularly breast, lung, gastric carcinomas.
      b. Leptomeningeal metastases are more common than dural metastases.
      c. Leptomeningeal metastases can result in sulcal-cisternal enhancement and ependymal-subependymal enhancement.
      d. Dural carcinomatosis or pachymeningeal metastases can result in convexity dural or tentorial enhancement. Dural carcinomatosis is usually associated with adjacent calvarial metastases. Isolated dural metastasis can mimic meningioma.

     e. Communicating hydrocephalus can be secondary complication of CSF involvement.

  4. Lymphoproliferative malignancies: Lymphoma or leukemia.
    a. Can have leptomeningeal enhancement.
    b. More often, CSF cytology will be positive without evidence of abnormal meninges.

E. Trauma, surgery, vascular.
  1. Chronic subdural hematoma (SDH): chronic SDH can develop a vascular fibrous neomembrane or capsule that enhances with contrast.
  2. Subarachnoid hemorrhage (SAH).
    a. Cisternal enhancement can occur in subacute SAH, up to several weeks after initial bleed. Possibly represents inflammatory response or increased vascular permeability secondary to arachnoiditis.
    b. Chronic repeated episodes of SAH can result in superficial pial siderosis, which may demonstrate abnormal leptomeningeal enhancement.
  3. Resolving parenchymal hematoma: meningeal enhancement may occur adjacent to resolving hematoma.
  4. Postsurgical changes: focal or diffuse dural enhancement can occur after craniotomy.
  5. Infarction.
    a. Mild meningeal enhancement adjacent to subacute infarction can occur.
    b. Not to be confused with gyriform enhancement, which is parenchymal and occurs later.

F. Metabolic, chemicals/toxins.
  1. Mucopolysaccharidoses: can cause dural thickening and enhancement due to infiltration.
  2. Medications: mechanism unknown.
    a. Antibiotics: e.g., penicillin, trimethoprim-sulphamethoxazole.
    b. Nonsteroidal antiinflammatories: e.g., ibuprofen.
    c. Antineoplastics: e.g., cytosine arabinoside.
  3. Intrathecal medications or contrast.
  4. Lead poisoning.

G. Miscellaneous.
  1. Benign intracranial hypotension.
    a. Diffuse dural thickening and enhancement may occur with decreased intracranial pressure and tonsillar descent, probably due to dural venous engorgement.
    b. May be caused by lumbar puncture, CSF leak, meningocele.

2. Idiopathic hypertrophic pachymeningitis.
   a. Rare idiopathic form of pachymeningitis for which no etiology can be found (diagnosis of exclusion).
   b. Biopsy or autopsy shows fibrotic dural thickening with infiltrates of lymphocytes, plasma cells, giant cells, and scattered necrosis.
   c. Common symptoms are headache and cranial nerve palsies.
   d. Does not respond very well to steroid therapy; 50% initial response rate but often progresses despite treatment. Immunosuppressive agents have also been tried with limited success.
   e. Imaging may show diffuse meningeal thickening and/or enhancement.

SUGGESTED READINGS

Cinnamon J, Sharma M, Gray D, et al: Neuroimaging of meningeal disease, *Sem US CT MRI* 15:466-498, 1994.

Greenberg RW, Lane EL, Cinnamon J, et al: The cranial meninges: anatomic considerations, *Semin US CT MRI* 15:454-465, 1994.

Osborn AG: Brain tumors and tumorlike processes. In *Diagnostic neuroradiology,* St Louis, 1994, Mosby, pp 399-528.

Prassopoulos P, Cavouras D, Golfinopoulos S, Nezi M: The size of the intra- and extraventricular cerebrospinal fluid compartments in children with idiopathic benign widening of the frontal subarachnoid space, *Neuroradiol* 37:418-421, 1995.

57

Ventricular Pathology

Key Concepts

1. Congenital causes of abnormal ventricular configuration include holo-prosencephaly, septo-optic dysplasia, schizencephaly, porencephaly, callosal dysgenesis, Chiari II malformation, Dandy-Walker malformation, heterotopias, and hamartomas.
2. Secondary deformation of ventricles can be caused by neurodegenerative diseases, herniations, or adjacent focal parenchymal masses.
3. Ventricular enlargement is due to four general processes.
   a. Physiologic.
   b. Atrophic.
   c. Obstructive.
   d. CSF overproduction.
4. Small ventricles may occasionally be seen with increased intracranial pressure, pseudotumor cerebri, or ventricular shunting. However, de-creased ventricular size is a less reliable indicator of increased intracra-nial pressure than effacement of subarachnoid spaces or basilar cisterns.
5. Intraventricular masses are uncommon but can be important cause of hydrocephalus, coma, or sudden death. Lesions can be grouped by pathology, age, or location.
6. Ependymal enhancement is most often associated with infection, inflam-mation, or neoplasm.

I. Abnormalities of ventricular configuration.
   A. Congenital.
      1. Holoprosencephaly.
         a. Alobar: large monoventricle with or without dorsal cyst.
         b. Semilobar: monoventricle partly divided superiorly by incomplete falx, rudimentary temporal and occipital horns.
         c. Lobar: absent septum pellucidum.
      2. Septo-optic dysplasia: absent septum pellucidum.
      3. Schizencephaly: ventricular wall contiguous peripherally with gray-matter-lined cleft.
      4. Porencephaly: focal encephalomalacia adjacent to and usually continuous with lateral ventricle.
      5. Callosal dysgenesis: high-riding third ventricle between parallel lateral ventricles.
      6. Chiari II malformation: "batwing" appearance of frontal horns and "hourglass" appearance of third ventricle on coronal images due to prominent massa intermedia, disproportionate enlargement of posterior portions of lateral ventricles (colpocephaly), slitlike fourth ventricle, may have hydrocephalus.
      7. Myelomeningocele (irrespective of Chiari II): may have colpocephaly, hydrocephalus.
      8. Dandy-Walker malformation: large posterior fossa cyst communicating with fourth ventricle, "keyhole" appearance on coronal or sagittal images if extends above tentorium, may have hydrocephalus.
      9. Congenital aqueductal stenosis: may have colpocephaly, hydrocephalus.
     10. Heterotopias and hamartomas: can deform ventricular margins.
     11. Hemimegalencephaly: ipsilateral ventricular enlargement.
     12. Unilateral atrophy: e.g., Dyke-Davidoff-Mason.
   B. Acquired.
      1. Neurodegenerative disease.
         a. Huntington's disease: although usually causes generalized cerebral atrophy, may initially see focal caudate atrophy resulting in flat or outwardly convex frontal horn margins.
         b. Pick's disease: selective frontotemporal atrophy; occasional involvement of basal ganglia and substantia nigra.
      2. Herniations (see Chapter 21).
      3. Focal masses: see p. 597.

II. Abnormalities of ventricular size.
  A. Increased ventricular size.
    1. Physiologic.
      a. Premature infants often have mildly enlarged ventricles.
      b. Slight gradual physiologic increase in ventricular size normally occurs with aging, with more rapid enlargement after 60 years of age.
    2. Atrophic.
      a. Congenital (TORCH) infections.
      b. Brain malformations: e.g., lissencephaly.
      c. Neurodegenerative disease (e.g., HIV encephalopathy, Alzheimer's disease, Pick's disease, Huntington's disease, multiinfarct dementia).
      d. Global ischemia/hypoxia.
      e. Posttraumatic.
      f. Postinflammatory.
      g. Alcohol and drug abuse.
      h. Iatrogenic (dilantin, steroids, radiation therapy, chemotherapy).
      i. Dehydration.
      j. Deprivational states.
    3. Obstructive.
      a. Noncommunicating or intraventricular hydrocephalus.
        (1) Congenital: e.g., aqueductal stenosis, Chiari malformation.
        (2) Infection.
          (a) Ventriculitis/ependymitis: obstruction due to inflammatory debris, edema or intraventricular loculations.
          (b) Neurocysticercosis: intraventricular cysts can cause ventricular obstruction.
        (3) Neoplastic: particularly tumors adjacent to foramen of Monro (e.g., colloid cyst, central neurocytoma) and posterior fossa tumors.
      b. Communicating or extraventricular hydrocephalus.
        (1) Meningitis.
        (2) Subarachnoid hemorrhage.
        (3) Neoplasm.
          (a) Leptomeningeal carcinomatosis.
          (b) Choroid plexus tumors: may impair CSF resorption by tumor cells, protein, or hemorrhage.
        (4) Dural sinus or cortical vein thrombosis.
        (5) Idiopathic (normal pressure hydrocephalus).

4. CSF overproduction: choroid plexus tumors (controversy whether hydrocephalus is due to overproduction or obstruction—see above).
B. Decreased ventricular size.
1. Diffuse cerebral edema (although is less reliable indicator of increased intracranial pressure than effacement of subarachnoid spaces or basilar cisterns).
2. Pseudotumor cerebri.
3. Ventricular shunting.
III. Intraventricular masses (for distribution by location and age see Fig. 57-1, boxes on p. 598-599).

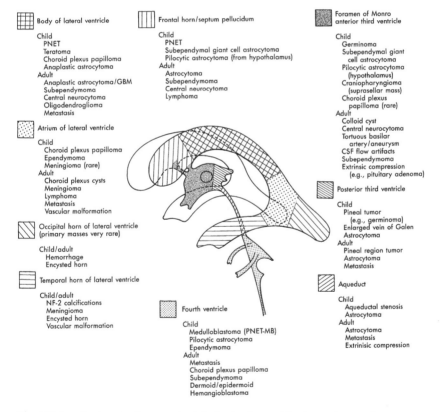

Body of lateral ventricle
Child
  PNET
  Teratoma
  Choroid plexus papilloma
  Anaplastic astrocytoma
Adult
  Anaplastic astrocytoma/GBM
  Subependymoma
  Central neurocytoma
  Oligodendroglioma
  Metastasis

Atrium of lateral ventricle
Child
  Choroid plexus papilloma
  Ependymoma
  Meningioma (rare)
Adult
  Choroid plexus cysts
  Meningioma
  Lymphoma
  Metastasis
  Vascular malformation

Occipital horn of lateral ventricle
(primary masses very rare)
Child/adult
  Hemorrhage
  Encysted horn

Temporal horn of lateral ventricle
Child/adult
  NF-2 calcifications
  Meningioma
  Encysted horn
  Vascular malformation

Frontal horn/septum pellucidum
Child
  PNET
  Subependymal giant cell astrocytoma
  Pilocytic astrocytoma (from hypothalamus)
Adult
  Astrocytoma
  Subependymoma
  Central neurocytoma
  Lymphoma

Fourth ventricle
Child
  Medulloblastoma (PNET-MB)
  Pilocytic astrocytoma
  Ependymoma
Adult
  Metastasis
  Choroid plexus papilloma
  Subependymoma
  Dermoid/epidermoid
  Hemangioblastoma

Foramen of Monro anterior third ventricle
Child
  Germinoma
  Subependymal giant cell astrocytoma
  Pilocytic astrocytoma (hypothalamus)
  Craniopharyngioma (suprasellar mass)
  Choroid plexus papilloma (rare)
Adult
  Colloid cyst
  Central neurocytoma
  Tortuous basilar artery/aneurysm
  CSF flow artifacts
  Subependymoma
  Extrinsic compression (e.g., pituitary adenoma)

Posterior third ventricle
Child
  Pineal tumor (e.g., germinoma)
  Enlarged vein of Galen
  Astrocytoma
Adult
  Pineal region tumor
  Astrocytoma
  Metastasis

Aqueduct
Child
  Aqueductal stenosis
  Astrocytoma
Adult
  Astrocytoma
  Metastasis
  Extrinisic compression

Fig. 57-1 Anatomic diagram depicts the brain ventricular system and common lesions encountered in each specific location. (From Osborn AG: *Diagnostic neuroradiology,* St Louis, 1994, Mosby.)

Intraventricular Masses in Adults

Lateral ventricles

Frontal horn
Astrocytoma (anaplastic, glioblastoma)
Subependymal giant cell astrocytoma (Tuberous sclerosis)
Central neurocytoma
Subependymoma
Cavum septi pellucidi and cavum vergae
Body
Astrocytoma
Central neurocytoma
Oligodendroglioma
Subependymoma
Atrium
Choroid plexus cysts/xanthogranulomas
Meningioma
Metastases
Occipital and temporal horns (rare)
Meningioma
Enlarged calcified choroid plexus with NF-2

Foramen of Monro/third ventricle

Foramen of Monro
Astrocytoma (anaplastic, glioblastoma)
Central neurocytoma
Oligodendroglioma
Subependymal giant cell astrocytoma (Tuberous sclerosis)
Third ventricle
Colloid cyst
Extrinsic mass (pituitary adenoma, aneurysm, glioma)
Sarcoid, germinoma (anterior recesses/hypothalamus/infundibular stalk)

Aqueduct/fourth ventricle

Aqueduct
Hemorrhage
Midbrain glioma
Metastasis
Fourth ventricle
Metastasis
Hemangioblastoma
Exophytic brainstem glioma
Subependymoma

(From Osborn AG: *Diagnostic neuroradiology,* St Louis, 1994, Mosby.)

Intraventricular Masses in Children

Lateral ventricles

Frontal horn
Cavum septi pellucidi and cavum vergae
Astrocytoma (usually low grade)
Subependymal giant cell astrocytoma (Tuberous sclerosis)
Body
PNET
Astrocytoma
Atrium
Choroid plexus papilloma
Ependymoma (rare)
Occipital and temporal horns (rare)
Meningioma
Enlarged calcified choroid plexus with NF-2

Foramen of Monro/third ventricle

Foramen of Monro
Subependymal giant cell astrocytoma
Astrocytoma
(N.B.—colloid cysts are rare in children; when they occur they are usually
   in older children and adolescents)
Third ventricle
Extrinsic mass (e.g., craniopharyngioma)
Astrocytoma (low grade, pilocytic)
Histiocytosis (anterior recesses/hypothalamus/infundibular stalk)
Germinoma

Fourth ventricle

Astrocytoma (usually pilocytic type)
Medulloblastoma
Ependymoma
Exophytic brainstem glioma

(From Osborn AG: *Diagnostic neuroradiology,* St Louis, 1994, Mosby.)

A. Congenital or developmental.
   1. Choroid plexus cyst: benign epithelial-lined cysts.
   2. Xanthogranuloma of choroid plexus: benign masses consisting
      of foam-filled cells with lymphocytes and macrophages.
   3. Ependymal cyst.
   4. Colloid cyst: typically occurs in anterior third ventricle, at
      foramen of Monro.

5. Subependymal nodule (Tuberous sclerosis).
6. Enlarged choroid plexus (Sturge-Weber disease): ipsilateral to affected hemisphere.
7. Dermoid/epidermoid: occasionally arise within fourth ventricle.

B. Neoplasm: intraventricular tumors are uncommon (10% of all intracranial neoplasms).
1. Medulloblastoma: arises from roof of fourth ventricle and grows into fourth ventricle.
2. Ependymoma.
   a. More common in children.
   b. Infratentorial (60%): typically fill fourth ventricle, may extrude through foramina of Lushka or Magendie.
   c. Supratentorial (40%): often involves parenchyma adjacent to lateral ventricles, purely intraventricular tumors less common but usually in atrium or frontal horn of lateral ventricle.
3. Subependymoma.
   a. More common in adults.
   b. Usually in fourth ventricle, may extrude through foramen of Magendie into cisterna magna or through foramen magnum (mimics Chiari I malformation).
   c. Less commonly occurs in lateral (frontal horn) or third ventricles.
4. Choroid plexus tumors.
   a. Most common in children: predilection for trigone of lateral ventricle.
   b. Occasionally in adults: third or fourth ventricles.
5. Central neurocytoma: usually in lateral ventricle, near foramen of Monro.
6. Subependymal giant-cell astrocytoma (Tuberous sclerosis): typically in lateral ventricle, at foramen of Monro.
7. Meningioma: 1% arise within ventricles, typically in atrium of lateral ventricle.
8. Oligodendroglioma: rarely intraventricular, occurs in lateral ventricles.
   a. Can arise from septum pellucidum or tela choroidea.
   b. More commonly arises from parenchyma, with intraventricular extension.

     9. Lymphoma.

       a. More commonly arises from parenchyma, with intraventricular extension.

       b. Can also cause diffuse nodular subependymal involvement.

    10. Craniopharyngioma: can occasionally arise from squamous epithelial rests in the region of the lamina terminalis and invaginate/grow into third ventricle.

C. Infectious/inflammatory.

    1. Neurocysticercosis: commonly in fourth ventricle, although can occur anywhere; cysts may be mobile.

    2. Loculations due to septations.

    3. Trapped ventricle.

D. Vascular.

    1. Vascular malformation.

       a. Dilated arterial feeders, draining veins, and venous varices may project into ventricles.

       b. Occasionally may arise in choroid plexus.

    2. Intraventricular hemorrhage.

       a. Germinal matrix hemorrhage in premature infants.

       b. Trauma.

       c. Basal ganglia hemorrhage (e.g., hypertension) with intraventricular extension.

E. Trauma/postsurgical.

    1. Intraventricular hemorrhage.

    2. Pneumocephalus.

F. Extrinsic compression and/or extension.

    1. From suprasellar masses.

       a. Pituitary macroadenoma.

       b. Craniopharyngioma.

       c. Germinoma.

       d. Hypothalamic-chiasmatic glioma.

       e. Neurosarcoidosis.

       f. Langerhans cell histiocytosis.

       g. Giant aneurysm.

    2. From posterior fossa masses.

       a. Pilocytic astrocytoma.

       b. Hemangioblastoma.

       c. Brainstem glioma.

    3. From cerebral hemispheric masses.

       a. Astrocytoma, GBM.

       b. Supratentorial PNET.

    4. From pineal region masses.

a. Germinoma.
b. Teratoma.
c. Pineoblastoma.
G. Artifacts: CSF flow artifact can mimic tumor, especially at foramen of Monro.
IV. Ependymal enhancement (box on p. 440).
A. Normal vascular structures.
   a. Subependymal veins.
   b. Choroid plexus.
B. Congenital/developmental.
   1. Tuberous sclerosis: subependymal nodules may enhance.
C. Vascular malformations.
   1. AVM: periventricular arteries and veins may become engorged.
   2. Venous angioma: enlarged medullary subependymal veins may drain into enlarged transcortical or deep vein.
   3. Dural sinus occlusion and cortical vein thrombosis: subependymal veins may enlarge due to collateral venous drainage pathway.
   4. Sturge-Weber syndrome: impaired cortical venous drainage may be associated with leptomeningeal angioma, with subsequent enlargement of subependymal and medullary veins.
D. Infectious/inflammatory.
   1. Ventriculitis/ependymitis (see Chapter 43).
   2. Neurosarcoidosis.
E. Neoplastic: tends to be nodular or diffuse; up to 35% falsely negative contrast-enhanced MR studies.
   1. Primary brain tumor.
      a. Pineal tumors (germinoma, pineoblastoma).
      b. PNET/medulloblastoma.
      c. Ependymoma.
      d. Choroid plexus tumors.
      e. Anaplastic astrocytoma, GBM.
   2. Lymphoma/leukemia.
   3. Metastases.
      a. Breast.
      b. Lung.
      c. Melanoma.

SUGGESTED READINGS

Jelinek J, Smirniotopoulos JG, Parisi JE, Kanzer M: Lateral ventricular neoplasms of the brain: differential diagnosis based on clinical, CT, and MR findings, *AJNR* 11:567-574, 1990.

Malm J, Kristensen B, Karlsson T, et al: The predictive value of cerebrospinal fluid dynamic tests in patients with the idiopathic adult hydrocephalus syndrome, *Arch Neurol* 52:783-789, 1995.

Morrison G, Sobel DE, Kelley WM, Norman D: Intraventricular mass lesions, *Radiol* 153:435-442, 1984.

Osborn AG: Brain tumors and tumorlike processes. In *Diagnostic neuroradiology,* St Louis, 1994, Mosby, pp 399-528.

Price AC, Babigian GV: MRI of intraventricular tumors, *MRI Decisions* May/June: 2-16, 1991.

Sotelo J, Rubalcava M, Gomez-Llata S: A new shunt for hydrocephalus that relies on CSF production rather than on ventricular pressure: initial clinical experiences, *Surg Neurol* 43:324-332, 1995.

Tien RD: Intraventricular mass lesions of the brain: CT and MR findings, *AJR* 157:1283-1290, 1991.

Van Roost D, Solymosi L, Funke K: A characteristic ventricular shape in myelomeningocele-associated hydrocephalus? A CT stereology study, *Neuroradiol* 37:412-417, 1995.

58

Sellar and Juxtasellar Lesions

Key Concepts

1. The pituitary gland is larger during puberty and during pregnancy. It may be up to 10 or 11 mm in height with upwardly convex superior margin in young females, and up to 7 or 8 mm in height in young males.
2. Up to 15% of asymptomatic patients have small low-signal foci in adeno-hypophysis on contrast-enhanced MRI, which may represent incidental microadenomas or benign cysts.
3. The posterior pituitary "bright spot" (T1 hyperintensity) is seen on MRI in 60% to 90% of the cases and is thought to be due to vasopressin-neurophysin complexes. Its absence may be normal or associated with alteration of ADH secretion or transport.
4. Pituitary adenoma is the most common sellar and suprasellar mass in adults.
5. Craniopharyngioma and hypothalamic-chiasmatic glioma are common suprasellar masses in children.
6. Infundibular masses in children include germinoma, Langerhans cell histiocytosis, lymphoma, and glioma.
7. Infundibular masses in adults include lymphoma, metastasis, sarcoidosis, hypophysitis, and granular cell tumor.
8. Juxtasellar masses are generally derived from the central skull base, cavernous sinus, or Meckel's cave.

I. Normal sella.
  A. Anatomy (Fig. 58-1).
    1. Sella.
      a. Bony components.
        (1) Sella turcica ("Turkish saddle"): concave depression in the superior basisphenoid.
        (2) Pituitary or hypophyseal fossa: deepest part of sella.
        (3) Tuberculum sella: anterior lip of sella.
        (4) Dorsum sella: posterior lip of sella.
        (5) Anterior and posterior clinoid processes: paired bony projections of the tuberculum and dorsum, respectively.
      b. Diaphragma sella: membranous roof of sella.
      c. Pituitary gland: situated within hypophyseal fossa of sella.
    2. Pituitary gland or hypophysis.
      a. Components.
        (1) Adenohypophysis.
          (a) Pars anterior or pars distalis (anterior lobe): 75% of gland and majority of adenohypophysis; derived from anterior wall of Rathke's pouch.
          (b) Pars intermedia: vestigial remnant of posterior wall of Rathke's pouch.
          (c) Pars tuberalis: extends partway along anterior and lateral surfaces of infundibulum.
        (2) Neurohypophysis.
          (a) Pars nervosa (posterior lobe).
          (b) Infundibulum or pituitary stalk: connects pituitary gland to tuber cinereum, through aperture in diaphragma sella.
          (c) Median eminence.
      b. Size.
        (1) Pituitary gland.
          (a) At birth and in neonatal period, gland is relatively rounder. Thereafter the superior margin becomes flat or concave while the gland grows in width.
          (b) Maximum height during puberty, pregnancy.
          (c) Females: up to 10 or 11 mm in height.
          (d) Males: up to 8 mm in height.
          (e) Pituitary size gradually decreases after 20 years of age.
        (2) Infundibulum.
          (a) 3 to 3.5 cm wide near median eminence, 2 mm wide near pituitary insertion.

(b) Tapers smoothly from hypothalamus to pituitary insertion.
3. Anatomic relations.
    a. Anteriorly and inferiorly.
        (1) Sphenoid sinus.
        (2) Nasopharynx.
    b. Superiorly.
        (1) Diaphragma sella.
        (2) Suprasellar subarachnoid space.
        (3) Optic chiasm.
        (4) Anterior recesses of third ventricle.

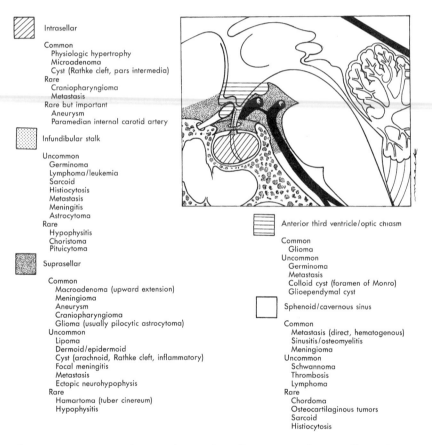

Intrasellar

Common
  Physiologic hypertrophy
  Microadenoma
  Cyst (Rathke cleft, pars intermedia)
Rare
  Craniopharyngioma
  Metastasis
Rare but important
  Aneurysm
  Paramedian internal carotid artery

Infundibular stalk

Uncommon
  Germinoma
  Lymphoma/leukemia
  Sarcoid
  Histiocytosis
  Metastasis
  Meningitis
  Astrocytoma
Rare
  Hypophysitis
  Choristoma
  Pituicytoma

Suprasellar

Common
  Macroadenoma (upward extension)
  Meningioma
  Aneurysm
  Craniopharyngioma
  Glioma (usually pilocytic astrocytoma)
Uncommon
  Lipoma
  Dermoid/epidermoid
  Cyst (arachnoid, Rathke cleft, inflammatory)
  Focal meningitis
  Metastasis
  Ectopic neurohypophysis
Rare
  Hamartoma (tuber cinereum)
  Hypophysitis

Anterior third ventricle/optic chiasm

Common
  Glioma
Uncommon
  Germinoma
  Metastasis
  Colloid cyst (foramen of Monro)
  Glioependymal cyst

Sphenoid/cavernous sinus

Common
  Metastasis (direct, hematogenous)
  Sinusitis/osteomyelitis
  Meningioma
Uncommon
  Schwannoma
  Thrombosis
  Lymphoma
Rare
  Chordoma
  Osteocartilaginous tumors
  Sarcoid
  Histiocytosis

Fig. 58-1 Anatomic diagram depicts the sella turcica and suprasellar region as seen from the lateral view. Common lesions and their differential diagnosis by location are indicated. (From Osborn AG: *Diagnostic neuroradiology*, St Louis, 1994, Mosby.)

        (5) Hypothalamus.
     c. Laterally: cavernous sinus and contents.
     d. Posteriorly.
        (1) Basilar artery.
        (2) Pons.
  4. Blood supply.
     a. Arteries.
        (1) Superior hypophyseal arteries: supply infundibular stalk.
        (2) Inferior hypophyseal arteries: supply pars nervosa.
        (3) Hypophyseal-portal plexus: capillary plexus derived from hypothalamic arteries and superior hypophyseal arteries that transport hormones from hypothalamus and also supply adenohypophysis.
     b. Veins: drain into cavernous sinuses with subsequent drainage into petrosal sinuses.
     c. *Note:* pituitary gland lacks blood-brain barrier.
B. Radiology (Table 58-1).
  1. CT: typically isodense with brain, uniform strong enhancement.
  2. MRI.
     a. Adenohypophysis.
        (1) Adenohypophysis is typically isointense with GM with strong uniform enhancement, although may be bright on T1WI in neonates.
        (2) Up to 15% of asymptomatic patients have small low-signal foci on contrast-enhanced MRI, which may represent incidental microadenomas or benign cysts.
        (3) Pars intermedia cysts: microscopic examination often demonstrates one or more small epithelial-lined cysts filled with proteinaceous fluid or cellular debris, thought to be embryologic remnants of Rathke cleft, probably precursor to Rathke cleft cyst.
     b. Neurohypophysis.
        (1) Posterior lobe typically appears hyperintense on T1WI (60% to 90%) and thought to result from neurosecretory vesicles containing vasopressin-neurophysin complexes.
        (2) Absence of "bright spot" can be normal or associated with alteration of ADH secretion or transport, including diabetes insipidus (central or nephrogenic), compressive pituitary gland lesions, hypophysectomy, traumatic stalk transection, infundibular infiltration such as sarcoidosis.
        (3) "Bright spot" can also be located in suprasellar location due to congenital ectopic neurohypophysis or due to disturbed transport of releasing hormones from hypothalamus.

Table 58-1 Typical MRI and CT Appearance of Common Suprasellar Lesions

Lesion	CT		MR Signal Compared to Brain		Comments
	Unenhanced	Enhanced	T1WI	T2WI	
Pituitary macroadenoma	Isodense	Modest uniform enhancement	Isointense; enhances strongly, sometimes inhomogeneously	Isointense or slightly hyperintense	Calcification is rare; displacement rather than invasion of adjacent structures; often lobulated (figure eight); mass indistinguishable from pituitary
Pituitary macroadenoma (hemorrhagic)	Inhomogeneously hyperdense	Hyperdense	Often complex mixed signal; iso/hyperintense	Complex mixed signal	Signal changes with age of clot
Meningioma	Sightly hyperdense	Strong uniform enhancement	Isointense (may be inconspicuous); enhances strongly	Variable: hypo- iso-, or slightly hyperintense	Smooth well-delineated lesion; calcification is common; look for dural "tail"; pituitary gland distinct from mass
Craniopharyngioma	Heterogeneous; cystic: hypodense; solid: iso- or slightly hyperdense	Variable; cystic: rim enhancement; solid: +/– enhancement	Variable; cystic: variable, often hyperintense; enhancement in rim of tumor nodule; solid: isointense	Variable; cystic: hyperintense; solid: hyperintense	Focal calcification is common (rim, globular) location: 70% intra and suprasellar; 20% suprasellar only; 10% intrasellar only

Lesion	CT	CT with contrast	MRI T1	MRI T2	Comments
Glioma (optico-chiasmatic-hypothalamic)	Isodense or slightly hypodense	+/− enhancement	Isointense; variable enhancement	Slightly hyperintense (may remain isointense)	May see chiasmal enlargement; calcification rare; retrochiasmatic extension is common (N.B.-occasionally compressive lesions such as craniopharyngioma or adenoma can cause hyperintensity in adjacent brain)
Aneurysm (patent)	Slightly hyperdense	Strong uniform enhancement	Flow void	Flow void	Turbulent flow may give inhomogeneous signal; ICA or ACoA are most common locations; may see rim calcification
Aneurysm (partially thrombosed)	Slightly hyperdense	Nonenhancing in area of thrombus; strongly enhancing patent lumen; may see rim enhancement	Thrombus: variable	Variable	Thrombus may appear heterogeneous (laminated blood products in different stages)

(From Osborn AG: *Diagnostic neuroradiology*, St Louis, 1994, Mosby.)

(4) T1 hyperintensity can also be caused by other lesions (box).

(5) Infundibulum lacks blood brain barrier and enhances strongly. May have central area of nonenhancement due to variable extension of infundibular recess of third ventricle.

II. Intrasellar pathology (see box on p. 611).

  A. Congenital and developmental.

    1. "Partial empty sella": normal variant in which sella is partially filled with CSF.

    2. Pars intermedia cyst, Rathke cleft cyst.

    3. Intrasellar arachnoid cyst: rare.

    4. Intrasellar dermoid/epidermoid: rare.

    5. Primary panhypopituitarism: small or absent gland.

  B. Vascular.

    1. Paramedian or "kissing" carotid arteries due to medially positioned cavernous segments (important surgical consideration).

    2. Intrasellar aneurysm.

    3. Pituitary apoplexy: typically due to hemorrhagic necrosis of

---

**Differential Diagnosis: Suprasellar "Hot Spot"
High Signal Focus on Unenhanced T1-Weighted MR Scans**

Common

Rathke's cleft cyst
Craniopharyngioma
Subacute hemorrhage
  Thrombosed aneurysm
  Hemorrhagic neoplasm (e.g., pituitary adenoma)
  Postoperative (hemorrhage, fat graft)

Uncommon

Lipoma
Dermoid
Congenital ectopic neurohypophysis
Disturbed transport of releasing hormones from hypothalamus to neural lobe
  Traumatic stalk transection
  Hypophysectomy
  Sarcoidosis, histiocytosis
  Pituitary or other tumor

(From Osborn AG: *Diagnostic neuroradiology,* St Louis, 1994, Mosby.)

pituitary adenoma; can also occur with peripartum pituitary necrosis (Sheehan's) or following bromocryptine therapy.
C. Neoplastic.
1. Pituitary microadenoma: most common intrasellar mass, tends to laterally displace internal carotid arteries, rather than encase arteries.
2. Intrasellar craniopharyngioma: only 5% to 10% are purely intrasellar.
3. Meningioma: purely intrasellar location rare, tends to encase internal carotid arteries.
4. Metastases: direct hematogenous spread to gland rare (more common in suprasellar location), but can occur from breast, lung, renal, or colon.
5. Granular cell tumor (choristoma, granular cell myoblastoma, or granular pituicytoma).
   a. Benign tumor of infundibulum or pars nervosa.
   b. Occurs more frequently in women.
D. Inflammatory/infectious.
1. Adenohypophysitis.
   a. Lymphocytic or lymphoid hypophysitis.
      (1) Rare lymphocytic inflammatory disorder typically involving adenohypophysis.

Intrasellar Masses

Common

Physiologic hyperplasia
Microadenoma
Nonneoplastic cyst (pars intermedia, colloid, Rathke's cleft)

Uncommon

Craniopharyngioma
Metastasis

Rare

Meningioma
Epidermoid or dermoid cyst

Rare but extremely important

Paramedian carotid arteries
Aneurysm

(From Osborn AG: *Diagnostic neuroradiology,* St Louis, 1994, Mosby.)

        (2) Usually occurs in women during late pregnancy or post-partum period, but has also been reported in premeno-pausal or postmenopausal women as well as men.

        (3) Enhancing intrasellar mass with suprasellar extension may mimic pituitary adenoma.

    b. Granulomatous hypophysitis.

        (1) Can be caused by syphilis, tuberculosis, sarcoidosis, or Langerhans cell histiocytosis.

        (2) Nonspecific appearance, may mimic macroadenoma.

  2. Pituitary abscess: rare.

E. Hyperplasia.

  1. Hypothalamic tumors or ectopic tumors secreting hypothalamic releasing factors.

  2. Central precocious puberty.

  3. End-organ failure (e.g., hypothyroidism, hypogonadism).

  4. Nelson syndrome (7% of adrenalectomy patients).

  5. Exogenous administration of estrogens.

F. Postoperative sella: fat, muscle, and dura used for packing can have heterogeneous, bizarre appearance.

G. Other: sellar expansion can be caused by increased intracranial pressure, obstructive hydrocephalus (e.g., dilated third ventricle).

III. Suprasellar pathology (for infundibular lesions, see box on p. 613).

A. Congenital and developmental.

  1. Ectopic neurohypophysis.

  2. Suprasellar arachnoid cyst.

  3. Rathke cleft cyst with suprasellar extension.

  4. Tuber cinereum hamartoma: resembles gray matter, nonenhanc-ing, noncalcifying.

  5. Dermoid/epidermoid cyst.

  6. Lipoma of infundibulum.

  7. Colloid cyst.

  8. Cephalocele.

B. Vascular.

  1. Suprasellar aneurysm.

  2. AVM.

  3. Dolichoectasia of ICA or basilar artery.

C. Neoplastic.

  1. Pituitary macroadenoma.

    a. Most common suprasellar mass.

    b. Typical "figure of eight" appearance due to constriction by diaphragma sellae.

  2. Craniopharyngioma.

  3. Meningioma: arise from sphenoid ridge, diaphragma sellae, or tuberculum sellae.

Infundibular Masses

Children

Common
Langerhans cell histiocytosis
Germinoma
Meningitis
Uncommon
Lymphoma
Glioma

Adults

Common
Sarcoidosis
Germinoma
Metastasis
Uncommon
Lymphoma
Glioma
Choristoma

(From Osborn AG: *Diagnostic neuroradiology,* St Louis, 1994, Mosby.)

4. Optico-chiasmatic-hypothalamic glioma.
5. Teratoma.
6. Germinoma: can have synchronous pineal lesion, CSF dissemination common.
7. Lymphoma/leukemia.
   a. Focal mass (granulocytic sarcoma or chloroma in AML).
   b. Infundibular enlargement.
8. Infundibuloma: rare glioma of pituitary stalk (usually pilocytic astrocytoma).
9. Granular cell tumor (choristoma or pituicytoma): rare benign tumor of infundibulum or pars nervosa.
10. Metastases: especially breast, lung, prostate, gastric.

D. Infectious.
   1. Tuberculous meningitis.
   2. Fungal meningitis.
   3. Bacterial meningitis.
   4. Neurocysticercosis: especially racemose cysts.

E. Inflammatory.
   1. Neurosarcoidosis: infundibular enlargement or rarely focal extraaxial or pituitary mass.
   2. Langerhans cell histiocytosis: infundibular enlargement.

IV. Juxtasellar (cavernous sinus, skull base) pathology (see also Chapter 61).
   A. Congenital or developmental.
      1. Arachnoid cyst.
      2. Dermoid/epidermoid.
   B. Vascular.
      1. Aneurysm.
      2. Carotid-cavernous fistula.
      3. Cavernous sinus thrombosis.
      4. AVM.
   C. Neoplasm.
      1. Meningioma.
      2. Chordoma.
      3. Osteocartilagenous tumors involving clivus.
      4. Nasopharyngeal tumors.
         a. Direct extension.
         b. Perineural extension.
      5. Schwannoma: involving trigeminal nerve (e.g., Meckel's cave).
      6. Metastases to clivus.
   D. Infection/inflammation.
      1. Sphenoid sinusitis, mucocele.
      2. Fungal: aspergilloma, mucormycosis.

SUGGESTED READINGS

Dietrich RB, Lis LE, Greensite FS, Pitt D: Normal MR appearance of the pituitary gland in the first 2 years of life, *AJNR* 16:1413-1419, 1995.

Elster AD: Modern imaging of the pituitary, *Radiol* 187:1-14, 1993.

Kollias SS, Ball WS, Prenger: Review of the embryologic development of the pituitary gland and report of a case of hypophyseal duplication detected by MRI, *Neuroradiol* 37:3-12, 1995.

Osborn AG: Brain tumors and tumorlike processes. In *Diagnostic neuroradiology,* St Louis, 1994, Mosby, pp 399-528.

Reul J, Weis J, Spetzger U, Isensee CH, Thron A: Differential diagnosis of truly suprasellar space-occupying masses: synopsis of clinical findings, CT, and MRI, *Eur Radiol* 5:224-237, 1995.

Sumida M, Uozumi T, Yamanaka M, et al: Displacement of the normal pituitary gland by sellar and juxtasellar tumors: surgical-MRI correlation and use in differential diagnosis, *Neuroradiol* 36:372-375, 1994.

Teramoto A, Hirakawa K, Sanno N, Osamura Y: Incidental pituitary lesions in 1,000 unselected autopsy specimens, *Radiol* 193:161-164, 1994.

59

Pineal Region

Key Concepts

1. Pineal region masses may arise from the pineal gland, posterior third ventricle, quadrigeminal cistern, tectum of midbrain, posterior thalamus, splenium of corpus callosum, or tentorial apex (Fig. 59-1, box on p. 617).
2. The majority of pineal region masses are neoplastic; more than two thirds are germ cell tumors.
3. Benign pineal cysts occur in up to 40% of routine autopsies and occasionally may be indistinguishable from cystic pinealoma.

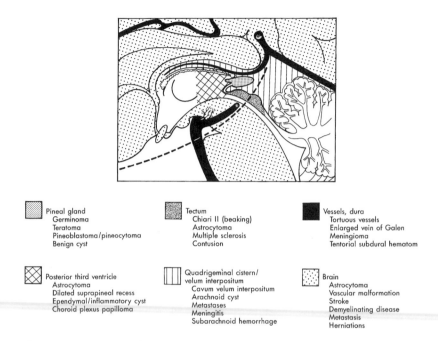

Fig. 59-1 Anatomic diagram depicts the pineal region and its common lesions. The approximate course of the tentorial incisura is shown by the dotted line. (From Osborn AG: *Diagnostic neuroradiology*, St Louis, 1994, Mosby.)

I. Anatomy.
  A. Morphology.
    1. Small midline glandular structure approximately 4 mm wide and 8 mm long.
    2. Derived from evagination of roof of third ventricle.
    3. Mostly composed of a neuronal type cell (pinealocyte) with dendritic processes (95%); with small areas of neuroglial supporting cells (5%).
  B. Function: regulation of certain circulating hormone levels and control of biorhythms (e.g., diurnal rhythm, puberty).
  C. Anatomic relations.
    1. Anteriorly.
      a. Posterior third ventricle.
      b. Posterior thalami.
      c. Posterior commissure.
    2. Inferiorly.
      a. Midbrain (tectum).
      b. Quadrigeminal cistern.

Common Pineal Region Masses

Germ cell tumors

Germinoma
Teratoma

Pineal parenchymal cell tumors

Pineocytoma
Pineoblastoma

Other cell tumors and neoplastic-like masses

Pineal cysts
Astrocytoma (pineal gland, thalamus, midbrain, tectum, corpus callosum)
Meningioma
Metastases
Vascular malformation (with or without enlarged vein of Galen)
Miscellaneous (lipoma, epidermoid, arachnoid cyst)

(Adapted from Osborn AG: *Diagnostic neuroradiology,* St Louis, 1994, Mosby.)

    3. Posteriorly.
       a. Quadrigeminal cistern.
       b. Vein of Galen.
       c. Tentorial apex.
    4. Superiorly.
       a. Suprapineal recess of third ventricle.
       b. Velum interpositum.
       c. Splenium of corpus callosum.
       d. Internal cerebral veins.
  D. Radiology.
    1. Normal pineal gland may not always be visualized due to small size.
    2. Plain film: may see midline pineal calcification, although usually not before age 10.
    3. CT.
       a. Isodense to gray matter.
       b. More sensitive in detecting calcification.
         (1) Approximately 10% of population at age 10.
         (2) Approximately 40% of population at age 20.
    4. MRI: isointense to gray matter; moderately enhancing with nodular, crescentic, or ring-like forms.
II. Pineal gland lesions.
  A. Neoplasms: majority of pineal gland masses; 1% to 2% of all intracranial tumors; 3% to 8% of pediatric intracranial tumors.

    1. Germ cell tumors: account for more than two thirds of all pineal region masses.
      a. Germinoma.
      b. Teratoma.
      c. Choriocarcinoma.
      d. Endodermal (yolk sac) tumor.
      e. Embryonal carcinoma.
      f. Mixed cell types.
    2. Pineal cell tumors: less than 15% of pineal region masses.
      a. Pineocytoma.
      b. Pineoblastoma.
    3. Pineal glioma (astrocytoma, glioblastoma multiforme): rare.
    4. Metastases: rare.
  B. Pineal cysts: up to 40% of routine autopsies.
    1. Failure of normal pineal development.
    2. Degenerative.
  C. Neurosarcoidosis: rarely causes focal pineal mass.
III. Posterior third ventricular lesions.
  A. Neoplasms.
    1. Choroid plexus papilloma.
    2. Meningioma.
    3. Metastases.
  B. Dilated suprapineal recess: may be due to aqueductal stenosis.
  C. Ependymal or inflammatory cysts: uncommon.
  D. Colloid cyst: although more common in foramen of Monro region, may occasionally occur in posterior third ventricle.
IV. Midbrain (tectal) lesions.
  A. Congenital/developmental.
    1. Dorsal mesencephalic or quadrigeminal plate lipoma.
  B. Neoplasms.
    1. Tectal glioma: usually low-grade astrocytoma.
    2. Lymphoma: occasionally involves tectum.
  C. Vascular.
    1. Cavernous angioma.
    2. Pial AVM.
  D. Demyelinating lesions: e.g., multiple sclerosis.
  E. Trauma: shearing injury or contusion.
  F. Infarct: from occlusion of thalamoperforating arteries or mesencephalic branches of posterior cerebral arteries.
  G. Neurodegenerative.
    1. Progressive supranuclear palsy.
      a. Occurs in older patients.
      b. Presents with axial rigidity, supranuclear ophthalmoplegia, and pseudobulbar palsy.

c. MRI may show T2 hyperintensity or focal atrophy of superior colliculi, periaqueductal gray T2 hyperintensity, or atrophy of the pars compacta of the substantia nigra.

V. Quadrigeminal cistern and velum interpositum lesions.
   A. Normal variant.
      1. Cavum velum interpositum.
         a. Typically triangular shaped, CSF-filled anterior extension of quadrigeminal plate cistern.
         b. May displace internal cerebral veins and pineal gland inferiorly.
   B. Congenital/developmental.
      1. Lipoma: up to one third are associated with other congenital anomalies.
      2. Arachnoid cyst: 8% of all arachnoid cysts occur in quadrigeminal cistern, rarely in velum interpositum.
      3. Dermoid/epidermoid.
   C. Vascular.
      1. Aneurysms: P2 or P3 posterior cerebral artery segments.
      2. Aneurysmal dilatation of vein of Galen due to choroidal artery fistula or mesencephalic AVM.
   D. Neoplasm: leptomeningeal metastases from primary or extracranial sources.

VI. Tentorial apex dura.
   A. Neoplasms.
      1. Meningioma.
      2. Metastases.

VII. Thalamic lesions.
   A. Neoplasms.
      1. Germinoma.
      2. Astrocytoma.
   B. Infarct.

VIII. Splenium lesions.
   A. Neoplasm.
      1. Lymphoma.
      2. Astrocytoma.
   B. Demyelinating: e.g., multiple sclerosis.
   C. Trauma: shearing injury.

SUGGESTED READINGS

Friedman DP: Extrapineal abnormalities of the tectal region: MR imaging findings, *AJR* 159:859-866, 1992.

Osborn AG: Brain tumors and tumorlike processes. In *Diagnostic neuroradiology,* St Louis, 1994, Mosby, pp 399-528.

Sener RN: The pineal gland: a comparative MR imaging study in children and adults with respect to normal anatomic variations and pineal cysts, *Pediatr Radiol* 25:245-248, 1995.

Smirniotopoulos JG, Rushing EJ, Mena H: Pineal region masses: differential diagnosis, *Radiographics* 12:577-596, 1992.

Tien RD, Barkovich AJ, Edwards MSB: MR imaging of pineal tumors, *AJNR* 11:557-565, 1990.

60

Cerebellopontine Angle Region

Key Concepts

1. Cerebellopontine angle region lesions can arise from structures in the cerebellopontine angle cistern, internal auditory canal, intraaxial posterior fossa masses, or extension from the fourth ventricle via the foramina of Lushka (Fig. 60-1).
2. Cerebellopontine angle "pseudotumors" include the cerebellar flocculus, choroid plexus, and prominent jugular tubercles.
3. The most common cerebellopontine angle mass is "acoustic" schwannoma, which actually arises from the vestibular division of CN VIII.

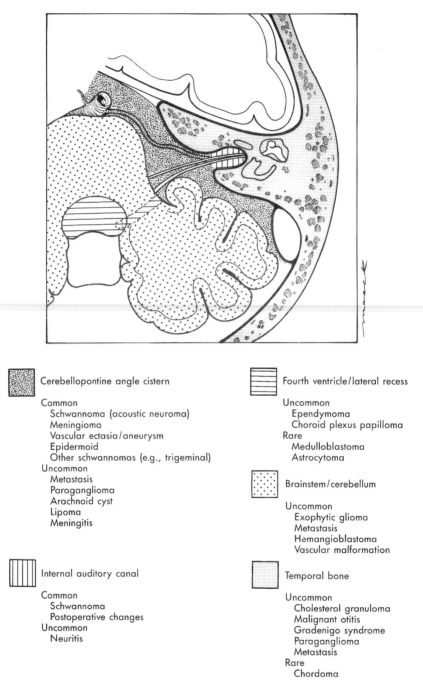

Fig. 60-1 Anatomic diagram depicts the cerebellopontine angle anatomy. Lesions that arise from each component are indicated. (From Osborn AG: *Diagnostic neuroradiology,* St Louis, 1994, Mosby.)

Table 60-1   Cerebellopontine Angle Cistern Masses

Frequency of Mass	Type of Mass	Percent (%)
Common	Acoustic schwannoma	75
	Meningioma	8 to 10
	Epidermoid	5
	Other schwannomas	2 to 5
	Vascular (vertebrobasilar ectasia, aneurysm, vascular malformation)	2 to 5
	Metastases	1 to 2
	Paraganglioma	1 to 2
	Ependymoma, choroid plexus papilloma (primary in CPA or extension from fourth ventricle)	1
Uncommon		= /<1
	Arachnoid cyst	
	Lipoma	
	Dermoid	
	Exophytic cerebellar/brainstem astrocytoma	
	Chordoma	
	Osteocartilagenous tumors	

(From Osborn AG: *Diagnostic neuroradiology,* St Louis, 1994, Mosby.)

I. Cerebellopontine angle lesions (Tables 60-1, 60-2).
  A. Normal structures (pseudotumors).
    1. Flocculus of cerebellum.
    2. Choroid plexus.
    3. Jugular tubercles.
  B. Congenital or developmental.
    1. Arachnoid cyst.
    2. Dermoid/epidermoid.
    3. Lipoma.
  C. Vascular.
    1. Vertebrobasilar dolichoectasia.
    2. Vessel loops: AICA, PICA, VA (can produce hemifacial spasm by impingement of CN VII).
    3. Aneurysm: SCA, PICA, VA.
  D. Infectious/inflammatory.
    1. Meningitis.
    2. Neurocysticercosis.
    3. Neurosarcoidosis.
    4. Langerhans cell histiocytosis.

Table 60-2 Comparative Imaging Findings of Common CPA Masses

| | MR (compared to brain) | | | | |
	T1	T2	Enhancement	Ca^{++}	Other
Acoustic schwannoma	Hypo/iso	Hyper	Intense	Very rare	"Ice cream cone" appearance; bilateral in NF-2; large tumors may have cystic degeneration
Meningioma	Hypo/iso	Iso	Strong	Common	Broad dural base; dural "tail"; may cause hyperostosis; may extend into IAC and mimic schwannoma
Epidermoid	Iso to CSF	Iso/hyper to CSF	Rare	Rare	Insinuates along CSF cisterns
Other schwannoma	Hypo/iso	Hyper	Strong	Very rare	CNV most common
Vascular (VBD, aneurysm)	Varies	Varies	Varies	Frequent	May have "flow void"; phase artifact common; MRA helpful; IAC normal
Metastasis	Iso	Iso	Moderate	None	Coexisting brain metastasis in 75%; multiple cranial nerve/meningeal lesions common

(From Osborn AG: *Diagnostic neuroradiology*, St Louis, 1994, Mosby.)

E. Neoplasm.
   1. Schwannoma.
      a. Acoustic (vestibulocochlear) schwannoma >> trigeminal or facial schwannomas.
      b. Typical "ice-cream" cone appearance with apex directed into IAC.
      c. Usually solid.
      d. Occasionally cystic.
   2. Meningioma.
      a. Typically dural based; globose or en-plaque.
      b. May have "dural tail" (although also seen in other lesions).
      c. Rarely cystic.
   3. Choroid plexus tumor.
      a. More commonly arises from fourth ventricle and extends into CPA cistern through foramina of Lushka.
      b. Occasionally arises within CPA cistern.
   4. Metastases.
      a. Leptomeningeal involvement.
      b. Perineural spread along trigeminal nerve.
      c. Parenchymal lesions.
II. Internal auditory canal lesions (box below).
   A. Congenital/developmental.
      1. Atresia.
      2. Lipoma.
   B. Vascular.
      1. Vascular loop: AICA.
      2. Vertebrobasilar dolichoectasia.

Internal Auditory Canal Masses

Common

Intracanalicular acoustic schwannoma
Postoperative fibrosis

Uncommon

Neuritis (e.g., Bell's palsy, Ramsay Hunt syndrome)
Hemangioma
Lymphoma
Metastasis
Sarcoidosis
Meningioma

(From Osborn AG: *Diagnostic neuroradiology,* St Louis, 1994, Mosby.)

C. Neoplasm.
1. Schwannoma: frequently extends into IAC, giving "ice-cream cone" appearance.
2. Meningioma: unlike schwannoma, rarely extends into IAC.
3. Hemangioma: vascular, enhancing lesion.
4. Melanoma: rare.
5. Lymphoma: rare.
6. Metastases: rare.
D. Inflammatory.
1. Neurosarcoidosis.
2. Langerhans cell histiocytosis.
3. Arachnoiditis.
4. Neuritis.
  a. Bell's palsy: idiopathic acute facial nerve palsy, probably related to nerve swelling due to viral neuritis or immune disease.
  b. Ramsay Hunt syndrome (herpes zoster otitis): involvement of vestibulocochlear ganglia and geniculate ganglion of facial nerve producing severe ear pain, hearing loss, vertigo, and facial nerve palsy.
5. Postoperative fibrosis: focal or diffuse dural enhancement may be due to vascular stasis.
III. Temporal bone lesions (box below).
A. Congenital/developmental.
1. Congenital malformations of inner, middle, or external ear.

Temporal Bone Lesions that may Involve the Cerebellopontine Angle Cistern

Uncommon

Gradenigo's syndrome
Malignant external otitis
Cholesterol granuloma
Paraganglioma
Metastasis

Rare

Chordoma
Mucocele
Plasmacytoma

(From Osborn AG: *Diagnostic neuroradiology,* St Louis, 1994, Mosby.)

2. Vascular pseudotumors.
   a. High or dehiscent jugular bulb.
   b. Aberrant internal carotid artery.
3. Primary cholesteotoma.
   a. Usually arises from aberrant epithelial rests.
   b. Occasionally associated with atresia of the external auditory canal.
   c. Most commonly occurs in epitympanum and is indistinguishable from acquired cholesteatoma.
   d. Typically see soft-tissue mass with erosion of adjacent bone and ossicles.
   e. Can also occur in petrous apex.
B. Infectious/inflammatory.
   1. Otitis/mastoiditis: typically see fluid in middle ear or mastoid air cells.
   2. Secondary cholesteatoma.
      a. Thought to arise from ingrowth of squamous epithelium through perforation of tympanic membrane or invagination of retraction pocket.
      b. Types.
         (1) Pars flaccida cholesteatoma.
             (a) Most common type.
             (b) Involves attic and herniates into Prussak's space in lateral attic. Can extend through aditus ad antrum into mastoid antrum.
         (2) Pars tensa cholesteatoma.
             (a) Less common type.
             (b) Usually due to posterosuperior retraction pockets.
             (c) Involves posterior mesotympanum, sinus tympani, and ossicles.
   3. Cholesterol granuloma or cholesterol cyst.
      a. Expansile cystic lesion of temporal bone (typically petrous apex) containing hemorrhage and cholesterol crystals.
      b. Typically hyperintense on T1WI and T2WI; non-enhancing.
      c. Even if lesion occurs in middle ear, ossicles remain intact.
   4. Petrous apicitis.
      a. Osteomyelitis of petrous apex often associated with fluid in middle ear and mastoid.
      b. Clinical presentation known as Gradenigo's syndrome: sixth nerve palsy, otorrhea, and retro-orbital pain.
   5. Malignant otitis externa.
      a. Temporal bone osteomyelitis seen in older diabetics and immunocompromised patients.

b. Usually caused by Pseudomonas aeroginosa.

c. Fulminant form can cause palsy of CNs VII, IX, X, or XI.

C. Neoplasm.

   1. Facial schwannoma.

   2. Ossifying hemangioma.

      a. Vascular mass with punctate ossification that occurs any-where in temporal bone, can resemble paraganglioma.

      b. May be associated with peripheral facial nerve palsy.

      c. CT: intensely enhancing mass with punctate foci of calcification, typical honeycomb, or spiculated appearance.

   3. Paraganglioma.

      a. Glomus tympanicum: usually very small, located on cochlear promontory in middle ear.

      b. Glomus jugulotympanicum: originates in jugular foramen but erodes through floor of middle ear and invades middle ear cavity.

      c. Glomus jugulare: confined to jugular foramen, typically erodes jugular spine.

   4. Chordoma: usually midline but occasionally can be off-axis and extend predominantly into CPA cistern.

   5. Metastases.

D. Trauma.

   1. Temporal bone fractures.

      a. Types.

         (1) Longitudinal: along axis of petrous temporal bone, most common.

         (2) Transverse: perpendicular to axis of petrous temporal bone.

      b. Often associated with blood in middle ear or mastoid air cells.

IV. Intraaxial or fourth ventricular lesions that may involve CPA cistern (see box on p. 629).

A. Neoplasms.

   1. Metastases.

   2. Exophytic brainstem or cerebellar astrocytoma.

   3. Hemangioblastoma.

   4. Ependymoma: usually arises in fourth ventricle and often extrudes through foramina of Lushka into CPA cistern, or through foramen of Magendie into cisterna magna.

   5. Choroid plexus papilloma: usually arises in fourth ventricle and can protrude into CPA cistern; occasionally arises directly in CPA cistern.

**Intraaxial Masses That May Involve the
Cerebellopontine Angle Cistern**

Common

Metastasis
Exophytic glioma

Uncommon

Hemangioblastoma
Extension from fourth ventricular neoplasm (ependymoma, choroid plexus
papilloma)

(From Osborn AG: *Diagnostic neuroradiology,* St Louis, 1994, Mosby.)

6. Medulloblastoma: usually midline but occasionally atypical
lesions (more likely in adults) can be off-midline with possible
extension into CPA cistern.

SUGGESTED READINGS

Harnsberger HR: The temporal bone: external, middle, and inner ear segments. In
Handbook of head and neck imaging, ed 2, St Louis, 1995, Mosby, pp 426-458.
Osborn AG: Brain tumors and tumorlike processes. In *Diagnostic neuroradiology,*
St Louis, 1994, Mosby, pp 399-528.

61

Skull Base Lesions

Key Concepts

1. Skull base lesions can be divided into anterior, central, and posterior skull base pathology (Fig. 61-1).
2. Anterior skull base lesions commonly originate from the head and neck with secondary extension or invasion; most commonly from sinonasal tumors (e.g., squamous cell carcinoma in adults, rhabdomyosarcoma in children).
3. Both fibrous dysplasia and Paget disease can involve the skull base. However, fibrous dysplasia is more likely to have facial and anterior skull base involvement than Paget disease. Fibrous dysplasia typically has "ground glass" appearance on plain film or CT, and low-signal intensity on T1WI and T2WI on MRI.
4. Central skull base lesions are also often derived from the head and neck, such as nasopharyngeal squamous cell carcinoma.
5. Metastasis from extracranial primary tumor is more likely to involve the central skull base than anterior or posterior skull base.
6. Common cavernous sinus lesions include schwannoma, meningioma, metastasis, and aneurysm.
7. Chordoma and osteocartilagenous tumors have predilection for central and posterior skull base.
8. Jugular foramen tumors include paraganglioma, schwannoma, and metastases.

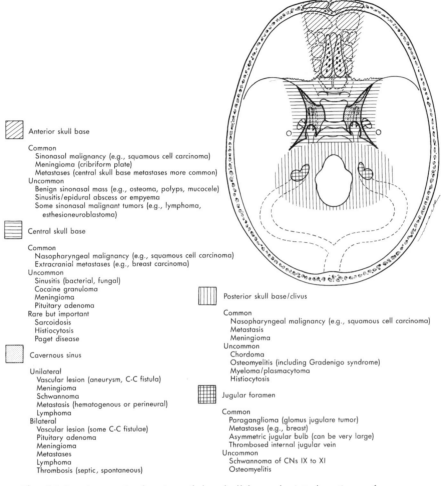

Anterior skull base

Common
  Sinonasal malignancy (e.g., squamous cell carcinoma)
  Meningioma (cribriform plate)
  Metastases (central skull base metastases more common)
Uncommon
  Benign sinonasal mass (e.g., osteoma, polyps, mucocele)
  Sinusitis/epidural abscess or empyema
  Some sinonasal malignant tumors (e.g., lymphoma,
    esthesioneuroblastoma)

Central skull base

Common
  Nasopharyngeal malignancy (e.g., squamous cell carcinoma)
  Extracranial metastases (e.g., breast carcinoma)
Uncommon
  Sinusitis (bacterial, fungal)
  Cocaine granuloma
  Meningioma
  Pituitary adenoma
Rare but important
  Sarcoidosis
  Histiocytosis
  Paget disease

Cavernous sinus

Unilateral
  Vascular lesion (aneurysm, C-C fistula)
  Meningioma
  Schwannoma
  Metastasis (hematogenous or perineural)
  Lymphoma
Bilateral
  Vascular lesion (some C-C fistulae)
  Pituitary adenoma
  Meningioma
  Metastases
  Lymphoma
  Thrombosis (septic, spontaneous)

Posterior skull base/clivus

Common
  Nasopharyngeal malignancy (e.g., squamous cell carcinoma)
  Metastasis
  Meningioma
Uncommon
  Chordoma
  Osteomyelitis (including Gradenigo syndrome)
  Myeloma/plasmacytoma
  Histiocytosis

Jugular foramen

Common
  Paraganglioma (glomus jugulare tumor)
  Metastases (e.g., breast)
  Asymmetric jugular bulb (can be very large)
  Thrombosed internal jugular vein
Uncommon
  Schwannoma of CNs IX to XI
  Osteomyelitis

Fig. 61-1 Anatomic drawing of the skull base depicts locations of common lesions in this area. (From Osborn AG: *Diagnostic neuroradiology,* St Louis, 1994, Mosby.)

I. Anterior skull base (Fig. 61-1, boxes on p. 632 and 640).
  A. Anatomy.
    1. Bony components include:
      a. Orbital plates of the frontal bones.
      b. Cribriform plate of the ethmoid.
      c. Planum sphenoidale.
    2. Anatomic relations.
      a. Anteriorly: frontal sinuses.
      b. Inferiorly.

Anterior Skull Base Lesions

Common

Malignant sinonasal tumor (e.g., squamous cell carcinoma, rhabdomyosarcoma)
Meningioma
Metastases

Uncommon

Mucocele
Osteoma
Polyposis
Inverted papilloma
Esthesioneuroblastoma
Lymphoma
Complicated sinusitis (bacterial, fungal, granulomatous)

Rare

Cephalocele
Dermoid cyst

(From Osborn AG: *Diagnostic neuroradiology,* St Louis, 1994, Mosby.)

(1) Nasal vault.
(2) Ethmoid sinuses.
(3) Medial orbits.
c. Superiorly.
(1) Meninges, extraaxial spaces.
(2) Frontal lobes.
d. Posteriorly: central skull base.
B. Congenital/developmental.
1. Nasoethmoidal cephalocele: 15% of cephaloceles.
2. Nasal dermoid with or without sinus tract: fusiform fat-density/signal mass.
3. Nasal cerebral heterotopia ("nasal glioma"): extracranial rest of glial tissue.
C. Inflammatory.
1. Complicated sinusitis: epidural/subdural empyema.
2. Sinonasal polyposis: occasionally can mimic aggressive skull base erosion.
3. Mucocele.
a. Frontal > ethmoid > maxillary > sphenoid sinuses.
b. Usually causes adjacent bone scalloping due to enlarging sinus, occasionally can mimic aggressive skull base erosion.

4. Wegener's granulomatosis: can cause aggressive sinonasal destruction that may extend to the anterior skull base.

5. Cocaine granulomatosis: can cause aggressive sinonasal destruction that may extend to the anterior skull base.

6. Midline ("lethal") granuloma: probably a lymphoma variant.

7. Sarcoidosis.

D. Trauma.

1. Anterior skull base fractures may be associated with facial fractures.

2. Acquired cephaloceles may be secondary to surgery or to trauma.

E. Neoplasm.

1. Head and neck (with adjacent extension).

a. Sinonasal carcinoma.

(1) Squamous cell carcinoma > adenoid cystic carcinoma.

(2) Typically appears as sinonasal mass with adjacent bone destruction and possible direct invasion intracranially.

(3) Can also extend intracranially through osseus foramina along neurovascular structures.

b. Inverting papilloma:

(1) Benign, slow-growing neoplasm that arises in nasal vault near junction of ethmoid and maxillary sinuses.

(2) Can occasionally extend cephalad with focal erosion of cribriform plate.

c. Esthesioneuroblastoma or olfactory neuroblastoma:

(1) Uncommon malignant tumor arising from bipolar sensory receptor cells in olfactory mucosa (neural crest origin).

(2) Can occur at any age, although bimodal peaks at second and fourth to fifth decades.

(3) Tumor usually located in high nasal vault but can extend into paranasal sinuses, orbit, or through cribriform plate.

(4) Variable density or signal with strong heterogeneous enhancement.

d. Osteoma.

(1) Benign bony tumor of cortical bone.

(2) Frontal sinus is most common location in the head and neck.

(3) Can expand and erode posterior sinus wall and protrude intracranially.

e. Rhabdomyosarcoma: most common pediatric soft-tissue sarcoma, usually found in head and neck (especially orbit, nasopharynx, paranasal sinuses, and middle ear).

      f. Lymphoma.
        (1) Soft-tissue masses may occur in orbits, nasal cavity, paranasal sinuses, or nasopharynx; with possible adjacent bone destruction.
        (2) May occasionally have isolated marrow infiltration.
    2. Intrinsic bony neoplasms.
      a. Osseus metastasis: less common than in central skull base.
      b. Intraosseus meningioma: rare, can mimic fibrous dysplasia or Paget disease; usually sclerotic, occasionally lytic.
    3. Intracranial.
      a. Meningioma.
        (1) Arising from planum sphenoidale and olfactory groove.
        (2) Typically broad-based anterior basal, subfrontal mass with strong uniform enhancement.
        (3) May see adjacent compressed cortex and white matter buckling indicative of extraaxial location.
        (4) Commonly see blistering and hyperostosis of adjacent bone. Less commonly see pneumosinus dilatans of ethmoid sinuses or frank bone destruction.
      b. Frontal lobe ganglioglioma: can cause pressure erosion of the adjacent skull.
      c. Frontal lobe anaplastic astrocytoma, GBM: can occasionally cause dural invasion or adjacent calvarial destruction.
  F. Other (see Chapter 55).
    1. Fibrous dysplasia.
      a. Can be monostoic or polyostotic.
      b. Frequently involves craniofacial region (20%).
      c. Typically "ground-glass" appearance on plain film or CT, low-signal intensity on T1WI and T2WI on MRI.
    2. Paget disease.
      a. Can be monostotic or polyostotic.
      b. Can have diffuse involvement of calvarium and skull base.
      c. Less frequently involves craniofacial region.
      d. Variable imaging appearance depending on phase of disease.
II. Central skull base (see boxes on p. 635, 636, and 640).
  A. Anatomy.
    1. Bony components include:
      a. Upper clivus.
      b. Sella turcica.
      c. Cavernous sinuses (see box on p. 636).
      d. Proximal sphenoid alae: including following important foramina.
        (1) Vidian canal.

**Destructive Central Skull Base Lesions
Differential Diagnosis**

Common

Metastases
 Nasopharyngeal malignancy
 Hematogenous

Uncommon

Osteomyelitis
Fungal sinusitis
Nonfungal granulomas
 Wegener granulomatosis
 Cocaine abuse
 Midline granuloma (probably a lymphoma variant)
Aggressive pituitary adenoma
Lymphoma
Myeloma
Meningioma
Juvenile nasopharyngeal angiofibroma
Chordoma

Rare

Leprosy
Rhinoscleroma
Syphilis
Sarcoidosis

(From Osborn AG: *Diagnostic neuroradiology,* St Louis, 1994, Mosby.)

       (2) Foramen rotundum.
       (3) Foramen ovale.
       (4) Foramen spinosum.
       (5) Foramen lacerum.
  2. Anatomic relations.
    a. Anteriorly: anterior skull base.
    b. Inferiorly: spheniod sinus.
    c. Superiorly: pituitary gland, suprasellar structures (see Chapter 58).
    d. Posteriorly: basilar artery, anterior brainstem, posterior skull base.
 B. Congenital/developmental.
  1. Cavernous sinus lipoma.
  2. Cavernous sinus epidermoid.

Cavernous Sinus Masses
Differential Diagnosis

Unilateral

Common
Schwannoma
Meningioma
Metastasis
Aneurysm (cavernous internal carotid artery)
Carotid-cavernous fistula
Uncommon
Chordoma
Lymphoma
Rare
Lipoma
Epidermoid
Cavernous hemangioma
Osteocartilagenous tumors
Plexiform neurofibroma (NF-1)

Bilateral

Common
Invasive pituitary adenoma
Meningioma
Metastases
Uncommon
Lymphoma
Cavernous sinus thrombosis

(From Osborn AG: *Diagnostic neuroradiology,* St Louis, 1994, Mosby.)

   C. Vascular.
      1. Aneurysm: cavernous ICA.
      2. Carotid-cavernous fistula.
      3. Cavernous sinus thrombosis.
   D. Neoplasms.
      1. Nasopharyngeal carcinoma.
         a. Squamous cell carcinoma > adenoid cystic carcinoma.
         b. Typically appears as a nasopharyngeal mass with adjacent bone destruction and possible direct invasion intracranially.
         c. Can also extend intracranially through osseus foramina along neurovascular structures.
         d. Often associated with serous otitis media due to obstruction of eustachian tube.

2. Pituitary adenoma: may extend into cavernous sinus or infero-posteriorly into sphenoid bone.
3. Meningioma: may involve sphenoid bone or cavernous sinus.
4. Nerve sheath tumors: can involve cavernous sinus or Meckel's cave.
   a. Plexiform neurofibromas: intracranial involvement rare but can occur from involvement of trigeminal nerve divisions (especially ophthalmic division) with central extension.
   b. Schwannoma involving central skull base is most likely to arise from trigeminal nerve.
      (1) Preganglionic or cisternal segment lesion appears as CPA cistern mass.
      (2) Ganglionic lesion may be confined to Meckel's cave or may be partly cisternal with "dumbbell" configuration due to constriction at entrance to Meckel's cave.
      (3) Peripheral nerve division lesion may have central extension.
5. Juvenile angiofibroma (JAF): highly vascular benign neoplasm that originates near sphenopalatine foramen and can spread along natural foramina/fissures into pterygopalatine fossa, orbit, middle cranial fossa, sphenoid sinus, and cavernous sinuses.
6. Chordoma: benign but locally invasive tumor of notochordal remnants that often arises in spheno-occipital region of clivus.
7. Osteocartilaginous tumors: skull base is derived from enchondral ossification and therefore can give rise to following tumors.
   a. Chondrosarcoma.
      (1) Rare, slow-growing locally invasive tumor.
      (2) Typically appears as soft-tissue mass that may or may not (50%) have matrix mineralization, and associated with focal bone destruction.
      (3) Typically low to intermediate signal on T1WI and hyperintense on T2WI.
      (4) Usually enhances strongly but heterogeneously.
   b. Osteosarcoma.
      (1) May arise de novo or in association with Paget disease or previous radiation therapy.
      (2) Typically appears as soft-tissue mass with tumor matrix mineralization and aggressive bone destruction.
   c. Enchondroma.
      (1) CT: expansile soft-tissue mass with scalloped endosteal bone resorption and curvilinear matrix mineralization.
      (2) MRI: isointense with muscle on T1WI and hyperintense on T2WI.

8. Lymphoma.
   a. In addition to many intracranial manifestations, may have marrow infiltration that results in focal or diffuse loss of normal fatty marrow T1 hyperintensity. Enhanced scans with fat suppression helpful to delineate tumor.
   b. May also involve cavernous sinuses: unilateral or bilateral soft-tissue masses.
9. Plasmacytoma, multiple myeloma.
   a. Multiple myeloma can produce diffuse skull base and calvarial vault destruction.
   b. Solitary plasmacytomas are uncommon but can occur in region of clivus/sphenoid sinus or calvarial vault.
10. Metastases.
    a. More common than primary bone neoplasms of the central skull base.
    b. Most common sources include prostate, lung, breast.
    c. Typically lytic destructive lesions.
    d. Prostate carcinoma has predilection for lateral orbital wall, may occasionally have sclerotic metastasis that can mimic meningioma.
E. Infection.
   1. Bacterial osteomyelitis: increased risk in immunocompromised population, potentially lethal.
   2. Complicated fungal sinusitis: aspergillosis, mucormycosis (see Chapter 47).
   3. Tuberculosis.
   4. Syphilis.
F. Inflammatory.
   1. Sarcoidosis.
   2. Wegener's granulomatosis.
   3. Cocaine granulomatosis.
   4. Midline ("lethal") granuloma: destructive lesions of midline face and upper aerodigestive tract (once thought to be within spectrum of Wegener's granulomatosis but now felt to be a T-cell lymphoma.)
G. Other.
   1. Fibrous dysplasia.
   2. Paget disease.
   3. Langerhans cell histiocytes.
III. Posterior skull base (see boxes on p. 639, 640).
   A. Anatomy.
      1. Bony components.

      a. Inferior clivus (below spheno-occipital synchondrosis).
      b. Petrous temporal bone.
      c. Pars lateralis and squamae of the occipital bones, including following important foramina:
        (1) Jugular foramen (box below).
        (2) Hypoglossal canal.
        (3) Foramen magnum (see Chapter 62).
   2. Anatomic relations.
      a. Anteriorly: central skull base.
      b. Inferiorly: foramen magnum.
      c. Posteriorly: basilar artery, anterior brainstem, CPA cisterns.
 B. Normal variants.
   1. Large jugular bulb.
   2. High jugular bulb.
 C. Congenital/developmental
   1. Primary cholesteatoma.
   2. Epidermoid cyst.
 D. Neoplasms (see box on p. 640).
   1. Paraganglioma.

Jugular Foramen Masses
Differential Diagnosis

Nonneoplastic masses

Common
Large jugular bulb (normal variant)
Jugular vein thrombosis
Uncommon
Osteomyelitis
Malignant external otitis

Neoplasms

Common
Paraganglioma
Metastasis
   Nasopharyngeal carcinoma
   Hematogenous
Uncommon
Schwannoma
Neurofibroma
Epidermoid tumor

(From Osborn AG: *Diagnostic neuroradiology,* St Louis, 1994, Mosby.)

Diffuse Skull Base Lesions

Nonneoplastic masses

Uncommon
Fibrous dysplasia
Paget's disease
Langerhans' cell histiocytosis

Neoplastic masses

Common
Metastases
Uncommon
Myeloma
Meningioma
Lymphoma
Rhabdomyosarcoma

(From Osborn AG: *Diagnostic neuroradiology,* St Louis, 1994, Mosby.)

---

      a. Glomus jugulare: typically soft-tissue mass that expands jugular foramen and erodes jugular spine.

      b. Glomus jugulotympanicum: involves both jugular foramen and typanic cavity with destruction of floor of middle ear.

  2. Nerve sheath tumors: may enlarge involved foramen but typically does not cause bone destruction, unlike paraganglioma.

      a. Schwannomas of CNs IX to XI may involve jugular foramen.

      b. Schwannoma of CN XII may involve hypoglossal foramen.

  3. Chordoma.

  4. Osteocartilaginous tumors (enchondroma, chondrosarcoma, osteosarcoma).

  5. Plasmacytoma, multiple myeloma.

  6. Metastases.

 E. Infectious/inflammatory (see Chapter 60).

  1. Cholesteatoma.

  2. Cholesterol granuloma.

  3. Osteomyelitis.

      a. Petrous apicitis.

      b. Malignant otitis externa.

 F. Other.

  1. Fibrous dysplasia.

  2. Paget disease.

  3. Langerhans cell histiocytosis.

SUGGESTED READINGS

Harnsberger HR: The skull base. In *Handbook of head and neck imaging,* ed 2, St Louis, 1995, Mosby, pp 399-425.

Madeline LA, Elster AD: Postnatal development of the central skull base: normal variants, *Radiol* 196:757-764, 1995.

Madeline LA, Elster AD: Suture closure in the human chondrocranium: CT assessment, *Radiol* 196:747-756, 1995.

Osborn AG: Brain tumors and tumorlike processes. In *Diagnostic neuroradiology,* St Louis, 1994, Mosby.

62

Foramen Magnum Lesions

Key Concepts

1. Foramen magnum lesions can be divided into intraaxial (cervicomedullary) masses, extramedullary intradural masses, and extradural (osseus or craniovertebral junction) masses (see box on p. 643).
2. 50% of brainstem gliomas (usually low-grade astrocytoma) occur at cervicomedullary junction.
3. Common cervicomedullary lesions include syringohydromyelia, demyelinating lesions, and glioma.
4. Common extramedullary intradural lesions include tonsillar herniation, ependymoma, subependymoma, and medulloblastoma.
5. Extradural lesions may arise from posterior skull base or from craniovertebral junction.

Foramen Magnum Masses

Cervicomedullary masses

Common
Syringohydromyelia
Demyelinating diseases
Glioma
Fourth ventricle tumor (e.g., medulloblastoma)
Uncommon
Hemangioblastoma
Metastasis

Anterior extramedullary intradural masses

Common
Vertebrobasilar dolichoectasia
Meningioma
Aneurysm (vertebral artery, posterior inferior cerebellar artery)
Uncommon
Schwannoma
Epidermoid tumor
Paraganglioma
Metastases
Arachnoid cyst
Dermoid cyst
Neurenteric cyst

Posterior extramedullary intradural masses

Common
Congenital/acquired tonsillar herniation
Ependymoma/subependymoma
Medulloblastoma
Uncommon
Arachnoid cyst
Dermoid/Epidermoid

Extradural masses

Craniovertebral junction
Trauma
Arthropathies
Congenital anomalies
Clivus and skull base
Metastases
Chordoma
Osteocartilagenous tumors

(Adapted from Osborn AG: *Diagnostic neuroradiology,* St Louis, 1994, Mosby.)

I. Anatomy (Fig. 62-1).
   A. The foramen magnum is a large aperture within the posterior skull base (see also Chapter 61) through which the brainstem continues into the upper cervical cord.
   B. Important structures transmitted.
      1. Cervicomedullary junction.
      2. Vertebral arteries.
      3. Spinal roots of hypoglossal nerve.
      4. Occasionally PICA loops inferiorly through foramen magnum.
   C. Anatomic relations.
      1. Anteriorly: inferior clivus.
      2. Superiorly: posterior fossa.
      3. Posteriorly: occipital squamae.
      4. Laterally: condylar portions (pars lateralis) of occipital bone.
      5. Inferiorly: cervical spine.
II. Cervicomedullary masses.
   A. Neoplasm.
      1. Astrocytoma. 50% of brainstem gliomas occur here (low-grade astrocytoma >> anaplastic astrocytoma).
      2. Hemangioblastoma.
      3. Metastases.
   B. Demyelinating lesions: e.g., multiple sclerosis.
   C. Syringomyelia and syringobulbia: e.g., with Chiari I, trauma, or neoplasm.
III. Anterior extramedullary intradural masses.
   A. Congenital/developmental.
      1. Epidermoid/dermoid cyst.
      2. Arachnoid cyst.
      3. Neurenteric cyst.
   B. Vascular.
      1. Vertebrobasilar dolichoectasia.
      2. Aneurysm: PICA, VA.
   C. Neoplasm.
      1. Meningioma.
      2. Schwannoma.
      3. Paraganglioma.
      4. Metastases.
      5. Extraosseous intradural chordoma: rare.
IV. Posterior extramedullary intradural.
   A. Congenital/developmental.
      1. Epidermoid/dermoid cyst.
      2. Arachnoid cyst.
      3. Occipitocervical cephalocele.

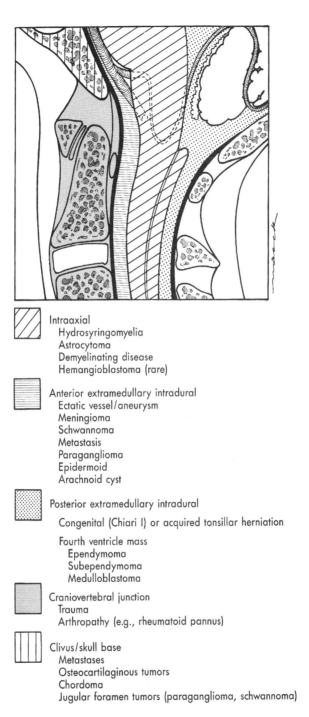

Fig. 62-1 Anatomic diagram depicts the foramen magnum and adjacent structures. Lesions and their locations are indicated. (From Osborn AG: *Diagnostic neuroradiology,* St Louis, 1994, Mosby.)

Intraaxial
Hydrosyringomyelia
Astrocytoma
Demyelinating disease
Hemangioblastoma (rare)

Anterior extramedullary intradural
Ectatic vessel/aneurysm
Meningioma
Schwannoma
Metastasis
Paraganglioma
Epidermoid
Arachnoid cyst

Posterior extramedullary intradural

Congenital (Chiari I) or acquired tonsillar herniation

Fourth ventricle mass
Ependymoma
Subependymoma
Medulloblastoma

Craniovertebral junction
Trauma
Arthropathy (e.g., rheumatoid pannus)

Clivus/skull base
Metastases
Osteocartilaginous tumors
Chordoma
Jugular foramen tumors (paraganglioma, schwannoma)

   B. Neoplasms: usually arising within fourth ventricle and extending into posterior perimedullary cistern, cisterna magna.
      1. Ependymoma.
      2. Subependymoma.
      3. Medulloblastoma.
   C. Tonsillar herniation: accounts for 5% to 10% of all foramen magnum masses.
      1. Congenital: Chiari I malformation.
      2. Acquired tonsillar herniation: due to increased intracranial pressure, intracranial mass lesion, or iatrogenic (lumboperitoneal shunting or lumbar puncture).
V. Extradural lesions: involving posterior skull base (see also Chapter 61) or craniovertebral junction.
   A. Congenital/developmental.
      1. Down syndrome: can be associated with atlanto-occipital or atlanto-axial subluxation.
      2. Mucopolysaccharidoses: can cause dural thickening and resulting spinal stenosis at craniovertebral junction.
      3. Congenital anomaly: spectrum of fusion, nonfusion, or rotational anomalies involving occiput/atlas/axis relationship can be associated with spinal stenosis.
   B. Neoplasm.
      1. Chordoma.
      2. Osteocartilaginous tumors.
      3. Metastases.
      4. Plasmacytoma, multiple myeloma.
   C. Trauma.
      1. Odontoid fractures.
      2. Epidural hematoma.
   D. Arthropathy.
      1. Rheumatoid arthritis: may result in atlanto-occipital or atlanto-axial subluxation, basilar invagination, or pannus.
      2. Osteoarthritis, calcium pyrophoshate deposition disease: uncommonly involves craniovertebral junction.
      3. Synovial cyst of atlanto-occipital joint.
   E. Infection: osteomyelitis with possible epidural abscess.
   F. Paget disease: can cause basilar invagination.

SUGGESTED READINGS

Harnsberger HR: The skull base. In *Handbook of head and neck imaging,* ed 2, St Louis, 1995, Mosby, pp 399-425.
Osborn AG: Brain tumors and tumorlike processes. In *Diagnostic neuroradiology,* St Louis, 1994, Mosby, pp 399-528.

Appendix:
Differential Diagnosis of Imaging Patterns

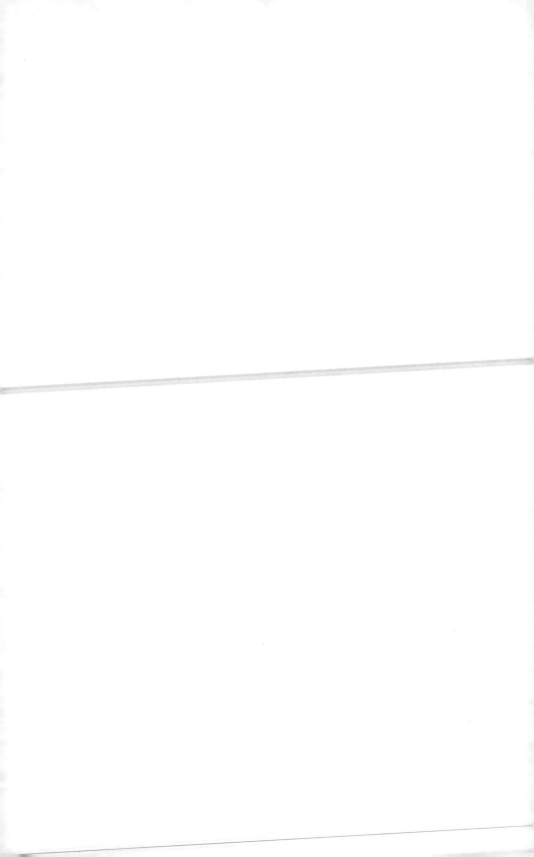

A: Morphologic Patterns

Diffuse Cerebral Atrophy

Congenital/developmental
    Congenital (TORCH) infections
    Brain malformations (e.g., lissencephaly)
    Inherited metabolic disorders, leukodystrophies
Neurodegenerative diseases
    HIV encephalopathy
    Alzheimer's disease
    Pick's disease
    Huntington's disease
    Multi-infarct dementia
    Jakob-Creutzfeldt disease
Acquired insult
    Global ischemia/hypoxia
    Post-traumatic
    Postinflammatory
    Alcohol and drug abuse
Iatrogenic
    Dilantin
    Steroids
    Radiation therapy
    Chemotherapy
Deprivational states
    Dehydration
    Malnutrition, anorexia nervosa
Age-related atrophy

Selective Cerebral Atrophy

Huntington's disease (caudate, putamen)
Pick's disease (frontotemporal)
Alzheimer's disease (cortical, mesial temporal)
Progressive supranuclear palsy (midbrain)
Shy-Drager syndrome (cerebellar hemispheres, vermis, and brainstem)
Olivopontocerebellar atrophy (inferior olives, pons, cerebellum)

Cerebellar Atrophy

Toxins
    Alcohol abuse
    Chronic toluene exposure

Iatrogenic
  Dilantin
  High-dose cytosine arabinoside
  Local radiotherapy
Neurodegenerative diseases
  Olivopontocerebellar atrophy
  Shy-Drager syndrome
Other
  Paraneoplastic cerebellar degeneration

Ventricular Enlargement (see Chapter 57)

Physiologic
Atrophic (see above)
Obstructive
  Noncommunicating or intraventricular hydrocephalus
  Communicating or extraventricular hydrocephalus
CSF overproduction

Decreased Ventricular Size (see Chapter 57)

Diffuse cerebral edema
Pseudotumor cerebri
Ventricular shunting

Ventricular Asymmetry

Normal variant
Unilateral obstruction of foramen of Monro (e.g., central neurocytoma, subependy-
  mal giant-cell astrocytoma)
Hemiatrophy (Sturge-Weber, Silver-Russell, Dyke-Davidoff-Mason)
Hemimegalencephaly

Nodularity of Ventricular Margins

Heterotopic gray matter
Tuberous sclerosis (subependymal hamartomatous nodules)
Subependymoma
Ependymal spread of tumor

Solid Lesions

Congenital/developmental
  Hamartoma
  Lipoma
Neoplasm
  Lymphoma
  Meningioma
  Schwannoma
  Germinoma
  Medulloblastoma

Choroid plexus papilloma
Diffuse fibrillary astrocytoma

Cystic Lesions

Congenital/developmental
    Dandy-Walker cyst
    Mega cisterna magna
    Porencephalic cyst
    Arachnoid cyst
    Epidermoid/dermoid
    Colloid cyst
    Pars intermedia cyst, Rathke cleft cyst
    Neurenteric cyst
Neuroepithelial or degenerative cysts
    Ependymal cyst
    Parenchymal cyst
    Choroid fissure cyst
    Choroid plexus cyst
    Pineal cyst
Infection
    Abscess
    Cysticercosis (vesicular stage or racemose form)
    Hydatid cyst
Perivascular or Virchow-Robin space

Partly Solid, Partly Cystic Lesions

Neoplasm with cystic components
    Pilocytic astrocytoma
    Hemangioblastoma
    Pleomorphic xanthoastrocytoma
    Ganglioglioma
    Craniopharyngioma
    Ependymoma
    PNET/medulloblastoma
    Pineocytoma
    Teratoma
    Metastasis (uncommon)
    Astrocytoma (rare)
    Pituitary adenoma (rare)
    Meningioma (rare)
    Schwannoma (rare)

B: Lesions by Location
(see also Chapters 55-62)

Cortical Lesions

Trauma
    Contusion
Vascular
    AVM
    Sturge-Weber (pial angioma, cortical atrophy/calcification)
Neoplasm
    Pleomorphic xanthoastrocytoma (mural nodule)
    Hemangioblastoma (mural nodule)
    Protoplasmic astrocytoma
    Dysembryoplastic neuroepithelial tumor (DNET)
Neurodegenerative
    Alzheimer's (cortical atrophy)

Corticomedullary Junction Lesions

Infection
    Septic emboli
    Cerebritis, abscess
    Toxoplasmosis (noncongenital)
Demyelinating
    PML
    ADEM
Vascular
    Bland embolic infarct
Neoplasm
    Oligodendroglioma
    Metastases
Trauma
    Shearing injury

Periventricular or Callosal Lesions

Congenital
    Lipoma
    Porencephaly
Neoplasm
    Ependymoma
    GBM

Lymphoma
Demyelinating disease
    Multiple sclerosis
    Marchiafava-Bignami disease
Trauma
    Shearing injury

Midline Lesions

Normal variant
    Cavum septi pellucidi
    Cavum vergae
    Cavum velum interpositum
    Mega cisterna magna
Congenital/developmental
    Cephalocele
    Dermoid
    Lipoma
    Rathke cleft cyst
    Hypothalamic hamartoma
    Colloid cyst
    Neurenteric cyst
Vascular
    Vein of Galen malformation
Neoplasm
    Pituitary adenoma
    Craniopharyngioma
    Hypothalamic-chiasmatic glioma
    Teratoma (suprasellar, pineal)
    Germinoma (suprasellar, pineal)
    Pineocytoma, pineoblastoma
    Medulloblastoma
Miscellaneous
    "Empty sella"
    Pineal cyst

Basal Ganglia Lesions

Physiologic
    Perivascular space
Vascular
    Lacunar infarct
    Hypertensive hemorrhage
Neoplasm
    Lymphoma
    Germinoma
Neurodegenerative
    Huntington's disease

Parkinson's disease
Toxin
Carbon monoxide intoxication
Methanol intoxication
Cyanide intoxication
Metabolic
Mitochondrial disorders
Methylmalonic or propionic acidemia
Wilson disease
Hallovorden-Spatz disease
Hypoxia

Posterior Fossa Lesions in Adults

Congenital/developmental
Dermoid/epidermoid
Arachnoid cyst
Mega cisterna magna
Neurenteric cyst
Chiari I malformation
Dysplastic gangliocytoma of cerebellum (Lhermitte-Duclos disease)
Vascular
Infarct
Vertebrobasilar dolichoectasia
Aneurysm
Cavernoma
Demyelinating disease
Multiple sclerosis
Central pontine myelinolysis
Neoplasm
Metastasis
Hemangioblastoma
Acoustic neuroma
Meningioma
Subependymoma
Choroid plexus papilloma
Brainstem glioma
Chordoma
Paraganglioma
Cerebellar astrocytoma (rare)
Medulloblastoma (rare)
Infectious/inflammatory
Abscess
Neurocysticercosis
Neurosarcoidosis
Miscellaneous
Syringobulbia

Posterior Fossa Lesions in Children

Congenital/developmental
> Occipital or occipitocervical cephalocele
> Chiari malformations
> Dandy-Walker malformation, other vermian-cerebellar hypoplasia syndromes
> Mega cisterna magna
> Dermoid/epidermoid
> Arachnoid cyst
> Lipoma

Neoplasm
> Medulloblastoma
> Cerebellar pilocytic astrocytoma
> Brainstem glioma
> Ependymoma

Infection/inflammatory
> Abscess
> Neurocysticercosis
> Langerhans cell histiocytosis

Miscellaneous
> Aqueductal stenosis
> Trapped fourth ventricle

C: Calcifications

Normal Intracranial Calcifications

Dura and arachnoid
    Falx
    Tentorium
    Petroclinoid, interclinoid ligaments
    Arachnoid granulations
Pineal gland (usually >10 years of age, <10 mm diameter)
Habenular region (actually tela choroidea of third ventricle)
Choroid (usually in glomus of lateral ventricular trigone, usually >10 years of age)
Basal ganglia (usually globus pallidus, bilateral > unilateral)
Dentate nuclei (usually with basal ganglia calcification)
Vascular (usually ICA, vertebrobasilar)

Abnormal Intracranial Calcifications by Pathologic Process

Congenital/developmental
    Tuberous sclerosis (>2 years of age, subependymal > parenchymal)
    Sturge-Weber (>2 years of age, gyriform, cortical)
    Basal cell nevus (falx, tentorial)
    Neurofibromatosis (choroid plexus, cerebellar hemispheres)
    Lipoma
    Dermoid
Infection/inflammatory
    TORCH infections (toxoplasmosis, CMV, herpes simplex, rubella)
    Tuberculosis (suprasellar, cisternal, parenchymal)
    Fungal (coccidiodomycosis, histoplasmosis)
    Parasitic (cysticercosis, echinococcus)
    Syphilitic gumma
Endocrine/metabolic/toxins
    Hypercalcemia
        Hyperparathyroidism (vascular, dural > parenchymal)
        Hypervitaminosis D (dural, pineal)
        Hypercalcemia of malignancy
        Idiopathic hypercalcemia of infancy (Williams syndrome)
    Hypoparathyroidism, pseudohypoparathyroidism,
        Pseudopseudohypoparathyroidism (basal ganglia, dentate nuclei)
    Lead encephalopathy
    Carbon monoxide intoxication

Vascular
   Aneurysm (5%)
   Vascular malformations (25%)
   Atherosclerosis
   Infarct (rare)
Trauma
   Chronic subdural hematoma
   Parenchymal hematoma
Neoplasm
   Craniopharyngioma (90%)
   Oligodendroglioma (90%)
   Central neurocytoma (50% to 70%)
   Supratentorial PNET (60%)
   Ependymoma (50%)
   Teratoma (common)
   Pineocytoma, pineoblastoma (common)
   Chordoma (20% to 70%)
   Osteocartilagenous tumors (chondrosarcoma, osteosarcoma)
   Metastases (osteosarcoma, mucinous adenocarcinoma of colon, carcinoid)
   Ganglioglioma (30%)
   Choroid plexus papilloma (25%)
   Meningioma (20% to 25%)
   Medulloblastoma (15% to 50%)
   Astrocytoma (15% to 25%)
Iatrogenic
   Radiation therapy (mineralizing microangiopathy)
   Chemotherapy: especially methotrexate (mineralizing microangiopathy)
   Pantopaque

Basal Ganglia Calcification

Physiologic
Congenital
   Tuberous sclerosis
   Neurofibromatosis
   Cockayne syndrome
   Down syndrome
Endocrine/metabolic/toxins
   Hyperparathyroidism
   Hypoparathyroidism, pseudohypoparathyroidism, pseudopseudohypopara-
      thyroidism
   Hypothyroidism
   Lead encephalopathy
   Carbon monoxide intoxication
   Mitochondrial disorders
   Fahr disease
   Hallovorden-Spatz disease

Infection
  Congenital (TORCH) infections
  Neurocysticercosis
Hypoxia
  Birth anoxia
  Cardiorespiratory collapse
Iatrogenic
  Radiation therapy
  Chemotherapy (especially methotrexate)
Idiopathic

Parasellar Calcification

Neoplasm
  Meningioma
  Craniopharyngioma
  Chordoma
  Osteocartilagenous tumors
  Hypothalamic-chiasmatic glioma
  Pituitary macroadenoma (rarely)
Vascular
  Aneurysm
  Atherosclerosis
Infection
  Tuberculosis (meningitis, granulomas)
  Neurocysticercosis

Multiple Small Nodular Calcifications

Congenital
  Tuberous sclerosis
Infectious/inflammatory
  Congenital (TORCH) infections
  TB/fungal granulomas
  Neurocysticercosis
Metabolic
  Hyperparathyroidism
Neoplastic
  Calcified metastasis (e.g., osteosarcoma)
Iatrogenic
  Pantopaque

Curvilinear or Ringlike Calcification

Congenital/developmental lipoma
Vascular
  Aneurysm
  Atherosclerosis
  AVM
  Hematoma

Neoplasm
    Cystic astrocytoma
    Cystic craniopharyngioma
    Teratoma
    Pineal germinoma (rarely)
Parasitic
    Hydatid cyst

D: Enhancement Patterns

Normally Enhancing Tissue

Vessels, dural sinuses (including cavernous sinuses)
Dura (falx, tentorium)
Choroid
Pituitary gland, infundibulum
Pineal gland
Area postrema (chemoreceptor zone, floor of fourth ventricle)
Nasal mucosa

Abnormal Meningeal Enhancement (see Chapter 56)

Infection
    Bacterial meningitis
    Tuberculous meningitis
    Fungal meningitis (especially cryptococcus, coccidiodomycosis)
    Syphilitic meningitis
    Viral meningitis (rarely)
Inflammation
    Neurosarcoidosis
    Langerhans cell histiocytosis
    Wegener's granulomatosis
    Rheumatoid pachymeningitis
Neoplastic
    Meningioma
    Medulloblastoma
    Ependymoma
    Germinoma
    Pineoblastoma
    Choroid plexus tumors
    High-grade astrocytoma/GBM
    Lymphoma/leukemia
    Leptomeningeal metastasis (especially breast, lung, gastric carcinoma)
Trauma
    Chronic SDH
    Subarachnoid hemorrhage (subacute SAH, superficial pial siderosis)
    Adjacent to resolving parenchymal hematoma
Metabolic
    Mucopolysaccharidoses
    Lead encephalopathy

Vascular
>   Adjacent to subacute infarction

Iatrogenic
>   Postcraniotomy
>   Postventricular shunt placement
>   Intrathecal medications or contrast
>   Systemic medications (e.g., antibiotics, NSAIDs, chemotherapeutic agents)

Miscellaneous
>   Benign intracranial hypotension
>   Idiopathic hypertrophic pachymeningitis

Gyriform Cortical Enhancement

Cerebral ischemia/infarct
Herpes encephalitis
Sturge-Weber disease
Subarachnoid hemorrhage
Leptomeningeal or subpial tumor spread
Seizure focus (during or immediately after)

Ependymal Enhancement

Infection/inflammation
>   Infectious ventriculitis/ependymitis (e.g., bacterial, CMV)
>   Iatrogenic (shunt placement, intrathecal chemotherapy)
>   Neurosarcoidosis

Neoplasm
>   High-grade astrocytoma, GBM
>   Germinoma
>   Pineoblastoma
>   PNET/medulloblastoma
>   Ependymoma
>   Choroid plexus tumor
>   Lymphoma/leukemia
>   Metastatic tumor (especially lung, breast, melanoma)

Vascular
>   Collateral venous drainage (Sturge-Weber, dural sinus occlusion, vascular malformation)

Solidly Enhancing Lesions

Vascular
>   Aneurysm

Neoplasm
>   Meningioma
>   Schwannoma
>   Germinoma
>   Choroid plexus papilloma
>   Lymphoma

Medulloblastoma
Metastasis (e.g., small lesions)
Infection/inflammatory
Fungal granuloma
Sarcoid granuloma

Ring-Enhancing Lesions

Neoplasm
High-grade astrocytoma, GBM
Primary lymphoma in AIDS
Cystic meningioma
Cystic schwannoma
Metastasis (e.g., large lesions)
Infection
Abscess (bacterial, tuberculous, toxoplasma, fungal)
Fungal granuloma
Demyelinating lesion
Multiple sclerosis (active lesion)
Vascular
Subacute infarct
Thrombosed aneurysm
Thrombosed vascular malformation
Resolving hematoma
Radiation necrosis

Cyst with Enhancing Mural Nodule

Pilocytic astrocytoma
Pleomorphic xanthoastrocytoma
Hemangioblastoma
Ganglioglioma

Multiple Enhancing Lesions

Neoplasm
Metastases
Multiple meningiomas
Lymphoma
Multifocal or multicentric GBM
Infection/inflammation
Septic emboli, multiple abscesses
Tuberculosis
Fungal granulomas (coccidiomycosis, aspergillosis, histoplasmosis)
Cysticercosis
Toxoplasmosis (noncongenital)
Sarcoidosis
Demyelinating disease
Multiple sclerosis (active lesions)
Subacute multiple infarctions

Enhancing "Dural Tail"

Neoplasm
    Meningioma
    Astrocytoma/GBM
    Oligodendroglioma
    Acoustic neuroma
    Lymphoma/leukemia
    Dural metastases (e.g., lung)
Inflammatory
    Neurosarcoidosis
    Langerhans cell histiocytosis
Infectious
    Cerebral aspergillosis

Enhancing Cranial Nerve

Viral neuritis (e.g., Bell's palsy)
Schwannoma
Perineural tumor spread (e.g., nasopharyngeal SCC)
Neurosarcoidosis

E: Miscellaneous CT Patterns

Hyperdense (Noncalcified) Focal Mass

Congenital/developmental
    Tuberous sclerosis (tubers or hamartomas)
    Colloid cyst
Neoplasm
    Meningioma
    Lymphoma
    Medulloblastoma
    Choroid plexus papilloma
Vascular
    Aneurysm
    Vascular malformation (AVM, cavernoma)
Acute or subacute hemorrhagic lesion (see below)

Parenchymal Hematoma

Trauma
    Contusion
    Hemorrhagic shearing injury
Coagulopathy
    Blood dyscrasia
    Anticoagulants
Hypertension
    Hypertensive vascular disease (basal ganglia > thalamus, pons, cerebellum, hemispheric white matter)
    Preeclampsia/eclampsia
    Renal failure
    Hemolytic-uremic syndrome
    Systemic lupus erythematosus
Vascular
    Aneurysm
    Vascular malformation (AVM, cavernoma)
    Amyloid angiopathy (corticomedullary junction)
    Vasculitis
Vascular occlusion
    Venous infarct (subcortical white matter)
    Embolic stroke with reperfusion hemorrhage (basal ganglia, cortex; at 3 to 14 days)
Infection
    Herpes encephalitis

Fungal cerebritis
Abscess (rarely)
Neoplasm
Hemorrhagic metastasis (melanoma, choriocarcinoma, renal cell carcinoma)
High-grade astrocytoma, GBM
Pituitary adenoma
Meningioma (rarely)
Schwannoma (rarely)
Miscellaneous
Neonatal hemorrhage (grade IV) of prematurity
Amphetamine abuse

Hyperdense Basilar Cisterns

Subarachnoid hemorrhage
Iodinated intrathecal contrast
Meningitis (tuberculous, fungal)
Sarcoidosis
Diffuse cerebral edema

Hyperdensity (Noncalcified) in Basal Ganglia

Hypertensive hemorrhage
Lymphoma
Krabbé's disease

Hypodensity in Basal Ganglia

Hypoxia
Toxins
Carbon monoxide intoxication (globus pallidus)
Methanol intoxication (putamen)
Cyanide intoxication
Metabolic
Mitochondrial disorders (e.g., Leigh's disease)
Methylmalonic or propionic acidemia (globus pallidus)
Wilson disease
Hallervorden-Spatz disease
Lacunar infarct
Perivascular space

Fat-Density Lesions

Lipoma
Dermoid
Teratoma
Surgical fat-packing

Pneumocephalus

Trauma
Iatrogenic (surgery, pneumoencephalography, ventriculography, myelography)
Neoplasm invading paranasal sinus
    Sinonasal carcinoma with intracranial invasion
    Osteoma of frontal or ethmoid sinus
    Pituitary adenoma
Infection with gas-forming organism (mastoiditis, sinusitis)
Air embolism

F: Miscellaneous MRI Patterns

Substances Bright on T1WI

Fat
    Lipoma
    Dermoid
    Teratoma
Subacute hemorrhage (methemoglobin)
    see Appendix E
Moderately proteinaceous fluid
    Colloid cyst
    Mucocele
Melanin
    Melanoma
Paramagnetic MR contrast agents
    Gadolinium
Mineralization or microcalcification
    Basal ganglia
Flow-related enhancement
    Normal vascular structures
Pantopaque

Substances Dark on T2WI

Air
    Postoperative
    Trauma
Minerals/metals
    Iatrogenic: surgical hardware
    Physiologic iron (basal ganglia, red nucleus, substantia nigra, dentate nucleus)
    Aspergillus or mucor mycetoma (manganese, iron or dense hyphae)
Dense calcification
    Neoplasm (e.g., meningioma, oligodendroglioma, osteosarcoma metastasis)
    Vascular (e.g., aneurysm, AVM, cavernoma)
    Infection (e.g., cysticercosis, TB/fungal granuloma)
Hemorrhage
    Acute and early subacute hemorrhage (deoxyhemoglobin, intracellular methemoglobin)
    Hemosiderin
Mucinous or dense proteinaceous material
    Colloid cyst

Mucocele
Mucinous adenocarcinoma of colon metastasis
Rapid vascular flow
Vascular (e.g., aneurysm, AVM)
Neoplasm (e.g., paraganglioma, hemangiopericytoma, angiomatous meningioma)

White Matter T2 Hyperintense Lesions

Physiologic
Perivascular spaces
White matter changes of aging
Congenital/developmental
Neurofibromatosis
Tuberous sclerosis
Metabolic/toxin
Amphetamine abuse
Phenylketonuria
Mucopolysaccharidoses
Dysmyelinating diseases or leukodystrophies
Adrenoleukodystrophy
Metachromatic leukodystrophy
Pelizaeus-Merzbacher disease
Canavan disease
Alexander disease
Demyelinating diseases
Multiple sclerosis
PML
ADEM
Marchiafava-Bignami
Infection
Viral encephalitis
PML
ADEM
SSPE
Cerebritis
Cryptococcoma
Vascular
Ischemia/infarct
Vasculitis (e.g., SLE, Behcet's)
Migraine-related
Iatrogenic
Chemotherapy: especially methotrexate (necrotizing leukoencephalopathy)
Radiation-induced (necrotizing leukoencephalopathy)
Miscellaneous
Parenchymal cyst

Brainstem T2 Hyperintense Lesions

Neoplasm
    Brainstem glioma
    Lymphoma
    Metastasis
    Perineural tumor spread (e.g., nasopharyngeal SCC)
Demyelinating disease
    Multiple sclerosis
    Central pontine myelinolysis
    ADEM
Vascular
    Cavernoma
    Hemorrhage
    Infarct
Trauma
    Shearing injury
Infection
    Abscess
    Encephalitis
Miscellaneous
    Syringobulbia
    Wallerian degeneration

Index

Page numbers followed by *f* indicate figures; those followed by *t* indicate tables.

A

Abducens nerve, 102*f*, 103*f*, 110
  apertures of skull base, 10*f*, 12*t*
  cavernous sinus, 78*f*
Abscess, 436–438, 651, 665
  increased intracranial pressure, 576
  corticomedullary junction, 652
  in differential diagnosis
    of glioblastoma multiforme, 237
    of lymphoma, 304
  enhancement patterns, 662
  epidural, 430–432
  foramen magnum region, 646
  fungal, 436, 460
  with HIV/AIDS, 458, 459, 460, 469, 470
  meningitis and, 427, 429
  MRI pattern, 669
  pyogenic, 436–439
  pituitary, 612
  posterior fossa, 654, 655
  ring-enhancing lesions, 439
  subarachnoid space enlargement, 588
  tuberculous, 460, 469, 470, 474, 475, 476
  white matter lesion differential diagnosis,
    546
Absent greater sphenoid wing, 583
Absent septum pellucidum, 595
Accessory falcine sinus, 73
Accessory (XI) nerve, 116–117
Achondrogenesis, 575
Achondroplasia, 575, 576
Acoustic artery, 42*f*
Acoustic (VIII) nerve, 102*f*, 103*f*, 113–114
Acoustic neuroma, or schwannoma, 314*t*, 315
  epidermoid tumor vs., 327
  enhancement pattern, 663
  posterior fossa, 654
  cerebellopontine angle, 623*t*, 624*t*, 625
  internal auditory canal, 625
  neurofibromatosis, type II, 168

Acquired Chiari I malformation, 128
Acromegaly, 575, 577, 578
Actinomycete infections, 430, 487–489
Acute cerebral ischemia and infarction,
  375–378
Acute disseminated encephalomyelitis
  (ADEM), 443, 450–451, 512
  and basal ganglia degeneration, 569
  corticomedullary junction, 652
  MRI patterns, 668, 669
Acute intracranial hemorrhage, 184–186, 184*f*,
  185*t*
Acute lymphocytic (aseptic) meningitis, 429
Addison disease, 522
Adenohypophysis
  inflammation, 611–612
  normal anatomy, 605, 606*f*
  pituitary adenomas, 245, 281–282, 610, 611
  radiology, 607
Adrenoleukodystrophy (ALD), 511, 512, 513,
  514, 515, 519, 521–523, 668
Adrenomyeloneuropathy (AMN), 522
Age-related changes, 512
  calvarial/skull abnormalities, 581, 582
  morphologic patterns, 649
  MRI patterns, T2 hyperintense lesions,
    668
  vascular, 411–412
Aging, normal, 538–543
  Alzheimer disease vs., 562
  grey matter, 542–543
  iron, 543
  sulci and cisterns, 538–539, 539*f*
  ventricles, 539–540, 539*f*, 596
  white matter, 540–542, 546–547
Agyria, 147
Aicardi syndrome, 136
AIDS; *see* HIV/AIDS
AIDS dementia complex, 457, 460
Air, MRI patterns, 667

671

Air embolism, 666
Alcohol abuse, 403
  calvarial/skull abnormalities, 575
  cerebellar atrophy, 649
  cerebral atrophy, 649
  subarachnoid space enlargement, 588
  ventricular pathology, 596
Alcohol toxicity
  and central pontine myelinolysis, 553
  encephalopathies, 552–553
Alexander disease, 519, 524, 525–526
  calvarial/skull abnormalities, 575
  inherited metabolic disorders, 514, 515
  MRI patterns, 668
Alpha fetoprotein, 276
Altlanto-axial subluxation, 646
Alzheimer disease, 512, 561–564
  cerebral atrophy, 649
  cortical atrophy, 652
  early-onset, 514, 515
  imaging, 562–563
  location, 562
  pathology, 561–562
  prevalence, inheritance, risk factors, 562
  subarachnoid space enlargement, 588
  ventricular pathology, 596
Ambient cistern, 23f, 25t
Aminoacidemias, 514, 515, 535
Amphetamine abuse, 665, 668
Amygdala, 91
  with Alzheimer disease, 562
Amyloid
  glioblastoma multiforme vs., 238
  and intracranial hemorrhage, 218
Amyloid angiopathy, 548, 664
Amyotrophic lateral sclerosis
  imaging, 556–557
  normal delayed myelination vs., 507t, 508
Anaplastic astrocytoma, 234–235
  arteriovenous malformation vs., 360
  ependymal enhancement, 602
  foramen magnum region, 644
  skull base lesions, 634
  ventricular mass lesions in adults, 598
Anastomoses
  carotid-vertebrobasilar, 41, 42f, 43, 44, 61
  extracranial to intracranial, 35
Anatomy
  of scalp, meninges, epi- and subdural space,
    587f
  skull base lesions
    anterior, 631–632
    central, 634–635
    posterior, 638–639
Anatomy, brain, 83–99
  mesencephalon, 93–94
  myelination, normal, 498–508

Anatomy, brain—cont'd
  prosencephalon, 84–93, 84f, 86–87f, 88f
    cerebrum, 84–91, 84f, 86–87f, 88f
    diencephalon, 91–93
  rhombencephalon, 93–99
    cerebellum, 95–98, 97f, 98f
    medulla, 98–99
    pons, 94–95
Anemia
  calvarial/skull abnormalities, 576, 578
  extramedullary hematopoiesis, 589
Aneurysm, 340–352, 664, 667, 668
  with arteriovenous malformations, 357
  calcification with, 657, 658
  cerebellopontine angle, 623, 623t, 624t
  circle of Willis, 41
  CT patterns, 664
  differential diagnosis
    meningiomas vs., 295
    schwannoma vs., 316
  dissecting, 351–352, 398
  enhancement patterns, 661
  extraaxial abnormalities, 599
  foramen magnum region, 643, 644, 645f
  fusiform, 351
  posterior cerebral artery, 619
  posterior fossa, 654
  ring-enhancing lesions, 439
  rupture of, 216
  saccular, 340–351
    age, 343
    angiography, 346, 348–349
    CT, 349–350
    etiology and pathogenesis, 340–342, 341f
    growth and flow dynamics, 345, 346f
    imaging, 346, 348–351
    incidence, 342–343
    location, 343, 344f
    MR, 350
    MR angiography, 350–351
    rupture of, 345, 346, 347–348f
  sellar/juxtasellar region
    cavernous sinus and skull base, 614
    intrasellar, 610
    sellar region, 610
    suprasellar, 609t, 612
  skull base lesions, 636
  traumatic, 210–211
  vein of Galen, 269, 359t, 365–366
  ventricular mass lesions in adults, 598
Angiography, 208f
Angiography; see also Computed tomography
    (CT) angiography
  aneurysms, 346, 348–349
  arterial occlusion, 400
  arteriovenous malformations, 357,
    358–359t, 362

Angiography—cont'd
  in atherosclerosis, 391
  cavernous angioma, 370
  cortical vein occlusion, 410
  deep cerebral vein thrombosis, 411
  dermoid tumors, 325
  dural sinus thrombosis, 408
  fungal infections, 484
  meningitis, 475
  sarcoid, 477
  in stroke, 376
  vein of Galen malformation, 366
Angioma; *see also* Venous angioma
  cortical, 652
  and intracranial hemorrhage, 216–217
  scalp, 574
Angiomatous meningioma, 290, 668
Angiosarcoma, meningeal, 298
Anorexia nervosa, 649
Anoxia; *see* Hypoxia/ischemia
Anterior cerebral artery, 50*f*, 52–54, 52*f*, 53*f*
  collateral circulation, 393
  idiopathic progressive arteriopathy of child-
    hood, 397
  stenosis, congenital causes, 396
  stroke, 379, 380–381*f*, 382
Anterior choroidal artery
  anatomy, 46
  stroke, 380–381*f*, 382
Anterior clinoid process, 76*f*
Anterior commissure, 91
Anterior communicating artery
  anatomy and variants, 50*f*, 52–53, 52*f*
  aneurysms, 343, 344*f*, 349
Anterior inferior cerebellar artery, 380–381*f*,
    384
  cerebellopontine angle abnormalities, 623
  internal auditory canal, 625
Anterior intercavernous sinus, 75*f*
Anterior pituitary; *see* Adenohypophysis
Anterior pontomesencephalic vein, 80, 81*f*
Anterior spinal artery, 66*f*
Antibiotics, abnormal meningeal enhancement,
    661
Anticoagulants, 218, 664
Antiphospholipid antibody syndrome (APLA),
    403
Aortic arch, 30, 31*f*
Apert disease, 576
Aqueduct, toxoplasmosis, 419
Aqueductal stenosis
  calvarial/skull abnormalities, 575, 576
  posterior fossa, 655
  ventricular pathology, 596
Aqueduct of Sylvius, 22
Arachnoid, 18, 587*f*
  anatomy, 16*f*, 17*t*, 18

Arachnoid—cont'd
  CSF circulation, 26*f*
Arachnoid calcification, 656
Arachnoid cyst, 651
  calvarial/skull abnormalities, 581, 582, 583
  cavernous angiomas with, 370
  cerebellopontine angle, 623*t*, 623
  congenital, 327–328
  in differential diagnosis
    of dermoid cyst, 323*t*, 325–327
  in differential diagnosis—cont'd
    of epidermoid tumor, 327
    of meningiomas, 295
    of neuroepithelial cysts, 330
    of pineal cyst, 332
    of pineocytoma, 268
    of Rathke's cleft cyst, 287
    of schwannomas, 317
  extraaxial fluid collections, 586
  foramen magnum region, 643, 644, 645*f*
  pineal, 616*f*, 617
  posterior fossa, 155*t*, 158–159, 654, 655
  quadrigeminal cistern and velum interposi-
    tum, 619
  sellar/juxtasellar region
    cavernous sinus and skull base, 614
    intrasellar, 610
    suprasellar, 612
Arachnoid granulations, 656
Arachnoiditis, internal auditory canal, 626
Arbovirus, 429, 443
Area postrema, enhancement patterns,
    660
Argyll-Robertson pupils, 468
Arrhinencephaly, 144
Arterial dissections, 207–209, 208*f*
Arterial stenosis and occlusion
  atherosclerotic, 387–393, 392*f*
  nonatheromatous, 396–403
    cell-mediated disorders, 401–402
    congenital causes, 396–397
    dissection, 398–399
    infections, 401
    ischemic stroke, 402–403
    vasculitis, 400–402
    vasculopathies, 399–400
    vasospasm, 399
Arteries; *see also specific vessels*
  age-related changes, 540
  apertures of skull base, 9, 10*f*, 11*f*, 12*t*
  cerebral; *see* Cerebral arteries
  internal carotid, 40–46, 40*f*, 42*f*
  normal white matter components, 512
  posterior fossa, 66–70, 66*f*, 67*f*
  scalp, 16*f*, 587*f*
  sellar/juxtasellar region, 606*f*, 607
  subarachnoid cisterns, 24–25*t*

Arteries—cont'd
  traumatic injury, 207
  vertebrobasilar circulation, 66–70, 66*f*, 67*f*
  white matter degenerative diseases, 547
Arteriosclerosis; *see* Atherosclerosis
Arteriovenous fistulae, traumatic, 211
Arteriovenous malformations, 355, 664, 667, 668
  calcification with, 657, 658
  cortical, 652
  CT patterns, 664
  dural, 360–363, 361*f*
  ependymal enhancement, 602
  glioblastoma multiforme vs., 238
  and intracranial hemorrhages, 216
  mesencephalic, 619
  midbrain, 618
  parenchymal (pial), 355–357, 358*t*, 360
  sellar/juxtasellar region, 612, 614
Arteritis, 401–402, 467
Arthropathy, foramen magnum region, 644, 645*f*, 646
Artifacts, CSF flow, 329, 602
Ascending pharyngeal artery, 33–34, 33*f*, 34*f*, 37
Aseptic meningitis, 429
  with HIV/AIDS, 458
  with poliovirus infection, 447
Aspergilloma, juxtasellar, 614
Aspergillosis, 483–484, 667
  enhancement patterns, 662
  with HIV/AIDS, 457, 458, 459
  meningitis, chronic, 430
  skull base lesions, 638
Asphyxia, neonatal, 516
Association fibers, normal anatomy, 90
Astroblastoma, with HIV/AIDS, 471
Astrocytes, 231
  normal white matter components, 512
  Rosenthal fibers, 525
Astrocytoma, 224, 225, 226*f*, 227, 228, 231–238, 650, 651, 665
  anaplastic (WHO grade III), 234–235
  basal ganglia degeneration, 569
  calcification with, 657, 659
  cerebellopontine angle, 623*t*
  cortical, 652
  CSF dissemination, 591
  in differential diagnosis
    of arteriovenous malformation, 360
    of choroid plexus tumors, 260
    of colloid cyst, 329
    of desmoplastic infantile gangliogliomas, 265
    of dysembryoplastic neuroepithelial tumor, 266
    of ependymomas, 256

Astrocytoma—cont'd
  in differential diagnosis—cont'd
    of gangliocytomas, 264
    of ganglioglioma, 264
    of lymphoma, 304
    of medulloblastomas, 273, 274
    of oligodendroglial tumors, 254
    of primary cerebral neuroblastomas, 275
    of schwannomas, 317
    of subependymomas, 258
  enhancement pattern, 661, 663
  ependymal enhancement, 440
  foramen magnum region, 644, 645*f*
  glioblastoma multiforme (WHO grade IV), 235–238, 236*f*
  histology and grading, 231–232
  with HIV/AIDS, 471
  leptomeningeal infiltration, 308
  low-grade (WHO grade II), 233–234
  morphologic pattern, 651
  neurofibromatosis type I, 165
  pineal, 616*f*, 617, 618
  pineal region, 619
  posterior fossa, 654, 655
  skull base lesions, 634
  suprasellar, 613
  tectal, 618
  temporal bone lesions, 628
  types, 232–233
  ventricular pathology, 598, 599, 600, 601
Astrocytoma variants, 241–250
  gliomatosis cerebri, 247–248
  gliosarcoma, 248–249
  pilocytic astrocytoma, 241–245
  pleomorphic xanthoastrocytoma, 245–246
  primary leptomeningeal gliomatosis, 249–250
  subependymal giant cell astrocytoma (SGCA), 171, 246–247
Astrocytosis, in disseminated encephalomyelitis, 450
Ataxia-telangiectasia (AT), 177–178
Atherosclerosis, 387–393
  calcification with, 657, 658
  collateral circulation, 393
  imaging, 389–393
  location, 388–389
  pathophysiology, 387–388, 387*f*
  and stroke, 402, 403
  white matter degenerative diseases, 547
  white matter lesion differential diagnosis, 546
Atrium, ventricular mass lesions in children, 599
Atrophy
  age-related changes, 542
  in Alzheimer disease, 561

Atrophy—cont'd
  cerebellar, 649–650
  cerebellorubral degeneration, 557
  cerebral, 649
  after herpes simplex encephalitis, 445
  with HIV, 461
  inherited metabolic disorders, 515
  meningitis and, 427, 430
  normal pressure hydrocephalus, 564
  olivopontocellular, 568
  Rasmussen encephalitis, 452
  tuberculosis and, 476
  ventricular pathology, 595, 596
Auditory association cortex, 88f, 89
Auditory canal atresia, 626
Auditory cortex, 88f, 89
Auditory pathway, 93, 94
Autoimmune demyelinating diseases, 512, 548–552
AZT, 460
Azygous anterior cerebral artery, 136

B

Bacterial infections
  parenchymal, 435–440
  ventriculitis and ependymitis, 439
Bacterial (pyogenic) meningitis, 426–427
  enhancement patterns, 660
  meningeal enhancement with, 590
  suprasellar, 613
Balo's disease, 548
Basal cell carcinoma, scalp, 574
Basal cell nevus (Gorlin) syndrome, 179, 656
Basal cisterns, 24t, 26–27
Basal ganglia
  calcification in, 656, 657–658
  collateral circulation, 393
  CT patterns, 665
  iron in, 539f, 667
  MRI patterns, 667
Basal ganglia abnormalities, 511, 568–569, 653–654
  diffuse necrotizing leukoencephalopathy, 555
  in disseminated encephalomyelitis, 451
  with HIV/AIDS
    neurosyphilis, 468
    toxoplasmosis, 462, 463t
    tuberculous, 470
  hypertensive vascular disease, 664
  with infections
    CMV, 417
    rubella, 423
  inherited metabolic and degenerative disorders, 514, 532–534
  Langerhans cell histiocytosis, 479
  in multiple sclerosis, 550
  Pick's disease, 595

Basal ganglia abnormalities—cont'd
  progressive multifocal leukoencephalopathy, 465
  ventricular mass lesions, 601
  white matter disorders, 519
Basal ganglia hemorrhage, 601
Basal nuclei, 91
Basal vein of Rosenthal, 74f, 77f, 78f, 80
Basilar artery, 50, 50f, 59f, 59f, 60f, 69–70, 66f, 67f
  aneurysms, 343, 344f, 349
  carotid-basilar anastomoses, 61
  dolichoectasia, 612
  idiopathic progressive arteriopathy of childhood, 397
  stroke, 380–381f, 383
Basilar cisterns
  ventricular pathology, 597
Basilar invagination, 580, 646
Basilar meningitis, with HIV/AIDS, 459
Basilar plexus, 75f
Basis pedunculi, 93
Batten disease, 514, 529
Behcet disease, 402
  MRI patterns, 668
  and vascular occlusion, 406, 407
Bell's palsy, 626
  enhancement patterns, 663
  internal auditory canal, 625
Benign hyperostosis, 578
Benign intracranial hypotension, 592, 661
Benign leptomeningeal fibrosis, 591
Benign pineal cyst, 268
Bithalamic astrocytomas, 569
Bland embolic infarct, corticomedullary junction, 652
Blastic metastasis, meningiomas vs., 294
Blistering hyperostosis, 579
Blood-brain barrier, in multiple sclerosis, 550
Blood dyscrasias; see Hematologic disorders
Blood flow patterns, 668
Blood vessels; see also Arteries; Vascular abnormalities; Vascular malformations; Veins; specific vessels
  age-related changes, 540
  calcification, 656
  congenital/developmental abnormalities; see Vascular malformations
  corpus callosum lipomas, 139, 140f
  enhancement patterns, 656, 660, 661
  ependymal enhancement, 602
  with HIV/AIDS, 459
  inflammation; see Vasculitis
  meningioma, 293f
  MRI patterns, 667
  normal white matter components, 512
  pineal region, 616f, 617
  scalp, 16f

Blood vessels—cont'd
  sellar/juxtasellar region, 606*f*, 607
  subarachnoid cisterns, 24–25*t*
  virus infections and, 443
Bone abnormalities; *see also* Calvarium;
    Skull; Spine
  calvarium/skull, 576, 577, 579, 580, 581
  Chiari I malformation, 126, 127*t*
  with corpus callosum abnormalities, 136
  inflammation; *see* Osteomyelitis
  metastases
    skull, 579
    vertebral, 308, 310
  neurofibromatosis type I, 166
  plasmacytomas, 306
  tuberculous spondylitis, 475
  tumors; *see* Osteocartilagenous tumors
Bone flap, 583
Bone marrow, 13, 14, 579; *see also* Fibrous
    dysplasia; Hematopoietic tissue
Bone scans; *see* Radionuclide imaging
Borrelia burghdorferi; *see* Lyme disease
Bourneville disease, 170
Brachium conjunctiva, 93
Brain
  anatomy; *see* Anatomy, brain
  normal development, 122–124
Brain death, 204
Brainstem, 196
  anatomy, 622*f*
  Chiari IV malformation, 127*t*, 131
  with Dandy-Walker malformation, 154
  in disseminated encephalomyelitis, 450, 451
  HIV involvement, 460
  MRI patterns, 669
  multiple sclerosis, 531
  progressive multifocal leukoencephalopathy,
    465
  tuberculomas, 475
Brainstem astrocytoma
  cerebellopontine angle, 623*t*
  temporal bone lesions, 628
Brainstem glioma, 227, 228
  foramen magnum region, 644
  MRI patterns, 669
  posterior fossa, 654, 655
  ventricular abnormalities, 598, 599, 601
Brain tumors; *see* Mass lesions; Neoplasms
Bright spot
  Langerhans cell histiocytosis, 480
  neurohyophysis, 607
Broca's area, 88*f*, 89
Bromocriptine, 282, 611
Brown tumor, 584
Bulbar polio, 447
Burns, 574, 583
Burr holes, 582, 583
Butterfly callosal lesions, 304

C

Caffey disease, 578
Calcarine artery, 59*f*
Calcification
  abnormal by pathologic process, 656–657
  basal ganglia, 569, 657–658
  calvarial/skull abnormalities, 577, 579
  chordomas, 320
  cortical, 652
  diffuse necrotizing leukoencephalopathy,
    555
  extraaxial abnormalities, 589
  with infections
    CMV, 417, 418
    cysticercosis, 492
    herpes simplex, 421, 445
    HIV/AIDS toxoplasmosis, 463
    meningitis, chronic, 430
    rubella, 422, 423
    toxoplasmosis, 419, 463
    tuberculosis, 475, 476
  metastases, 309, 658
  MRI patterns, 667
  multiple small nodules, 658
  normal intracranial, 656
  parasellar, 658
  posterior fossa, 655
  ringlike, 658–659
  ventricular mass lesions in children,
    599
Callosal agenesis, 136–140, 137*f*, 138*f*, 139*f*,
    140*f*, 595
Callosal lesions, 652–653
Calvarium; *see also* Scalp and calvarium; Skull
  fontanelles, 8, 8*f*
  Langerhans cell histiocytosis, 307, 478
  mega cisterna magna, 586
  meninges and, 16–17, 16*f*
    anatomy of meninges, epi- and subdural
      space, 587*f*
    dural carcinomatosis, 591
  plasmacytomas, 638
Canavan disease, 514, 515, 519, 524, 525
  calvarial/skull abnormalities, 575
  MRI patterns, 668
Candida infection, 486–487
  with HIV/AIDS, 457, 458, 459
  meningitis, chronic, 430
Capillary hemangioblastoma, 296–298
Capillary malformations, 358*t*, 366–368
Capillary telangiectasias, 358*t*, 366–367, 370,
    371
Caput succedaneum, 574
Carbon monoxide intoxication, 665
  and basal ganglia degeneration, 568
  basal ganglia lesions, 654
  calcification in, 656, 657
  toxic encephalopathy, 554–555

Carcinoma; *see also specific sites and tissue*
    dural carcinomatosis, 591
    head and neck, 320, 574
    leptomeningeal infiltration, 308
Carcinomatous meningitis; *see*
        Leptomeningeal metastases
Caroticotympanic artery, 41
Carotid arteries; *see also* Common carotid
        artery; External carotid artery and
        branches; Internal carotid artery
    paramedian, 610
    stroke risk, 375
Carotid artery dissection, 208*f*
Carotid-basilar anastomoses, 61
Carotid body tumor, 319
Carotid canal, 11*f*, 13*t*
Carotid-cavernous fistula, 211, 636
Carotid siphon, 43
Carotid space, 13*t*
Carpenter disease, 576
Caudate nucleus, 91
    inherited metabolic disorders affecting, 514,
        516
    iron in, 543
Cavernomas, 358t, 365, 368–370, 369*f*, 371,
        664, 667
    CT patterns, 664
    glioblastoma multiforme vs., 238
    MRI patterns, 669
    posterior fossa, 654
    and intracranial hemorrhages, 216
    midbrain, 618
    schwannoma vs., 316
Cavernous internal carotid artery, 40*f*, 43–44,
        393
Cavernous malformations, 368
Cavernous sinus, 13*t*, 44, 74*f*, 75*f*, 78–79, 75*f*,
        76*f*, 78*f*, 211, 614, 634
    arteriovenous malformations, 361
    enhancement patterns, 660
    epidermoid, 635, 636
    lipoma, 635, 636
    nerve sheath tumors, 637
    pituitary adenomas, 282, 283
    skull base lesions, 636
    suprasellar region anatomy, 606, 606*f*,
        607
    venous system, 76*f*
Cavernous sinus malformations, 370
Cavum septi pellucidi and cavum vergae, 20,
        598, 599, 653
Cavum velum interpositum, 26, 619
    midline lesions, 653
    pineal cyst vs., 332
    pineocytoma vs., 268
CECT
    aneurysm, 350
    arteriovenous malformations, 358*t*, 359*t*

CECT—cont'd
    in atherosclerosis, 390
    brain death, 204
    cortical vein occlusion, 410–411
    deep cerebral vein thrombosis, 411
    dural sinus thrombosis, 409
    epidermoid versus dermoid tumors, 323*t*
    white matter disease, 555
Cellular migration disorders, 147–151, 148*f*,
        149*f*, 150*f*
Cellulitis, scalp, 574
Central cord syndrome, 126, 127*t*
Central gray matter, 94
Central neurocytoma, 247, 267; *see also* Neu-
        rocytoma
    calcification with, 657
    in differential diagnosis
        of colloid cyst, 329
        of ependymomas, 257
        of subependymomas, 258
    ventricular pathology, 596, 598, 600
Central pontine myelinolysis (CPM), 512, 553
    MRI patterns, 669
    posterior fossa lesions, 654
Central precocious puberty, 612
Central sulcus, normal anatomy, 84, 85
Central tegmental hemorrhages, 203
Centrum semiovale, autoimmune demyelina-
        tion, 551
    carbon monoxide poisoning, 554
    HIV involvement, 460
    toxoplasma lesions, HIV/AIDS-related, 462
Cephalocele, 134–140, 137*f*, 138*f*, 139*f*, 140*f*
    calvarial/skull abnormalities, 582, 583
    Chiari III malformations, 127*t*, 131
    with Dandy-Walker malformation, 154
    midline, 653
    nasoethmoidal, 632
    skull base lesions, 633
    suprasellar, 612
Cephalohematoma, 574
    calvarial/skull abnormalities, 575, 577,
        579
    in infants, 215
Cerebellar arteries, vertebrobasilar circulation,
        66–70, 66*f*, 67*f*
Cerebellar astrocytoma
    ependymomas vs., 256
    posterior fossa, 654, 566, 655
    temporal bone lesions, 628
Cerebellar ataxia, Creutzfeldt-Jakob disease,
        454
Cerebellar atrophy, 568
Cerebellar gangliocytoma, dysplastic, 161,
        265, 655
Cerebellar syndrome, Chiari I malformation,
        126, 127*t*
Cerebellar tonsils, 20*f*, 22

Cerebellomedullary cisterns, 23, 23*f*, 24*t*
Cerebellopontine angle cistern
   anatomy, 23, 23*f*, 24*t*, 622*f*
   mass lesions, 623*t*, 624*t*, 628, 629
   temporal bone lesions involving, 626
Cerebellopontine angle, 622–629, 622*f*, 623*t*
   cerebellopontine angle lesions, 623–625,
      623*t*, 624*t*
   internal auditory canal lesions, 625–626
   intraaxial or fourth ventricle lesions,
      628–629
   temporal bone lesions, 626–628
Cerebellorubral degeneration, 557
Cerebellum, 95–97, 96*f*, 97*f*
   age-related changes, 539
   anatomy, 622*f*
   atrophy, 649–650
   calcification, 656
   Chiari I malformation, 126, 127*t*
   Chiari II malformations, 127*t*, 129
   Chiari IV malformation, 127*t*, 131
   Creutzfeldt-Jakob disease, 453
   in disseminated encephalomyelitis, 450,
      451
   HIV involvement, 460
   hypertensive vascular disease, 664
   multiple sclerosis, 531
   neoplasms, 242–245, 243–244*f*; *see also*
      specific cerebellar mass lesions
   normal development, 122, 123
   toxoplasma lesions, HIV/AIDS-related, 462
   tuberculomas, 475
Cerebral amyloid angiopathy (CAA), 218
Cerebral aqueduct of Sylvius, 22, 94
Cerebral arteries, 50–62, 50*f*, 52*f*, 53*f*
   anterior, 52–54, 52*f*, 53*f*
   circle of Willis, 50–52, 50*f*
   with holoprosencephaly, 144
   idiopathic progressive arteriopathy of child-
      hood, 397
   middle, 54–58, 55*f*, 56*f*, 57*f*, 58*f*
   posterior, 58–62, 59*f*, 60*f*, 62*f*
   subarachnoid cisterns, 25*t*
Cerebral aspergillosis, 663
Cerebral atrophy, 575; *see also* Atrophy
   diffuse, 649
   selective, 649
Cerebral cortex
   normal anatomy, 85–90
   normal development, 123
Cerebral edema, 202, 203–204, 650
   diffuse, 665
   ventricular pathology, 597
Cerebral gigantism, 575
Cerebral hemiatrophy, 575
Cerebral hemispheres
   Chiari II malformations, 130
   Langerhans cell histiocytosis, 479

Cerebral hemispheres—cont'd
   normal development, 122
   ventricular abnormalities from mass lesions
      of, 601
Cerebral herniations, 199–202, 200*f*
Cerebral heterotopia, nasal, 632
Cerebral hyperemia, 202
Cerebral infarction, 202, 203, 428, 661; *see
   also* Infarct
Cerebral ischemia, 202, 661; *see also* Stroke
   acute, 375–378
   aneurysm rupture and, 345, 347–348*f*
Cerebral neuroblastoma, 263
Cerebral palsy, 575
Cerebral peduncle, 93
Cerebral PNET, 228, 265
Cerebral veins, 79
Cerebral vein thrombosis, 411
Cerebritis, 435–440
   abscess, 436–439
   calvarial/skull abnormalities, 576
   corticomedullary junction, 652
   meningitis and, 427
   MRI patterns, 668
   ventriculitis/ependymitis, 439–440
Cerebrohepatorenal (Zellweger) syndrome,
   514, 515, 516, 575
Cerebro-oculo-muscular syndrome, 158
Cerebrospinal fluid, 12*t*
   anatomy, 16*f*
   Chiari II malformations, 131
   CT, 184*f*
   dissemination of tumors, 501, 613
   normal development, 123
   normal pressure hydrocephalus, 564
   overproduction, 597, 650
   ventricular pathology, 597
Cerebrospinal fluid flow
   fourth ventricle, 22
   ventricle system, 20*f*
Cerebrospinal fluid flow artifact, 329, 602
Cerebrovascular disorders; *see*
   Atherosclerosis; Vascular abnormalities
Cerebrum
   normal anatomy, 84–91, 84*f*, 86–87*f*,
     88*f*
   tuberculomas, 475
Ceroid lipofuscinoses, 514, 529–530
Cervicomedullary junction, 644
Cervicomedullary masses, 643
Charcot-Bouchard aneurysm, 217
Chemical toxins, 592
Chemodectoma, 318–319
Chemoreceptor zone, enhancement patterns,
   660
Chemotherapy
   and basal ganglia degeneration, 569
   calcification with, 657, 658

Chemotherapy—cont'd
  cerebral atrophy, 649
  enhancement patterns, 661
  and intracranial hemorrhage, 218
  MRI patterns, 668
  subarachnoid space enlargement, 588
  ventricular pathology, 596
  white matter damage, 555–556
Chiari I malformation, 126, 127*t*, 128,
  128*f*
  foramen magnum region, 644, 645*f*, 646
  posterior fossa, 654
Chiari II malformation, 127*t*, 129–131, 129*f*
  calvarial/skull abnormalities, 580
  with corpus callosum abnormalities, 136
  ventricular pathology, 595
Chiari III malformation, 127*t*, 131
Chiari IV malformation, 127*t*, 131, 160
Chiari malformations
  calvarial/skull abnormalities, 575, 576
  posterior fossa, 654, 655
Chiasmatic (suprasellar) cistern, 23*f*, 24*t*
Chiasmatic-hypothalamic glioma
  craniopharyngioma vs., 286
  germ cell tumor differential diagnosis, 278
  hypothalamic hamartoma vs., 334
  pituitary adenoma vs., 284
Chickenpox, 450
Choristoma, pituitary, 611
Chloroma, 305, 613
Cholesteatoma
  secondary, 627
  skull base lesions, 639, 640
  temporal bone, 626
Cholesterol granuloma, 626
  schwannomas vs., 317
  skull base lesions, 640
  temporal bone, 627
Chondrodysplasia, calvarial/skull abnormalities, 576, 577
Chondroma, 298
Chondrosarcoma
  calcification with, 657
  calvarial/skull abnormalities, 584
  cavernous sinus and skull base, 614
  meningeal, 298
  skull base lesions, 637, 640
Chordoma, 319–320
  calcification with, 657, 658
  cerebellopontine angle, 623*t*
  foramen magnum region, 643, 644, 645*f*,
  646
  posterior fossa, 654
  skull base lesions, 614, 635, 637, 640
  temporal bone lesions, 626
Choriocarcinoma, 276, 277, 278, 665
  hemorrhage with, 309
  pineal, 618

Chorioretinitis
  cytomegalovirus, 467
  toxoplasmosis, 419
Choristoma, 613
Choroid
  calcification, 656
  enhancement patterns, 660
Choroidal artery anatomy, 60,–61, 60*f*
Choroidal artery fistula, 619
Choroid fissure cyst, 266, 651
Choroid plexitis, MRI, 438
Choroid plexus
  anatomy, 19, 20*f*, 21
  calcification, 656
  cerebellopontine angle, 623
  CSF circulation, 26*f*
  ependymal enhancement, 602
  hemorrhage in, 196
  normal development, 123
Choroid plexus cyst, 651
  ventricular mass lesions, 599
  ventricular mass lesions in adults, 598
Choroid plexus papilloma, 227, 228
  calcification with, 657
  cerebellopontine angle, 623*t*
  CT patterns, 664
  enhancement patterns, 661
  in differential diagnosis
    of ependymomas, 256, 257
    of germ cell tumor differential diagnosis,
    278
    of medulloblastomas, 274
    of meningiomas, 295
    of pineoblastoma, 269
    of schwannoma, 316
    of subependymomas, 258
  morphologic patterns, 651
  posterior fossa, 654
  temporal bone lesions, 628
  third ventricle, 618
  ventricular mass lesions in children, 599
Choroid plexus tumors, 224, 225, 226*f*, 228,
  231, 258–260
  cerebellopontine angle, 625
  CSF dissemination, 591
  enhancement patterns, 660, 661
  ependymal enhancement, 440, 602
  leptomeningeal infiltration, 308
  ventricular pathology, 596, 597, 600
Chronic hemorrhage, 187
Chronic meningitis, 426
Chronic progressive ophthalmoplegia (CPEO),
  534, 535
Chronic subdural hematoma
  calcification in, 657
  enhancement patterns, 660
  enhancement with, 592
Cine-mode phase-contrast velocity MRI, 128

Cingulate herniation, 199
Cingulate sulcus, 23*f*
Circle of Willis, 41, 50–52, 50*f*, 50*f*, 59*f*,
    398
    aneurysms, 343
    dissection, 398
Cisterna magna, 22, 23, 23*f*, 24*t*, 586, 628,
    644
Cisterns
    age-related changes, 538–539, 539*f*
    CSF circulation, 27
    normal pressure hydrocephalus, 564
    subarachnoid, 23–27, 23*f*, 24–25*t*, 26*f*
Claustrum, 91
Cleidocranial dysplasia, 576, 577, 583
Clival venous plexus, 74*f*
Clivus, 637
    anatomy, 645*f*
    chondrosarcoma of, 614
    inferior, 639, 644
    plasmacytomas, 638
    upper, 634
Cloverleaf skull, 576
Coagulation necrosis, 555
Coagulopathies, 664
    and intracranial hemorrhage, 218
    and stroke, 403
    and vascular occlusion, 406, 407
Coats disease, 179
Cocaine granulomatosis, 633, 635,
    638
Coccioidomycosis, 487, 590
    calcification, 656
    chronic meningitis, 426, 430
    enhancement patterns, 660, 662
    with HIV/AIDS, 457, 458
Cochlear nuclei, 95
Cockayne syndrome, 657
Collagenosis, periventricular venous, 411–412,
    411–412, 546, 547
Collateral circulation
    enhancement patterns, 661
    ependymal enhancement, 440
    moya-moya, 397
Colloid cyst, 247, 328–329, 651, 667
    central neurocytoma vs., 267
    CT patterns, 664
    ependymomas vs., 257
    midline, 653
    subependymomas vs., 258
    suprasellar, 612
    ventricular pathology, 596, 598, 599, 618
Colpocephaly, 127*t*, 131, 595
Commissural fibers, normal anatomy, 90–91
Common carotid artery
    internal carotid artery origin, 40, 40*f*
    left, 31*f*, 32
    right, 30, 31*f*

Common carotid artery bifurcation, 31*f*, 32,
    40, 40*f*
Communicating hydrocephalus, 650
    with HIV/AIDS-associated tuberculosis,
        469
    malignancy and, 592
    ventricular pathology, 596
Computed tomography; *see also*
        Single-photon emission computed tomog-
        raphy
    arteriovenous malformations, 358–359*t*
    cortical contusions, 196
    dermoid tumors, 325
    diffuse axonal injury, 195
    emergency, indication for, 189
    epidermoid tumors, 326
    epidural hematoma, 191
    of intracranial hemorrhage, 184–185, 184*f*,
        184*t*, 186, 187
    post-infectious syndromes, 445
    sarcoid, 477
    subdural empyema, 430
    subdural hematoma, 193
Computed tomography (CT) angiography
    aneurysm, 350
    atherosclerosis, 390
Computed tomography patterns, 664–666
Concentric sclerosis, 548
Confluens sinuum, 73, 74*f*, 77*f*
Congenital/developmental abnormalities
    aqueductal stenosis, 596
    arachnoid cyst, 327–328
    brain malformations, 123
    calcification with, 656, 657, 658
    callosal, 135–140, 137*f*, 138*f*, 139*f*, 140*f*,
        652
        cephaloceles, 134
        with holoprosencephaly, 144
    calvarial/skull abnormalities, 575, 577, 580,
        583
    cephaloceles and corpus callosum abnor-
        malities, 134–140
    cerebellar tonsillar ectopia, 126, 127*t*, 128,
        128*f*
    cerebellopontine angle, 623
    cerebral atrophy, 649
    classification of, 123–124
    CT patterns, 664
    Dandy-Walker complex, 154–161
    ependymal enhancement, 602
    extraaxial fluid collections, 586, 588
    foramen magnum region, 643, 644, 646
    holoprosencephaly, 142–144
    internal auditory canal, 625
    and intracranial hemorrhages, 216
    mass lesions, 224; *see also* Cysts and
        tumor-like lesions; Mass lesions
    midbrain, 618

Congenital/developmental abnormalities—
    cont'd
  midline lesions, 653
  morphologic patterns, 650, 651
  MRI patterns, 668
  neural tube disorders and Chiari malforma-
    tions, 126–131
  neurocutaneous syndromes, 164–168,
    170–179
  neurofibromatosis, 164–168
  periventricular, 652
  pineal region, 616f
  posterior fossa, 154–161, 654, 655
  quadrigeminal cistern and velum interposi-
    tum, 619
  sellar/juxtasellar region
    cavernous sinus and skull base, 614
    sellar region, 610
  skull
    calvarium, 575, 577, 578
    temporal bone lesions, 626–627
  skull base lesions
    anterior, 632
    central, 635
    posterior, 639
  sulcation and cellular migration disorders,
    147–151
  suprasellar, 612
  tumors, 124, 224; see also Mass lesions
  ventricular pathology, 596, 597, 599–600
    configuration abnormalities, 595
    ependymal enhancement, 602
    mass lesions, 597, 599–600
Congenital ectopic neurohypophysis, 610
Congenital and neonatal infections
  cytomegalovirus, 416–418
  herpes simplex virus, 420–422
  HIV, 423–424
  rubella, 422–423
  subarachnoid space enlargement, 588
  TORCH; see also TORCH infections
    calcification with, 658
    cerebral atrophy, 649
    ventricular pathology, 596
  toxoplasmosis, 418–420
Contrast agents, 592, 665
  with cysticercosis, 492
  enhancement patterns, 661
  MRI, 667
Contusions, 195–196, 195f, 652, 664
Cornelia de Lange syndrome, 575
Corpus callosum
  agenesis, 136–140, 137f, 138f, 139f,
    140f
  carbon monoxide poisoning, 554
  developmental abnormalities, 135–140,
    137f, 138f, 139f, 140f, 652
  cephaloceles, 134

Corpus callosum—cont'd
  developmental abnormalities—cont'd
    with holoprosencephaly, 144
  HIV/AIDS-related lymphoma, 463t
  holoprosencephaly, 143
  lesions of, 652–653
  normal, 137f
  normal anatomy, 90–91
  normal development, 123
  normal pressure hydrocephalus, 563
  progressive multifocal leukoencephalopathy,
    465
Corpus callosum cistern, 25t, 27
Corpus striatum, 91
  inherited metabolic disorders affecting, 514
  projection fibers, 91
Cortical atrophy, 564, 652; see also Atrophy
Cortical contusions, 195–196, 195f
Cortical dementias, 564–567
Cortical enhancement, gyriform, 661
Cortical hamartoma, 579; see also Hamartoma
Cortical veins
  anatomy, 16f
  occlusion, 410–411
  thrombosis
    ependymal enhancement, 602
    and intracranial hemorrhage, 217
    meningitis and, 427
    ventricular pathology, 596
Corticobulbar tract, 94
Corticomedullary junction, 652, 664
  HIV/AIDS-related toxoplasmosis, 463t
  tuberculomas, 475, 476
Corticospinal tract, 94, 95, 99, 514
Corticosteroids; see Steroids
Corticotroph adenoma, 282
Cowden disease, 161, 179, 265
Coxsackievirus, 443, 450
CPA lesions, meningiomas vs., 295
Cranial involvement; see Cranium
Cranial nerve abnormalities; see Cranial
    neuropathies; specific cranial nerves
Cranial nerve enhancement
  with neurosyphilis, 468
  sarcoid, 477
Cranial nerve palsies; see also specific cranial
    nerves
  calvarial/skull abnormalities, 580
  idiopathic hypertrophic pachymeningitis, 593
  with malignant otitis externa, 628
Cranial nerves, 94, 95, 99, 102f, 103f
  abducens (VI), 110
  accessory (XI), 116–117
  acoustic (VIII), 113–114
  apertures of skull base, 12–13t
  cavernous sinuses, 78
  in disseminated encephalomyelitis, 451
  enhancing, 663

Cranial nerves—cont'd
  external carotid artery and branches, innervation of, 37
  facial (VII), 111–113, 623
  foramina, 6f, 9–14, 10f, 11, 11f, 12–13t
  fourth ventricle region, 22
  glossopharyngeal (IX), 114–115
  with HIV/AIDS
    cytomegalovirus, 466
    neurosyphilis, 468
  hypoglossal (XII), 117–118
  Langerhans cell histiocytosis, 479
  meningitis and, 427
  neurofibroma, 317, 318
  oculomotor (III), 105–106
  olfactory (I), 102–103
  optic (II), 103–105
  with poliovirus infection, 447
  sarcoid, 477
  schwannomas, 314t, 315
  spinal accessory (xi), 116–117
  subarachnoid cisterns, 24–25t
  trigeminal (V), 107–110
  trochlear (IV), 106–107
  vagus (X), 115–116
  venous system, 76f
  vestibulocochlear (VIII), 113–114
Cranial nerve schwannomas
  neurofibromatosis type II, 168
  skull base lesions, 614, 640
Cranial nerve tumors, 314
Cranial neuropathies
  aneurysm and, 344–345
  with calvarial/skull abnormalities, 580
  in Lyme disease, 446
  with malignant otitis externa, 628
Craniocerebral trauma; see Trauma
Craniofacial dysostosis, 576
Craniolacuna, 580
Craniometaphyseal dysplasia, 575
Craniopharyngioma, 224, 225, 226f, 228, 284–286, 651
  calcification with, 657, 658, 659
  in differential diagnosis
    of astrocytomas, 245
    of choroid plexus tumors, 260
    of germ cell tumors, 278
    of hypothalamic hamartoma, 334
    of pituitary adenomas, 283
    of Rathke's cleft cyst, 287
  midline, 653
  sellar/juxtasellar region, 608t, 611, 612
  ventricular abnormalities, 599, 601
Craniostenosis, 575
Craniosynostosis, 575
Craniotomy
  calvarial/skull abnormalities, 583
  enhancement patterns, 661

Craniovertebral junction, 645f
Craniovertebral junction abnormalities, 646
Craniovertebral junction masses, 643
Cranium
  anatomy, 4–7, 5f, 6f
  inherited metabolic disorders affecting, 514
  Langerhans cell histiocytosis, 479
  metastases, 307–310
  Wegener's granulomatosis, 478
Creutzfeld-Jakob disease, 443, 453–454, 512, 566
  basal ganglia degeneration, 569
  cerebral atrophy, 649
Cribriform plate, 12t
Crouzon disease, 576
Crus cerebri, 93
Cryptococcoma
  with HIV/AIDS, 460
  MRI patterns, 668
Cryptococcosis, 485–486, 590
  basal ganglia degeneration, 569
  enhancement patterns, 660
  with HIV/AIDS, 457, 458, 463–464
Curvilinear calcification, 658–659
Cushing disease, 581
Cyanide intoxication, 654, 665
Cyclops, 142
Cyclosporin A, 555
Cystic acoustic neuroma, 327
Cystic astrocytoma, 659
Cystic craniopharyngioma, 659
Cysticercosis, 489–492, 651, 667
  calcification with, 656, 658
  cerebellopontine angle, 623
  enhancement patterns, 662
  epidermoid tumor vs., 327
  posterior fossa, 654, 655
  Rathke's cleft cyst vs., 287
  subarachnoid space enlargement, 588
  suprasellar, 613
  ventricular pathology, 596, 601
  white matter lesion differential diagnosis, 546
Cystic meningioma, 327, 662
Cystic schwannoma, 295, 662
Cysts and tumor-like lesions, 323–334; see also Congenital/developmental abnormalities; Mass lesions; Neoplasms; specific lesions
  arachnoid cyst, congenital, 327–328
  calcification with, 659
  choroid plexus, 599
  colloid cyst, 328–329
  dermoid (inclusion) cyst, 323–325, 323t
  enhancement patterns, 662

Cysts and tumor-like lesions—cont'd
  in differential diagnosis
    of epidermoid tumor, 327
    of meningiomas, 295
    of neuroepithelial cysts, 330
    of pineal cyst, 332
  endodermal cysts, 330–331
  epidermoid tumor, 323*t*, 325–327
  hypothalamic hamartoma, 333–334
  lipoma, 332–333
  morphologic patterns, 651
  neuroepithelial cysts, 329–330
  pineal, 331–332, 616*f*, 617, 618
  posterior fossa, 156*t*
  temporal bone, 627
  third ventricle, 618
  ventricular pathology, 596
Cytarabine, 555
Cytogenesis, 124
Cytomegalovirus
  calcification, 656
  congenital and neonatal, 416–418
  with HIV/AIDS, 457, 458, 466–467
  Rasmussen encephalitis, 452
  ventriculitis and ependymitis, 439
Cytomegalovirus ependymitis, 470
Cytosine arabinoside, 650

D

Dandy-Walker malformation, 136, 154, 155*t*,
    157, 157*f*, 158*f*, 160, 651
  astrocytomas vs., 245
  calvarial/skull abnormalities, 575, 576
  cephaloceles with, 134
  with corpus callosum abnormalities,
    136
  posterior fossa, 655
  ventricular pathology, 595
Dandy-Walker variant, 154, 157–158,
    157*f*
  differential diagnosis, 155–156*t*
  mega cisterna magna, 586
  posterior fossa, 655
Decreased intracranial pressure, 128, 592
Decussation of superior cerebellar peduncles,
    93
Degenerative cysts, 651
Degenerative disorders; *see also* Myelination,
    normal development
  acquired
    of gray matter, 561–569
    of white matter, 511–512, 546–557
  basal ganglia lesions, 653–654
  cerebellar atrophy, 650
  cerebral atrophy, 649
  cortical, 652
  inherited
    classification, 511–516

Degenerative disorders—cont'd
  inherited—cont'd
    of gray matter, 514–516, 528–535,
      528–535
    of white matter, 511–516, 518–526
  subarachnoid space enlargement, 588
  tectal/midbrain involvement, 618–619
  ventricular pathology, 595, 596
Degenerative spine disorders, and arterial oc-
    clusion, 399
Dehydration
  cerebral atrophy, 649
  and vascular occlusion, 406, 407
  ventricular pathology, 596
Delayed encephalopathy, 554
Delayed myelination, 422, 507–508, 507*t*
Dementias; *see also* Alzheimer disease; Gray
    matter disorders, acquired
  AIDS, 457, 460
  cortical, 564–567
  neurosyphilis, 468
  subcortical, 567–568
de Morsier syndrome, 144
Demyelinating disease, 511–512
  acquired, 546–557
    autoimmune, 548–552
    toxic, 552–555
  corticomedullary junction, 652
  in differential diagnosis
    of astrocytomas, 234, 235
    of neuroepithelial cysts, 330
  enhancement patterns, 662
  foramen magnum lesions, 643, 644,
    645*f*
  inherited, 512, 518–526
  MRI patterns, 668, 669
  periventricular/callosal, 653
  posterior fossa lesions, 654
  ring-enhancing lesions, 439
  splenium, 619
  subacute necrotizing encephalomelopathy,
    532
  tectal, 618
Dentate nuclei
  calcification in, 656
  cerebellorubral degeneration, 557
  iron in, 538, 543, 667
Deoxyhemoglobin, 667
Deprivational states
  calvarial/skull abnormalities, 577
  cerebral atrophy, 649
  scalp abnormalities with, 574
  subarachnoid space enlargement, 588
  ventricular pathology, 596
Dermoid/epidermoid, 227, 323–327, 651, 654,
    665
  calcification, 656
  calvarial/skull abnormalities, 574, 582, 583

Dermoid/epidermoid—cont'd
  cerebellopontine angle, 623*t*, 623
  dermoid vs. epidermoid, 323*t*
  in differential diagnosis
    of astrocytomas, 245
    of congenital arachnoid cyst, 328
    of meningiomas, 295
    of neuroepithelial cysts, 330
    of pineal cyst, 332
    of pineocytoma, 268
    of Rathke's cleft cyst, 287
    of schwannomas, 317
  foramen magnum region, 643, 644, 645*f*
  midline, 653
  MRI patterns, 667
  nasal, 632
  pineal, 616*f*, 617
  posterior fossa, 156*t*, 654, 655
  quadrigeminal cistern and velum interpositum, 619
  sellar/juxtasellar region
    cavernous sinus and skull base, 614
    intrasellar, 610
    sellar region, 610
    suprasellar, 612
  skull base lesions, 635, 636, 639
  ventricular pathology, 600
Descending transtentorial herniation, 199, 201
Desmoplastic infantile ganglioglioma (DIG), 263, 264, 265
Development; *see also* Fetal development; Myelination, normal development
  myelination, normal, 498–508
  normal, 122–123
Developmental abnormalities; *see* Congenital/developmental abnormalities
Developmental tumors, 224; *see also* Cysts and tumor-like lesions; Mass lesions
Devic's disease, 548, 549
Diabetes
  and atrophy, 542
  temporal bone osteomyelitis, 627
Diaphragma sellae, 18, 76*f*
Diastematomyelia, 127*t*, 131
Diencephalon, 91
  normal development, 122
  projection fibers, 91
Diffuse axonal injury (DAI), 194–195, 194*f*
Diffuse cerebral atrophy, 649
Diffuse cerebral edema, 597, 650, 665
Diffuse meningeal enhancement, 660–661
Diffuse necrotizing leukoencephalopathy (DNL), 555–556
Dilantin
  calvarial/skull abnormalities, 577, 578
  cerebellar atrophy, 650
  cerebral atrophy, 649
  subarachnoid space enlargement, 588
  ventricular pathology, 596

Diploic channels, calvarial/skull abnormalities, 582
Diploic veins, 587*f*
Dissecting aneurysm, 208*f*, 351–352, 398, 403
Disseminated necrotizing leukoencephalopathy (DML), 512
Dolichocephaly, 576
Dolichoectasia
  suprasellar arteries, 612
  vertebrobasilar; *see* Vertebrobasilar dolichoectasia
Doppler ultrasound
  arterial occlusion, 400
  brain death, 204
  in stroke, 376
Dorsal root ganglia, 468
Dorsomedial nucleus, 92
Down syndrome
  calcification with, 657
  calvarial/skull abnormalities, 576, 577, 580
  foramen magnum abnormalities, 646
Drug abuse, 403, 665
  cerebral atrophy, 649
  cocaine granulomatosis, 633
  MRI patterns, 668
  subarachnoid space enlargement, 588
  toxic encephalopathy, 555
  ventricular pathology, 596
Drugs; *see* Chemotherapy; Medications
Dura, 12*t*
  anatomy, 16*f*, 17–18, 17*t*, 587*f*
  calcification, 656
  Chiari II malformations, 129
  enhancement patterns, 660
  with HIV/AIDS-associated neurosyphilis, 467
  metastasis, 308, 310
    enhancement patterns, 663
    hemangiopericytomas vs., 296
  tentorial apex, 619
Dural carcinomatosis, 591
Dural lesions
  arteriovenous malformations, 358*t*, 360–363, 362*f*
  foramen magnum region, 643
  neurofibromatosis, type I, 166
Dural plaques, 656
Dural sinuses, 73–79, 74*f*, 75*f*, 76*f*, 77*f*, 78*f*
  anatomy of, 587*f*
  enhancement patterns, 660
Dural sinus thrombosis, occlusion, 406–410
  enhancement patterns, 661
  ependymal enhancement, 440, 602
  ventricular pathology, 596
Dural tail, 316, 327, 501
  cerebellopontine angle meningioma, 625
  enhancing, 663
  meningiomas, 294

Duret hemorrhage, 203
Dyke-Davidoff-Masson syndrome, 452, 650
  calvarial/skull abnormalities, 575, 578
  ventricular pathology, 595
Dysembryoplastic neuroepithelial tumor
    (DNET), 265–266
  cortical, 652
  ganglioglioma vs., 264
Dysmyelinating diseases, 512, 518–526; *see
    also* Leukodystrophies
  calvarial/skull abnormalities, 575
  MRI patterns, 668
Dysplasias
  calvarial/skull abnormalities, 575, 577, 580
  gray matter, 150
Dysplastic gangliocytoma of cerebellum, 161,
    265, 655

E

Ear
  congenital malformations, 626
  internal auditory canal anatomy, 6*f*, 9, 622*f*
  internal auditory canal lesions, 625–626
  malignant otitis externa, 626, 627–628, 639,
      640
  otitis media, 627, 636
  skull base lesions, 639, 640
Echinococcosis, 492–493, 656
Echovirus, 443
Eclampsia, 217, 548, 568, 664
Ectopic neurohypophysis, 610, 612
Edema
  with abscess, 437
  deep white matter, 548
  meningiomas, 294
  scalp, 574
  toxoplasma lesions, 462
Electrical injury, 574, 583
Electrolyte disorders
  and basal ganglia degeneration, 568–569
  and myelinolysis, 553–554
Emboli; *see also* Infarct
  corticomedullary junction, 652
  septic, 652, 662
  and stroke, 402
    aneurysm and, 346
    with reperfusion hemorrhage, 664
  white matter degenerative diseases, 546, 547
Embryonal carcinoma, 276, 277, 278, 618
Embryonal remnants, 224
Embryonic circulation, persistent, 41, 42*f*
Empty delta sign, 211
Empty sella, 653
  partial, 610
  pituitary adenomas vs., 283
  Rathke's cleft cyst vs., 287
Empyema, subdural, 430–432
Encephalitis, 443–454, 551
  astrocytomas vs., 234

Encephalitis—cont'd
  basal ganglia degeneration, 569
  Creutzfeldt-Jakob disease, 453–454
  defined, 443
  with HIV/AIDS, 459, 460
    cytomegalovirus, 466
    toxoplasmosis, 462
    tuberculous, 469
  Lyme disease, 445–446
  MRI patterns, 669
  Rasmussen encephalitis, 451–452
  Reye's syndrome, 452–453
  secondary (post-infectious)
    acute disseminated encephalomyelitis,
        450–451
    progressive multifocal leukencephalopa-
        thy (PML), 449–450
    subacute sclerosing panencephalitis
        (SSPE), 448–449
  tuberculous, 474
  viral
    herpes simplex (non-neonatal), 443–445
    poliovirus, 447
Encephalomalacia
  focal, 595
  after herpes simplex encephalitis, 445
  with HIV/AIDS-associated toxoplasmosis,
      463
  meningitis and, 427
Encephalomyelitis
  acute disseminated; *see* Acute disseminated
      encephalomyelitis
  and basal ganglia degeneration, 569
Encephalomyelopathy, subacute necrotizing,
    532
Encephalopathy
  and basal ganglia degeneration, 568
  cerebral atrophy, 649
  cytomegalovirus, 466
  delayed, with carbon monoxide poisoning,
      554
  with HIV/AIDS, 459, 466
  hypertensive, 548
  hypoxic-ischemic, 547
  toxic, 552–555
  Wernicke, 552
Enchondroma, skull base lesions, 637–638,
    640
Endocrine disorders, calcification with, 656,
    657
Endodermal cyst, 330–331
Endodermal sinus (yolk sac) tumor, 276, 277,
    278
Enhancement, 656, 660–663
  calvarial/skull abnormalities, 580
  in disseminated encephalomyelitis, 451
  ependymal, 602; *see also* Ependymal en-
      hancement
  with hemorrhage and hematoma, 592

Enhancement—cont'd
  with HIV/AIDS, 458
    lymphomas, 471
    neurosyphilis, 468
    tuberculous, 470
  with infections
    herpes simplex encephalitis, 445
    with tuberculosis, 470, 476
  Langerhans cell histiocytosis, 480
  leptomeningeal metastases, 591
  meningeal, 589–591, 660–661
  in multiple sclerosis, 550
  normally enhancing tissue, 660
  sarcoid, 477, 478
Enterogenous cyst, 156t, 330–331
Entorhinal complex, Alzheimer disease, 562
Eosinophilic granuloma, 582
Ependyma, sarcoid, 477
Ependymal cells, 231
Ependymal cyst, 651
  third ventricle, 618
  ventricular mass lesions, 599
Ependymal enhancement, 602, 661
  differential diagnosis of, 440
  with HIV/AIDS-associated tuberculous,
    470
  with sarcoid, 478
  ventricles, 602
Ependymal tumors, 254–258, 255f
Ependymitis, 661; see also
    Ventriculitis/ependymitis
  cytomegalovirus, 466
  enhancement patterns, 602, 661
  HIV/AIDS, 459, 466
  toxoplasmosis, 419
Ependymoblastoma, 275–276
Ependymoma, 224, 225, 226f, 225, 227, 228,
    231, 247, 254–257, 255f, 651
  calcification with, 657
  cerebellopontine angle, 623t
  CSF dissemination, 591
  in differential diagnosis
    of astrocytomas, 242
    of choroid plexus tumors, 260
    of medulloblastomas, 273, 274
    of meningiomas, 295
    of primary cerebral neuroblastomas, 275
    of schwannoma, 316
    of subependymomas, 258
  enhancement patterns, 660, 661
  ependymal enhancement, 440, 602
  foramen magnum region, 643, 645f, 646
  fourth ventricular, 244f
  leptomeningeal infiltration, 308
  periventricular/callosal, 652
  posterior fossa, 655
  temporal bone lesions, 628
  ventricular pathology, 599, 600
Epidermal nevus syndromes, 179

Epidermoid, 323t, 325–327, 227, 651, 654,
    655; see also Dermoid/epidermoid
Epidural abscess, 430–432
  foramen magnum region, 646
  meningitis and, 427
Epidural empyema, 427
Epidural hematoma (EDH), 190–192, 191f
  foramen magnum region, 646
  subarachnoid space enlargement, 588
Epidural space
  anatomy of, 17, 18–19, 587f
  tuberculomas, 475
Epithalamus, 93
Epithelial membrane antigen (EMA), 290
Epstein Barr virus, 450
  meningitis, 429
  Rasmussen encephalitis, 452
Equine encephalitis, 443
Esthesioneuroblastoma, 633
Ethmoid foramina, anatomy, 6f, 10f, 14
Ethmoid sinuses, 666
Ewing's osteosarcoma, 584
Exophytic brainstem glioma, 598, 599
Exophytic cerebellar/brainstem astrocytoma,
    623t
External auditory canal, 9
External auditory canal atresia, 626
External carotid artery and branches, 31f,
    32–37, 33f, 34f, 40
  anastomoses, 35
  ascending pharyngeal artery, 33–34, 33f,
    34f
  collateral circulation, 393
  facial artery, 33f, 34f, 35
  innervation, 37
  lingual artery, 33f, 34–35, 34f
  maxillary artery, 33f, 34f, 36–37
  occipital artery, 33f, 34f, 35–36
  posterior auricular artery, 33f, 34f, 36
  superficial temporal artery, 33f, 34f, 36
  superior thyroid artery, 32–33, 33f, 34f
External hydrocephalus, 586, 588
External jugular bulb, 77f
External jugular vein, 77f
Extraaxial pathology, 586–593, 587f
  fluid collections, 586–588, 587f
  mass lesions, 587f, 588–589
  meningeal pathology, 589–593
    enhancement, 589–590
    infection, 590
    inflammation, 590–591
    metabolic, chemical, toxins, 592
    miscellaneous, 592–593
    neoplasia, 591–592
    trauma, surgery, vascular, 592
Extradural lesions, foramen magnum region,
    643, 646
Extradural space, 18–19
Extramedullary intradural mass lesions, 643

Extraosseus intradural chordoma, 644
Extrapontine myelinolysis, 553–554
Eye
  infections
    HIV/AIDS-associated cytomegalovirus,
      467
    HIV/AIDS-associated neurosyphilis,
      468
    rubella, 422, 423
    toxoplasmosis, 419
  motor cortex, 88f, 89
  neurofibromatosis, type I, 166
  sarcoid, 477
  Sturge-Weber syndrome, 172, 173
  von Hippel-Lindau syndrome, 174
  Wilson's disease, 533

F

Facial anomalies
  with corpus callosum abnormalities, 136
  holoprosencephalies, 142, 142t, 143, 144
Facial artery
  anatomy, 33f, 34f, 35
  collateral circulation, 393
Facial nerve, 102f, 103f, 111–113, 623, 626
  apertures of skull base, 12t
  foramina, 10f
  sarcoid, 477
Facial nerve palsy, 626
Facial schwannoma, 315
  cerebellopontine angle, 625
  temporal bone lesions, 628
Fahr disease, 657
Falx, enhancement patterns, 660
Falx cerebelli, 17–18
Falx cerebri, 16f, 17, 587f
  Chiari II malformations, 129
  holoprosencephalies, 142t
Familial degeneration of striatum, 569
Fasciitis, scalp, 574
Fat
  MRI patterns, 667
  sarcoid, 477
Fat-Density Lesions, 665
Fat graft, 610
Ferritin, 543
Fetal circulation
  persistent, 41, 42f, 43, 44
  posterior communicating artery, 51
Fetal development
  abnormal, 123–124
  myelination, normal, 498–499, 501f
  normal, 122–123
Fibrillary astrocytomas, 232, 245
  ependymomas vs., 256
  morphologic patterns, 651
Fibrinoid leukodystrophy; see Alexander dis-
    ease
Fibroma, meningeal, 298

Fibromuscular dysplasia, 342, 398, 399, 403
Fibrosarcoma
  calvarial/skull abnormalities, 580, 584
  meningeal, 298
Fibrous dysplasia
  calvarial/skull abnormalities, 575, 577, 578,
    579, 584
  meningiomas vs., 294
  skull base lesions, 634, 638, 640
Fibrous histiocytoma, meningeal, 298
Fibroxanthoma, meningeal, 298
Figure of eight appearance, pituitary adenoma,
    612
Fistulas, cavernous sinus and skull base, 614
Flap failure, 583
Flexures, normal development, 122
Flow dynamics, aneurysm, 345, 346f
Flow-related enhancement, 667
Flow-related vasculopathy, and arterial steno-
    sis, 400
Fluid attenuated inversion recovery (FLAIR),
    216
Fluid collections, extraaxial, 586–588, 587f
Fluorosis, 578
5-Fluorouracil, 555
Focal encephalomalacia, 595
Fontanelles
  anatomy, 8, 8f
  calvarial/skull abnormalities, 581, 583
Foramen lacerum, 11f, 13t
Foramen magnum, 13t
  Chiari II malformations, 129
  lesions of, 643–646, 645f
Foramen of Luschka (lateral aperture), 20f,
    22, 26f, 625, 628
Foramen of Magendie (median aperture), 20f,
    22, 26f, 628
Foramen of Monro, 595
  anatomy, 19, 20f, 21
  CSF circulation, 26f, 27
  mass lesions in adults, 598
  obstruction of, 199, 200f, 650
  subependymal giant-cell astrocytoma, 171,
    246
  ventricular mass lesions in children, 599
Foramen ovale, 6f, 10f, 11f, 12t
Foramen ovale plexus, 75f
Foramen rotundum, 6f, 10f, 12t, 13t
Foramen spinosum, 6f, 10f, 11, 11f, 12t
Foramina
  anatomy, 6f, 9–14, 10f, 11f, 12–13t
  calvarial/skull abnormalities, 580, 581
  central skull base, 635
  CSF circulation, 26f, 27
Forebrain
  anatomy, 84–93, 84f, 86–87f, 88f
  normal development, 122
Fourth ventricle, 595
  anatomy, 22, 622f

Fourth ventricle—cont'd
  aneurysms, 349
  communications, 21
  CSF circulation, 26*f*
  enhancement patterns, 660
Fourth ventricle lesions, 628–629
  astrocytomas, 243*f*
  cerebellopontine angle involvement, 625,
    628, 629
  cisternal involvement, 644
  differential diagnosis of posterior fossa ab-
    normalities, 155*t*, 655
  ependymoma, 244*f*, 255*f*
  foramen magnum region, 643, 645*f*
  mass lesions in adults, 598
  mass lesions in children, 599
  subependymomas, 257
  temporal bone involvement, 628
Fractures
  calvarial/skull abnormalities, 575, 582, 583
  foramen magnum region, 646
  skull base lesions, 633
  surgical defect, 582
  temporal bone, 628
  and vascular occlusion, 399
Frontal bone
  anatomy, 4, 5*f*, 6*f*
  foramina, 9
Frontal eye area, 88*f*, 89
Frontal horn
  mass lesions in adults, 598
  mass lesions in children, 599
Frontal lobe
  Alexander disease, 519
  inherited metabolic disorders, 514
  normal anatomy, 84*f*, 85
  toxoplasma lesions, HIV/AIDS-related, 462
Frontal lobe ganglioma, bone destruction, 634
Frontal sinus, 580, 666
Frontal sinus osteoma, 633
Fukuyama syndrome, 147
Fungal abscess, 436, 460
Fungal cerebritis, 665
Fungal granuloma, 662, 667
Fungal infection, 483–487
  and abscess, 436, 460
  and arterial occlusion, 401
  aspergillosis, 483–484
  calcification, 656
  calcification with, 658
  calvarial/skull abnormalities, 583
  candidiasis, 486–487
  cavernous sinus and skull base, 614
  coccidiomycosis, 487
  cryptococcosis, 485–486
  enhancement patterns, 590, 660, 662
  with HIV/AIDS, 457, 459, 460
  mucormycosis, 485
  skull base lesions, 635, 638

Fungal meningitis, 665
  enhancement patterns, 660
  meningeal enhancement with, 590
  suprasellar, 613
Fungal sinusitis, 635, 638
Fungal vasculitis, 401
Fusiform aneurysms, 351

G

Gadolinium, 667
Galea aponeurotica, 16*f*, 587*f*
Gangliocytoma
  astrocytomas vs., 234
  dysembryoplastic neuroepithelial tumor vs.,
    266
  dysplastic, of cerebellum, 161, 265, 655
  Lhermitte-Duclos syndrome, 161
  posterior fossa, 161
Ganglioglioma, 651
  calcification with, 657
  calvarial/skull abnormalities, 584
  in differential diagnosis
    of astrocytomas, 245
    of dysembryoplastic neuroepithelial tu-
      mor, 266
    of hemangioblastoma, 298
    of oligodendroglial tumors, 254
    of pleomorphic xanthoastrocytoma, 246
  enhancement patterns, 662
Ganglioma
  frontal lobe, 634
  skull base lesions, 634
Ganglion cell tumors, 263–265
Gangliosidoses, 516
Genetic disorders; *see also* Inherited metabolic and degenerative disorders
  brain malformations, 123
  multiple sclerosis vs., 551
Geniculate ganglion, 626
Germ cell tumors, 224, 226*f*, 276–279
  germinoma vs., 278
  pineal, 616*f*, 617, 618
Germinal matrix hemorrhage, 214–215, 601
Germinoma, 224, 226*f*, 228, 276, 277–278
  astrocytomas vs., 245
  basal ganglia, 653
  CSF dissemination, 591
  in differential diagnosis
    of craniopharyngioma vs., 286
    of germ cell tumor, 278
    of hypothalamic hamartoma, 334
    of pineoblastoma, 269
    of pineocytoma, 268
    of pituitary adenoma, 284
  enhancement patterns, 660, 661
  ependymal enhancement, 440, 602
  midline, 653
  morphologic patterns, 650
  pineal, 616*f*, 617, 618, 619

Germinoma—cont'd
  suprasellar, 613
  ventricular abnormalities, 598, 599, 601,
    602
Gerstmann-Straussler-Schenker syndrome,
    454, 566
Giant aneurysm, ventricular abnormalities
    from, 601
Giant-cell astrocytoma, 650
  calvarial/skull abnormalities, 580
  colloid cyst vs., 329
  subependymal, 171, 246–247
  subependymomas vs., 258
  ventricular pathology, 598, 599, 600
Giant MS plaque, 238
Glial fibrillary acidic protein (GFAP), 232
Glial tumors, 224; *see also specific tumors*
  astrocytic; *see* Astrocytomas; *specific tu-
    mor types*
  nonastrocytic, 253–260, 255f
    choroid plexus tumors, 258–260
    ependymomas, 254–257, 255f
    oligodendroglial, 253–254
    subependymomas, 257–258
Glioblastoma multiforme, 235–238, 236f, 298,
    598, 665
  arteriovenous malformation vs., 360
  enhancement patterns, 660, 661, 662, 663
  ependymal enhancement, 440, 602
  gliosarcomas vs., 249
  with HIV/AIDS, 458, 459, 460, 471
  periventricular/callosal, 653
  pineal, 618
  skull base lesions, 634
  ventricular abnormalities from, 598, 601
Glioma, 224, 225, 226f; *see also* Astrocyto-
    mas
  cerebellopontine angle cistern involvement,
    628, 629
  foramen magnum region, 643, 644
  germ cell tumor vs., 278
  with HIV/AIDS, 471
  midline, 653
  MRI patterns, 669
  nasal, 135
  neurofibromatosis type I, 165
  pineal, 618
  pineocytoma vs., 268
  pontine, 244f
  posterior fossa, 654, 655
  sellar/juxtasellar region, 609t, 613
  tectal, 618
  ventricular abnormalities from, 598, 599,
    601
  white matter lesion differential diagnosis,
    546
Gliomatosis, primary leptomeningeal, 249–
    250
Gliomatosis cerebri, 247–248

Gliosarcoma, 248–249, 298
Gliosis
  with abscess, 437
  chemotherapeutic agents and, 555
Global ischemia/hypoxia, 383
  calcification with, 658
  cerebral atrophy, 649
  ventricular pathology, 596
Globoid cell leukodystrophy (GLD)/Krabbe'
    disease, 511, 512, 513, 514, 515, 519,
    520–521, 534
Globus pallidus, 91, 665
  calcification, 656
  carbon monoxide poisoning, 554
  iron in, 538, 543, 543
Glomus jugulare, 628, 640
Glomus jugulotympanicum, 319, 628
Glomus of lateral ventricular trigone, calcifi-
    cation, 656
Glomus tumor, 318–319
  skull base lesions, 640
  temporal bone lesions, 628
Glomus tympanicum, 319, 628
Glomus vagale, 319
Glossopharyngeal (IX) nerve, 102f, 103f,
    114–115
  apertures of skull base, 12t
  foramina, 10f
Glutaric acidemias, 535
Glycogen storage disease, 511, 514, 515
Gonadotroph adenoma, 282
Gorlin syndrome, 179, 656
Gradenigo syndrome, 626, 627
Granular cell tumor, 611, 613
Granulocytic sarcoma, 305
  germ cell tumor differential diagnosis, 278
  suprasellar, 613
Granulomas, 667
  calcification with, 658
  enhancement patterns, 662
    meningeal enhancement, 591
    ring-enhancing lesions, 439
  with HIV/AIDS-associated infections
    neurosyphilis, 467
    tuberculosis, 469
Granulomatous angiitis, 402
Granulomatous disease, 474–480
  Langerhans cell histiocytosis, 479–480
  meningitis, chronic, 430
  neurosarcoid, 476–478
  skull base lesions, 633, 635, 638
  tuberculosis, 474–476
  Wegener's granulomatosis, 478–479
Granulomatous hypophysitis, 612
GRASS sequences, 185
Gray matter
  age-related changes, 538, 542–543
  heterotopic, 144, 147–151, 650
  in multiple sclerosis, 549

Gray matter disorders, 511
  acquired, 561–569
    Alzheimer disease, 561–564
    basal ganglia disorders, 568–569
    cortical atrophy, 564
    Creutzfeld-Jakob disease, 566
    ischemic vascular dementia, 564–565
    miscellaneous cortical dementias,
      564–567
    normal pressure hydrocephalus, 563–564
    Parkinson disease, 566–567
    Pick disease, 565
    subcortical dementias, 567–568
  inherited, 514–516, 528–535
    globoid cell leukodystrophy, 534
    Hallerworden-Spatz disease, 534
    Huntington disease, 532–533
    Leigh disease, 532
    mitochondrial disorders, 534–535
    neuronal ceroid-lipofuscinosis, 529–530
    organic acidurias and acidemias, 535
    Wilson disease, 533–534
    Zellweger syndrome, 531–532
Great cerebral vein, 80
Great vessels, 30–37, 31*f*, 33*f*
  aortic arch, 30, 31*f*
  common carotid artery, left, 31*f*, 32
  common carotid artery bifurcation, 31*f*, 32
  external carotid artery and branches, 31*f*,
    32–37, 33*f*, 34*f*
  innominate artery, 30, 31*f*
  nerve supply, 37
  subclavian artery, left, 31*f*, 32
"Ground glass" appearance, calvarial/skull ab-
    normalities, 579
Group B streptococcus meningitis, 428
Growth hormone adenoma, 282
Guillain-Barre syndrome, 466
Gyral enhancement, 445, 589
Gyri
  anatomy, 84–87, 84*f*, 85*f*
  Chiari II malformations, 130
  normal development, 123
Gyriform cortical enhancement, 661

H

Habenular calcification, 656
Habenular commissure, 91
Hallervorden-Spatz disease, 511, 515, 534,
    665
  basal ganglia lesions, 654
  calcification with, 657
Hamartoma, 224
  calvarial/skull abnormalities, 579
  CT patterns, 664
  dysplastic cerebellar gangliocytoma, 265
  gangliocytomas vs., 264
  hypothalamic, 333–334
  hypothalamic, astrocytomas vs., 245

Hamartoma—cont'd
  morphologic patterns, 650
  with neurofibromatosis, 166
  scalp, 574
  in tuberous sclerosis complex, 170–171
  ventricular abnormalities, 650
  ventricular pathology, 595
Hand-Schuller-Christian disease, 307,
    479–480, 574
Head and neck tumors, 314–320
  carcinoma, 320, 669
  chordoma, 319–320
  enhancement patterns, 663
  neurofibroma, 314*t*, 317
  parasympathetic paraganglioma, 318–319
  peripheral nerve sheath tumors, 318
  schwannoma, 314–317, 314*t*
  enhancement patterns, 663
  sellar/juxtasellar region, cavernous sinus
    and skull base, 614
  skull base lesions, 633, 635, 636, 639
Hemangioblastoma, 225, 226*f*, 227, 296–298,
    651
  cerebellopontine angle cistern involvement,
    629
  cortical, 652
  in differential diagnosis
    of astrocytomas, 245
    of choroid plexus tumors, 260
    of medulloblastomas, 274
  enhancement patterns, 662
  foramen magnum masses, 643
  foramen magnum region, 644, 645*f*
  posterior fossa, 654
  temporal bone lesions, 628
  ventricular abnormalities from, 601
  ventricular mass lesions in adults, 598
  von Hippel-Lindau syndrome, 173–174
Hemangioma
  calvarial/skull abnormalities, 582, 584
  internal auditory canal, 625, 626
  scalp, 574
Hemangiopericytoma, 295–296, 588, 668
  calvarial/skull abnormalities, 584
  in differential diagnosis
    of gliosarcomas, 249
    of meningeal mesenchymal tumors, 299
    of meningiomas, 294
    of plasmacytoma, 307
Hematologic disorders, 664
  calvarial/skull abnormalities, 576, 577, 578
  and intracranial hemorrhage, 218
  malignancies, 303–307; *see also* Leukemia;
    Lymphoma
  and stroke, 403
  and vascular occlusion, 406, 407
Hematoma
  aneurysm rupture and, 345, 347–348*f*
  calcification with, 657, 658

Hematoma—cont'd
  calvarial/skull abnormalities, 579
  CT, 184*f*, 185
  enhancement patterns, 660, 662
  extraaxial abnormalities, 589
  foramen magnum region, 646
  glioblastoma multiforme vs., 237
  paravascular, 208*f*
  parenchymal, 664–665
  ring-enhancing lesions, 439
  scalp, 574
  subarachnoid space enlargement, 588
Hematopoietic tissue, 13, 14
  extramedullary, 589
  fibrous dysplasia; *see* Fibrous dysplasia
  skull base, lymphoma infiltration of, 638
Hemiatrophy, ventricular, 650
Hemimegalencephaly, 150, 248, 650
  calvarial/skull abnormalities, 575
  ventricular pathology, 595
Hemispheric veins, 80, 81*f*
Hemolytic-uremic syndrome, 664
  and basal ganglia degeneration, 568
  and intracranial hemorrhage, 217
Hemorrhage, 667; *see also* Hematoma; Intra-
    cranial hemorrhage; *specific sites*
  aneurysm rupture and, 347–348*f*, 350
  with arteriovenous malformations, 357
  basal ganglia, 653
  with cavernous angioma, 370
  CT patterns, 664
  enhancement patterns, 660, 661
  with HIV/AIDS, 463
  hypertensive, 665
  with infection
    herpes simplex, 421, 445
    toxoplasmosis, 463
  MRI patterns, 667, 669
  reperfusion, 664
  sellar/juxtasellar region, 610
  subarachnoid space enlargement, 588
  ventricular mass lesions, 598, 601
  white matter degenerative diseases, 547
Hemorrhagic infarct
  glioblastoma multiforme vs., 238
  and intracranial hemorrhage, 217
Hemorrhagic metastasis, 665
Hemorrhagic necrosis, pituitary adenoma, 610
Hemorrhagic shearing injury, 664
Hemosiderin, 543, 667
Hepatolenticular degeneration, 533–534
Hepatorenal (Zellweger) syndrome, 514, 515,
    516, 575
Hereditary hemorrhagic telangiectasia (HHT),
    177, 368
Hereditary spherocytosis, 578
Herniation
  cerebral, 199–202, 200*f*, 203
  meningeal, 583

Herniation—cont'd
  tonsillar, 202, 643, 645*f*, 646
  ventricular pathology, 595
Heroin, 555
Herpes simplex viruses, 241, 443
  calcification, 656
  congenital and neonatal infections, 420–422
  encephalitis, non-neonatal, 248, 443–445,
    664
    enhancement patterns, 661
    with HIV/AIDS, 457
    Rasmussen encephalitis, 452
  meningitis, 429
Herpes simplex virus type 2, 457
Herpesviruses; *see also* Cytomegalovirus;
    Epstein-Barr virus; Varicella-zoster
    virus
  meningitis, 429
  Rasmussen encephalitis, 452
Herpes zoster otitis, 626
Heterotopias
  gray matter, 147–151, 148*f*, 149*f*, 150*f*, 151*f*
  with corpus callosum abnormalities, 136
  ventricular margins, 650
  ventricular pathology, 595
High-grade astrocytoma, 665
  CSF dissemination, 591
  enhancement patterns, 660, 661, 662
  primary cerebral neuroblastomas vs., 275
  ring-enhancing lesions, 439
Hindbrain (rhombencephalon)
  anatomy, 94–99
    metencephalon, 94–97, 96*f*, 98*f*
    myencephalon, 98–99
  Chiari II malformations, 129
  normal development, 122, 123
Hippocampal commissure, 91
Hippocampus
  Alzheimer disease, 562, 563
  normal pressure hydrocephalus, 564
Histiocytoma, malignant fibrous, 298
Histiocytosis
  Langerhans cell, 245, 307; *see also* Langer-
    hans cell histiocytosis
  sellar/juxtasellar region, 610
  ventricular mass lesions in children, 599
Histogenesis, 124
Histoplasmosis
  calcification, 656
  enhancement patterns, 662
  with HIV/AIDS, 457, 458
HIV/AIDS
  autoimmune demyelination disorders vs.,
    552
  congenital, 423–424
  enhancement patterns, 662
  encephalopathy, 443, 457, 459–461
    AIDS dementia complex, 457, 460
    cerebral atrophy, 649

HIV/AIDS—cont'd
  encephalopathy—cont'd
    parenchymal involvement, 458
    progressive multifocal leukoencephalopa-
        thy, 449
    subarachnoid space enlargement, 588
    ventricular pathology, 596
  meningitis, 429
HIV infection, manifestations of, 457–471
  agents causing infections with, 457–458
    cryptococcosis, 463–464
    cytomegalovirus, 466–467
    mycobacterial infections, 468–470
    neurosyphilis, 467–468
    toxoplasmosis, 461–463, 463t
  AIDS dementia complex, 457, 460
  HIV infection of CNS, 459–461
  neoplastic diseases, 458–459
    glioma, 471
    lymphoma, 470–471
  progressive multifocal leukoencephalopathy,
      464–466
Holoprosencephaly, 142–144, 142t, 143f
  calvarial/skull abnormalities, 575
  cephaloceles with, 134
  with corpus callosum abnormalities, 136
  ventricular pathology, 595
Horner syndrome, 398
Hot spots, suprasellar, 610
Human chorionic gonadotropin, 276
Hunter disease, 513
Huntington disease, 515, 532–533
  basal ganglia lesions, 654
  cerebral atrophy, 649
  juvenile, 511
  subarachnoid space enlargement, 588
  ventricular pathology, 595, 596
Hurler disease, 513
Hyaline eosinophilic rods (Rosenthal fibers),
    525
Hydatid disease, 492–493, 651, 659
Hydrocephalus, 650
  aneurysm and, 350
  calvarial/skull abnormalities, 575, 576, 577,
      580, 581
  Chiari I malformations, 126, 127t
  Chiari II malformations, 127t, 131
  with choroid plexus tumors, 258–259
  with Dandy-Walker malformation, 154, 155t
  extraaxial abnormalities, 586, 588, 599
  with infection
    HIV/AIDS-associated tuberculous, 469
    meningitis, 427
    meningitis, chronic, 430
    meningitis, neonatal, 429
    toxoplasmosis, 419
    tuberculosis, 475, 476
  with malignancy
    meningeal malignant melanoma, 299

Hydrocephalus—cont'd
  with malignancy—cont'd
    metastases, 309–310
  normal pressure, 563–564, 596
  with sarcoid, 478
  sellar expansion, 612
  with subarachnoid hemorrhage, 216
  ventricular pathology, 440, 596, 597
  with vermian-cerebellar hypoplasia,
      158
Hydromyelia, 126, 127t
Hydrosyringomelia, 643, 645
Hypercalcemia
  calcification, 656
  calvarial/skull abnormalities, 576
  of malignancy, 656
Hyperdense basilar cisterns, 665
Hyperdense (noncalcified) focal mass, 664,
    665
Hyperostosis, blistering, 579
Hyperostosis frontalis interna, 577, 578
Hyperparathyroidism
  calcification with, 656, 657, 658
  calvarial/skull abnormalities, 576, 578, 581,
      582, 584
Hyperphosphatasia, 575
Hypertension, 664
  and atrophy, 542
  and basal ganglia degeneration, 568
  eclampsia, 217, 548, 568, 664
  intracranial; see Increased intracranial pres-
      sure
  and intracranial hemorrhage, 217, 665
Hypertensive encephalopathy, 548
Hypertensive hemorrhage, 665
  basal ganglia, 653
  glioblastoma multiforme vs., 238
Hypertensive vascular disease, 664
Hyperthyroidism, 576
Hypervitaminosis A, 576
Hypervitaminosis D, 576, 578, 656
Hypodensity in basal ganglia, 665
Hypoglossal artery, 42f
Hypoglossal canal, 6f, 10f, 11f, 13t
Hypoglossal (XII) nerve, 102f, 103f,
    117–118
  apertures of skull base, 10f, 12t
  spinal roots, 644
Hypoglycemia, and basal ganglia degenera-
    tion, 569
Hypomelanosis of Ito, 151
Hypoparathyroidism
  calcification with, 656, 657
  calvarial/skull abnormalities, 576, 578
Hypophosphatasia, 576, 577, 581
Hypophysectomy, 610
Hypophysis; see Pituitary gland
Hypophysitis, granulomatous, 612
Hypotension, intracranial, 128, 592

Hypothalamic-chiasmatic glioma; *see also* opticochiasmatic-hypothalamic glioma, 228, 245, 260
  calcification with, 658
  midline, 653
  ventricular abnormalities from, 601
Hypothalamic glioma, 609*t*
Hypothalamic hamartoma, 245, 333–334
  craniopharyngioma vs., 286
  germ cell tumor differential diagnosis, 278
  midline, 653
Hypothalamic hormone transport disturbances, 610
Hypothalamic-pituitary dysfunction, with holoprosencephaly, 144
Hypothalamic releasing factors, 612
Hypothalamus, 92, 607
  Langerhans cell histiocytosis, 307, 479
  neoplasms and mass lesions, 260, 601, 609*t*, 653, 658
    developmental abnormalities, 245, 286, 333–334
    germ cell tumor, 276–279
    hamartoma; *see* Hypothalamic hamartoma
    ventricular mass lesions, 598, 599
  normal development, 122
  venous system, 76*f*
Hypothyroidism
  calcification with, 657
  calvarial/skull abnormalities, 576, 577
Hypoxia/ischemia, 202–203, 665; *see also* Infarct
  acute cerebral ischemia and infarction, 375–378
  basal ganglia lesions, 654
  calcification with, 658
  cerebral atrophy, 649
  MRI patterns, 668
  subarachnoid space enlargement, 588
  ventricular pathology, 596
  white matter degenerative diseases, 547
Hypoxic/ischemic encephalopathy, 547
  and basal ganglia degeneration, 568
  with HIV/AIDS, 459

I

Iatrogenic lesions, 666
  basal ganglia degeneration, 569
  calcification with, 657, 658
  calvarial/skull abnormalities, 575, 578
  cerebellar atrophy, 650
  cerebral atrophy, 649
  enhancement patterns, 661
  epidermoid tumor, 325
  infection, postoperative, 431
  MRI patterns, 667, 668
  pituitary apoplexy, 611
  pituitary hyperplasia, 612
  and Reyes syndrome, 452

Iatrogenic lesions—cont'd
  subarachnoid space enlargement, 588
  and tonsillar herniation, 646
  ventricular pathology, 596
  white matter disorders, 555–556
Ibuprofen, 592
Ice-cream cone appearance, schwannomas, 624*t*, 625, 626
I-cell disease, 513
Idiopathic hypertrophic pachymeningitis, 593, 661
Idiopathic megalencephaly, 575
Idiopathic micrencephaly, 575
Idiopathic progressive arteriopathy of childhood, 397, 403
Immune complexes
  and arterial occlusion, 401
  in Lyme disease, 445
Immunization
  and acute disseminated encephalomyelitis, 450
  autoimmune demyelination, 551–552
  white matter lesion differential diagnosis, 546
Immunoblastic lymphoma, 470
Immunosuppression
  and infection, 436
  progressive multifocal leukoencephalopathy with, 449
  skull base lesions, 638
  and temporal bone osteomyelitis, 627
Inborn errors of metabolism, 511–516
Inclusion cyst, calvarial/skull abnormalities, 583
Increased intracranial pressure
  calvarial/skull abnormalities, 576, 580, 581
  sellar expansion, 612
  and tonsillar herniation, 646
  ventricular pathology, 597
Infantile cortical hyperostosis, 578
Infants; *see also* Neonates; Premature infants
  basal ganglia degeneration, 569
  fontanelles, 8, 8*f*
  intracranial hemorrhages, 214–215
  normal myelination, 503–507, 504*f*, 506*f*
  ventriculitis/ependymitis, 440
  watershed infarctions, 547
Infarct, 664; *see also* Stroke
  acute cerebral ischemia, 375–378
  aneurysm rupture and, 345, 347–348*f*
  basal ganglia lesions, 568, 653
  calcification in, 657
  cerebral, 203
  corticomedullary junction, 652
  in differential diagnosis
    of astrocytomas, 234, 235
    of dysplastic cerebellar gangliocytoma, 265
  enhancement patterns, 661, 662

Infarct—cont'd
  with HIV/AIDS
    neurosyphilis, 468
    tuberculous, 470
  lacunar, 665
  meningeal enhancement with, 592
  with meningitis, 427, 429, 430
  MRI patterns, 668, 669
  posterior fossa, 654
  ring-enhancing lesions, 439
  with sarcoid, 477, 478
  tectal, 618
  venous; *see* Venous infarct
  virus infections and, 443
  white matter degenerative diseases, 547
Infection, 651, 667; *see also* Encephalitis;
      Granulomatous disease; Virus infections
  actinomycetes, 487–489
  congenital and neonatal, 416–423; *see also*
        TORCH infections
    cytomegalovirus, 416–418
    herpes simplex virus, 420–422
    HIV, 423–424
    rubella, 422–423
    toxoplasmosis, 418–420
  fungal, 483–487
  gray matter disorders, acquired, 566
  with HIV/AIDS, 457–458
    cryptococcosis, 463–464
    cytomegalovirus, 466–467
    mycobacterial infections, 468–470
    neurosyphilis, 467–468
    toxoplasmosis, 461–463, 463*t*
  meningitis and complications, 426–432, 590
  parasite, 489–493
Infection/inflammation, 664; *see also*
      Encephalitis; Inflammation
  abscess, 436–439
  and aneurysm, 341
  and autoimmune demyelinating disorders,
      551–552
  and basal ganglia degeneration, 569
  brain malformations, 123
  calcification with, 656, 658
  calvarial/skull abnormalities, 579, 583
  cerebellopontine angle, 623
  cerebritis, 435–436
  corticomedullary junction, 652
  enhancement patterns, 660, 661, 662, 663
  ependymal enhancement, 602
  foramen magnum region, 646
  meningeal enhancement with, 590
  MRI patterns, 668, 669
  pneumocephalus, 666
  post-infectious encephalopathies, 448–451
  posterior fossa, 654, 655
  scalp, 574
  sellar/juxtasellar region, 606*f*
    cavernous sinus and skull base, 614

Infection/inflammation—cont'd
  sellar/juxtasellar region—cont'd
    pituitary, 611–612
    suprasellar, 613
  skull base lesions
    anterior, 632–633
    central, 638
    posterior, 640
  and stroke, 403
  subarachnoid space enlargement, 588
  temporal bone lesions, 627–628
  toxoplasma lesions, 462
  and vascular occlusion, 401, 406, 407
  ventricular pathology, 596, 601
  ventriculitis/ependymitis, 661; *see also*
        Ependymitis; Ventriculitis/ependymitis
Infectious mononucleosis, 450
Inferior cerebellar arteries, stroke, 380–381*f*,
      383–384
Inferior colliculus, 93, 94
Inferior olive
  atrophy, 649
  cerebellorubral degeneration, 557
Inferior ophthalmic vein, 75*f*
Inferior petrosal sinus, 74*f*, 75*f*, 79
Inferior sagittal sinus (ISS), 73, 74*f*, 77*f*
Inferior vermian vein, 80, 81*f*
Inflammation; *see also* Granulomatous
      disease; Infection/inflammation
  and basal ganglia degeneration, 569
  cerebral atrophy, 649
  enhancement patterns, 660
  internal auditory canal, 626
  meningeal enhancement with, 590–591
  subarachnoid space enlargement, 588
  suprasellar, 613
  and vascular occlusion, 400–402
  ventricular pathology, 596
  white matter lesion differential diagnosis,
      546
Inflammatory bowel disease, 406, 407
Inflammatory cyst, posterior fossa, 156*t*
Infratentorial lesions, tuberculomas, 475
Infundibular nucleus, 92
Infundibular stalk lesions, 598, 599
Infundibuloma, 613
Infundibulum
  enhancement patterns, 660
  Langerhans cell histiocytosis, 479
  lipoma, 612
  mass lesions, 613
  normal anatomy, 605–606, 606*f*
  stalk resection, 611
  venous system, 76*f*
Inherited metabolic and degenerative disor-
      ders, 511–516
  and basal ganglia degeneration, 569
  cerebral atrophy, 649
  dys- vs. *de*myelination, 512

Inherited metabolic and degenerative
    disorders—cont d
gray matter, 528–535
inherited vs. acquired, 511–512
of organelles, 512–514
    lysosomes, 512–513
    mitochondria, 514
    peroxisomes, 513–514
patterns of involvement, 514–516
white matter, 518–526
white matter lesion differential diagnosis,
    546
Innervation, carotid artery and branches, 37
Innominate artery, 30, 31*f*
Interclinoid ligament calcification, 656
Internal auditory canal anatomy, 6*f*, 9, 622*f*
Internal auditory canal lesions, 625–626
Internal carotid artery, 40–46, 40*f*, 42*f*, 42*f*,
    52*f*, 56*f*, 60*f*
aberrant, 626
anastomoses, 35
aneurysms, 343, 344*f*
atherosclerosis, 388
calcification, 656
cavernous, 43–44
cavernous sinuses, 77*f*, 78
cervical, 40–41
circle of Willis, 50, 50*f*
dissection, 398
dolichoectasia, 612
embryonic anastomoses, 41, 42*f*
foramina, 10*f*
idiopathic progressive arteriopathy of child-
    hood, 397
innervation, 37
intracranial, 44–46
left, 50, 50*f*
petrous, 41–43
posterior fossa artery variants, 70
right, 50, 50*f*
sellar meningiomas and, 611
skull base lesions, 636
stenosis, congenital causes, 397
traumatic injury, 209
Internal cerebral veins (ICV), 80
anatomy, 74*f*, 80, 77*f*, 78*f*
thrombosis, 411
Internal jugular bulb, 78*f*
Internal jugular vein, 75*f*, 78*f*
Internal maxillary artery, 41
Interpeduncular cistern, 23*f*, 24*t*, 26
Interpeduncular fossa, 93
Intraaxial lesions, 194, 628–629
Intracanalicular acoustic schwannoma, 625
Intracranial hemorrhage
aneurysm rupture and, 347–348*f*
CT vs. MR appearance
    acute, 184–186, 184*f*, 185*t*
    chronic, 186

Intracranial hemorrhage—contd
CT vs. MR appearance—cont'd
    subacute, 185
nontraumatic
    elderly adults, 217–219
    perinatal, 214–215
    young, middle-aged adults, 216–217
Intracranial hypotension, 128, 592
Intracranial pressure
decreased, 128, 592
increased; *see* Increased intracranial pressure
Intradural chordoma, 644
Intradural masses, foramen magnum region,
    643
Intramural hematoma, dissecting, 210
Intraosseus meningioma, 579
Intrathecal medications, 592, 661
Intrauterine exposure; *see*
    Congenital/developmental abnormalities
Intraventricular hemorrhage, 196, 601
Intraventricular hydrocephalus, 650
Inverting papilloma, skull base lesions, 633
Ion imbalance
and basal ganglia degeneration, 568–569
and myelinolysis, 553–554
Iron, 554
age-related changes, 538, 539*f*, 543
MRI patterns, 667
Iron deficiency anemia, calvarial/skull abnor-
    malities, 578
Ischemia, 202–203; *see also* Hypoxia/
    ischemia; Infarct; Stroke
Ischemic vascular dementia; *see* Multiinfarct
    dementia
Ischemic vasculopathy, with rubella, 422

J

Jakob-Creutzfeldt disease; *see* Creutzfeldt-
    Jakob disease
Joubert syndrome, 158, 160
Jugular bulb, 77*f*, 78*f*, 639
Jugular bulb dehiscence, 627
Jugular foramen, 639
Jugular foramen anatomy, 6*f*, 10*f*, 11*f*, 13*t*
Jugular foramen tumors, 645*f*
Jugular tubercles, cerebellopontine angle, 623
Jugular vein thrombosis, skull base lesions,
    639
Juvenile Huntington disease, 511
Juvenile nasopharyngeal angiofibroma, 635,
    637
Juxtacortical tumor, 579
Juxtasellar aneurysm, 284
Juxtasellar internal carotid artery, 40*f*, 43–44
Juxtasellar lesions, 614

K

Kallmann syndrome, 144
Kaposi's sarcoma, 458, 460, 574

Kearns-Sayre syndrome (KSS), 534, 535
Keyser-Fleischer rings, 533
Kleebattschadel, 576
Klippel-Feil syndrome, 126, 127t
Klippel-Trenaunay syndrome, 173
Korsakoff's psychosis, 552
Krabbe' disease (globoid cell leukodystrophy),
    511, 512, 513, 514, 515, 516, 519,
    520–521, 665
Kufs disease, 529

L

Labyrinthitis, 428
Lacunar infarct, 665
    basal ganglia lesions, 653
    neuroepithelial cysts vs., 330
    white matter degenerative diseases, 547
Lacunar skull, 580, 581
Lambdoidal suture defect, 583
Laminar heterotopia, 147–148, 149f
Lamina terminalis cistern, 23f, 25t, 27
Langerhans cell histiocytosis, 307, 479–480,
    588
    astrocytomas vs., 245
    calvarial/skull abnormalities, 584
    cerebellopontine angle, 623
    enhancement patterns, 660, 663
    and hypophysitis, granulomatous, 612
    hypothalamic hamartoma vs., 334
    internal auditory canal, 626
    meningitis, chronic, 430
    posterior fossa, 655
    scalp, 574
    skull base lesions, 638, 640
    suprasellar, 613
    ventricular abnormalities from, 601
Lateral lemniscus, 94
Lateral lenticulostriate artery, 54, 56f
Lateral nucleus, 92
Lateral spinothalamic tract, 94
Lateral sulcus cistern, 27
Lateral superior cisterns, 27
Lateral ventricle, 595
    anatomy, 19–21, 20f
    calcification, 656
    CSF circulation, 26f, 27
    mass lesions in adults, 598
    mass lesions in children, 599
Lead poisoning, 592
    calcification in, 656, 657
    calvarial/skull abnormalities, 576
    enhancement patterns, 660
Leigh disease, 513, 514, 515, 516, 532, 665
    and basal ganglia degeneration, 569
Leiomyoma, meningeal, 298
Lenticulostriate arteries, 50–51, 52, 52f, 54, 56f
    microaneurysm, and intracranial hemor-
        rhage, 217
    stroke, 380–381f, 382

Lentiform nucleus, 91
Leprosy, 635
Leptomeningeal angioma
    ependymal enhancement, 602
    Sturge-Weber syndrome, 172
Leptomeningeal carcinomatosis, ventricular
    pathology, 596
Leptomeningeal cyst, calvarial/skull abnor-
    malities, 581, 582, 583
Leptomeningeal enhancement, 589
    with HIV/AIDS, 458, 468
    Langerhans cell histiocytosis, 480
    with neurosyphilis, 468
    normal, 18
    tumors with, 592
Leptomeningeal fibrosis, benign, 591
Leptomeningeal gliomatosis, primary, 249–250
Leptomeningeal metastases, 309–310, 587f,
    591, 619
    enhancement patterns, 660
    imaging, 309–310
Leptomeningeal sarcomatosis, 292, 298
Leptomeninges
    anatomy, 17t, 18
    cerebellopontine angle tumors, 625
    in cysticercosis, 492
    Langerhans cell histiocytosis, 479
    Sturge-Weber syndrome, 172
    tumor infiltration, 308
Leptomeningitis, MRI, 438
Lethal midline granuloma, 478
Letterer-Siwe disease, 574
Leukemia, 305, 588
    calvarial/skull abnormalities, 576, 578, 584
    enhancement patterns, 660, 661, 663
        ependymal enhancement, 440, 602
        leptomeningeal enhancement, 592
    progressive multifocal leukoencephalopathy
        with, 449
Leukoaraiosis, 411
Leukodystrophies, 248, 511
    adrenoleukodystrophy (ADL), 521–523
    cerebral atrophy, 649
    fibrinoid (Alexander disease), 525–526; see
        also Alexander disease
    globoid cell (GLD), 520–521
    metachromatic (MLD), 518–520
    MRI patterns, 668
    organic acid disorders, 523–524
    spongiform (Canavan disease), 525; see
        also Canavan disease
Leukoencephalopathies
    diffuse necrotizing (DNL), 555–556
    with HIV/AIDS, 460
    inherited, 524–526
    MRI patterns, 668
    nonspecific, 541
    progressive multifocal (PML), 443,
        449–450

Leukoencephalopathies—cont'd
white matter lesion differential diagnosis, 546
Levamisole, 555
Lewy-body disease, 561
Lhermitte-Duclos disease, 161, 265, 655
Lhermitte's sign, 550
Linear sebaceous nevus syndrome, 151
Lingual artery
innervation, 37
Lipidoses, 513, 516
Lipids, organic toxins and, 554
Lipid storage disorders, 516
Lipofucsinosis, 529–530
Lipoma, 224, 332–333, 665
calcification, 656
cerebellopontine angle, 623t, 623
corpus callosum, 139, 140f
internal auditory canal, 625
meningeal, 298
midbrain, 618
midline, 653
morphologic patterns, 650
MRI patterns, 667
periventricular/callosal, 652
pineal, 616f, 617
posterior fossa, 655
quadrigeminal cistern and velum interpositum, 619
scalp, 574
sellar/juxtasellar region
sellar region, 610
skull base lesions, 635, 636
suprasellar, 612
Lisch nodules, 165
Lissencephaly, 147, 148, 418
calvarial/skull abnormalities, 575
cerebral atrophy, 649
subarachnoid space enlargement, 588
ventricular pathology, 596
Locus ceruleus, 95
Louis-Bar syndrome, 177–178
Low-grade astrocytoma
dysembryoplastic neuroepithelial tumor vs., 266
foramen magnum region, 644
gangliocytomas vs., 264
lymphoma vs., 304
Lukenshadel, 580
Lumbar puncture
and Chiari I malformation, 128
and tonsillar herniation, 646
Lumboperitoneal shunts
and tonsillar herniation, 646
Lyme disease, 443, 445–446, 552
Lymphangioma, scalp, 574
Lymphocytic/lymphoid hypophysitis, 284, 611–612
Lymphocytic meningitis, 426

Lymphoma, 225, 226f, 227, 588, 665
basal ganglia, 653
calvarial/skull abnormalities, 576, 578, 584
CSF dissemination, 591
CT patterns, 664
in differential diagnosis
of germ cell tumor, 279
of glioblastoma multiforme, 237
of glioma multiforme, 238
of hypothalamic hamartoma, 334
of white matter lesion, 546
enhancement patterns, 661, 662, 663
ependymal enhancement, 440, 602
leptomeningeal enhancement, 592
hemorrhage with, 463
with HIV/AIDS, 458, 459, 460, 470–471
toxoplasmosis vs., 463, 463t
internal auditory canal, 625, 626
leptomeningeal infiltration, 308
and meningitis, 458
morphologic patterns, 650
MRI patterns, 669
periventricular/callosal, 653
pineal region, 619
primary CNS, 303–304
progressive multifocal leukoencephalopathy with, 449
scalp, 574
secondary CNS, 304–305
skull base lesions, 634, 635, 638, 640
suprasellar masses, 613
tectal, 618
ventricular mass lesions, 601
Lysosomal disorders
globoid cell leukodystrophy, 520–521
inherited, 512–513
metachromatic leukodystrophy, 518–520

M

Macrocephaly, 519, 575
Magnetic resonance angiography
aneurysm, 350–351
arteriovenous malformations, 360
in atherosclerosis, 391
brain death, 204
deep cerebral vein thrombosis, 411
dural sinus thrombosis, 410
Magnetic resonance imaging, 203, 216, 667–669
arteriovenous malformations, 358–359t
Chiari I malformations, 128
cortical contusions, 196
dermoid tumors, 325
diffuse axonal injury, 195
epidermoid tumors, 326–327
epidural hematoma, 191
intracranial hemorrhage, 185, 185t, 186, 187
myelination, normal, 498–508
post-infectious syndromes, 445

Magnetic resonance imaging—cont'd
  sarcoid, 477
  subdural hematoma, 193
Magnetic resonance spectroscopy, 203
  Canavan disease, 525
  gray matter disease, 563
  Leigh disease, 532
  myelination, 498, 501, 503, 505, 507
Magnetization transfer (MT) MR scans, 557
Malignant fibrous histiocytoma (MFH), 298
Malignant melanoma, meningeal, 299
Malignant otitis externa, 626, 627–628, 639,
    640
Malnutrition, and cerebral atrophy, 649
Maple syrup urine disease, 523–524, 535
Marburg-type multiple sclerosis, 548
Marchiafava-Bignami disease, 653, 668
Marrow; see Bone marrow; Hematopoietic
    tissue
Mass lesions; see also Granulomatous disease;
    Neoplasms
  calvarial/skull abnormalities, 581
  extraaxial, 587f, 588–589
  foramen magnum, 643, 644, 645f, 646
  foramen magnum region, 645f
  with HIV/AIDS, 458, 460
    neurosyphilis, 468
    tuberculous, 469
  internal auditory canal, 625
  midline, 653
  morphologic patterns, 650–651
  pineal, 616f, 617–618
  scalp, 574
  sellar/juxtasellar region, 608–609t, 610,
      613, 616f
  and tonsillar herniation, 646
  ventricles, 597–602
    congenital/developmental, 597, 599–600
    extrinsic, 601–602
    inflammation/infection, 601
    neoplasia, 600–601
    from suprasellar masses, 601
    trauma/surgery, 601
    vascular, 601
Mastoid air cells , 628
Mastoiditis, 627, 666
  and abscess, 436
  calvarial/skull abnormalities, 583
Maxillary artery, 33f, 34f, 35, 36–37
Measles, 450
Meckel's cave, 12t, 614, 637
Medial lemniscus, 94, 99
Medial lenticulostriate arteries, 50–51, 52, 52f
Median cerebellar hypoplasia, 160
Medications
  and atrophy, 542
  calvarial/skull abnormalities, 577
  chemical vasculitis, 402
  enhancement patterns, 661

Medications—cont'd
  meningeal enhancement, 592
  neurotoxicity with HIV/AIDS, 459
  pituitary apoplexy, 611
  and Reyes syndrome, 452
  and venous occlusion, 406, 407
Medulla
  apertures of skull base, 13t
  normal anatomy, 98–99
  normal development, 122, 123
Medullary cistern, 23, 23f, 24t
Medullary veins, 79
  ependymal enhancement, 602
  venous angioma, 359t, 363, 364f
Medulloblastoma, 224, 225, 226f, 228, 243f,
    651
  calcification with, 657
  cerebellopontine angle cistern involvement,
      629
  CSF dissemination, 591
  CT patterns, 664
  in differential diagnosis
    of astrocytomas vs., 242
    of choroid plexus tumors vs., 260
    of ependymomas vs., 256
  enhancement patterns, 660, 661, 662
  ependymal enhancement, 440, 602
  foramen magnum region, 643, 645f, 646
  leptomeningeal infiltration, 308
  midline, 653
  morphologic patterns, 650
  posterior fossa, 654, 655
  ventricular mass lesions in children, 599
  ventricular pathology, 600
Medulloepithelioma, 275
Medusa head, venous angioma, 359t, 363,
    364f
Mega cisterna magna, 586, 651
  midline lesions, 653
  posterior fossa, 654, 655
  with vermian-cerebellar hypoplasia, 155t,
      158
Megalencephaly, unilateral, 150
Melanin, 314, 667
Melanocytoma, 299
Melanoma, 665, 667
  hemorrhage with, 309
  internal auditory canal, 626
  meningeal, 299
Melanosis, 299
Melanosis, neurocutaneous, 178
MELAS (mitochondrial encephalopathy with
    lactic acidosis and strokelike episodes),
    513, 514, 515, 516, 534, 535
Meningeal carcinomatosis; see
    Leptomeningeal metastases
Meningeal enhancement, 589–591, 660–661
Meningeal pathology, 589–593; see also Men-
    ingitis

Meningeal pathology—cont'd
  enhancement, 589–590
    with HIV/AIDS-related lymphomas, 470,
      471
  infection, 590
  inflammation, 590–591
  Langerhans cell histiocytosis, 479
  metabolic, chemical, toxins, 592
  miscellaneous, 592–593
  neoplasia, 591–592; *see also* Meningeal tu-
    mors
  neurofibromatosis, type II, 168
  trauma, surgery, vascular, 592
Meningeal spaces, 16*f*, 17, 17*t*, 18–19
Meningeal tumors, 290–299, 591–592
  hemangioblastoma, 296–298
  hemangiopericytoma, 295–296
  leukemias, 305
  lymphomas, 305
  malignant melanoma, 299
  meningioma; *see* Meningioma
  miscellaneous mesenchymal tumors,
    298–299
  primary melanocytic neoplasms, 297
  sarcomas, 298, 584
Meninges
  anatomy, 16–18, 16*f*, 17*t*, 587*f*
  herniation of with calvarial/skull abnormali-
    ties, 583
Meningioangiomatosis (MA), 178
Meningioma, 224, 225, 226*f*, 227, 290–295,
    292*f*, 293*f*, 588, 651, 665, 667, 668
  calcification with, 657, 658
  calvarial/skull abnormalities, 577, 579, 582,
    584
  cerebellopontine angle, 623*t*, 624*t*, 625
  CT patterns, 664
  in differential diagnosis
    of dural metastasis, 310
    of ependymomas, 257
    of glioma multiforme, 238
    of gliosarcomas, 249
    of hemangiopericytomas, 296
    of meningeal mesenchymal tumors, 299
    of pineocytoma, 268
    of pituitary adenoma, 284
    of plasmacytoma, 307
    of pleomorphic xanthoastrocytoma,
      246
    of schwannoma, 316
    of subependymomas, 258
  enhancement patterns, 660, 661, 663
  foramen magnum, 643, 644, 645*f*
  imaging, 501
  internal auditory canal, 625, 626
  morphologic patterns, 650
  neurofibromatosis type II, 168
  pineal region, 268, 616*f*, 617, 619
  posterior fossa, 654

Meningioma—cont'd
  sellar/juxtasellar region
    cavernous sinus and skull base, 614
    sellar region, 611
    suprasellar, 608*t*, 612
  skull base lesions, 634, 635, 636, 640
  ventricular, 598, 599, 600
    in adults, 598
    in children, 599
    third ventricle, 618
Meningiomatosis (NF-2), 168, 290
Meningitis, 426–432, 443, 665
  aseptic, 429
  calcification with, 658
  calvarial/skull abnormalities, 575,
    576
  cerebellopontine angle, 623
  chronic, 429–430
  enhancement patterns, 660
  fungal; *see specific agents*
  with HIV/AIDS, 458, 459, 460
    neurosyphilis, 467, 468
    tuberculous, 469
  HIV/AIDS-related cryptococcosis, 464
  with Lyme disease, 446
  meningeal enhancement with, 590
  with poliovirus infection, 447
  pyogenic, 426–429
    categories (agents causing), 425
    clinical course, 427–428
    imaging, 428–429
    pathophysiology, 426–427
  sellar/juxtasellar region, 613
  tuberculous, 474, 475, 475, 476
  ventricular pathology, 596
  ventriculitis and ependymitis, 439
Meningocele, defined, 134
Meningococcal meningitis, 427
Meningoencephalitis
  with Lyme disease, 446
  with rubella, 422
Meningoencephalocele, defined, 134
Meningomyelitis, with HIV/AIDS-associated
  neurosyphilis, 468
Meningothelial tumors, 225
Meningovasculitis, with HIV/AIDS-associated
  neurosyphilis, 467
Menke's syndrome, 575, 577
Mesencephalic arteriovenous malformation,
  619
Mesencephalic cisterns, 25*t*, 26
Mesencephalon (midbrain), 93–94; *see also*
  Midbrain lesions
  anatomy, 93–94
  Creutzfeldt-Jakob disease, 453
  normal development, 122–123
Mesenchymal tumors, 225
Mesial temporal sclerosis, 266
Metabolic demyelination, 512

Metabolic disorders, 665
  and basal ganglia degeneration, 568–569
  basal ganglia lesions, 654
  calcification with, 656, 657, 658
  calvarial/skull abnormalities, 575, 576, 577,
      578, 581, 584
  cellular enzyme deficiency, 512–513
  cerebral atrophy with, 649
  enhancement patterns, 660
  foramen magnum abnormalities, 646
  inherited, 511–516
    of gray matter, 528–535
    of white matter, 518–526
  meningeal pathology, 592
  MRI patterns, 668
Metabolic encephalopathy, 459, 515
Metachromatic leukodystrophy (MLD), 511,
    512, 513, 514, 515, 518–520, 668
Metals, MRI patterns, 667
Metastases, 225, 226f, 227, 227, 667
  basal ganglia degeneration, 569
  calcification with, 657, 658
  calvarial/skull abnormalities, 577, 578, 579,
      582, 584
  cerebellopontine angle, 623t, 624t, 625
  corticomedullary junction, 652
  cranial, 307–310
  CSF spread, 591
  in differential diagnosis
    of choroid plexus tumors, 260
    of glioblastoma multiforme, 237
    of glioma multiforme, 238
    of hemangioblastoma, 298
    of hemangiopericytomas, 296
    of lymphoma, 304
    of medulloblastomas, 274
    of meningiomas, 295
    of pineocytoma, 268
    of pituitary adenoma, 284
    of plasmacytoma, 307
    of schwannoma, 316
    of subependymomas, 258
    of white matter lesions, 546
  enhancement patterns, 660, 661, 662,
      663
    ependymal enhancement, 440, 602
    ring-enhancing lesions, 439
  foramen magnum region, 643, 644, 646
  internal auditory canal, 625, 626
  and intracranial hemorrhage, 219
  leptomeningeal, 591
  MRI patterns, 669
  pineal region, 616f, 617, 618, 619
  posterior fossa, 654
  sellar/juxtasellar region
    sellar region, 611
    suprasellar, 613
  skull base lesions, 634, 635, 636, 638, 639,
      640

Metastases—cont'd
  subarachnoid space enlargement, 588
  temporal bone, 626, 628
  third ventricle, 618
  ventricular mass lesions in adults, 598
Metathalamus, 93
Metencephalon
  anatomy, 94–97, 96f, 98f
  normal development, 122, 123
Methanol intoxication, 665
  and basal ganglia degeneration, 569
  basal ganglia lesions, 654
Methemoglobin, 667
Methotrexate, 555
  calcification with, 657, 658
  MRI patterns, 668
Methylmalonic acidemia, 515, 535, 654, 665
MIBI, glioblastoma multiforme, 237
Microadenoma, pituitary, 611
Microangiopathy
  calcification with, 657
  mineralizing, 555
Microcalcification, MRI patterns, 667
Microcephaly, 575
  calvarial/skull abnormalities, 576, 577
  with infections, 419
    CMV, 417
    rubella, 422, 423
    toxoplasmosis, 419
Microglial cells, 231
Midbrain; see Mesencephalon
Midbrain lesions, 618–619
  Chiari II malformations, 130
  glioma, ventricular mass lesions in adults,
      598
Middle cerebral artery
  anatomy, 50f, 52f, 54–58, 55f, 56f, 57f, 58f
  aneurysms, 343, 344f, 349
  with HIV/AIDS-associated neurosyphilis,
      468
  idiopathic progressive arteriopathy of child-
      hood, 397
  stroke, 376, 379, 380–381f
Middle cerebral artery bifurcation, 56f
Middle meningeal artery
  anastomosis, 35
  foramina, 9, 10f
  innervation, 37
Midline (lethal) granuloma, 633, 635, 638
Midline lesions, 653
Migraine, 403, 548, 668
Migration disorders, with corpus callosum ab-
    normalities, 136
Miliary tuberculosis, 475, 476
Miller-Dieker syndrome, 147
Mineralization, MRI patterns, 667
Mineralizing microangiopathy, 555, 657
Mitochondrial disorders, 513, 534–535, 665
  basal ganglia lesions, 654

Mitochondrial disorders—cont'd
  calcification with, 657
  of deep gray and white matter, 534–535
  inherited, 514
  subacute necrotizing encephalomelopathy, 532
Mitochondrial encephalopathy with lactic acidosis and strokelike episodes (MELAS), 513, 514, 515, 516, 534, 535
Mixed germ cell tumors, 276
Morphologic patterns, 649–651
Motor cortex, normal anatomy, 85–86, 88f
Motor (expressive) speech area, 88f, 89
Motorfacial (VII) nerve, 111–113, 623; *see also* Facial nerve
Moyamoya sign, 167, 397
Mucinous proteinaceous material, 667
Mucocele, 667, 668
  juxtasellar, 614
  skull base lesions, 632
  temporal bone lesions, 626
Mucolipidoses, 511, 513
Mucopolysaccharidoses, 513, 516, 519
  calvarial/skull abnormalities, 575, 576
  enhancement with, 592, 660
  foramen magnum abnormalities, 646
  MRI patterns, 668
Mucormycetoma, 667
Mucormycoses, 485
  juxtasellar, 614
  skull base lesions, 638
Multiinfarct (ischemic vascular) dementia, 564–565
  cerebral atrophy, 649
  subarachnoid space enlargement, 588
  ventricular pathology, 596
Multiple enhancing lesions, 662
Multiple hamartoma syndrome, 161, 179
Multiple myeloma, 305–306, 588; *see also* Myeloma
  in differential diagnosis
    of hemangiopericytomas, 296
    of meningeal mesenchymal tumors, 299
    of plasmacytoma, 307
  foramen magnum region, 646
  skull base lesions, 638, 640
Multiple sclerosis, 511, 512, 548–552
  in differential diagnosis
    of autoimmune demyelination disorders, 551–552
    of normal delayed myelination, 507t
  enhancement patterns, 662
  foramen magnum region, 644
  MRI patterns, 668, 669
  periventricular/callosal lesions, 653
  posterior fossa lesions, 654
  white matter lesion differential diagnosis, 546

Multiple system atrophies (MSA), 567–568
Mumps virus, 429, 443
Mural nodule, cortical, 652
Mycobacterial infections; *see also* Tuberculosis
  actinomycetaceae and, 487
  with HIV/AIDS, 457, 468–470
  skull base lesions, 635
Myelencephalon
  normal anatomy, 98–99
  normal development, 122, 123
Myelinated axons, 512
Myelination, 418; *see also* Demyelinating disease; Dysmyelinating disease; Leukodystrophies
  dys- versus *de*myelination, 512
  delayed
    normal, 507–508, 507t
    with rubella, 422
  normal development, 123, 498–508, 512
    birth, 499–502, 500f, 502f
    delayed, areas of, 507–508, 507t
    fetal brain, 498–499, 501f
    postnatal months, 503–507, 504f, 506f
Myelinolysis
  central pontine, 553
  extrapontine, 553–554
Myelitis, 443
Myelofibrosis, 589
Myelography, 666
Myeloma; *see also* Multiple myeloma
  calvarial/skull abnormalities, 582, 584
  skull base lesions, 635, 640
Myelomeningocele, Chiari II malformations, 127t, 131
Myelopathy; *see* Spinal cord lesions
Myoblastoma, granular cell, 611
Myoclonic epilepsy with ragged red fibers (MERRF), 534, 535

N

Nasal glioma, 135
Nasal mucosa, enhancement patterns, 660
Nasopharyngeal angiofibroma, 635, 637
Nasopharyngeal cancers, 669
  enhancement patterns, 663
  sellar/juxtasellar region, cavernous sinus and skull base, 614
  skull base lesions, 635, 636, 639
Nasopharyngeal cephaloceles, 135
Necrosis
  calvarial/skull abnormalities, 583
  pituitary, 611
  toxoplasma lesions, 462
Necrotizing leukoencephalopathy, MRI patterns, 668
NECT
  arteriovenous malformations, 358t, 359t
  atherosclerosis, 390

NECT—cont'd
  cortical vein occlusion, 410
  deep cerebral vein thrombosis, 411
  dural sinus thrombosis, 408–409
  epidermoid versus dermoid tumors, 323*t*
  meningitis, 475
  stroke, 377
  white matter disease, 555
Nelson syndrome, 612
Neonatal asphyxia, 516
Neonatal hemorrhage of prematurity, 665
Neonatal infections, 416–423, 428, 435
Neonates
  abscesses, 436
  intracranial hemorrhages, 214–215
  iron in brain of, 538, 543
  meningitis, 427, 429
  myelination state, 499–502, 500*f*, 502*f*
  pituitary anatomy, 605
  scalp disorders, 574
  ventriculitis and ependymitis, 439, 440
Neoplasms, 665, 668; *see also* Metastases;
    specific tumor types
  Alzheimer disease workup, 562
  astrocytomas, 231–238
  astrocytoma variants, 241–250
  basal ganglia, 653
  basal ganglia degeneration, 569
  calcification with, 657, 658, 659
  calvarial/skull abnormalities, 575, 576, 578,
    579, 581, 583
  cerebellopontine angle, 625
  classification
    by age and location, 227–228
    by histology, 224–225
    by prevalence, 225–227, 226*f*
  cortical, 652
  corticomedullary junction, 652
  CT patterns, 664
  with cystic components, 651
  enhancement patterns, 660, 661, 662, 663
  ependymal enhancement, 602
  foramen magnum region, 644, 645*f*, 646
  glial tumors
    neuronal, mixed neuronal-glial, and pi-
      neal tumors, 263–269
    nonastrocytic, 253–260, 255*f*
  head and neck tumors, 314–320
  hematopoietic and reticuloendothelial tu-
    mors, 303–307
  with HIV/AIDS, 458–459, 458, 459
    glioma, 471
    lymphoma, 470–471
  internal auditory canal, 626
  and intracranial hemorrhage, 217, 219,
    219–220
  meningeal pathology, 591–592
  meningeal tumors, 290–299
  midline, 653

Neoplasms—cont'd
  morphologic patterns, 650–651
  MRI patterns, 667, 669
  multiple sclerosis vs., 550
  neurofibromatosis, 164*t*, 165, 166
    type I, 165
    type II, 168
  paranasal sinus-invading, 666
  periventricular/callosal, 652–653
  pineal, 616*f*, 617–618
  pituitary adenoma and Rathke's pouch tu-
    mors, 281–287*t*
  posterior fossa, 156*t*, 654, 655
  primitive neuroepithelial and germ cell tu-
    mors, 272–279
  sellar/juxtasellar region
    cavernous sinus and skull base, 614
    sellar region, 611
    suprasellar, 612–613
    anterior, 633–634
    central, 636–638
  subarachnoid space enlargement, 588
  temporal bone, 628
  third ventricle, 618
  in tuberous sclerosis complex, 170–171
  and vascular occlusion
    arterial, 399
    venous, 406, 407
  ventricles, 596, 600–601, 618; *see also*
      specific ventricles
  von Hippel-Lindau syndrome, 173–175
  white matter lesion differential diagnosis,
    546
Nephrotic syndrome, and basal ganglia degen-
    eration, 568
Nerve roots; *see* Radiculopathies; Spinal nerve
    roots
Nerve sheath tumors, 224–225
  schwannomas; *see* Schwannomas
  skull base lesions, 637, 640
Neural crest cell tumors, 314, 633
Neural tube development, 122
Neural tube abnormalities, 124
  cephaloceles, 134–140, 137*f*, 138*f*, 139*f*,
    140*f*
  Chiari malformations, 126–131, 127*t*, 128*f*
Neurenteric cyst, 651
  epidermoid tumor vs., 327
  foramen magnum region, 643, 644
  midline, 653
  posterior fossa, 654
Neurilemmoma, 314–317
Neurinoma, 314–317
Neuritis
  internal auditory canal, 625, 626
  viral, 663
Neuroblastoma, 588
  calvarial/skull abnormalities, 576, 577, 578,
    584

Neuroblastoma—cont'd
  primary cerebral, 274–275
  skull base lesions, 633
Neurocutaneous syndromes, 124
  arterial stenosis with, 397
  ataxia-telangiectasia syndrome, 177–178
  basal cell nevus syndrome, 179
  Cowden disease, 179
  epidermal nevus syndromes, 179
  meningioangiomatosis, 178
  neurocutaneous melanosis, 178
  neurofibromatosis, 164–168, 164*t*
  Rendu-Osler-Weber disease, 177
  Sturge-Weber syndrome, 172–173
  tuberous sclerosis complex, 170–172
  von Hippel-Lindau disease, 173–175
  white matter lesion differential diagnosis,
    546
  Wyburn-Mason syndrome, 177
Neurocysticercosis, 489–492; *see also* Cys-
    ticerosis
Neurocytoma, 650
  central, 267; *see also* Central neurocytoma
  choroid plexus tumors vs., 260
  ventricular pathology, 598, 600
Neurodegenerative disorders; *see* Degenerative
    disorders
Neuroectodermal tumors; *see* Primitive neu-
    roepithelial tumors
Neuroenteric cyst, 330–331
Neuroepithelial cysts, 329–330, 651
Neuroepithelial tumors
  dysembryonic neuroepithelial tumors
    (DNET), 265–266
  primitive (PNET); *see* Primitive neuroepi-
    thelial tumors
Neurofibroma, 225, 317
  scalp, 574
  schwannoma vs., 314*t*
  skull base lesions, 637, 639
Neurofibromatosis, 164–168, 164*t*
  arterial stenosis with, 397
  calcification with, 656, 657
  calvarial/skull abnormalities, 575, 583
  MRI patterns, 668
  type I, 164*t*, 164–167, 397
  type II, 164*t*, 167–168, 599, 624*t*
  ventricular mass lesions in adults, 598, 599
  white matter lesion differential diagnosis,
    546
Neurohypophysis, 281
  ectopic, 610, 612
  Langerhans cell histiocytosis, 480
  normal anatomy, 605, 606*f*
  radiology, 607
Neuromyelitis optica, 548, 549
Neuronal ceroid-lipofuscinosis, 529–530
Neuronal migration disorders, 147–151, 148*f*,
    149*f*, 150*f*, 154

Neuronal organization abnormalities, 151
Neuronal tumors, 224
Neurons, normal development, 123
Neuron-specific enolase (NSE), 318
Neurosarcoidosis; *see* Sarcoidosis
Neurosecretory granules, 607
Neurosyphilis; *see* Syphilis
Neurulation, normal development, 122
Niemann-Pick disease, 513
Nocardiosis, 457, 460, 487–488
Nodular heterotopias, 148–149, 149*f*
Nonaccidental trauma (child abuse), 196
Noncommunicating hydrocephalus, ventricular
    pathology, 596
Non-Hodgkins lymphoma, 470
Nonspecific leukoencephalopathy (NSLE),
    541
Nonsteroidal antiinflammatory agents
    (NSAIDS), 592, 661
Nontropical sprue, 449
Normal anatomy; *see* Anatomy, brain
Normal pressure hydrocephalus, 563–564, 596
Normal structures (pseudotumors), cerebel-
    lopontine angle, 623
Normal variants, midline, 653
Notochord, 637
Nuclear medicine; *see* Positron emission
    tomography; Radionuclide imaging
Nuclei, anatomy, 95, 99
Nucleus ambiguus, 99
Nucleus cuneatus, 99
Nucleus gracilis, 99
Nucleus solitarius, 99

O
Obstruction, ventricular, 596
Obstructive hydrocephalus, 599
  calvarial/skull abnormalities, 581
  sellar expansion, 612
  ventricular pathology, 596
Occipital artery, 33*f*, 34*f*, 35–36, 60*f*
  anastomosis, 35
  collateral circulation, 393
  innervation, 37
Occipital bone
  anatomy, 5*f*, 6*f*, 7
  apertures of skull base, 13*t*
  foramen magnum region, 644
  foramina, 9
  skull base lesions, 639
Occipital cephalocele, posterior fossa, 655
Occipital eye area, 89
Occipital lobe
  Creutzfeldt-Jakob disease, 453
  inherited metabolic disorders, 514
  normal anatomy, 84*f*, 85
  toxoplasma lesions, HIV/AIDS-related,
    462
Occipital sinus, 74*f*, 77, 78*f*

Occipital squamae, calvarial/skull abnormalities, 581
Occipital white matter, adrenoleukodystrophy, 519
Oculomotor (III) nerve, 102f, 103f, 105–106
  apertures of skull base, 10f, 12t
  venous system, 76f
Oculomotor nerve palsy, aneurysm and, 344
Olfactory bulbs, 144
Olfactory cortex, 90
Olfactory (I) nerve, 102–103, 102f, 103f
  apertures of skull base, 12t
  foramina, 10f
  venous system, 76f
Olfactory neuroblastoma, 633
Oligodendrocytes, 231, 512
Oligodendroglia, progressive multifocal leukoencephalopathy, 465
Oligodendroglioma, 224, 225, 226f, 227, 231, 253–254, 667
  astrocytomas vs., 234
  calcification with, 657
  calvarial/skull abnormalities, 584
  corticomedullary junction, 652
  dysembryoplastic neuroepithelial tumor vs., 266
  enhancement patterns, 663
  ganglioglioma vs., 264
  pleomorphic xanthoastrocytoma vs., 246
  ventricular mass lesions in adults, 598
  ventricular pathology, 600
Olivary nuclei, 99
Olivopontocerebellar atrophy (OPCA), 568, 649, 650
Ophthalmic artery, 40f, 44–45, 393
Optic canal, 12t
Optic chiasm, 50f
  pituitary adenomas, 282
  venous system, 76f
Optic glioma, 165
Optic nerve, 50f, 102f, 103–105, 103f
Optic (II) nerve, 103–105, 150
  apertures of skull base, 12t
  in disseminated encephalomyelitis, 451
  foramina, 10f
  with HIV/AIDS-associated neurosyphilis, 468
  with holoprosencephaly, 144
  in multiple sclerosis, 549
  sarcoid, 478
Optic nerve enhancement, 451, 477, 478
Opticochiasmatic-hypothalamic glioma, 228, 245, 609t
Orbit
  calvarial/skull abnormalities, 580
  sarcoid, 477
Organic acid disorders, 523–524, 535
Organic toxins, 554
Osmotic myelinolysis, 568–569

Osseous anomalies; see Bone abnormalities
Ossifying hemangioma, 628
Osteoblastic metastasis, 579
Osteocartilagenous tumors, 298, 645f
  calcification with, 657, 658
  cerebellopontine angle, 623t
  foramen magnum region, 643, 646
  meningeal, 298
  skull base lesions, 640
Osteochrondroma, 298
Osteogenesis imperfecta, 576, 577, 580, 581
Osteoma, 666
  calvarial/skull abnormalities, 577, 579
  frontal sinus, 633
  meningiomas vs., 294
Osteomyelitis
  calvarial/skull abnormalities, 579, 582, 583
  foramen magnum region, 646
  skull base lesions, 635, 638, 639, 640
  temporal bone, 627
Osteopetrosis, 577, 578
Osteoporosis, 582, 584
Osteoporosis circumscripta, 580, 581, 582, 584
Osteosarcoma, 667
  calcification with, 657, 658
  calvarial/skull abnormalities, 579, 580
  meningeal, 298
  skull base lesions, 637, 640
Osteosclerosis, 578
Otic artery, 42f, 43
Otitis externa
  malignant, 626, 627–628, 639, 640
  skull base lesions, 639, 640
Otitis media, 627, 636
Otomastoid infection, and abscess, 436
Otorrhea, 627
Oxycephaly, 576

P

Pacchionian (arachnoid) granulations, 16f, 581, 582
Pachydermoperiostosis, 576, 577
Pachygyria, 147, 248
Pachymeninges
  anatomy, 16–18, 16f, 17t
  metastasis, 591
Pachymeningitis
  enhancement patterns, 661
  idiopathic hypertrophic, 593
  rheumatoid, 591
Paget disease
  calvarial/skull abnormalities, 575, 577, 578, 580, 584
  foramen magnum region, 646
  skull base lesions, 634, 637, 638, 640
Panencephalitis, subacute sclerosing (SSPE), 443, 448–449
Panhypopituitarism, 610

Pannus, 646
Pantopaque, 657, 658, 667
Papilloma
  choroid plexus; *see* Choroid plexus papil-
    loma
  skull base lesions, 633
  temporal bone lesions, 628
Papovavirus infection, 457, 464–466
Para-aortic sympathetic paraganglioma, 318
Paracavernous internal carotid artery, 388
Paradoxic embolism, and stroke, 402
Paraganglioma, 626, 668
  cerebellopontine angle, 623*t*
  foramen magnum region, 643, 644, 645*f*
  parasympathetic, 318–319
  posterior fossa, 654
  schwannoma vs., 316
  skull base lesions, 639
  temporal bone lesions, 628
Paramagnetic MRI contrast agents, 667
Paranasal sinuses
  calvarial/skull abnormalities, 579
  Wegener's granulomatosis, 478
Paraneoplastic cerebellar degeneration, 650
Paraneoplastic syndrome, and vascular occlu-
    sion, 406, 407
Parasellar calcification, 658
Parasite infections, 489–493
  calcification with, 656, 659
  subarachnoid space enlargement, 588
Parasympathetic paraganglioma, 318–319
Paraventricular nucleus, 92
Parenchyma; *see also* White matter
  inflammation/infection; *see also* Encephal-
    itis
  Langerhans cell histiocytosis, 479
  meningitis and, 427
  metastasis, 308
  myelination; *see also* Myelination, normal
    development
  sarcoid, 477
  trauma, and cerebral edema, 203
Parenchymal cysts, 651, 668
Parenchymal hematoma, 592, 664–665
  calcification with, 657
  enhancement patterns, 660
Parenchymal lesions
  cerebellopontine angle, 625
  with HIV/AIDS, 459
Parenchymal metastasis, 309
Parietal bone
  anatomy, 4, 5*f*, 6*f*
  calvarial/skull abnormalities, 581, 582
  foramina, 9
Parietal lobe
  normal anatomy, 84*f*, 85
  toxoplasma lesions, HIV/AIDS-related, 462
Parkinson disease, 512, 566–567, 654
Parkinson plus disorders, 567–568

Pars flaccida cholesteatoma, 627
Pars intermedia cyst, 606*f*, 607, 610, 651
Pars nervosa, 13*t*
Pars tensa cholesteatoma, 627
Partial empty sella, 610
Pediatric patients
  basal ganglia degeneration, 569
  congenital and neonatal infections, 416–423
  intraventricular masses, 599
  neoplasms, 227–228
  pineal tumors, 617
  posterior fossa lesions, 655
  Reyes syndrome, 452
  scalp masses, 574
  sellar/juxtasellar region, 613
  tuberculosis, 474, 475
Peduncular hemorrhage, 203
Pelizaeus-Merzbacher disease, 514, 519, 524
  calvarial/skull abnormalities, 575
  MRI patterns, 668
Penicillin, 592
Periaqueductal gray matter, 94
Pericallosal cistern, 23*f*, 24*t*
Periclival venous plexus, 78
Perinatal hemorrhage, 214–215
Perineural tumor spread, 669
Periosteum, 16*f*
Peripartum pituitary necrosis, 611
Peripheral nerves
  cytomegalovirus infections, 466, 467
  sarcoid, 477
Peripheral neuropathy, with HIV/AIDS, 460
Perivascular inflammation
  in disseminated encephalomyelitis, 450
  with HIV/AIDS-associated neurosyphilis,
    467
Perivascular necrosis, with rubella, 422
Perivascular space; *see* Virchow-Robin spaces
Periventricular calcifications, 417, 418
Periventricular lesions, 652–653
  with CMV infection, 417, 418
  with HIV/AIDS
    HIV involvement, 460
    lymphoma, 463*t*
    tuberculous, 470
  Langerhans cell histiocytosis, 307
  in multiple sclerosis, 549
  tuberculomas, 475
Periventricular leukomalacia (PVL), 215, 507*t*,
    508
Periventricular nodular heterotopia, 149
Periventricular venous collagenosis, 411–412,
    546, 547
Periventricular white matter
  age-related changes, 541–542
  carbon monoxide poisoning, 554
  inherited metabolic disorders affecting, 514
Peroxisomal disorders, 516
  adrenoleukodystrophy, 521–522

Peroxisomal disorders—cont'd
  inherited, 513–514
  Zellweger syndrome, 531–532
Persistent embryonic circulation, 41, 42f, 43, 44
Persistent trigeminal artery, 41, 42f
Pertussis immunization, 450
Petroclinoid ligament calcification, 656
Petrous apex cholesteatomas, 626
Petrous apicitis, 627, 640
Pharyngeal artery
  anastomosis, 35
  collateral circulation, 393
Phentoin; see Dilantin
Phenylketonuria, 523, 535, 668
Pheochromocytoma, 174, 175, 318
Physiologic abnormalities
  basal ganglia lesions, 568–569, 653
  and demyelination, 553–554
  and MRI hyperintense lesions, 668
Pial angioma, cortical, 652
Pial arteriovenous malformations, 355–357, 358t, 360
Pial collaterals, 393
Pial siderosis, enhancement patterns, 660
Pia mater, 18
  anatomy, 16f, 17t
  CSF circulation, 27
  HIV/AIDS-associated neurosyphilis, 467
Pick disease, 512, 565
  cerebral atrophy, 649
  subarachnoid space enlargement, 588
  ventricular pathology, 595, 596
Pilocytic astrocytoma, 231, 241–245, 651
  in differential diagnosis
    of astrocytomas, 235
    of choroid plexus tumors, 260
    of ependymomas, 256
    of ganglioglioma, 264
    of hemangioblastoma, 297
    of medulloblastomas, 273, 274
    of pleomorphic xanthoastrocytoma, 246
    of schwannomas vs., 317
  enhancement patterns, 662
  suprasellar, 613
  ventricular abnormalities from, 601
  ventricular mass lesions in children, 599
Pineal cyst, 331–332, 651, 653
Pineal gland, 616–619
  anatomy, normal, 616–617, 616f
  calcification of, 656
  enhancement patterns, 660
Pineal gland tumors, 224, 225, 226f, 228, 278, 613, 617–619; see also Pineoblastoma; Pineocytoma
  calcification with, 657, 659
  differential diagnosis, 269
  ependymal enhancement, 440, 602
  germ cell, 276–279, 613, 659

Pineal gland tumors—cont'd
  midline, 653
  parenchymal, 268–269
  ventricular abnormalities from, 601–602
Pineal stalk, 91
Pineoblastoma, 228, 268–269, 616f, 617, 618
  calcification with, 657
  CSF dissemination, 591
  enhancement patterns, 660, 661
  ependymal enhancement, 440, 602
  germ cell tumor differential diagnosis, 278
  leptomeningeal infiltration, 308
  midline, 653
  ventricular abnormalities from, 602
Pineocytoma, 224, 226f, 268, 269, 616f, 617, 618, 651
  calcification with, 657
  midline, 653
  pineal cyst vs., 332
Pituicytoma, 611, 613
Pituitary adenoma, 224, 225, 226f, 227, 281–284, 651, 665, 666
  astrocytomas vs., 245
  calcification with, 658
  craniopharyngioma vs., 286
  midline, 653
  MRI and CT appearance, 608t
  Rathke's cleft cyst vs., 287
  skull base lesions, 635, 636, 637
  suprasellar hot spots, 610
  ventricular, 598, 601
Pituitary apoplexy, 610
Pituitary gigantism, 575
Pituitary gland, 44, 635
  enhancement patterns, 660
  Langerhans cell histiocytosis, 307, 479, 480
  myelination, 505
  normal anatomy, 605–607, 606f
  venous system, 76f
Pituitary hyperplasia, pituitary adenomas vs., 283
Pituitary macroadenoma, 601, 658
Pituitary neuroendocrine tumors, 224, 226f
Plagiocephaly, 576
Plain film studies
  dermoid tumors, 325
  epidermoid tumor, 326
  infections, 419
  lipoma, 333
Plasmacytoma, 305–306, 588
  calvarial/skull abnormalities, 584
  foramen magnum region, 646
  hemangiopericytomas vs., 296
  with HIV/AIDS, 458
  meningeal mesenchymal tumors vs., 299
  skull base lesions, 640
  temporal bone lesions, 626

Pleomorphic xanthoastrocytoma, 245–246,
    651
    cortical, 652
    enhancement patterns, 662
    hemangioblastoma vs., 297
    oligodendroglial tumors vs., 254
Plexiform neurofibroma
    scalp, 574
    skull base lesions, 637
PNETs; *see* Primitive neuroepithelial tumors
Pneumocephalus, 666
    subarachnoid space enlargement, 588
    ventricular mass lesions, 601
Pneumoencephalography, 666
Pneumosinus dilatans, 634
Poliodystrophies, 511
Poliovirus, 443, 447
Polyarteritis nodosa (PAN), 401
Polymicrogyria/pachygyria complex, 151
Polyoma virus, 457, 464–466
Polyradiculopathy; *see* Radiculopathies
Pons, 94–95
    atrophy, 649
    hypertensive vascular disease, 664
    normal development, 122, 123
Pontine cavernous angioma, 369*f*
Pontine cistern, 23, 23*f*, 24*t*
Pontine nuclei, 95
Pontine paramedian reticular formation, 95
Pontine tumors
    astrocytoma, ependymomas vs., 256
    glioma, 244*f*
Porencephalic cyst, 651
Porencephaly
    periventricular/callosal, 652
    ventricular pathology, 595
Positron emission tomography (PET)
    Alzheimer disease, 563
    glioblastoma multiforme, 237
    multiinfarct dementia, 565
    normal pressure hydrocephalus, 564
    Pick disease, 565
Posterior auricular artery, 33*f*, 34*f*, 36
Posterior cerebral artery, 40*f*, 50*f*, 58–62, 59*f*,
    60*f*, 62*f*, 70
    idiopathic progressive arteriopathy of child-
        hood, 397
    stenosis, congenital causes, 396
    stroke, 379, 380–381*f*
Posterior cerebral artery aneurysms, 619
Posterior cerebral artery occlusion, 618
Posterior choroidal artery, 60–61, 60*f*
Posterior commissure, 91
Posterior communicating artery
    anatomy, 40*f*, 41, 42*f*, 45–46, 50*f*, 51, 59,
        59*f*, 60*f*
    aneurysms, 343, 349
Posterior communicating artery infundibulum,
    51, 349

Posterior fossa anatomy, 13*t*, 644
    apertures of skull base, 13*t*
    arteries, 66–70, 66*f*, 67*f*
        basilar arteries, 69–70, 66*f*, 67*f*
        vertebral arteries, 66–69, 66*f*, 67*f*
    cisterns, 23, 23*f*, 24*t*, 26, 27
    veins, 80, 81*f*
Posterior fossa cyst, 595
Posterior fossa lesions, 595
    in adults, 654
    autoimmune demyelination, 551
    in children, 655
    tumors, 241–245, 243–244*f*, 291, 596
    ventricular pathology, 596
    von Hippel-Lindau syndrome, 174
Posterior fossa malformations, 154–161,
    155–156*t*, 157*f*, 595
    Chiari II, 129
    Chiari IV, 127*t*, 131
Posterior inferior cerebellar artery
    aneurysm, 643
    stroke, 380–381*f*, 383–384
Posterior intercavernous sinus, 75*f*
Posterior interior carotid artery, 46
    aneurysms, 349, 644
    cerebellopontine angle abnormalities, 623
    foramen magnum region, 644
Posterior nucleus, 92
Posterior pituitary; *see* Neurohypophysis
Postventricular shunt placement, enhancement
    patterns, 661
Pott's disease, 475
Precentral cerebellar vein (PCV), 80, 81*f*
Preeclampsia/eclampsia, 217, 548, 568, 664
Prefrontal cortex, 90
Pregnancy
    eclampsia, 217, 548, 568, 664
    and stroke, 403
    and venous occlusion, 406
Premature closure of fontanelles, 575–576
Premature infants
    intracranial hemorrhage, 214–215
    neonatal hemorrhage of prematurity, 665
    ventricular enlargement, 596
    ventricular mass lesions, 601
Premotor area, 86, 88*f*
Preoptic nucleus, 92
Primary auditory area, 88*f*, 89
Primary leptomeningeal gliomatosis,
    249–250
Primary motor area, 85–86, 88*f*
Primary (lateral) olfactory area, 90
Primary somesthetic area, 86, 88*f*
Primary visual area, 88*f*, 89
Primitive neuroepithelial tumors, (PNETs),
    224, 226*f*, 228, 272–276, 651
    calcification with, 657
    cerebral neuroblastomas, 274–275
    choroid plexus tumors vs., 260

Primitive neuroepithelial tumors, (PNETs)—
  cont'd
  desmoplastic infantile ganglioglioma and,
    263, 265
  enhancement patterns, 661
  ependymal enhancement, 440, 602
  ependymoblastomas, 275
  ependymomas vs., 256
  leptomeningeal infiltration, 308
  medulloblastomas, 272–274
  medulloepitheliomas, 275
  ventricular abnormalities from, 601
  ventricular mass lesions in children, 599
Proatlantal intersegmental artery, 42
Progeria, 577
Progressive multifocal leukoencephalopathy
    (PML), 443, 449–450
  corticomedullary junction, 652
  with HIV/AIDS, 458, 459, 464–466
  MRI patterns, 668
Progressive supranuclear palsy, 618–619,
    649
Projection fibers, 91
Prolactinoma, 282
Propionic acidemias, 535, 654, 665
Prosencephalon; see Forebrain
Protoplasmic astrocytoma, 232–233, 652
Pseudoaneurysm, 208f
Pseudobulbar palsy, 618
Pseudo empty delta sign, 211
Pseudohypoparathyroidism, 656, 657
Pseudopseudohypoparathyroidism, 656, 657
Pseudotumor
  cerebellopontine angle, 623
  schwannoma vs., 316
Pseudotumor cerebri, 650
  calvarial/skull abnormalities, 576
  ventricular pathology, 597
Pterygoid canal, 11, 41
Pterygoid plexus, 12t, 75f
Pterygopalatine fossa, 12t
Purely granulomatous Wegener's granulomato-
    sis (PGWG), 478
Putamen, 91, 665
  carbon monoxide poisoning, 555
  inherited metabolic disorders affecting, 514,
    516
  iron in, 538, 543
Pyknodysostosis, 576, 577
Pyogenic infections, parenchymal, 435–440
Pyrimethamine, 462

Q

Quadrigemina, 93
Quadrigeminal cistern, 23f, 25t, 26, 616, 616f,
    617, 618, 619

R

Racemose cysts, suprasellar, 613

Radiation
  and basal ganglia degeneration, 569
  calcification with, 657, 658
  and calvarial/skull abnormalities, 575
  and cerebellar atrophy, 650
  and cerebral atrophy, 649
    subarachnoid space enlargement, 588
  and vascular occlusion, 399
  ventricular pathology, 596
  white matter injury, 556
Radiation-induced necrotizing leukoencephal-
    opathy, 668
Radiation necrosis, 668
  calvarial/skull abnormalities, 583
  enhancement patterns, 662
  glioma multiforme vs., 238
  lymphoma vs., 304
  ring-enhancing lesions, 439
Radiation vasculopathy, 367–368, 399
Radiculopathies; see also Spinal nerve roots
  with HIV/AIDS
    cytomegalovirus, 466
    neurosyphilis, 468
  in Lyme disease, 446
Radionuclide imaging
  abscess, 438
  brain death, 204
  glioblastoma multiforme, 237
  post-infectious syndromes, 445
  lymphoma, 462
  multiple myeloma, 306
Ramsay Hunt syndrome, 625, 626
Rasmussen encephalitis, 443, 451–452
Rathke cleft cyst, 286–287, 606f, 607, 610,
    610, 651
  midline, 653
  pituitary adenomas vs., 283
  pituitary adenoma vs., 284
  suprasellar extension, 612
Rathke pouch lesions, 284–287
  craniopharyngioma, 284–286; see also
    Craniopharyngioma
  Rathke cleft cyst, 286–287
Reactive sclerosis, calvarial/skull abnormali-
    ties, 583
Rebound growth, calvarial/skull abnormalities,
    577
Recurrent artery of Huebner, 52f, 53
Red nucleus, 94
  cerebellorubral degeneration, 557
  iron in, 538, 543, 667
Regional head and neck tumors, 314–320
Renal cell carcinoma, 665
Renal failure, 664
  and basal ganglia degeneration, 568
  and intracranial hemorrhage, 217
Renal osteodystrophy, calvarial/skull abnor-
    malities, 578
Rendu-Osler-Weber disease, 177, 356, 368

Reperfusion hemorrhage, 664
Reticular formation, 94, 95, 99
Reticuloendothelial tumors, 225, 303–307
Reye syndrome, 443, 452–453
Rhabdomyoma, meningeal, 298
Rhabdomyosarcoma, 298, 633, 640
Rheumatoid arthritis, 646
Rheumatoid pachymeningitis, 430, 591, 660
Rhinencephalon, 102
Rhinoscleroma, 635
Rhombencephalon; see Hindbrain
Rhombencephalosynapses, 160
Rickets, 576, 581
Ring-enhancing lesions, 662
    differential diagnosis of, 439
    in disseminated encephalomyelitis, 451
    lymphoma vs., 304
    in multiple sclerosis, 550
    parenchymal metastasis, 309
    with tuberculosis, 470, 476
Ringlike calcification, 658–659
Rocky Mountain spotted fever, 443
Rosenthal fibers, 525
Rubella, 443, 450
    calcification with, 656
    congenital and neonatal, 422–423

S

Saccular aneurysms, 340–351, 341f, 344f,
    346f, 347–348f
Saggital sinus anatomy, 16f, 17, 17t
Salivary gland tumors, 320
San Filippo disease, 513
Sarcoid granuloma, 662
Sarcoidosis, 402, 476–478, 588, 633, 665
    cerebellopontine angle, 623
    enhancement patterns, 660, 661, 662, 663
        ependymal, 440, 602
        meningeal, 590–591
    germ cell tumor vs, 279
    and hypophysitis, granulomatous, 612
    hypothalamic hamartoma vs., 334
    internal auditory canal, 625, 626
    meningitis, chronic, 430
    pineal, 618
    posterior fossa, 654
    progressive multifocal leukoencephalopathy
        with, 449
    sellar/juxtasellar region, 610, 613
    skull base lesions, 635, 638
    ventricular abnormalities from, 601
    ventricular mass lesions in adults, 598
Sarcomas, 292, 588
    calvarial/skull abnormalities, 584
    desmoplastic infantile gangliogliomas vs.,
        265
    gliosarcomas, 248–249
    granulocytic, 305
    hemangiopericytomas vs., 296

Sarcomas—cont'd
    with HIV/AIDS, 458
    leptomeningeal, 298–299
    plasmacytoma vs., 307
    primary cerebral neuroblastomas vs.,
        275
Scalp and calvarium, 574–584; see also
    Calvarium; Skull
    anatomy, 4, 16f
    anatomy of meninges, epi- and subdural
        space, 587f
    basal cell carcinoma, 320
    cranial size, 575
    suture abnormalities, 575–577
    thickness abnormalities, 577–584
SCALP (mnemonic), 4
Scaphocephaly, 576
Schizencephaly, 149–150, 150f
    with holoprosencephaly, 144
    ventricular pathology, 595
Schwannoma, 224, 225, 226f, 225, 227,
    314–317, 651, 665
    cerebellopontine angle, 623t, 624t, 625
    enhancement patterns, 661, 663
    foramen magnum region, 643, 644, 645f
    internal auditory canal, 625, 626
    meningiomas vs., 295
    morphologic patterns, 650
    neurofibromatosis type II, 168
    skull base lesions, 614, 636, 637, 639
    temporal bone lesions, 628
Secondary auditory area, 88f, 89
Secondary hemorrhage, 203
Secondary (medial) olfactory area, 90
Secondary visual area, 88f, 89
Secondary white matter disorders, 556–557
Seizure
    with aneurysm, 345
    enhancement patterns, 661
    with HIV/AIDS-associated toxoplasmosis,
        462
    Rasmussen encephalitis, 452
Sellar/juxtasellar lesions, 605–614
    anatomy, 605–607, 606f
    aneurysm, 349
    calvarial/skull abnormalities, 578
    normal, 605–607, 605f
    pathology, 608–614
        intrasellar, 610–612
        juxtasellar, 614
        MRI and CT appearance, 608–609t
        suprasellar, 612–613
    radiology, 607, 610
    ventricular abnormalities, 601
Sella turcica, 76f, 634
Senile plaques, 561
Sensory cortex, 86, 88f
Sensory (receptive) speech area, 87, 88f, 89
Septal vein, 74f, 77f, 78f, 80

Septic emboli, 652, 662
Septooptic dysplasia, 144, 595
Septum pellucidum, 150
  holoprosencephalies, 142t
  with holoprosencephaly, 144
  oligodendroglioma, 600
SGCA; see Subependymal giant-cell astrocy-
  toma
Shear injury, 194–195, 194f
  corticomedullary junction, 652
  hemorrhagic, 664
  MRI patterns, 669
  periventricular/callosal, 653
Sheehan's pituitary necrosis, 611
Short-inversion time inversion-recovery
  (STIR), 498
Shunts
  calvarial/skull abnormalities, 577, 583
  and Chiari I malformation, 128
  enhancement patterns, 661
  and tonsillar herniation, 646
  ventriculitis and ependymitis, 439
Shy-Drager syndrome, 568, 649, 650
Sickle cell disease, 397, 578
Siderosis, 216, 660
Sigmoid sinus
  anatomy, 76–77, 74f, 75f, 77f, 78f
  arteriovenous malformations, 361
Sigmoid sinus thrombosis, 429
Silver-Russell, 575, 578, 650
Single-photon emission computed tomography
  (SPECT), 203
  abscess, 438
  Alzheimer disease, 563
  glioblastoma multiforme, 237
  lymphoma, 462
  multiinfarct dementia, 565
  normal pressure hydrocephalus, 564
  Pick disease, 565
  post-infectious syndromes, 445
Sinonasal carcinoma
  with intracranial invasion, 666
  skull base lesions, 633
Sinus confluence, 73, 74f, 77f, 365
Sinusitis, 436, 632, 666
  calvarial/skull abnormalities, 583
  skull base lesions, 638
  and subdural empyema, 431
Sinus lesions
  calvarial/skull abnormalities, 578, 579,
    582
  pneumocephalus, 666
Sixth nerve palsy, 627
Skeletal lesions; see Bone abnormalities
Skull; see also Calvarium; Scalp and calvarium
  anatomy, 4–14, 16f
    cranial bones, 4–7, 5f, 6f
    fontanelles, 8, 8f

Skull—cont'd
  anatomy—cont'd
    foramina, apertures and contents, 9–14,
      10f, 11f, 12–13t
    marrow, 13
    meninges, epi- and subdural space, 587f
    suture intersections, 9
    sutures, 5f, 6f, 7
    synchondrosis, 6f, 7–8
  Chiari II malformations, 129
  craniovertebral junction abnormalities, 646
  Langerhans cell histiocytosis, 307
  magna cisterna magna, 586
  meningeal anatomy, 17t
  metastasis, 225, 308, 310
  plasmacytomas, 638
  scalp and calvarium, 574–584
Skull base
  anatomy, 4, 5f, 6f, 7, 10f, 645f
  apertures, 12–13t
  foramen magnum region, 646
  synchondrosis, 6f, 7–8
Skull base lesions, 614, 631–640, 631f
  anterior, 631–634
    anatomy, 631–632
    congenital/developmental abnormalities,
      632
    infection/inflammation, 632–633
    neoplasms, 633–634
    trauma, 633
  central, 634–638
    anatomy, 634–635
    congenital/developmental abnormalities,
      635
    infection/inflammation, 638
    neoplasms, 636–638
    vascular abnormalities, 636
  foramen magnum, 643–646
  posterior, 638–640
    anatomy, 638–639
    congenital/developmental abnormalities,
      639
    infection/inflammation, 640
    neoplasms, 639–640
Smallpox, 450
Somesthetic association area, 86, 88f
Sonography; see Ultrasonography
Soto syndrome, 575
Spaces, meningeal, 16f, 17, 17t, 18–19
Speech cortex, 87, 88f, 89
Sphenoid bone
  anatomy, 5f, 7
  apertures of skull base, 13t
  foramina, 9
Sphenoid sinus
  plasmacytomas, 638
  suprasellar region anatomy, 606, 606f
  venous system, 76f
Sphenoid sinusitis, 614

Sphenoparietal sinus, 74f, 75f, 79
Spina bifida
    Chiari I malformation, 126, 127t
    Chiari II malformations, 129
Spinal accessory nerve, 102f, 103f, 116–117
    apertures of skull base, 12t
    foramina, 10f
Spinal cord
    CSF circulation, 27
    normal development, 122
Spinal cord lesions
    autoimmune demyelination, 551
    Chiari I malformations, 126, 127t
    Chiari II malformations, 129, 131
    in disseminated encephalomyelitis, 451
    hemangioblastoma, 174
    with HIV/AIDS, 458, 460
    multiple sclerosis, 531, 549
    neurofibromatosis type II, 167, 168
    sarcoid, 477
    von Hippel-Lindau syndrome, 174
Spinal lemniscus, 99
Spinal nerve roots
    neurofibromatosis
        type I, 165
        type II, 167, 168
    radiculopathies; see Radiculopathies
Spinal nerves
    cytomegalovirus, 466
    schwannoma vs. neurofibroma, 314t
    tumors, 314
Spinal poliomyelitis, 447
Spine
    arthropathies, 643, 645f, 646
    Chiari II malformations, 127t, 129,
        131
    neurofibromatosis type II, 167, 168
    tuberculous spondylitis, 475
    vertebral metastasis, 308, 310
Splenial artery, 60f
Splenium lesions, 619
Spondylitis, tuberculous, 475
Spongiform leukodystrophy (Canavan disease), 525; see also Canavan disease
Squamous cell carcinomas (SCC), regional,
    320
Stapedial artery, persistent, 53
Steroids
    cerebral atrophy, 649
    with HIV/AIDS
        toxoplasmosis, 462
        tuberculous, 470
    subarachnoid space enlargement, 588
    with tuberculosis, 470, 475
    ventricular pathology, 596
Straight sinus (SS), 73, 74f, 77f, 78f, 81f
Straight sinus thrombosis, 429
Striated cerebellum, 161
Striatonigral degeneration, 567

Striatum
    Creutzfeldt-Jakob disease, 453
    necrosis, and basal ganglia degeneration,
        569
Stroke, 374–384
    acute cerebral ischemia and infarction,
        375–378
    aneurysm, 345
    causes of in children and young adults,
        402–403
    demographic, 374–375
    with HIV/AIDS, 459
    infratentorial infarcts, 380–381
    subacute chronic infarction, 378–379
    supratentorial infarcts, 379–383, 380–381f
Sturge-Weber syndrome (SWS), 172–173
    calcification, 656
    calvarial/skull abnormalities, 575, 578
    cortica lesions, 652
    enhancement patterns, 661
    ependymal enhancement, 440, 602
    ventricular abnormalities, 600, 650
Styloid foramen, 11f
Stylomastoid foramen, 13t
Subacute encephalitis, with tuberculous, 469
Subacute hemorrhage
    imaging, 186
    MRI patterns, 667
Subacute infarction
    enhancement patterns, 662
    glioblastoma multiforme vs., 237
Subacute necrotizing encephalomyelopathy, 532
Subacute necrotizing leukoencephalopathy,
    513
Subacute sclerosing panencephalitis (SSPE),
    443, 448–449
    autoimmune demyelination disorders vs., 552
    imaging, 668
Subadventitial dissection, 208f
Subarachnoid cisterns, 23–27, 23f, 24–25t, 26f
Subarachnoid hemorrhage (SAH), 193–194,
    665
    aneurysm and, 216, 343–344, 347–348f
    enhancement patterns, 592, 660, 661
    subarachnoid space enlargement, 588
    ventricular pathology, 596
Subarachnoid space, 12t, 19
    age-related changes, 539
    anatomy, 16f, 17t, 587f
    CSF circulation, 27
    external hydrocephalus, 586
    in Lyme disease, 446
    suprasellar, 606
    tuberculomas, 475
    ventricular pathology, 597
Subarachnoid space abnormalities, 588
Subclavian artery
    left, 31f, 32
    right, 30, 31f

Subclavian steal syndrome, 393
Subcortical dementias, 567–568
Subcortical focal heterotopias, 150f
Subdural effusion, meningitis and, 427, 429
Subdural empyema, 427, 430–432
Subdural hematoma (SDH), 192
  Alzheimer disease workup, 562
  aneurysm and, 350
  calcification in, 657
  calvarial/skull abnormalities, 575, 577, 579
  enhancement with, 592, 660
  in infants, 215
  subarachnoid space enlargement, 588
Subdural space, 19
  anatomy of, 17t, 587f
  tuberculomas, 475
Subependymal giant cell astrocytoma (SGCA),
    171, 232, 246–247, 650
  in differential diagnosis
    of central neurocytoma, 267
    of choroid plexus tumors, 260
    of colloid cyst, 329
    of ependymomas, 257
    of subependymomas, 258
  ventricular pathology, 600
    in adults, 598
    in children, 599
Subependymal hamartoma
  in tuberous sclerosis complex, 170–171
  ventricular abnormalities, 650
Subependymal nodules, 171, 599, 600, 650
Subependymal veins
  anatomy, 79–80
  ependymal enhancement, 602
Subependymoma, 247, 257–258
  in differential diagnosis
    of central neurocytoma, 267
    of choroid plexus tumors, 260
    of colloid cyst, 329
  foramen magnum region, 643, 645f, 646
  posterior fossa, 654
  ventricular pathology, 598, 600, 650
Subfalcine herniation, 199
Subgaleal hematoma, 574
Subgaleal space, 16f
Subintimal dissection, 208f
Subintimal hematoma, 208f
Substantia nigra, 94
  iron in, 538, 543, 667
  Pick's disease, 595
  progressive supranuclear palsy, 619
Subthalamus, 93
Sulci, 147–151, 148f, 149f, 150f
  age-related changes, 538–539, 539f
  Alzheimer disease, 561
  Chiari II malformations, 130
  normal anatomy, 84–87, 84f, 85f
  normal development, 123
  normal pressure hydrocephalus, 564

Sulfadiazine, 462
Superficial middle cerebral (sylvian) vein, 74f,
    79
Superficial temporal artery, 33f, 34f, 36
Superior cerebellar artery
  cerebellopontine angle abnormalities, 623
  vertebrovasilar circulation, 67–68, 67f, 70
Superior cerebellar artery stroke, 380–381f,
    383
Superior cerebellar cistern, 23f, 24t
Superior colliculus, 93, 94
Superior ophthalmic vein, 75f
Superior orbital fissure, 12t
Superior petrosal sinus, 75f, 79
Superior sagittal sinus, 16f, 73, 74f, 77f, 408,
    587f
Superior thyroid artery, 32–33, 33f, 34f
Superior vermian vein, 80, 81f
Supracallosal herniation, 199
Supraclinoid ICA dissection, 398
Supraoptic nucleus, 92
Suprasellar (basal) cistern, 24t, 26–27, 76f
Suprasellar lesions, 612–613
  germ cell tumor differential diagnosis, 278
  midline, 653
  ventricular mass lesions, 601
Supratentorial ependymoma, 265, 275
Supratentorial PNET, 274–275
  calcification with, 657
  ventricular abnormalities from, 601
Supratentorial tuberculomas, 475
Surgery, 666
  calvarial/skull abnormalities, 575, 583,
    592
  cerebellorubral degeneration, 557
  and infection, 431, 436
  meningeal pathology, 592
  postoperative fibrosis, 625, 626
  sella, 610, 612
  ventricular mass lesions, 601
Surgical fat-packing, 665
Suture abnormalities, 575–577
Suture anatomy, 5f, 6f, 7, 9
Sylvian cistern, 27
Sylvian fissure, 25t, 27
  Alzheimer disease, 562
  middle cerebral artery, 56f, 57f
Sylvian point, 56f, 57f
Sylvian vein, 74f, 79
Synchondrosis, 6f, 7–8
Syphilis
  calcification, 656
  calvarial/skull abnormalities, 579, 583
  enhancement patterns, 660
  with HIV/AIDS, 457, 458, 459, 460,
    467–468
  and hypophysitis, granulomatous, 612
  skull base lesions, 635, 638
Syphilitic meningitis, 590, 660

Syringobulbia, 669
    foramen magnum region, 644
    posterior fossa, 654
Syringohydromelia, 127*t*, 131, 643, 645
Syringomelia, foramen magnum region, 644
Systemic lupus erythematosus, 664
    and aneurysm, 342
    and intracranial hemorrhage, 217
    MRI patterns, 668
    progressive multifocal leukoencephalopathy
        with, 449
    and stroke, 403
    and vascular occlusion
        arterial, 401
        venous, 406, 407

T

Takayasu arteritis, 402
Tapeworm, 489–493
Target-like lesions, in multiple sclerosis, 550
Taste cortex, 88*f*, 90
Tectal lesions, 618–619
Tectum, 94
    Chiari II malformations, 130
    normal development, 122, 123
Tegmentum, 93
Tela choroidea
    calcification, 656
    oligodendroglioma, 600
Telencephalon
    normal anatomy, 84–91, 84*f*, 86–87*f*, 88*f*
    normal development, 122
Temporal arteritis, 401–402
Temporal bone
    anatomy, 4, 5*f*, 6*f*, 622*f*
    foramina, 9
    skull base apertures, 13*t*
Temporal bone lesions, 581, 626–628
    Chiari II malformations, 129
    skull base lesions, 639
Temporal lobe
    Alzheimer disease, 561
    normal anatomy, 84*f*, 85
    toxoplasma lesions, HIV/AIDS-related, 462
    venous system, 76*f*
Tentorial apex dura, 619
Tentorial sinuses, 73, 74*f*, 76
Tentorium
    arteriovenous malformations, 361
    enhancement patterns, 660
Teratoma, 228, 276, 277, 278, 651, 665
    calcification with, 657, 659
    desmoplastic infantile gangliogliomas, 265
    in differential diagnosis
        of astrocytomas, 245
        of craniopharyngioma, 286
        of germ cell tumor, 278
        of pineoblastoma, 269
        of primary cerebral neuroblastomas, 275

Teratoma—cont'd
    midline, 653
    MRI patterns, 667
    pineal, 616*f*, 617, 618
    suprasellar, 613
    ventricular abnormalities from, 602
Tetanus immunization, 450
Thalamogeniculate arteries, 51
Thalamoperforating artery, 45, 51, 60*f*,
        380–381*f*, 382
Thalamoperforating artery occlusion,
        618
Thalamostriate vein, 74*f*, 77*f*, 78*f*, 80
Thalamotuberal artery, 380–381*f*, 382
Thalamus, 91–92, 619
    carbon monoxide poisoning, 555
    holoprosencephalies, 142*t*, 143
    hypertensive vascular disease, 664
    infections
        CMV, 417
        Creutzfeldt-Jakob disease, 453
        disseminated encephalomyelitis, 451
        toxoplasmosis, HIV/AIDS-related, 462
    inherited metabolic disorders affecting, 514,
        516
    normal development, 122
    progressive multifocal leukoencephalopathy,
        465
    rhombencephalosynapses, 160
Thalassemia, 578
Thanatophoric dysplasia, 575, 576
Thermal injury, scalp, 574, 583
Third ventricle, 595, 619
    Alzheimer disease, 562
    anatomy, 19, 20*f*, 21–22
        CSF circulation, 26*f*
        pineal, 616*f*, 617
        subarachnoid cisterns, 25*t*
        suprasellar region, 606, 606*f*, 607
        venous system, 76*f*
    calcification, 656
    mass lesions in adults, 598
    mass lesions in children, 599
    sellar expansion, 612
Thrombophlebitis, meningitis and, 427
Thrombosis
    atherosclerosis and, 389
    enhancement patterns, 662
    meningitis and, 427, 429
    sellar/juxtasellar region
        cavernous sinus and skull base, 614
        sellar region aneurysm, 610
        suprasellar aneurysm, 609*t*
    vascular malformation, 371, 662
    venous occlusions, 406–411
    ventricular pathology, 596
Thyrotroph adenomas, 282
Tick-borne pathogens, 443
Toluene, 649

Tonsillar ectopia, Chiari I malformation, 126, 127*t*, 128*f*
Tonsils, cerebellar
  anatomy, 20*f*, 22
  herniation of, 202, 643, 645*f*, 646
Top of basilar syndrome, 568
TORCH infections, 416–423
  calcification with, 656, 658
  calvarial/skull abnormalities, 575
  subarachnoid space enlargement, 588
  ventricular pathology, 596
Torcular herophili (sinus confluence), 73, 74*f*, 77*f*, 157*f*
Torulosis, 485–486
Toxic demyelination, 512
  carbon monoxide intoxication, 554–555
  central pontine myelinolysis, 553
  drug abuse, 555
  extrapontine myelinolysis, 553–554
  organic toxins, 554
Toxic encephalopathies, white matter disorders, 552–555
Toxins, 665
  basal ganglia lesions, 568–569, 654
  calcification with, 656, 657
  cerebellar atrophy, 649–650
  meningeal pathology, 592
  MRI patterns, 668
  and Reyes syndrome, 452
Toxoplasmosis, 418–420
  basal ganglia degeneration, 569
  calcification, 656
  enhancement patterns, 662
  with HIV/AIDS, 457, 458, 460, 461–463, 463*t*
  lymphoma vs., 304
  noncongenital, corticomedullary junction, 652
Transalar herniation, 201–202
Transfalcial herniation, 199
Transtentorial herniation, 199, 201
Transverse sinuses (TS), 73, 74*f*, 74*f*, 77*f*
  arteriovenous malformations, 361, 361*f*
  thrombosis, 429
Trapped ventricle, 601, 655
Trauma, 664, 666
  and calcification, 657
  calvarial, scalp and skull, 574, 575, 579, 582, 583
    anterior skull base lesions, 633
    temporal bone lesions, 628
  cerebellorubral degeneration, 557
  cerebral atrophy, 649
  cortical, 652
  corticomedullary junction, 652
  enhancement patterns, 660
  extraaxial abnormalities, 589
  foramen magnum region, 643, 644, 645*f*, 646

Trauma—cont'd
  and infection, 436
  meningeal pathology, 592
  MRI patterns, 667, 669
  periventricular/callosal, 653
  pineal region, 619
  primary manifestations, 189–196
    cortical contusions, 195–196, 194*f*
    CT indications and protocol, 189–190
    diffuse axonal injury, 194–195, 194*f*
    epidural hematoma, 190–192, 191*f*
    subarachnoid hemorrhage, 193–194
    subdural hematoma, 192–193
  secondary effects, 199–204
    brain death, 204
    cerebral edema, 203–204
    cerebral herniation, 199–202, 200*f*, 203
    ischemic/infarction, 202–203
    secondary hemorrhage, 203
  subarachnoid space enlargement, 588
  tectal, 618
  vascular effects, 190–194, 207–211, 208*f*
    aneurysm, 341
    arterial occlusion, 399
    venous occlusion, 406, 407
  ventricular pathology, 596, 601
  white matter lesion differential diagnosis, 546
Traumatic stalk transection, 610
Trigeminal artery, persistent, 44
Trigeminal (V) nerve, 102*f*, 103*f*, 107–110
  apertures of skull base, 12*t*
  foramina, 10*f*
  schwannomas, 315
  tumor spread along, 625
  veins, 76*t*
Trigeminal schwannoma, cerebellopontine angle, 625
Trigonocephaly, 576
Triphyllocephaly, 576
Trisomies, calvarial/skull abnormalities, 575, 576
Trochlear (IV) nerve, 102*f*, 103*f*, 106–107
  apertures of skull base, 12*t*
  foramina, 10*f*
  venous system, 76*f*
Trimethoprim-sulfamethoxazole, 592
Tuberculoma, 460, 469, 474, 475, 476
Tuberculosis, 474–476, 667
  calcification with, 656, 658
  calvarial/skull abnormalities, 579, 583
  chronic meningitis, 426, 430
  enhancement patterns, 662
  with HIV/AIDS, 457, 460, 468–470
  and hypophysitis, granulomatous, 612
  progressive multifocal leukoencephalopathy with, 449
  skull base lesions, 635, 638
Tuberculous abscess, 460, 469, 470, 474, 475, 476

Tuberculous arteritis, 401
Tuberculous meningitis, 665
    enhancement patterns, 660
    with HIV/AIDS, 458
    meningeal enhancement with, 590
    suprasellar, 613
Tuberomammillary nucleus, 92
Tuberous sclerosis, 148
    arterial stenosis with, 397
    calcification with, 656, 657, 658
    calvarial/skull abnormalities, 579
    CT patterns, 664
    ependymal enhancement, 602
    MRI patterns, 668
    subependymal giant cell astrocytomas in,
        246–247
    ventricular pathology, 600, 650
    white matter lesion differential diagnosis,
        546
Tuberous sclerosis complex (TSC), 170
Tumoral multiple sclerosis, 550
Turricephaly, 576

U

Ultrasonography
    arterial occlusion, 398–400
    atherosclerosis, 389–390
    Canavan disease, 525
    Chiari II malformations, 129
    choroid plexus cystes, 330
    dural sinus thrombosis, 408
    infections, 417, 419, 421, 423
    lipoma, 333
    in stroke, 376
    vein of Galen malformation, 366

V

Vaccines
    sequelae, 450
    white matter lesion differential diagnosis,
        546
Vagus (X) nerve, 102f, 103f, 115–116
    apertures of skull base, 12t
    foramina, 10f
Varicella-zoster virus, 443, 450
    with HIV/AIDS, 457, 458, 459
    meningitis, 429
    herpes zoster otitis, 626
Vascular abnormalities, 664
    aneurysms, 340–352
    arterial stenosis and occlusion,
        396–403
    atherosclerosis, 387–393
    and atrophy, 542
    basal ganglia lesions, 568, 653
    calcification with, 656, 657, 658
    of calvarium/scalp/skull, 574, 582
        central skull base lesions, 636
        internal auditory canal, 625

Vascular abnormalities—cont'd
    cerebellopontine angle, 623t, 623
    congenital/developmental; see Vascular mal-
        formations
    cortical, 652
    corticomedullary junction, 652
    CT patterns, 664
    enhancement patterns, 661, 662
    extraaxial abnormalities, 599
    foramen magnum region, 643, 644,
        645f
    with infections
        HIV/AIDS-associated neurosyphilis, 467,
            468
        rubella, 422, 423
    leukemia and, 305
    meningeal pathology, 592
    midbrain, 618
    midline, 653
    mineralizing microangiopathy, 555
    MRI patterns, 667, 668, 669
    neurofibromatosis type II, 167
    pineal, 616f, 617
    posterior fossa, 654
    quadrigeminal cistern and velum interposi-
        tum, 619
    sellar/juxtasellar region, 606f, 610
        cavernous sinus and skull base, 614
        suprasellar, 612
    stroke, 374–384
    venous occlusion, 406–412
    ventricles, 601
    white matter lesion differential diagnosis,
        546
Vascular causes of white matter disorders,
    546–548
Vascular disease; see Atherosclerosis
Vascular dementia, 512
Vascular ectasia
    meningiomas vs., 295
    schwannoma vs., 316
Vascular inflammation; see Vasculitis
Vascularity, toxoplasma lesions, 462
Vascular loops, 349
    cerebellopontine angle, 623
    internal auditory canal, 625
Vascular malformations, 355–371, 664
    arteriovenous; see Arteriovenous malforma-
        tions
    calcification in, 657
    capillary, 358t, 366–368
    cavernous, 358t, 368–370, 369f
    cerebellopontine angle, 623t
    cryptic/occult, 370–371
    CT patterns, 664
    enhancement patterns, 661, 662
    ependymal enhancement, 440, 602
    and intracranial hemorrhages,
        216–217

Vascular malformations—cont'd
  with neurocutaneous syndromes; see Neuro-
    cutaneous syndromes
  ring-enhancing lesions, 439
  Sturge-Weber syndrome, 172
  thrombosis, enhancement patterns, 662
  venous, 363–366
    vein of Galen malformation, 359t,
      365–366
    venous angioma, 359t, 363–365, 364f
  ventricular mass lesions, 601
Vascular occlusion; see also Infarct; Thrombosis
  arterial; see Arterial stenosis and occlusion
  venous, 406–412; see also Venous infarct
Vascular pseudotumors, temporal bone lesions,
  627
Vascular structures; see Arteries; Blood
  vessels; Veins; specific vessels
Vascular trauma, 207–211, 208f
Vasculitis, 548, 664
  arteritis, 401–402, 467
  and basal ganglia degeneration, 568
  in disseminated encephalomyelitis, 450
  with HIV/AIDS, 459
    cytomegalovirus, 466
    neurosyphilis, 467, 468
  with infections
    rubella, 423
    viral, 443
  MRI patterns, 668
  with sarcoid, 477
  and stroke, 403
  and vascular occlusion
    arterial, 400–402
    venous, 406, 407
  Wegener's granulomatosis, 478
  white matter lesion differential diagnosis,
    546
Vasculopathy; see Atherosclerosis; Vascular
  abnormalities
Vasospasm
  aneurysm rupture and, 347–348f
  meningitis and, 427
Vein of Galen, 77f, 78f, 80, 81f, 617
  aneurysm, 269, 359t, 365–366
  aneurysmal dilatation, 619
  midline malformation, 653
  straight sinus formation, 73, 74f
  thrombosis, 411, 429
Vein of Labbe, 74f, 79
Vein of Labbe thrombosis, 429
Vein of Rolando, 79
Vein of Trolard, 74f, 79
Veins; see also Thrombosis
  age-related changes, 540
  apertures of skull base, 12t
  intracranial, 73–91, 74f

Veins—cont'd
  intracranial—cont'd
    cerebral veins, 74f, 76f, 77f, 78f, 79–80
    dural sinuses, 73–79, 74f, 76f, 77f, 78f
    posterior fossa vein, 80, 81f
  normal white matter components, 512
  scalp, 16f, 587f
  sellar/juxtasellar region, 606f, 607
  subarachnoid cisterns, 24–25t
  traumatic injury, 207, 211
  ventricular mass lesions, 601
Velum interpositum, 23f, 25t, 26, 616f
Velum interpositum lesions, 619
Venous angioma, 359t, 363–365, 364f, 371
  cavernous angiomas with, 370
  ependymal enhancement, 602
  and intracranial hemorrhages, 216
Venous collagenosis
  periventricular, 411–412, 546, 547
  white matter degenerative diseases, 547
Venous drainage, 151
Venous infarct, 429, 664; see also Infarct
  and basal ganglia degeneration, 568
  and intracranial hemorrhage, 217
  meningitis and, 427
Venous lakes, calvarial/skull abnormalities,
  582
Venous occlusion, 406–412
  collagenosis, 411–412
  cortical vein, 410–411
  deep cerebral vein thrombosis, 411
  dural sinus thrombosis, 406–410
Venous sinus anatomy, 587f
Venous sinus anomalies, 582
Venous sinus occlusive disease (VSOD),
  406–411
Venous sinus thrombosis, 429
Venous stasis, meningitis and, 427
Venous varices, 365
  extraaxial abnormalities, 599
  imaging, 359t
  ventricular mass lesions, 601
Ventral spinothalamic tract, 94
Ventricles
  age-related changes, 539–540, 539f,
    541–542
  anatomy, 19–20, 20f
  calcification, 656
  CSF circulation, 26f, 27
  myelination; see Myelination, normal devel-
    opment
  normal pressure hydrocephalus, 563, 564
  subarachnoid cisterns, 24–25t
Ventricular abnormalities, 595–602
  Alzheimer disease, 561, 562
  cerebellopontine angle cistern involvement,
    625
  Chiari II malformations, 127t, 131

of configuration, 595, 650
Ventricular abnormalities—cont'd
  with cysticercosis, 492
  ependymal enhancement, 602
  HIV/AIDS-related lymphoma, 463t
  holoprosencephalies, 142t, 144
  with infections, 419
  mass lesions, 329, 597–602, 650–651
    congenital/developmental, 597, 599–600
    extrinsic, 601–602
    inflammation/infection, 601
    neoplasia, 600–601
    trauma/surgery, 601
    vascular, 601
  pineal region, 619
  with sarcoid, 478
  sellar expansion, 612
  of size, 595–597, 650; see also Ventricu-
    lomegaly
  temporal bone involvement, 628
  tuberculomas, 475
Ventricular shunting, 597, 650
Ventriculitis/ependymitis, 439, 661; see also
  Ependymitis
  ependymal enhancement, 602
  with meningitis, 427, 428
  MRI, 438
  ventricular pathology, 596
Ventriculography, 666
Ventriculomegaly, 418, 596–597
  with holoprosencephaly, 144
  with infections, rubella, 423
Ventromedial nucleus, 92
Vermian-cerebellar hypoplasia; see Dandy-
  Walker variant
Vermian pilocytic astrocytoma, 273
Vermis, posterior fossa abnormalities, 155t
Vertebral artery, 59f, 66–69, 66f, 67f, 644
  anastomosis, 35
  aneurysms, 643, 644
  cerebellopontine angle abnormalities, 623
  dissection, 398
  innervation, 37
  right, 30, 31f
  stenosis of, congenital causes, 396
  traumatic injury, 209–210
Vertebral metastasis, 308, 310
Vertebrobasilar dolichoectasia, 643, 644
  cerebellopontine angle, 623, 623t, 624t
  internal auditory canal, 625
  posterior fossa, 654
Vertebrobasilar system
  anastomosis, persistent, 41, 42f, 43, 44
  anatomy, 66–70, 66f, 67f
  aneurysms, 344f
  atherosclerosis, 388
  calcification, 656
Vesicles, normal development, 122

Vessel loops; see Vascular loops
Vestibular nuclear complex, 95
Vestibular nucleus, schwannomas, 315
Vestibulocochlear ganglia, 626
Vestibulocochlear (VII) nerve, 102f, 103f,
  113–114
  apertures of skull base, 10f, 12t
  with HIV/AIDS-associated neurosyphilis,
    468
Vidian artery, 13t, 35, 41
Vidian canal, 11, 13t, 634
Viral encephalitis
  congenital and neonatal, 416–418, 420–423
  herpes simplex (non-neonatal), 443–445
  MRI patterns, 668
  poliovirus, 443, 447
  secondary; see Encephalitis, secondary
Viral meningitis, 429
  enhancement patterns, 660
  meningeal enhancement with, 590
Viral neuritis, enhancement patterns, 663
Virchow-Robin (perivascular) spaces, 587f,
  651
  abnormalities of, 665
  age-related changes, 538, 540, 546
  anatomy, 16f, 18
  basal ganglia lesions, 653
  MRI patterns, T2 hyperintense lesions, 668
  neuroepithelial cysts vs., 330
  sarcoid, 477
Virus infections, 443–445; see also specific viruses
  and autoimmune demyelinating disorders,
    551–552
  congenital and neonatal, 416–418, 420–423
  with HIV/AIDS, 457, 459
    cytomegalovirus, 466–467
    progressive multifocal leukoencephalopa-
      thy, 464–466
  meningitis; see Viral meningitis
  post-infectious encephalitides; see also En-
    cephalitis, secondary
  ventriculitis and ependymitis, 439
  white matter lesion differential diagnosis,
    546
Visual cortex, 88f, 89
Visual reflexes, superior colliculi, 93
Vitamin A excess, 576
Vitaminosis D excess, 576, 578, 656
von Hippel-Lindau syndrome (VHL),
  173–175, 296, 297
von Recklinghausen neurofibromatosis, 164t,
  167–168, 397

W

Walker-Warburg syndrome, 147, 158
Wallerian degeneration, 557, 669
Watershed, collateral circulation, 393

Watershed infarcts, 382, 547
Wegener granulomatosis, 402, 478–479, 588
  enhancement patterns, 660
  meningeal enhancement with, 591
  meningitis, chronic, 430
  skull base lesions, 633, 635, 638
Wernicke encephalopathy, 552
Wernicke's area, 88*f*, 89
Whipple's disease, 449
White matter; *see also* Parenchyma
  age-related changes, 538, 539*f*, 540, 538,
    540–542
  with holoprosencephaly, 144
  hypertensive vascular disease, 664
  MRI patterns, T2 hyperintense lesions, 668
  myelination, delayed, 507–508
  normal anatomy, 90–91
  normal components, 512
White matter disorders
  acquired, 511–512, 546–557
    HIV/AIDS, 459, 470
    iatrogenic, 555–556
    miscellaneous, 554–555
    multiple sclerosis and autoimmune demy-
      elinating diseases, 548–552
    secondary, 556–557
    toxic encephalopathies, 552–555
    vascular causes, 546–548

White matter disorders—cont'd
  amyotrophic lateral sclerosis, 556–557
  cerebellorubral degeneration, 557
  inherited, 511–516, 518–526; *see also* Leu-
    kodystrophies
    leukodystrophies affecting deep white
      matter, 518–524
    leukoencephalopathies affecting periph-
      eral white matter, 524–526
  Wallerian degeneration, 557
White matter spongiosis, 411
Williams syndrome, 656
Wilson disease, 515, 516, 533–534, 654,
  665
Wormian bones, 577, 583
Wyburn-Mason syndrome (WMS), 177,
  356

X

Xanthoastrocytoma, 245–246, 297, 651, 652,
  662
Xanthogranuloma, 598, 599

Z

Zellweger (cerebrohepatorenal) syndrome,
  514, 515, 516, 575
Zidovudine (AZT), 460